T0073054

Cognitive Informatics in Biomedicine and Healthcare

Series Editor
Vimla L. Patel, Ctr Cognitive Studies in Med & PH
New York Academy of Med, Suite 454, New York, NY, USA

Enormous advances in information technology have permeated essentially all facets of life. Although these technologies are transforming the workplace as well as leisure time, formidable challenges remain in fostering tools that enhance productivity, are sensitive to work practices, and are intuitive to learn and to use effectively. Informatics is a discipline concerned with applied and basic science of information, the practices involved in information processing, and the engineering of information systems.

Cognitive Informatics (CI), a term that has been adopted and applied particularly in the fields of biomedicine and health care, is the multidisciplinary study of cognition, information, and computational sciences. It investigates all facets of computer applications in biomedicine and health care, including system design and computer-mediated intelligent action. The basic scientific discipline of CI is strongly grounded in methods and theories derived from cognitive science. The discipline provides a framework for the analysis and modeling of complex human performance in technology-mediated settings and contributes to the design and development of better information systems for biomedicine and health care.

Despite the significant growth of this discipline, there have been few systematic published volumes for reference or instruction, intended for working professionals, scientists, or graduate students in cognitive science and biomedical informatics, beyond those published in this series. Although information technologies are now in widespread use globally for promoting increased self-reliance in patients, there is often a disparity between the scientific and technological knowledge underlying healthcare practices and the lay beliefs, mental models, and cognitive representations of illness and disease. The topics covered in this book series address the key research gaps in biomedical informatics related to the applicability of theories, models, and evaluation frameworks of HCI and human factors as they apply to clinicians as well as to the lay public.

Trevor A. Cohen • Vimla L. Patel
Edward H. Shortliffe

Editors

Intelligent Systems in Medicine and Health

The Role of AI

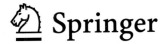 Springer

Editors
Trevor A. Cohen
University of Washington
Seattle, WA, USA

Vimla L. Patel
New York Academy of Medicine
New York, NY, USA

Edward H. Shortliffe
Columbia University
New York, NY, USA

ISSN 2662-7280   ISSN 2662-7299   (electronic)
Cognitive Informatics in Biomedicine and Healthcare
ISBN 978-3-031-09107-0   ISBN 978-3-031-09108-7   (eBook)
https://doi.org/10.1007/978-3-031-09108-7

This Springer imprint is published by the registered company Springer Nature Switzerland AG
The registered company address is: Gewerbestrasse 11, 6330 Cham, Switzerland

We wish to dedicate this volume to three giants of science who greatly inspired and influenced us while helping to lay the groundwork for artificial intelligence in medicine, even though each of them made their primary contributions in other fields. Furthermore, each has been a personal friend of at least one of us and we look back fondly on their humanity and their contributions.

Herbert Simon (Carnegie Mellon University) won the Nobel Prize in Economics (1978) for his pioneering research into the decision-making process within economic organizations. He is also known as an early innovator in the field of artificial intelligence, whose long partnership with Allen Newell led to early work on the Logic Theory Machine and General Problem Solver. As a psychologist who studied human and machine problem solving, he pioneered notions of bounded rationality and satisficing.

Joshua Lederberg (Stanford and Rockefeller Universities) won the Nobel Prize in Physiology or Medicine (1958) for his discoveries of genetic transfer in bacteria. A computer scientist as well as a geneticist, he was instrumental in devising the notion of capturing expert knowledge in computers. His Dendral Project led to a body of work that dealt with the interpretation of mass spectral data to identify organic compounds, and he created the first national resource to support research on artificial intelligence in medicine (SUMEX-AIM).

vi

Walter Kintsch (University of Colorado Boulder) is a psychologist and cognitive scientist who used both experimental and computational modeling techniques to study how people understand language. He reformulated discourse comprehension as a constraint satisfaction process. His work on latent semantic analysis demonstrated how machine learning could be used to construct a high-dimensional semantic space. His writing has influenced research on natural language understanding as well as the cognitive informatics focus reflected in this volume.

T.C., V.L.P., E.H.S.—March 2022

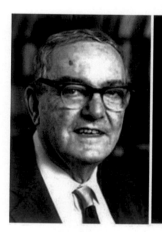 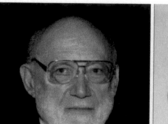 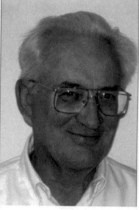

Herbert Simon
1916 - 2001

Joshua Lederberg
1925 - 2008

Walter Kintsch
1932 -

Photograph of Herbert Simon provided courtesy of Carnegie Mellon University.

Photograph of Joshua Lederberg provided courtesy of EH Shortliffe.

Photograph of Walter Kintsch provided by Professor Kintsch.

Foreword

Delivering quality, affordable health care to large populations is one of humankind's greatest challenges.

There are so many facets to health care, however, that talking about "the problem" is a gross understatement. George Polya's heuristic (from Descartes) of dividing problems into subproblems[1] remains one of the best tools in our cognitive toolkit—human or artificial intelligence (AI).[2] This book explores many of those subproblems from the perspective of using computing—AI in particular—to meet them.

The idea of automating solutions to specific human problems is rooted in Greek mythology but actual implementations of automated problem solving with mechanical or electronic computers were initially restricted to single-purpose applications. For example, wartime uses included decoding encrypted messages and calculating trajectories of artillery shells; business uses included payroll accounting, information retrieval, and process automation. Medical uses included keeping medical records, recording physiological data, and calculating drug doses.

Modern medicine is grounded in data from observations as well as measurements. But the machines running initial applications of computers to medicine were so restricted in size and scope that demonstrations beyond single-purpose problems were severely limited.

Around 1950 Turing introduced the audacious idea that computers could be intelligent and could be used on problems that required reasoning, understanding,

---

[1] Polya G. *How to Solve It: A New Aspect of Mathematical Method*. Princeton, NJ: Princeton University Press, 2014 (originally published 1945).

[2] Two memorable examples of identifying key subproblems are cited in McCullough's book on building the Panama Canal [McCullough, D. *The Path between the Seas: The Creation of the Panama Canal, 1870-1914*. New York: Simon & Schuster, 1978]. First, after several years of failure, a new engineer put in charge of the project rethought the steps of digging a huge trench and recognized that the most rate-limiting step was getting rid of the dirt. Second, the same engineer recognized another rate-limiting step was keeping workers healthy. Neither was "the problem" per se; solving both subproblems made the difference.

and learning—to work smarter, not harder. Acquiring measurements is one thing, interpreting the data is another. Importantly, early AI research introduced a conceptual framework that includes two critical differences from mathematical computation: symbolic reasoning and heuristic reasoning. Reasoning with symbols, as opposed to numeric quantities, carries with it the essential link human beings made when they invented language between words and the world, i.e., semantics. Heuristic reasoning is even older than humankind, being bound up with the Darwinian notion of survival. A decision to fight or flee does not leave time to consider the consequences of all possible options,[3] and most decisions in everyday life have no algorithm that guarantees a correct answer in a short time (or often not in any amount of time).

The importance of human health quickly attracted early pioneers to the possibility of using computers to assist physicians, nurses, pharmacists, and other health-care professionals.

The initial applications of AI limited their scope so they could be dealt with successfully in single demonstration projects on the small computers of the day. Cognitive psychologists recognized that clinicians *reason* about the available data in medicine just as they do in other fields like chess. The process of diagnostic reasoning became the focus of work on expert systems, with early programs becoming convincing examples that AI could replicate human reasoning in this area on narrowly defined problems.

An important part of this demonstration was with Bayesian programs that used statistics to reason in a mathematically rigorous way for clinical decision support. However, those initial applications of Bayes' Theorem to medicine were also limited until means were found to reduce their complexity with heuristic reasoning. Another important set of demonstrations encoded knowledge accumulated by human experts, along the lines suggested by cognitive science. One of the shortcomings of the expert systems approach, however, is the time and effort it takes to acquire the knowledge from experts in the first place, and to maintain a large knowledge base thereafter.

In practice, medical professionals are faced with several inconvenient truths, which further complicate efforts to use computers in health care. The chapters of this book address many of them. For example:

- The body of knowledge in, and relevant to, medicine is growing rapidly. E.g., diagnosis and treatment options for genetic diseases in the last few decades, and of viral infections in the last few years, have come into the mainstream.
- Complete paradigm shifts in medicine require rethinking whole areas of medicine. E.g., prion diseases have forced a reconceptualization of the mechanisms of pathogen transmission.

---

[3] Herb Simon, one of the founding fathers of AI, received a Nobel Prize in Economics in 1978 for elucidation of this concept in the world of decision making. His term for it was "Bounded Rationality." See https://www.cmu.edu/simon/what-is-simon/herbert-a-simon.html (accessed August 11, 2022).

- Medical knowledge is incomplete and there are no good treatment options, and sometimes no good diagnostic criteria, for some conditions. E.g., Parkinson's disease can be managed, but is still not curable after decades of research.
- Information about an individual patient is often erroneous and almost always incomplete. E.g., false positive and false negative test results are expected for almost every diagnostic test.
- Patients' medical problems exist within a larger emotional, social, economic, and cultural context. E.g., the most effective treatment options may be unaffordable or unacceptable to an individual.
- Professionals are expected to learn from their own, and others', experience (both positive and negative). E.g., continuing to recommend a failed treatment modality is reason for censure.
- Professionals at the level of recognized specialists are expected to deal with unique cases for which there are neither case studies nor established diagnostic or treatment wisdom. E.g., primary care providers refer recalcitrant cases to specialists for just these reasons.
- Communication between patients and professionals is imperfect. E.g., language is full of ambiguity, and we all have biases in what we want to hear or fear most.

Collectively, these issues are more than merely "inconvenient," but are humbling reminders that "the problem" of providing health care is overwhelming in the large. They also represent significant barriers to harnessing the presently available power of computers to actual healthcare delivery. The perspectives offered in this book summarize current approaches to these issues and highlight work that remains to be done. As such it is valuable as a textbook for biomedical informatics and as a roadmap for the possibilities of using AI for the benefit of humankind.

The book's emphasis on reasoning provides a central focus not found in other collections. The chapters here deal with transforming data about patients, once acquired, to actionable information and using that information in clinical contexts. With today's understanding, AI offers the means to augment human intelligence by making the accumulated knowledge available, suggesting possible options, and considering consequences. We are betting that computers can help to overcome human limitations of imperfect memory, reasoning biases, and sheer physical stamina. We are betting on the power of knowledge over the persistent forces of random mutations. Most of all we are betting that the synergy of human and computer intelligence will succeed in the noble quest of improving the quality of human lives.

University of Pittsburgh
Pittsburgh, PA, USA
August 2022

Bruce G. Buchanan

Preface

The State of AI in Medicine

Recent advances in computing power and the availability of large amounts of training data have spurred tremendous advances in the accuracy with which computers can perform tasks that were once considered the exclusive province of human intelligence. These include perceptual tasks related to medical diagnosis, where deep neural networks have attained expert-level performance for the diagnosis of diabetic retinopathy and the identification of biopsy-proven cases of skin cancer from dermatological images. These accomplishments reflect an increase in activity in Artificial Intelligence (AI), both in academia and industry. According to the 2021 AI Index report assembled and published at Stanford University, there was a close to twelvefold increase in the total number of annual peer-reviewed AI publications between 2000 and 2019, and a close to fivefold increase in annual private investment in funded AI companies between 2015 and 2020, with commercial applications of AI technologies such as speech-based digital assistants and personalized advertising and newsfeeds by now woven deeply into the threads of our everyday lives. These broad developments throughout society have led to a resurgence of public interest in the role of AI in medicine[1] (AIM), reviving long-standing debates about the nature of intelligence, the relative value of data-driven predictive models and human decision makers, and the potential for technology to enhance patient safety and to disseminate expertise broadly.

Consequently AIM is in the news, with frequent and often thoughtful accounts of the ways in which it might influence—and hopefully improve—the practice of medicine appearing in high visibility media venues such as *The New York Times* [1, 2], *The Atlantic* [3], *The New Yorker* [4], *The Economist* [5], and others [6, 7]. As biomedical informaticians with long-standing interests in AIM, we are encouraged to see this level of attention and investment in the area. However, we are also aware

---

[1] We consider the scope of AIM to include public health and clinically driven basic science research, as well as clinical practice.

that this is by no means the first time that the promise of AIM has emerged as a focus of media attention. For example, a 1977 *New York Times* article [8] describes the MYCIN system (discussed in Chap. 2), noting the ability of this system to make medical diagnoses, to request missing information, and to explain how it reaches conclusions. The article also mentions the extent of government funding for AI research at the time at $5 million a year, which when adjusted for inflation would be around $23 million annually. The question arises as to what has changed between then and now, and how these changes might affect the ongoing and future prospects for AI technologies to improve medical care. Some answers to this question are evident in this 1977 article, which is critical of the potential of the field to accomplish its goals of championship-level chess performance and machine translation ("neither has been accomplished successfully, and neither is likely to be any time soon") and face recognition ("they cannot begin to distinguish one face from another as babies can"). Today all of these tasks are well within the capabilities of contemporary AI systems, which is one indication of the methodological advances that have been made over the intervening four decades. However, translating methods with strong performance on tightly constrained tasks to applications with positive impact in health care is not (and has never been) a straightforward endeavor, on account of the inherent complexities of the healthcare system and the prominent role of uncertain and temporarily unavailable information in medical decision making, among other factors. While AI technologies do have the potential to transform the practice of medicine, computer programs demonstrating expert-level performance in diagnostic tasks have existed for decades, but significant challenges to realizing the potential value of AI in health care—such as how such AI systems might best be integrated into clinical practice—remain unresolved.

It is our view that the discipline of Cognitive Informatics (CI) [9], which brings the perspective of the cognitive sciences to the study of medical decision making by human beings and machines, is uniquely positioned to address many of these challenges. Through its roots in the study of medical reasoning, CI provides a sound scientific basis from which to consider the relationship between current technologies and human intelligence. CI has extended its area of inquiry to include both human-computer interaction and the study of the effects of technology on the flow of work and information in clinical settings [10]. Accordingly, CI can inform the integration of AI systems into clinical practice. In recent years, patient safety has emerged as a research focus of the CI community, providing new insights into the ways in which technology might mitigate or, despite best intentions, facilitate medical error. Consequently, a volume describing approaches to AIM from a CI perspective seemed like an excellent fit for the Springer Nature Cognitive Informatics book series led by one of us (VLP). We fondly recall that this volume is a project that we first discussed several years ago over a bottle of Merlot in proximity to a conference in Washington, DC.

However, as our discussions developed over the course of subsequent meetings, it became apparent that there was a need for a more comprehensive account of the field. As educators, we considered the knowledge and skills that future researchers and practitioners in the field might need in order to realize the transformative potential of AI methods for the practice of health care. We were aware of books on the subject, such as cardiologist Eric Topol's cogent account of the implications of contemporary machine learning approaches for the practice of medicine [11], and the development of pediatric cardiologist Anthony C. Chang's excellent clinician-oriented introduction to AI methods with a focus on their practical application to problems in health care and medicine [12].[2] Books drawing together the perspectives of multiple authors were also available, including a compendium of chapters in which authors focus on their research interests within the field [13], and an account of the organizational implications of "big data" and predictive models that can be derived from such large collections of information [14]. However, none of the books we encountered was developed with the focused intention to provide a basis for curricular development in AIM, and we were hearing an increasing demand for undergraduate, graduate, and postgraduate education from our own trainees—students and aspiring physician-informaticians.

Consequently, we pivoted from our original goal of a volume primarily concerned with highlighting the role of CI in AIM, to the goal of developing the first comprehensive coauthored textbook in the AIM field, still with a CI emphasis. We reached out to our friends and colleagues, prominent researchers with deep expertise in the application of AI methods to clinical problems, several of whom have been engaged with AIM since the inception of the field. This was a deliberate decision on our part, as we felt that in addition to lacking a cognitive perspective (despite the emergence of the term "cognitive computing" as a catch-all for AI methods), much work we encountered was presented without apparent consideration of the history of the field. Our concern with this disconnect was not only a matter of the academic impropriety of failure to acknowledge prior work. We were also concerned that work conducted from this perspective would not be informed by the many lessons learned from decades of work and careful consideration of the issues involved in implementing AI at the point of care. Thus, in developing our ideas for the structure of this volume, and in our selection of chapter authors, we endeavored to make sure that presentations of current methods and applications were contextualized in relation to the history of the field, and informed by a CI perspective.

Introducing Intelligent Systems in Medicine and Health: The Role of AI

The result of these efforts is the current volume, a comprehensive textbook that takes stock of the current state of the art of AIM, places current developments in their historical context, and identifies cognitive and systemic factors that may help or hinder their ability to improve patient care. It is our intention that a reader of this

---

[2] A trained data scientist, Dr. Chang also contributed a chapter on the future of medical AI and data science in this volume.

volume will attain an accurate picture of the strengths and limitations of these emerging technologies, emphasizing how they relate to the AI systems that preceded them, to the intelligence of human decision makers in medicine, and to the needs and expectations of those who use the resulting tools and systems. This will lay a foundation for an informed discussion of the potential of such technology to enhance patient care, the obstacles that must be overcome for this to take place, and the ways in which emerging and as-yet-undeveloped technologies may transform the practice of health care.

With increasing interest and investment in AIM technologies will come the recognition of the need for professionals with the prerequisite expertise to see these technologies through to the point of positive impact. Progress toward this goal will require both advancement of the state of the science through scholarly research and measurably successful deployment of AIM systems in clinical practice settings. As the first comprehensive coauthored textbook in the field of AIM, this volume aims to define and aggregate the knowledge that researchers and practitioners in the field will require to advance it. As such, it draws together a range of expert perspectives to provide a holistic picture of the current state of the field, to identify opportunities for further research and development, and to provide guidance to inform the successful integration of AIM into clinical and public health practice.

We intend to provide a sound basis for a seminar series or a university level course on AIM. To this end, authors have been made aware of the context of their chapters within the logical flow of the entire volume. We have sought to assure coordination among authors to facilitate cross-references between chapters, and to minimize either coverage gaps or redundancies. Furthermore, all chapters have followed the same basic organizational structure, which includes explicit learning objectives, questions for self-study, and annotated suggestions for further reading. Chapters have been written for an intended audience of students in biomedical informatics, AI, machine learning, cognitive engineering, and clinical decision support. We also offer the book to established researchers and practitioners of these disciplines, as well as those in medicine, public health, and other health professions, who would like to learn more about the potential for these emerging technologies to transform their fields.

Structure and Content

The book is divided into four parts. They are designed to emphasize pertinent *concepts* rather than technical detail. There are other excellent sources for exploring the technical details of the topics we introduce. The **Introduction** provides readers with an overview of the field. Chapter 1 provides an introduction to the fields of Artificial Intelligence and Cognitive Informatics and describes how they relate to one another. Chapter 2 provides a historical perspective, drawing attention to recurring themes, issues, and approaches that emerged during the course of the development of early AI systems, most of which remain highly relevant today. Chapter 3 provides an overview of the landscape of biomedical data and information, to familiarize readers with the resources AIM systems can draw upon for training and evaluation, and as sources of structured knowledge. This chapter also serves as a bridge to subsequent parts in the book, introducing some of the methods, applications, and issues that will be covered in greater detail later.

The **Approaches** part covers methods used by AIM systems. Chapter 4 commences this part with a discussion of knowledge-based approaches, spanning from knowledge modeling efforts, used in expert systems at the inception of AIM as a field, to contemporary efforts to infuse machine learning models with structured biomedical knowledge. Chapter 5 considers the idea of AIM from a cognitive perspective, beginning with an account of the parallel development of the two fields, and advancing an argument for the development of complementary human/AI systems with superior clinical utility when compared with either of these components alone. Chapter 6 introduces the machine learning approaches that have come to predominate in the current wave of AIM systems, with the intention of providing readers with a conceptual understanding of some key algorithms, and issues that may arise during their application to modeling medical data. Chapter 7 considers Natural Language Processing (NLP), which has been intertwined with AI at least since Turing's proposal of the ability to conduct a passably human conversation as an observable surrogate for "thinking" [15]. The chapter focuses on biomedical NLP, giving an account of the main problems to be addressed in this area, and the methods that predominate at present, from rule-based methods through to deep learning approaches. Chapter 8 considers approaches to the explanation of decisions recommended by AIM models, with an emphasis on its importance in clinical settings in which "black box" predictions may not—and arguably should not—be taken at face value without some justification to earn trust and to permit detection of predictions made on tenuous grounds. Chapter 9 revisits the issue of language, with a focus on methods that support human-like conversational interactions with the goal of supporting health care.

Having introduced the fundamental methods of the field, the book focuses in the third part on **Applications**. Chapter 10 describes those in which AIM methods are applied to support decision making in clinical care, through integration with existing platforms and workflows. Chapter 11 focuses on the prediction of clinical outcomes, such as near-term readmission, with an emphasis on dynamic models of variables and outcomes that change over time. Chapter 12 describes what is arguably the most successful area of application of contemporary AIM methods to date—the interpretation of medical images. Chapter 13 shifts from a focus on methods to support the care of individual patients to the population level, with a discussion of the emerging role of AI in the field of public health. Chapter 14 then describes AI applications at the molecular level: methods that yield clinically actionable insights from -omics data. Chapter 15 discusses AIM applications that are of administrative importance to a healthcare system, such as approaches to optimize the use of resources. This chapter also includes a discussion of the practical concerns that may arise when attempting to implement AI solutions in the context of an operational healthcare system. Finally, Chap. 16 focuses on AI applications in medical education, including the roles of cognitive and learning sciences in informing how clinicians-in-training should be educated about AIM, and how AI might support the education of clinicians in their chosen fields.

The final part in the volume considers **the road ahead** for AIM. It addresses issues that are likely to be of importance for the successful progression of the field, including two potential stumbling blocks: inadequate evaluation, and failure to consider the ethical issues that may accompany the deployment of AI systems in healthcare settings. Accordingly, the first chapter in this part, Chap. 17, is focused on evaluation of AIM systems, including enabling capabilities such as usability and the need to move beyond "in situ" evaluations of accuracy toward demonstrations of acceptance and clinical utility in the natural world. Chapter 18 concerns the need for a robust ethical framework to address issues proactively such as algorithmic bias, and exacerbation of healthcare inequities due to limited portability of methods and algorithms. Chapter 19 projects from the trajectory of current trends to anticipate the future of AI in medicine with an emphasis on data science, and how broader deployment of AI systems may affect the practice of medicine. Finally, Chap. 20 provides a summary and synthesis of the volume, including the editors' perspectives on the prospects and challenges for the field. The final part is then followed by a detailed glossary that provides definitions of all terms displayed in bold throughout the body of the book (with an indication of the chapter(s) in which each term was used). The book closes with a subject index for the entire volume.

Guide to Use of This Book

This book is written as a textbook, such that it can be used in formal courses or seminars. For this purpose, we would anticipate curricular design to follow the overall structure of the book, with a logical progression from introduction through approaches to applications and projections for the future. For example, this structure could support an undergraduate or graduate level course in a Computer Science, Biomedical Informatics, or Cognitive Engineering program that aims to provide students with a comprehensive survey of current applications and concerns in the field. At the graduate level, this could be coupled to a student-led research project. Alternatively, one might imagine an MS level course that aims to provide clinical practitioners seeking additional training in clinical informatics with the knowledge they will need to be informed users of AIM systems, in which case content could be drawn from the book selectively with an emphasis on introductory content, and clinical applications and issues that relate to them directly (Chaps. 1–3, 10–12, 15, and 17–19). Of course, the book may be used for self-study and reference, and readers may wish to explore particular topics in greater detail—starting with a particular chapter (say, machine learning methods) and then exploring the cross-references in this chapter to find out more about how this topic features in the context of particular applications, or issues that are anticipated to emerge as the field progresses.

This is an exciting time to be working in the field of AIM, and an ideal time to enter it. There is increasing support for AIM work, both through federal funding initiatives such as the NIH-wide Bridge to Artificial Intelligence program[3] and in light of an acceleration in private investment in digital health technologies. Such support has been stimulated in part by the field's demonstrated utility and acceptance as a way to diagnose disease, to deliver care, and to support public health efforts during the COVID-19 pandemic. On account of the pervasiveness of AI technologies across industries outside of health care, skepticism about the ability of these technologies to deliver meaningful improvements is balanced by enthusiasm for their potential to improve the practice of medicine. It is our goal that readers of this volume will emerge equipped with the knowledge needed to realize this potential and to proceed to lead the advancement of health care through AIM.

References

1. Metz C. A.I. shows promise assisting physicians. The New York Times. 2019. [cited 2021 Apr 15]. https://www.nytimes.com/2019/02/11/health/artificial-intelligence-medical-diagnosis.html.
2. O'Connor A. How artificial intelligence could transform medicine. The New York Times. 2019. [cited 2021 Apr 15]. https://www.nytimes.com/2019/03/11/well/live/how-artificial-intelligence-could-transform-medicine.html.
3. Cohn J. The robot will see you now. The Atlantic. 2013. [cited 2021 Jun 14]. https://www.theatlantic.com/magazine/archive/2013/03/the-robot-will-see-you-now/309216/.
4. Mukherjee S. A.I. versus M.D.. The New Yorker. [cited 2021 Apr 15]. https://www.newyorker.com/magazine/2017/04/03/ai-versus-md.
5. Artificial intelligence will improve medical treatments. The Economist. 2018. [cited 2021 Jun 16]. https://www.economist.com/science-and-technology/2018/06/07/artificial-intelligence-will-improve-medical-treatments.
6. Aaronovitch D. DeepMind, artificial intelligence and the future of the NHS. [cited 2021 Jun 16]. https://www.thetimes.co.uk/article/deepmind-artificial-intelligence-and-the-future-of-the-nhs-r8c28v3j6.
7. Artificial intelligence has come to medicine. Are patients being put at risk?. Los Angeles Times. 2020. [cited 2021 Jun 16]. https://www.latimes.com/business/story/2020-01-03/artificial-intelligence-healthcare.
8. Experts argue whether computers could reason, and if they should. The New York Times. [cited 2021 Apr 15]. https://www.nytimes.com/1977/05/08/archives/experts-argue-whether-computers-could-reason-and-if-they-should.html.
9. Patel VL, Kaufman DR, Cohen T, editors. Cognitive informatics in health and biomedicine: case studies on critical care, complexity and errors. London:

---

[3] https://commonfund.nih.gov/bridge2ai (accessed August 11, 2022).

Springer; 2014. [cited 2021 Jun 16]. (Health Informatics). https://www.springer.com/gp/book/9781447154891.

10. Patel VL, Kaufman DR. Cognitive science and biomedical informatics. In: Shortliffe EH, Cimino JJ, editors. Biomedical informatics: computer applications in health care and biomedicine. 5th ed. New York: Springer; 2021. p. 133–85.

11. Topol E. Deep medicine. How artificial intelligence can make healthcare human again. Hachette UK; 2019.

12. Chang AC. Intelligence-based medicine: artificial intelligence and human cognition in clinical medicine and healthcare. Academic Press; 2020.

13. Agah A, editor. Medical applications of artificial intelligence. Boca Raton: CRC Press; 2013. 526 p.

14. Natarajan P, Frenzel JC, Smaltz DH. Demystifying big data and machine learning for healthcare. Boca Raton: CRC Press; 2017. 210 p.

15. Turing AM. Computing machinery and intelligence. Mind : a quarterly review of psychology and philosophy. 1950;LIX:433.

Seattle, WA, USA   Trevor A. Cohen
New York, NY, USA   Vimla L. Patel
New York, NY, USA   Edward H. Shortliffe
August 2022

Acknowledgments

While my coeditors are well known for their prescience in anticipating (and influencing) the evolution of AIM, I think it is safe to say that none of us envisioned developing a textbook together when we first met at the annual retreat of Columbia University's Department of Medical Informatics in the Catskills in 2002. At the time, I had just joined the program as an incoming graduate student, attracted in part by what I had learned of Ted's work in medical AI and Vimla's in medical cognition. As these topics have remained core components of my subsequent research, it is especially encouraging to see the upsurge in interest in the field. The expanding pool of talented graduate students and physician-informaticians excited about the potential of AIM was a key motivator for our development of this volume, as was our recognition of the need for a textbook in the field that represented historical and cognitive perspectives, in addition to recent methodological developments. However, given the breadth of methods and biomedical applications that by now fall under the AIM umbrella, it was apparent to us that we would need to draw upon the expertise of leaders in relevant fields to develop a multiauthored textbook. Our efforts to weave the perspectives of these authors into a coherent textbook benefited considerably from Ted's experience as lead editor of a multiauthored textbook in biomedical informatics (fondly known as the "blue bible" of BMI, and now in its fifth edition). We modeled both our approach to encouraging the integration of ideas across chapters and the key structural elements of each chapter on the example of that book. We were aided in this endeavor by our authors, who were highly responsive to our suggestions for points of reference between chapters, as well as our recommendations to reduce overlap. We especially appreciated our correspondence with authors during the editing process, which broadened our own perspectives on AIM, and influenced the themes we focused on when developing the final chapter (Reflections and Projections). We owe additional gratitude to Grant Weston, Executive Editor of Springer's Medicine and Life Sciences division, for his steadfast support and guidance throughout the development of this volume. We would also like to acknowledge our Production Editor Rakesh Jotheeswaran, Project Manager Hashwini Vytheswaran, and Editorial Assistant Leo Johnson for their assistance in keeping the project on track. Special thanks also go to Bruce Buchanan (an AI luminary, key mentor for Ted's work in the 1970s, and his long-term collaborator and colleague) for his willingness to craft the foreword for this volume. The development of this volume coincided with a global pandemic. Many involved in the project were affected by this in a professional capacity through their practice of medicine, their role in an informatics response at their institutions, or the position of their professional home within a healthcare system under siege. We trust the development of their chapters provided a welcome respite for these authors, as ours did for us, and hope that readers of this volume will be inspired to develop AIM solutions that equip us to anticipate and manage global health crises more effectively in the future.

Seattle, WA, USA   Trevor A. Cohen
August 2022

Contents

Contributors

Emily Alsentzer Massachusetts Institute of Technology, Cambridge, MA, USA

Riccardo Bellazzi Department of Electrical, Computer and Biomedical Engineering, University of Pavia, Pavia, Italy

Laboratory of Informatics and Systems Engineering for Clinical Research, Istituti Clinici Scientifici Maugeri, Pavia, Italy

Timothy Bickmore Khoury College of Computer Sciences, Northeastern University, Boston, MA, USA

Bethene D. Britt UW Medicine, University of Washington, Seattle, WA, USA

David L. Buckeridge McGill University, Montreal, QC, Canada

Anthony C. Chang Medical Intelligence and Innovation Institute (MI3), Children's Health of Orange County, Orange, CA, USA

Jake Y. Chen Informatics Institute, University of Alabama at Birmingham, Birmingham, AL, USA

Trevor A. Cohen University of Washington, Seattle, WA, USA

Gregory F. Cooper Department of Biomedical Informatics, University of Pittsburgh, Pittsburgh, PA, USA

Arianna Dagliati Department of Electrical, Computer and Biomedical Engineering, University of Pavia, Pavia, Italy

Dev Dash Stanford University School of Medicine, Stanford, CA, USA

Parvati Dev SimTabs LLC, Los Altos Hills, CA, USA

Kenneth W. Goodman Institute for Bioethics and Health Policy, University of Miami, Miami, FL, USA

Michael B. Gotway Mayo Clinic, Scottsdale, AZ, USA

Tina Hernandez-Boussard Stanford University School of Medicine, Stanford, CA, USA

Andrew J. King Department of Critical Care Medicine, University of Pittsburgh, Pittsburgh, PA, USA

Diane M. Korngiebel Department of Biomedical Informatics and Medical Education, University of Washington, Seattle, WA, USA

Ron C. Li Stanford University School of Medicine, Stanford, CA, USA

Jianming Liang Arizona State University, Phoenix, AZ, USA

Naveen Muthu University of Pennsylvania School of Medicine, Philadelphia, PA, USA

Children's Hospital of Philadelphia, Philadelphia, PA, USA

Thanh M. Nguyen Informatics Institute, University of Alabama at Birmingham, Birmingham, AL, USA

Giovanna Nicora Department of Electrical, Computer and Biomedical Engineering, University of Pavia, Pavia, Italy

Vimla L. Patel The New York Academy of Medicine, New York, NY, USA

Kirk Roberts The University of Texas Health Science Center at Houston, Houston, TX, USA

Martìn-Josè Sepùlveda Florida International University, Miami, FL, USA

Nigam H. Shah Stanford University School of Medicine, Stanford, CA, USA

Edward H. Shortliffe Vagelos College of Physicians and Surgeons, Columbia University, New York, NY, USA

Ida Sim University of California San Francisco, San Francisco, CA, USA

Marina Sirota University of California San Francisco, San Francisco, CA, USA

Anthony Solomonides Research Institute, NorthShore University HealthSystem, Evanston, IL, USA

Devika Subramanian Rice University, Houston, TX, USA

Peter Szolovits Massachusetts Institute of Technology, Cambridge, MA, USA

Shyam Visweswaran Department of Biomedical Informatics, University of Pittsburgh, Pittsburgh, PA, USA

Byron Wallace Khoury College of Computer Sciences, Northeastern University, Boston, MA, USA

Adam B. Wilcox Washington University in St. Louis School of Medicine, St. Louis, MO, USA

Hua Xu The University of Texas Health Science Center at Houston, Houston, TX, USA

Zongwei Zhou Johns Hopkins University, Baltimore, MD, USA

Part I
Introduction

Chapter 1
Introducing AI in Medicine

Trevor A. Cohen, Vimla L. Patel, and Edward H. Shortliffe

After reading this chapter, you should know the answers to these questions:
- How does one define artificial intelligence (AI)? What are some ways in which AI has been applied to the practice of medicine and to health care more broadly?
- How does one define cognitive informatics (CI)? How can the CI perspective inform the development, evaluation and implementation of AI-based tools to support clinical decision making?
- What are some factors that have driven the current wave of interest in AI methods?
- How can one compare and contrast knowledge-based systems with machine learning models? What are some of the relative advantages and disadvantages of these approaches?
- Considering the current state of progress, where is research and development most urgently needed in the field and why?

T. A. Cohen (✉)
University of Washington, Seattle, WA, USA
e-mail: cohenta@uw.edu

V. L. Patel
New York Academy of Medicine, New York, NY, USA

E. H. Shortliffe
Columbia University, New York, NY, USA

T. A. Cohen et al. (eds.), *Intelligent Systems in Medicine and Health*, Cognitive Informatics in Biomedicine and Healthcare,
https://doi.org/10.1007/978-3-031-09108-7_1

The Rise of AIM

Knowledge-Based Systems

The term "artificial intelligence" (AI) can first be found in a proposal for a conference that took place at Dartmouth College in 1956, which was written by John McCarthy and his colleagues [1]. The research to be conducted in this two-month conference was built upon the "conjecture that every aspect of learning or any other feature of intelligence can in principle be so precisely described that a machine can be made to simulate it." This conference is considered a seminal event in AI, and was followed by a steady growth of interest in the field that is reflected by the frequency with which the term 'artificial intelligence' appeared in books of this era (Fig. 1.1). There was a first peak of activity in the mid-1980s that followed a period of rapid progress in the development of knowledge-based **expert systems**, systems that were developed by eliciting knowledge from human experts and rendering this content in computer-interpretable form. Diagnostic reasoning in medicine was one of the first focus areas for the development of such systems, providing proof that AI methods could approach human performance in tasks demanding a command of a rich base of knowledge [3]. This shows that medical decision making has long been considered a paradigmatic example of intelligent human behavior, and has been a focus of—and has had an influence on—AI research for decades.

The historical trend in term usage in Fig. 1.1 also reveals a dip in enthusiasm and in support for AI endeavors following the peak in the 1980s (one of the so-called 'AI Winters'), for reasons that are discussed in Chap. 2. For the purpose of this introduction, we focus on the events of recent years, which have seen rapid growth in interest in AIM applications driven by media attention to AI in general (evident to the right of Fig. 1.1), coupled with high profile medical demonstrations of diagnostic

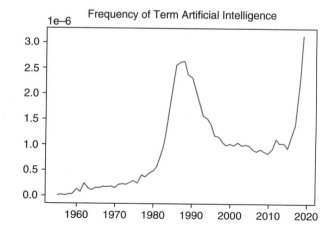

Fig. 1.1 Frequency with which the term 'artificial intelligence' appears in books published between 1950 and 2019 and digitized by Google (data obtained from the Google Books n-gram viewer website [2]). 1e-6 indicates the order of frequency of occurrence of the term (e.g. approximately 2.5 occurrences per million bigrams at the peak in the late eighties)

accuracy, particularly in image recognition. This growth is part of a larger picture in which the capabilities of **artificial neural networks**—originally conceived as models of human information processing and learning [4, 5]—have been enhanced through a convergence of the availability of large data sets for training, refinements in training approaches, and increases in computational power.

Neural Networks and Deep Learning

Loosely inspired by the interconnections between neurons in the human brain, artificial neural networks consist of interconnected functional units named neurons, each producing an output signal determined by their input data, weights assigned to incoming connections, and an **activation function** that transforms cumulative incoming signals into an output that is passed on to a next layer of the network. The weights of a neural network serve as parameters that can be altered during training of a model, so that the output of the neural network better approximates a desired result, such as assigning a high probability to the correct diagnostic label for a radiological image. When used in this way, neural networks exemplify the paradigm of **supervised machine learning**, in which models learn from labels (such as diagnoses) assigned to training data. This approach is very different in nature from the deliberate engineering of human knowledge that supported the expert systems in the first wave of AIM (see Chap. 2 and, for detailed accounts of knowledge modeling and machine learning methods, see Chaps. 4 and 6 respectively).

While machine learning models can learn to make impressively accurate predictions, especially when large data sets are available for training, systems leveraging explicitly modeled human knowledge—systems intended to reason *as humans do*—are much better positioned to explain themselves (for an example, see Box 1.1) than systems that have been developed to optimize accuracy without considering human cognition. Explanation has long been recognized as a desirable property of AI systems for automated diagnosis, and as a prerequisite for their acceptance by clinicians [6] (and see Chap. 8). However, the general trend in machine learning has been that accuracy comes at the cost of interpretability, to the point at which restoring some semblance of interpretability to the predictions made by contemporary machine learning models has emerged as a field of research in its own right—explainable AI—with support from the Defense Advanced Research Projects Agency (DARPA),[1] the same agency that initiated the research program on network protocols that ultimately led to a consumer-accessible internet.

---

[1] See https://www.darpa.mil/program/explainable-artificial-intelligence (accessed August 18, 2022) for details.

Box 1.1 An explanation provided by the MYCIN system in response to a user entering "WHY": From Shortliffe et al. 1974 [7]

- **WHY
- [1.0] It is important to find out whether there is therapeutically significant disease associated with this occurrence of ORGANISM-1.
- It has already been established that:
- [1.1] the site of the culture is not one of those which are normally sterile, and
- [1.2] the method of collection is sterile
- Therefore, if:
- [1.3] the organism has been observed in significant numbers
- Then: there is strongly suggestive evidence (.9) that there is therapeutically significant disease associated with this occurrence of the organism
- [Also: there is strongly suggestive evidence (.8) that the organism is not a contaminant]

This trend toward accurate but opaque predictions has accelerated with the advent of **deep learning** models—neural networks that have multiple intervening layers of neurons between input data and output predictions. While deep neural network architectures are not new phenomena (see for example the important paper by Hinton et al. [8]), their performance when trained on large data sets has produced dramatic improvements in results attained across fundamental tasks such as speech recognition, question answering and image recognition.

Figure 1.2 shows the extent of recent improvements for three key benchmarks: the Stanford Question Answering Dataset (SQUAD [9])—over 100,000 comprehension questions related to short articles; ImageNet—over 14 million images each assigned one of two hundred possible class labels [10]; and LibriSpeech—over 1000 hours of speech with matching text from audiobooks [11]. Of note, with both SQUAD and ImageNet, human performance on the tasks concerned has been estimated, and superseded by deep learning models.

Conceptually, the advantages of deep learning models over previous machine learning approaches have been attributed to their capacity for **representation learning** [12]. With prior machine learning approaches, performance generally advanced through engineering ways to represent incoming data (such as pixels of an image representing a handwritten digit) that led to better downstream machine learning performance (representations such as a count of the number of loops in a handwritten digit [13]). With deep learning models, the lower layers of a network can learn to represent incoming data in ways that facilitate task performance automatically.[2] Of particular importance for domains such as medicine, where large labeled data

---

[2] While deep learning models excel at learning representations that lead to better predictive modeling performance, representation learning is broader than deep learning and includes a number of previously established methods. For a review of developments up to 2013, see [14].

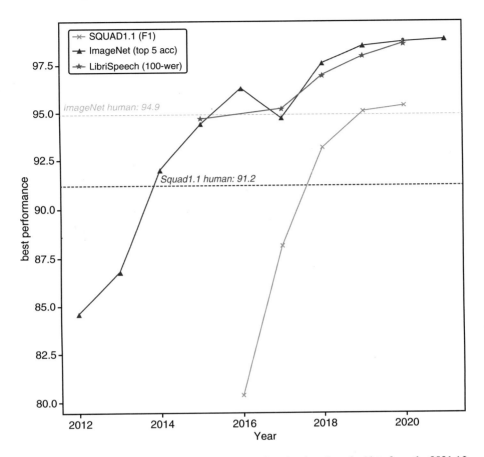

Fig. 1.2 Best documented performance, by year, on three key benchmarks (data from the 2021 AI Index Report [15, 16]). (1) SQUAD1.1 = Stanford Question Answering Dataset (version 1.1). Performance metric is "F1" (the balanced f-measure; see Chap. 6); (2) ImageNet - performance metric is "top 5 acc" (the percent of images in which the correct label, among 200 possibilities, appeared in the top 5 predictions); (3) LibriSpeech - performance metrics is "100-wer" (a transformation of the word error rate, with 100 indicating every word in a recording was recognized correctly). Dashed lines indicate documented human performance on the task concerned, which has been superseded by AI in both cases

sets are relatively difficult to obtain, the ability to extract useful representations for one task can often be learned from training on another related one. This ability to apply information learned from one task or data set to another is known as **transfer learning**, and is perhaps best exemplified by what has become a standard approach to classifying medical images (see Chap. 12): adding a classification layer to a deep neural network that has been pretrained on the task of recognizing non-medical images in ImageNet [17]. Similarly, fine-tuning of models such as Google's **BERT** and Open-AI's GPT series, which were originally trained to predict held-out words in large amounts of text from a range of digital data sources, has advanced performance across a broad range of **natural language processing (NLP)** tasks [18, 19].

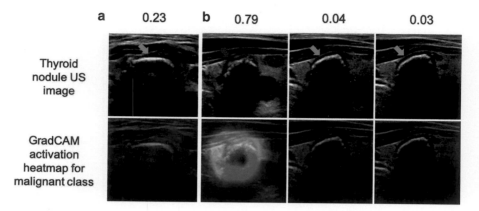

Fig. 1.3 Recognition of a subtle diagnostic cue by a deep neural network trained to detect thyroid cancer in different ultrasound images of the same nodule. Each image (top row) is annotated with the probability of malignancy according to the model, and is paired with a visualization of the pixels attended to by the deep learning model when making a prediction for whether an image is in the "malignant class", developed using the GradCam method [20]. Only the second image from the left exhibits the diagnostic feature of interrupted eggshell calcification, in which the rim of the opaque "shell" of calcification (blue arrows in the top row) is disrupted (red arrow). The GradCam visualization reveals the model has learned to attend to this subtle diagnostic feature. Image courtesy of Dr. Nikita Pozdeyev

Machine Learning and Medical Practice

Of course, outperforming humans on the repetitive and mundane task of selecting among hundreds of possible labels for a given image, or surpassing their accuracy in answering multiple choice questions about particular passages, does not necessarily provide an indication that deep neural networks could meet the requirements for flexibility, prioritization and adaptive decision making under uncertainty needed to *replace* medical practitioners in a busy clinical environment (audiobooks are also far less challenging to transcribe than recordings captured in a naturalistic environment—see Chap. 9 for a related discussion of automated medical transcription).

Nonetheless, the ability to recognize diagnostically important features is a fundamental task in interpreting medical images (as illustrated in Fig. 1.3—see also Chap. 12). A system capable of answering clinical questions accurately on the basis of written notes would make the information that these notes contain amenable to downstream computational processing for decision support or observational research (methods to achieve such ends are discussed in detail in Chap. 7). Furthermore, similar advances in performance have been achieved by predictive models in medicine, due in part to the large volume of digitized medical data that has accompanied the adoption of **electronic health record** (EHR) systems,[3] and the widespread use of digital platforms for image storage and retrieval (see Chap. 3) [22].

---

[3] In the United States this increase in adoption is attributable to the incentivization structures provided by the Health Information Technology for Economic and Clinical Health (HITECH) act of 2009 [21].

For example, a 2016 paper in the *Journal of the American Medical Association* describes an impressively accurate deep learning system for the diagnosis of diabetes-related eye disease in images of the retina [23]. Similarly, a widely-cited 2017 paper in *Nature* describes the application of deep learning to detect skin cancer [24], with the resulting system performing as well as 21 board-certified dermatologists in identifying two types of neoplastic skin lesions. These systems leveraged recent advances in AI, including deep neural network architectures and approaches to train them efficiently, as well as large sets of labeled data that were used to train the networks—*over 125,000 images* in each study. The dermatology system benefitted further from pre-training on over *1.25 million non-medical images* labeled with 1000 object categories. Beyond imaging, deep learning models trained on EHR data have learned to predict in-hospital mortality, unplanned readmission, prolonged length of stay, and final discharge diagnosis—in many cases outperforming traditional predictive models that are still widely used in clinical practice [25]. In this case, models were trained on data from over 200,000 hospitalized adult patients from two academic medical centers, considering *over 40 billion sequential data points* collectively.

These advances have attracted a great deal of press attention, with frequent articles in prominent media outlets considering the potential of AI to enhance—or disrupt—the practice of medicine [26–28]. As we have discussed in the preface to this volume, neither AI systems with physician-level performance nor media attention to such systems are without precedent, even in the days before advances in computational power and methodology mediated the current explosive interest in machine learning. However, the convergence of an unprecedented availability of clinical data with the maturation of machine learning models (and the computational resources to train them at scale) has allowed the rapid development of AI-based predictive models in medicine. Many demonstrate impressive results beyond those we have briefly described here. Furthermore, the proven commercial viability and public acceptance of such models in other areas have offset some of the skepticism with which AI models were greeted initially. Having seen the effectiveness with which machine learning models leverage data to deliver our entertainment and shopping recommendations on a daily basis, why would we not wish such systems to assist our clinicians in their medical practice? A strong indicator of the commercial potential of AI-based systems in medicine is the emergence of regulatory frameworks for their application in practice (see also Chap. 18) [29], with a number of AI systems already approved for medical use in the United States (Fig. 1.4) and Europe [30].

The Scope of AIM

A fundamental question in the study (and regulation) of AIM systems concerns the definition of the term "Artificial Intelligence". Given the breadth of approaches that have been categorized as related to AI, it is perhaps not surprising that there is no universally-accepted definition of this term, and that the extent to which contemporary deep learning approaches constitute AI is still vigorously debated [32, 33]. A representative sample of AI definitions is provided in Box 1.2. While there are

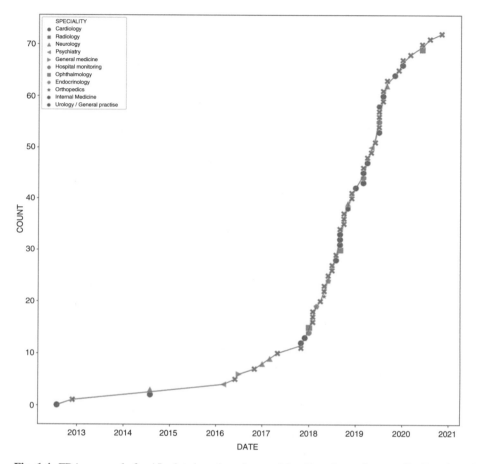

Fig. 1.4 FDA approvals for AI-related products by specialty (data drawn from medicalfuturist. com [30, 31]) with radiology systems (X) the most common category

---

Box 1.2 Sample Definitions of Artificial Intelligence

- *"The study of complex information processing problems that often have their roots in some aspect of biological information processing" (Marr, 1977)* [34]
- *"...the study of ideas that enable computers to do the things that make human beings seem intelligent: the ability to reason symbolically, the ability to acquire and apply knowledge, and the ability to manipulate and communicate ideas" (Winston, 1977)* [35]
- *"....the part of computer science concerned with designing intelligent computer systems, that is, systems that exhibit the characteristics we associate with intelligence in human behavior – understanding, language, learning, reasoning, solving problems and so on" (Barr et al., vol 1, 1981, p. 3)* [36]

- *"The branch of computer science that is concerned with the automation of intelligent behavior" (Luger and Stubblefield, 1993)* [37]
- *"It is the science and engineering of making intelligent machines, especially intelligent computer programs. It is related to the similar task of using computers to understand human intelligence, but AI does not have to confine itself to methods that are biologically observable". (McCarthy, 2007)* [38]

clearly common threads that run among them, notably the emphasis on intelligence (loosely defined by Barr as exhibiting the characteristics we associate with intelligence in human behavior, or by Winston as emphasizing the use of knowledge and an ability to communicate ideas), the definitions also reflect a departure from the cognitive motivations of AI at its inception—performance of tasks as humans do— to the more pragmatic motivations of the performance-oriented systems that are commonly termed AI today. Note that McCarthy in particular asserts explicitly that biological constraints need not apply. Of course, motivations for understanding how machines might solve a problem presumed to require human intelligence are not exclusively pragmatic, as this topic is also of considerable academic interest.

As one might anticipate given the fluidity of definitions of AI in general, the notion of what qualifies as AI in medicine is also in flux. At the inception of the field, the focus was on systems that could reason, leveraging encoded knowledge (including probabilistic estimates or uncertainty) derived from clinical experts. Such formalization of knowledge to render it computable also underlies the clinical decision support rules embedded in contemporary EHR systems. However, few would argue that the individual rules firing alerts in such systems constitute AI, even when considered collectively (see the discussion of warnings and alerts in Chap. 17). It seems, therefore, that the perceived difficulty of the tasks accomplished by a system determine whether it is thought to have exhibited intelligent behavior. Today, machine learning approaches (including deep neural networks) are strongly associated with the term AI. These systems are not designed to reason, but instead learn to recognize patterns, such as diagnostic features of radiology images, leading to performance on constrained tasks that is comparable to that of highly trained physicians. As such it is easy to argue that they exhibit intelligent human behavior, at least in the context of a task for which large amounts of labeled training data are readily available. Furthermore, such models can make predictions that are beyond the capabilities of human experts at times, such as prediction of cardiovascular risk factor status from retinal fundus photographs [39], or prediction of 3-D protein structure from an amino acid sequence [40]. Perhaps as a consequence of the lack of funding for research associated with the term AI during periods in which it was out of favor (see Chap. 2), a great deal of machine learning work in the field was not framed as AI research, but would be perceived this way in retrospect. Analogous to the case with rule-based models, this raises the question of how sophisticated a machine learning model is required to qualify as AI. For example, would a system based on a logistic regression model trained on a handful of features, with less than ten trainable parameters constitute AI? Perhaps, as with rules, the main question concerns the nature of the task that the model is able to accomplish, with a benchmark for AIM being the automated accomplishment of tasks that would be challenging for a highly trained human.

From Accurate Predictions to Clinically Useful AIM

However, irrespective of whether the engineers of AIM systems attempt to emulate human-like problem-solving processes, the ultimate goal of such efforts is often to support decision making by human clinicians at the point of care. The role of AIM in improving the quality, efficiency and safety of clinical practice exists within a larger system that includes human decision makers [41]. As such, both the remarkable capabilities and recognized constraints of human information processing must also be considered when designing and deploying AI-based systems, even if the systems concerned do not explicitly attempt to emulate human information processing methods. The consideration of the broader context in which AI-based systems must operate to influence patient care reveals a number of challenges that must be overcome in order to bridge the gulf between systems that perform well in the context of a constrained reference set, and systems that provide clinical utility at the point of care. Many of these challenges have been recognized since the inception of the field. In a 1975 paper, Shortliffe and Davis identified a series of seven considerations for expert system evaluation that suggest a path from conception of a system to clinical utility (Table 1.1; see also Chap. 17).

Of note, most of the work on accurate automated medical image interpretation we have discussed addresses only the second consideration in Table 1.1, and improving the ability of machine learning models to approach (or even surpass) the accuracy of expert clinicians has remained the focus of much recent work [43]. However, such models must be embedded in systems that are both usable and acceptable to clinicians if they are to exert an effect on management to improve outcomes for patients or to advance institutional or societal priorities such as cost-effectiveness. Furthermore, the design of AI systems should be motivated by the needs of clinicians, which are best understood in the context of the processes and environmental constraints in which they work [41].

Table 1.1 Overview: seven considerations for system evaluation [42]

	Demonstration		Impact
1	Need	5	Management
2	Expert-level performance	6	Patient outcome
3	Usability	7	Cost-effectiveness
4	Acceptance by clinicians		

The Cognitive Informatics Perspective

Why CI?

It is our view that the discipline of *cognitive informatics* (CI) [44–46], which brings the perspective of the cognitive sciences to the study of medical decision making by human beings and machines, is uniquely positioned to address these challenges. Through its roots in the study of medical reasoning [47–49], CI provides a sound scientific basis from which to consider the relationship between current technologies and human intelligence. CI has extended its area of inquiry to include both human-computer interaction and the study of the effects of technology on the flow of work and information in clinical settings [50–53]. Accordingly CI is well-positioned to inform the integration of AIM systems into clinical practice, and more broadly to inform the design of AI systems that complement the cognitive capabilities of human decision makers, in alignment with seminal ideas concerning the potential of cooperative human-machine systems [54].

The Complementarity of Human and Machine Intelligence

As is discussed in Chap. 5, evaluations in the context of image processing tasks have demonstrated that the performance of human beings and machines working in concert can result in better diagnostic accuracy than either machines or human beings alone [55–57]. In some ways this is not surprising, given the different strategies human experts and machines employ to achieve diagnostic accuracy. Cognitive studies of radiologists have shown that experts in this domain integrate their knowledge of anatomical structures and their projections onto two-dimensional images, with their knowledge of general physiology and specific disease processes. This allows radiologists to generate initial hypotheses that narrow the focus of their search for a definitive diagnosis [47]. In contrast, contemporary neural network models learn to identify radiological abnormalities by training two-dimensional "feature detectors" to recognize regions that are useful in distinguishing between diagnostic categories in the training data (as illustrated previously, in Fig. 1.3), irrespective of where within an image these regions may occur [58]. Differences in the processes through which neural networks and human experts interpret images can also be detected empirically. Recent work has shown that human beings and machines focus on different features when interpreting histology slides [59].

Acknowledgment of these differences leads naturally to the conclusion that a human/AI collaborative team has the potential to make better decisions than those that would emerge from a fully automated or exclusively manual process (see, for example, the discussion of QMR in Chap. 2). However, many open questions remain regarding how best to realize this potential. A promising proposal concerns deliberately designing AI systems to compensate for known "blind spots" in clinical

decision making [60], such as biases in diagnostic reasoning that have been identified through cognitive research [61], or distracted attention in busy clinical settings
[62]. Alternatively, one might envision developing ways to distribute labor across a
human/AI collaborative system to maximize the expected utility of this system, taking into account both the accuracy of model predictions and the time required for a
human actor to reassess them. Recent work has developed an approach to optimizing collaborative systems in this way, resulting in some experiments in systems that
increase high-confidence predictions (i.e. predictions to which the model assigns
extremely high or low probability) at the expense of its accuracy in edge cases (i.e.
predictions close to the model's decision boundary), where human input could
resolve model uncertainty [63].

Mediating Safe and Effective Human Use of AI-Based Tools

CI methods are already well established as means to evaluate the **usability** of decision support tools [45, 46]. Findings from this line of research have led to recommendations that the usability of clinical systems should be prioritized as a means
to enhance their acceptability and safety [64]. In contrast to system-centric methods of usability evaluation, such as heuristic evaluations by usability experts [65],
CI approaches attempt to understand the thought process of a user, which is particularly important in knowledge-rich domains, such as medicine, where both
knowledge of the system being used and of the domain are required to perform
tasks correctly [66]. This can be accomplished through analysis of a **think-aloud
protocol**, collected by prompting users to verbalize their thoughts during the process of completing representative tasks [67]. This approach is similarly well-suited
to the study of clinician interactions with AI-based systems, where users must
make clinical decisions on the basis of their estimation of the veracity of system output.

Critical questions concerning the nature of these interactions remain to be
answered. One such question concerns how best to represent model predictions. For
example, recent work in dermatology diagnosis found that advantages in performance for a human-computer collective were contingent upon the granularity (probabilities of all of the diseases in the differential diagnosis vs. a single global risk of
malignancy) and cognitive demand of the representation used to convey predictions
to physicians [57]. Analysis of verbal protocols collected during interactions with
interfaces, using alternative representations of the same predictions, could inform our
understanding of *why* this is the case by revealing the reasoning dermatologists use
when deciding whether to accept a particular recommendation. Another important
question concerns the role of explanations provided by a system in influencing human
decision making. Intriguingly, recent research has shown that revealing the influence
of input features (here, words in a passage of text) on model predictions increases the
likelihood that users will accept the validity of these predictions, irrespective of
whether they are accurate [68]. This suggests that displaying feature salience may not

be adequate to support the fault detection procedures that are a prerequisite to safe and resilient human/AI collaborative systems. CI methods are well-suited to identify the thought processes through which faulty AI decisions are (or are not) identified when considering explanations, to inform the development of effective systems in which process are *both* highly automated *and* subject to human control. This should arguably be the case for systems making critical medical decisions, where mistakes have irreversible consequences [69].

Concluding Remarks

In this chapter, we have provided an introduction to AIM, with a focus on recent developments. In doing so, we have highlighted some key challenges that AI models must meet if they are to achieve the goal of improving the efficiency, safety and quality of health care. We have argued that the field of CI is well-suited to address these challenges, by providing greater insight into the role of the human component of human/AI collaborative systems, to inform their design and evaluation. Consideration of the cognitive processes through which human beings evaluate, interpret and act upon the recommendations made by AI systems is fundamental to the development of solutions that enhance the capabilities of clinicians and researchers in the biomedical domain. Accordingly, one of our goals in developing this volume has been to provide a resource to support the multidisciplinary training required to design and implement AI methods with the potential to enhance the practice of medicine as well as life science research in human biology.

Questions for Discussion

- What is an example of a recent technological advancement in AIM, and what are its implications for clinical practice?
- Provide your own definition of AIM that reflects the discussion in this chapter (i.e., do not simply pick one from Box 1.2). Do any aspects of the field of which you are aware fall outside the scope of this definition?
- What are the main application areas and techniques for AIM?
- AI in medicine has a long history, and AIM technologies have been proposed as a potential disruptor of the healthcare industry before. What current contextual factors might increase or limit the potential for broad adoption?

Further Reading

Chang, AC. Intelligence-Based Medicine: Artificial Intelligence and Human Cognition in Clinical Medicine and Healthcare. Academic Press (Elsevier); July 8th 2020.

- This book provides a survey of AI methods from clinical and data science perspectives, with an emphasis on their implementation in, and impact upon, medicine and its subspecialties.

Miotto R, Wang F, Wang S, Jiang X, Dudley JT. Deep learning for healthcare: review, opportunities and challenges. Briefings in Bioinformatics. 2018 Nov 27;19 (6):1236–1246.

- This paper provides an overview and of deep learning applications in healthcare up to 2018, and introduces a number of issues that are addressed in the current volume.

Patel VL, Kannampallil TG. Cognitive informatics in biomedicine and healthcare. Journal of biomedical informatics. 2015 Feb 1;53:3–14.

- This paper provides a definition and overview of the field of cognitive informatics, with a focus on biomedical applications.

Topol EJ. High-performance medicine: the convergence of human and artificial intelligence. Nature Medicine. Nature Publishing Group; 2019 Jan;25 (1):44–56.

- This paper provides an overview of AI applications in healthcare, including a thoughtful account of challenges that distinguish this domain from others in which AI applications have established their value.

Zhang D, Mishra S, Brynjolfsson E, Etchemendy J, Ganguli D, Grosz B, Lyons T, Manyika J, Niebles JC, Sellitto M, Shoham Y, Clark J, Perrault R. The AI Index 2021 Annual Report. arXiv:210306312 [cs] [Internet]. 2021 Mar 8 [cited 2021 Apr 24]; Available from: http://arxiv.org/abs/2103.06312

- Stanford's AI Index Report provides an overview of national and global AI trends in research and industry.

References

1. McCarthy J, Minsky ML, Rochester N, Shannon CE. A proposal for the Dartmouth summer research project on artificial intelligence, August 31, 1955. AIMag. 2006;27(4):12.
2. Google Books Ngram Viewer [Internet]. [cited 2021 June 25]. Available from: https://books.google.com/ngrams.
3. Yu VL, Buchanan BG, Shortliffe EH, Wraith SM, Davis R, Scott AC, Cohen SN. Evaluating the performance of a computer-based consultant. Comput Programs Biomed. 1979;9(1):95–102.
4. Rosenblatt F. The perceptron: a probabilistic model for information storage and organization in the brain. Psychol Rev. 1958;65(6):386.
5. McClelland JL, Rumelhart DE, Group PR. Parallel distributed processing. Boston, MA: MIT Press; 1986. p. 1.
6. Swartout WR. Explaining and justifying expert consulting programs. Computer-assisted medical decision making. Springer; 1985. p. 254–71.
7. Shortliffe EH, Davis R, Axline SG, Buchanan BG, Green CC, Cohen SN. Computer-based consultations in clinical therapeutics: explanation and rule acquisition capabilities of the MYCIN system. Comput Biomed Res. 1975;8(4):303–20.
8. Hinton GE, Osindero S, Teh Y-W. A fast learning algorithm for deep belief nets. Neural Comput. 2006;18(7):1527–54.

9. Rajpurkar P, Zhang J, Lopyrev K, Liang P. Squad: 100,000+ questions for machine comprehension of text. In Proceedings of the 2016 Conference on Empirical Methods in Natural Language Processing, pages 2383–2392, Austin, Texas. Association for Computational Linguistics.

10. Deng J, Dong W, Socher R, Li L-J, Li K, Fei-Fei L. Imagenet: a large-scale hierarchical image database. 2009 IEEE conference on computer vision and pattern recognition. IEEE; 2009. p. 248–55.

11. Panayotov V, Chen G, Povey D, Khudanpur S. Librispeech: an ASR corpus based on public domain audio books. 2015 IEEE international conference on acoustics, speech and signal processing (ICASSP). 2015. p. 5206–5210.

12. LeCun Y, Bengio Y, Hinton G. Deep learning. Nature. 2015;521(7553):436–44.

13. Kumar G, Bhatia PK. A detailed review of feature extraction in image processing systems. 2014 fourth international conference on advanced computing communication technologies. 2014. p. 5–12.

14. Bengio Y, Courville A, Vincent P. Representation learning: a review and new perspectives. IEEE Trans Pattern Anal Mach Intell. 2013;35(8):1798–828.

15. Zhang D, Mishra S, Brynjolfsson E, Etchemendy J, Ganguli D, Grosz B, Lyons T, Manyika J, Niebles JC, Sellitto M, Shoham Y, Clark J, Perrault R. The AI Index 2021 annual report. arXiv:210306312 [cs] [Internet]. 2021 Mar 8 [cited 2021 Apr 24]. Available from: http://arxiv.org/abs/2103.06312.

16. AI Index 2021 [Internet]. Stanford HAI. [cited 2021 June 25]. Available from: https://hai.stanford.edu/research/ai-index-2021.

17. Shin H-C, Roth HR, Gao M, Lu L, Xu Z, Nogues I, Yao J, Mollura D, Summers RM. Deep convolutional neural networks for computer-aided detection: CNN architectures, dataset characteristics and transfer learning. IEEE Trans Med Imaging. 2016;35(5):1285–98.

18. Devlin J, Chang M-W, Lee K, Toutanova K. BERT: pre-training of deep bidirectional transformers for language understanding. Proceedings of the 2019 conference of the North American Chapter of the Association for computational linguistics: human language technologies, Vol. 1 (Long and Short Papers). 2019. p. 4171–4186.

19. Radford A, Wu J, Child R, Luan D, Amodei D, Sutskever I. Language models are unsupervised multitask learners. OpenAI Blog. 2019;1(8):9.

20. Selvaraju RR, Cogswell M, Das A, Vedantam R, Parikh D, Batra D. Grad-cam: Visual explanations from deep networks via gradient-based localization. Proceedings of the IEEE international conference on computer vision. 2017. p. 618–626.

21. Adler-Milstein J, Jha AK. HITECH act drove large gains in hospital electronic health record adoption. Health Aff. 2017;36(8):1416–22.

22. Bauman RA, Gell G, Dwyer SJ. Large picture archiving and communication systems of the world--part 1. J Digit Imaging. 1996;9(3):99–103.

23. Gulshan V, Peng L, Coram M, Stumpe MC, Wu D, Narayanaswamy A, Venugopalan S, Widner K, Madams T, Cuadros J. Development and validation of a deep learning algorithm for detection of diabetic retinopathy in retinal fundus photographs. JAMA. 2016;316(22):2402–10.

24. Esteva A, Kuprel B, Novoa RA, Ko J, Swetter SM, Blau HM, Thrun S. Dermatologist-level classification of skin cancer with deep neural networks. Nature. 2017;542(7639):115–8.

25. Rajkomar A, Oren E, Chen K, Dai AM, Hajaj N, Hardt M, Liu PJ, Liu X, Marcus J, Sun M, Sundberg P, Yee H, Zhang K, Zhang Y, Flores G, Duggan GE, Irvine J, Le Q, Litsch K, Mossin A, Tansuwan J, Wang D, Wexler J, Wilson J, Ludwig D, Volchenboum SL, Chou K, Pearson M, Madabushi S, Shah NH, Butte AJ, Howell MD, Cui C, Corrado GS, Dean J. Scalable and accurate deep learning with electronic health records. NPJ Digit Med. 2018;1(1):1–10.

26. Mukherjee S. A.I. versus M.D. [Internet]. The New Yorker. [cited 2021 Apr 15]. https://www.newyorker.com/magazine/2017/04/03/ai-versus-md.

27. Metz C. A.I. shows promise assisting physicians. The New York Times [Internet]. 2019 Feb 11 [cited 2021 Apr 15]. https://www.nytimes.com/2019/02/11/health/artificial-intelligence-medical-diagnosis.html.

28. O'Connor A. How artificial intelligence could transform medicine. The New York Times [Internet]. 2019 Mar 11 [cited 2021 Apr 15]. https://www.nytimes.com/2019/03/11/well/live/how-artificial-intelligence-could-transform-medicine.html.
29. Health C for D and R. Artificial intelligence and machine learning in software as a medical device. FDA [Internet]. FDA; 2021 Jan 11 [cited 2021 Apr 19]. https://www.fda.gov/medical-devices/software-medical-device-samd/artificial-intelligence-and-machine-learning-software-medical-device.
30. Benjamens S, Dhunnoo P, Meskó B. The state of artificial intelligence-based FDA-approved medical devices and algorithms: an online database. NPJ Digit Med. 2020;3(1):1–8.
31. The Medical Futurist [Internet]. The Medical Futurist. [cited 2021 Apr 19]. Available from: https://medicalfuturist.com/fda-approved-ai-based-algorithms.
32. Marcus G. Deep learning: a critical appraisal. arXiv preprint arXiv:180100631. 2018.
33. Zador AM. A critique of pure learning and what artificial neural networks can learn from animal brains. Nat Commun. 2019;10(1):1–7.
34. Marr D. Artificial intelligence—a personal view. Artif Intell. 1977;9(1):37–48.
35. Winston PH. Artificial Intelligence. Reading, MA: Addison-Wesley; 1977.
36. Barr A, Feigenbaum EA. The handbook of artificial intelligence (Vol. 1). Los Altos, CA: William Kaufman; 1981.
37. Luger GF, Stubblefield WA. Artificial intelligence (2nd ed.): structures and strategies for complex problem-solving. USA: Benjamin-Cummings Publishing Co., Inc.; 1993.
38. McCarthy J. What is artificial intelligence? [Internet]. What is artificial intelligence? 2007 [cited 2021 Apr 20]. http://www-formal.stanford.edu/jmc/whatisai/whatisai.html.
39. Poplin R, Varadarajan AV, Blumer K, Liu Y, McConnell MV, Corrado GS, Peng L, Webster DR. Prediction of cardiovascular risk factors from retinal fundus photographs via deep learning. Nat Biomed Eng. 2018;2(3):158–64.
40. Jumper J, Evans R, Pritzel A, Green T, Figurnov M, Ronneberger O, Tunyasuvunakool K, Bates R, Žídek A, Potapenko A, Bridgland A, Meyer C, Kohl SAA, Ballard AJ, Cowie A, Romera-Paredes B, Nikolov S, Jain R, Adler J, Back T, Petersen S, Reiman D, Clancy E, Zielinski M, Steinegger M, Pacholska M, Berghammer T, Bodenstein S, Silver D, Vinyals O, Senior AW, Kavukcuoglu K, Kohli P, Hassabis D. Highly accurate protein structure prediction with AlphaFold. Nature. 2021;15:1–11.
41. Berg M. Patient care information systems and health care work: a sociotechnical approach. Int J Med Inform. 1999;55:87–101.
42. Shortliffe T, Davis R. Some considerations for the implementation of knowledge-based expert systems. SIGART Bull. 1975;55:9–12.
43. Topol EJ. High-performance medicine: the convergence of human and artificial intelligence. Nat Med. 2019;25(1):44–56.
44. Wang Y. The theoretical framework of cognitive informatics. Int J Cogn Inform Nat Intell. 2007;1(1):1–27.
45. Patel VL, Kaufman DR. Cognitive science and biomedical informatics. In: Shortliffe EH, Cimino JJ, editors. Biomedical informatics: computer applications in health care and biomedicine. 5th ed. New York: Springer; 2021. p. 133–85.
46. Patel VL, Kannampallil TG. Cognitive informatics in biomedicine and healthcare. J Biomed Inform. 2015;53:3–14.
47. Lesgold A, Rubinson H, Feltovich P, Glaser R, Klopfer D, Wang Y. Expertise in a complex skill: diagnosing x-ray pictures. In: Chi MTH, Glaser R, Farr MJ, editors. The nature of expertise. Hillsdale, NJ: Lawrence Erlbaum; 1988. p. 311–42.
48. Elstein AS, Shulman LS, Sprafka SA. Medical problem solving: an analysis of clinical reasoning. Cambridge, MA: Harvard University Press; 1978.
49. Patel VL, Arocha JF, Kaufman DR. Diagnostic reasoning and medical expertise. Psychol Learn Motiv. 1994;31:187–252.
50. Kushniruk AW, Patel VL, Cimino JJ. Usability testing in medical informatics: cognitive approaches to evaluation of information systems and user interfaces. Proceedings/AMIA annual fall symposium. 1997. p. 218–222.

51. Kushniruk AW, Patel VL. Cognitive and usability engineering methods for the evaluation of clinical information systems. J Biomed Inform. 2004;37:56–76.
52. Malhotra S, Jordan D, Shortliffe E, Patel VL. Workflow modeling in critical care: piecing together your own puzzle. J Biomed Inform. 2007;40:81–92.
53. Cohen T, Blatter B, Almeida C, Shortliffe E, Patel V. A cognitive blueprint of collaboration in context: distributed cognition in the psychiatric emergency department. Artif Intell Med. 2006;37:73–83.
54. Licklider JC. Man-computer symbiosis. IRE transactions on human factors in electronics. IEEE. 1960;1:4–11.
55. Patel BN, Rosenberg L, Willcox G, Baltaxe D, Lyons M, Irvin J, Rajpurkar P, Amrhein T, Gupta R, Halabi S, Langlotz C, Lo E, Mammarappallil J, Mariano AJ, Riley G, Seekins J, Shen L, Zucker E, Lungren MP. Human–machine partnership with artificial intelligence for chest radiograph diagnosis. NPJ Digit Med. 2019;2(1):1–10.
56. Hekler A, Utikal JS, Enk AH, Hauschild A, Weichenthal M, Maron RC, Berking C, Haferkamp S, Klode J, Schadendorf D, Schilling B, Holland-Letz T, Izar B, von Kalle C, Fröhling S, Brinker TJ, Schmitt L, Peitsch WK, Hoffmann F, Becker JC, Drusio C, Jansen P, Klode J, Lodde G, Sammet S, Schadendorf D, Sondermann W, Ugurel S, Zader J, Enk A, Salzmann M, Schäfer S, Schäkel K, Winkler J, Wölbing P, Asper H, Bohne A-S, Brown V, Burba B, Deffaa S, Dietrich C, Dietrich M, Drerup KA, Egberts F, Erkens A-S, Greven S, Harde V, Jost M, Kaeding M, Kosova K, Lischner S, Maagk M, Messinger AL, Metzner M, Motamedi R, Rosenthal A-C, Seidl U, Stemmermann J, Torz K, Velez JG, Haiduk J, Alter M, Bär C, Bergenthal P, Gerlach A, Holtorf C, Karoglan A, Kindermann S, Kraas L, Felcht M, Gaiser MR, Klemke C-D, Kurzen H, Leibing T, Müller V, Reinhard RR, Utikal J, Winter F, Berking C, Eicher L, Hartmann D, Heppt M, Kilian K, Krammer S, Lill D, Niesert A-C, Oppel E, Sattler E, Senner S, Wallmichrath J, Wolff H, Gesierich A, Giner T, Glutsch V, Kerstan A, Presser D, Schrüfer P, Schummer P, Stolze I, Weber J, Drexler K, Haferkamp S, Mickler M, Stauner CT, Thiem A. Superior skin cancer classification by the combination of human and artificial intelligence. Eur J Cancer. 2019;120:114–21.
57. Tschandl P, Rinner C, Apalla Z, Argenziano G, Codella N, Halpern A, Janda M, Lallas A, Longo C, Malvehy J, Paoli J, Puig S, Rosendahl C, Soyer HP, Zalaudek I, Kittler H. Human–computer collaboration for skin cancer recognition. Nat Med. 2020;26(8):1229–34.
58. Soffer S, Ben-Cohen A, Shimon O, Amitai MM, Greenspan H, Klang E. Convolutional neural networks for radiologic images: a Radiologist's guide. Radiology. 2019;290(3): 590–606.
59. Kimeswenger S, Tschandl P, Noack P, Hofmarcher M, Rumetshofer E, Kindermann H, Silye R, Hochreiter S, Kaltenbrunner M, Guenova E, Klambauer G, Hoetzenecker W. Artificial neural networks and pathologists recognize basal cell carcinomas based on different histological patterns. Mod Pathol. 2020;13:1–9.
60. Horvitz E. One hundred year study on artificial intelligence: reflections and framing. Microsoft com. 2014
61. Chapman GB, Elstein AS. Cognitive processes and biases in medical decision-making. In: Chapman GB, Sonnenberg FS, editors. Decision-making in health care: theory, psychology, and applications. Cambridge: Cambridge University Press; 2000. p. 183–210.
62. Franklin A, Liu Y, Li Z, Nguyen V, Johnson TR, Robinson D, Okafor N, King B, Patel VL, Zhang J. Opportunistic decision making and complexity in emergency care. J Biomed Inform. 2011;44(3):469–76.
63. Bansal G, Nushi B, Kamar E, Horvitz E, Weld DS. Is the Most accurate AI the best teammate? Optimizing AI for teamwork. Proc AAAI Conf Artif Intell. 2021;35(13):11405–14.
64. Middleton B, Bloomrosen M, Dente MA, Hashmat B, Koppel R, Overhage JM, Payne TH, Rosenbloom ST, Weaver C, Zhang J. Enhancing patient safety and quality of care by improving the usability of electronic health record systems: recommendations from AMIA. J Am Med Inform Assoc. 2013;20(e1):e2–8.
65. Nielsen J, Molich R. Heuristic evaluation of user interfaces. Proceedings of the SIGCHI conference on human factors in computing systems. 1990. p. 249–256.

66. Horsky J, Kaufman DR, Oppenheim MI, Patel VL. A framework for analyzing the cognitive complexity of computer-assisted clinical ordering. J Biomed Inform. 2003;36:4–22.
67. Ericsson KA, Simon HA. Protocol analysis: verbal reports as data. Cambridge, MA: MIT Press; 1993.
68. Bansal G, Wu T, Zhou J, Fok R, Nushi B, Kamar E, Ribeiro MT, Weld D. Does the whole exceed its parts? The effect of AI explanations on complementary team performance. Proceedings of the 2021 CHI conference on human factors in computing systems. New York, NY: Association for Computing Machinery; 2021. p. 1–16. https://doi.org/10.1145/3411764.3445717.
69. Shneiderman B. Human-centered artificial intelligence: reliable, safe & trustworthy. Int J Hum Comput Interact. 2020;36(6):495–504.

Chapter 2
AI in Medicine: Some Pertinent History

Edward H. Shortliffe and Nigam H. Shah

After reading this chapter, you should know the answers to these questions:
- What are the roots of artificial intelligence in human history, even before the general introduction of digital computers?
- How did computer science emerge as an academic and research discipline and how was AI identified as a component of that revolution?
- How did a medical focus on AI applications emerge from the early general principles of the field?
- How did the field of cognitive science influence early work on AI in Medicine (AIM) and how have those synergies evolved to the present?
- What were the early medical applications of AI and how were they received in the clinical and medical research communities?
- How has the focus of medical AI research and application evolved in parallel with AI itself, and with the progress in computing power, communications technology, and interactive devices?
- To what extent are the early problems and methods developed by early AIM researchers still relevant today? What has been lost and what has been gained?
- How have the advances in hardware and the availability of labeled data made certain forms of AI popular? How can we combine these recent advances with what we learned from the previous 40 years?
- How might we anticipate the further evolution of AI in medicine in light of the way the field has evolved to date and its likely trajectory?

E. H. Shortliffe (✉)
Vagelos College of Physicians and Surgeons, Columbia University, New York, NY, USA
e-mail: ted@shortliffe.net

N. H. Shah
Stanford University School of Medicine, Stanford, CA, USA
e-mail: nigam@stanford.edu

© The Author(s), under exclusive license to Springer Nature
Switzerland AG 2022
T. A. Cohen et al. (eds.), *Intelligent Systems in Medicine and Health*, Cognitive
Informatics in Biomedicine and Healthcare,
https://doi.org/10.1007/978-3-031-09108-7_2

21

Introduction

The history of artificial intelligence in medicine (AIM) is intimately tied to the history of AI itself, since some of the earliest work in applied AI dealt with biomedicine. In this chapter we provide a brief overview of the early history of AI, but then focus on AI in medicine (and in human biology), providing a summary of how the field has evolved since the earliest recognition of the potential role of computers in the modeling of medical reasoning and in the support of clinical decision making. The growth of medical AI has been influenced not only by the evolution of AI itself, but also by the remarkable ongoing changes in computing and communication technologies. Accordingly, this chapter anticipates many of the topics that are covered in subsequent chapters, providing a concise overview that lays out the concepts and progression that are reflected in the rest of this volume.

Artificial Intelligence: The Early Years

As was discussed in Chap. 1, AI is a diverse field that addresses a wide variety of topics regarding human intelligence and expertise, with an emphasis on how to model and simulate these topics in computer systems. Thus studies of how human beings reason are part of AI, but so are the creation of devices (such as robots) that incorporate human-like features. Viewed in this framework, notions relevant to AI emerged early in human history as people studied the workings of the human mind or imagined creations that might duplicate those capabilities.

For example, fantastical non-human intelligent entities were imagined as far back as Greek mythology. Hephaestus was a mythical blacksmith who manufactured mechanical servants, and there were even early tales that involved the concept of intelligent robots. But perhaps the most important early harbinger of AI was Aristotle's invention of **syllogistic logic** (a formal deductive reasoning system) in the fourth century BC.

Mechanical inventions that attempted the creation of human-like machines are known to have existed as early as the thirteenth century, when talking heads were created as novelty items and Al-Jazari, an Arab inventor, designed what is believed to be the first programmable humanoid robot (a boat carrying four mechanical musicians, powered by water flow). There are many other examples that could be mentioned from periods prior to the twentieth century.[1]

---

[1] For more discussion, see "A Brief History of AI" at https://aitopics.org/misc/brief-history (accessed August 13, 2022) and "History of Artificial Intelligence" at https://en.wikipedia.org/wiki/History_of_artificial_intelligence. (accessed August 13, 2022).

In the early twentieth century Bertrand Russell and Alfred North Whitehead published *Principia Mathematica*, which revolutionized formal logic [1]. Subsequent philosophers pursued the logical analysis of knowledge. The first use of the word "robot" in English occurred in a play by Karel Capek that was produced in 1921.[2] Thereafter a mechanical man, Electro, was introduced by Westinghouse Electricat at the New York World's Fair in 1939 (along with a mechanical dog named Sparko). It was a few years earlier (1936–37) that Alan Turing proposed the universal **Turing Machine** concept and proved notions of computability.[3] Turing's analysis imagined an abstract machine that can manipulate symbols on a strip of tape, guided by a set of rules. He showed that such a simple machine was capable of simulating the logic of any computer algorithm that could be constructed. Also relevant (in 1943) were the introduction of the term **cybernetics**, the publication by McCulloch and Pitts of *A Logical Calculus of the Ideas Immanent in Nervous Activity* (an early stimulus to the notion of **artificial neural networks**) [2], and Emil Post's proof that **production systems** are a general computational mechanism [3].

Especially important for AI was George Polya's 1945 book *How to Solve It*, which introduced the notion of **heuristic** problem solving [4]—a key influential concept in the AI community to this day. That same year Vannevar Bush published *As We May Think*, which offered a remarkable vision of how, in the future, computers could assist human beings in a wide range of activities [5]. In 1950, Turing published *Computing Machinery and Intelligence*, which introduced the **Turing Test** as a way of defining and testing for intelligent behavior [6]. In that same year, Claude Shannon (of **information theory** fame) published a detailed analysis showing that chess playing could be viewed as **search** (*Programming A Computer to Play Chess*) [7]. The dawn of computational artificial intelligence was upon us as computers became viable and increasingly accessible devices.

Modern History of AI

The history of AI, as we think of it today, began with the development of **stored-program** digital computers and the ground-breaking work of John von Neumann and his team at Princeton University in the 1950s. As the potential of computers

---

[2] Čapek K. *Rossumovi Univerzální Roboti* (Rossum's Universal Robots). It premiered on 25 January 1921 and introduced the word "robot" to the English language and to science fiction as a whole. https://en.wikipedia.org/wiki/R.U.R. (accessed August 13, 2022).

[3] Turing submitted his paper on 31 May 1936 to the London Mathematical Society for its *Proceedings*, but it was published in early 1937. https://en.wikipedia.org/wiki/Turing_machine. (accessed August 13, 2022).

began to be appreciated, academic engineering scientists began to pursue concepts that would evolve to be known as computer science. The history and capabilities of AI have subsequently been tied to the evolution of computers and their associated technologies.

As is mentioned in Chap. 1, it was at a conference at Dartmouth University in 1956 that a group of early computer scientists gathered to discuss the notion of simulating human reasoning by computer. One attendee, John McCarthy from Massachusetts Institute of Technology (MIT) (who later spent most of his professional life at Stanford University), coined a name for the developing field: *artificial intelligence*. At Carnegie Mellon University (then known as Carnegie Tech), psychologist Allen Newell, economist/psychologist Herbert Simon, and systems programmer (from the Rand Corporation) John Clifford Shaw introduced the Logic Theorist system[4]—arguably the first AI program—which was followed by their General Problem Solver in 1957.[5] At about the same time (1958), Frank Rosenblatt invented the **perceptron algorithm** at the Cornell Aeronautical Laboratory [8]. This introduced the notion of **connectionism** in AI, where networks of circuits or connected units were used to simulate intelligent behavior.

The notion of **machine learning** was first explored by Arthur Samuel (IBM) between 1958 and 1962 [9]. He developed a checker-playing program that learned strategy and novel methods by having it mounted on two machines and then having it play against itself thousands of times—resulting in a program that was able to beat the world champion. Another key development during that era (1958) was John McCarthy's creation of the **LISP** programming language[6]—which dominated as the basis for AI research and development for several decades (including in the medical AI community).

During the 1960s there was an explosion in creative AI work, initially at MIT and Carnegie Mellon, but later in the decade at other universities in the US. International explorations of AI were also underway, especially in the United Kingdom (where the first **Machine Intelligence** workshop was held in Edinburgh in 1966). By the end of the decade, as early computer science departments began to be formed, AI groups began to appear more broadly (with notable efforts underway at the University of California Berkeley and Stanford University). The first industrial robot company was formed (1962) and a series of influential AI PhD

---

[4] http://shelf1.library.cmu.edu/IMLS/MindModels/logictheorymachine.pdf. (accessed August 13, 2022).

[5] http://bitsavers.informatik.uni-stuttgart.de/pdf/rand/ipl/P-1584_Report_On_A_General_Problem-Solving_Program_Feb59.pdf. (accessed August 13, 2022).

[6] McCarthy's original paper is available at http://www-formal.stanford.edu/jmc/recursive.html. (accessed August 13, 2022).

dissertations emerged—particularly at MIT where the students of Marvin Minsky had a huge impact on the evolving field [10]. Also noteworthy was the invention of the mouse pointing device by Doug Engelbart at Stanford Research Institute (SRI[7]), which was to revolutionize the way in which human beings would interact with computers. In 1969, also at SRI, scientists developed "Shakey", a mobile robot that had a problem-solver embedded in addition to locomotion (wheels) and perception (cameras with image processing).[8] The first International Joint Conference on Artificial Intelligence (IJCAI) was held in Washington, DC in 1969. Meanwhile, that same year at MIT, Minsky and Seymour Papert published *Perceptrons* [11], an influential book that discussed the computational approach that Rosenblatt had introduced a decade earlier, outlining the limits of what perceptrons could do. This led to a decrease in interest in connectionist concepts and arguably held back the pace of development for what eventually became known as neural networks in the 1980s and in turn led to today's **deep learning** approaches (see Chap. 6).

AI research topics in the 1960s seem remarkably similar to those that dominate today. Machine learning, natural language processing, speech understanding, image analysis, robotics, and simulation of human problem solving were all major areas of research focus. Much of the funding for such research in the US came from the **Department of Defense (DOD)**, which envisioned eventual military applications of AI but provided extensive support for basic methodology development that had no immediate military application. The DOD also supported communications research, which in turn became a great facilitator of AI development work. Perhaps most notable was the introduction of a nationwide network for interconnecting major research computers that were located at academic institutions and in research centers for military contractors. The DOD's **Advanced Research Projects Agency (ARPA)**[9] supported much of the AI and communications research in the country. This network for research computers, was built on the notion of **packet switching** and became known as the ARPA Network or, simply, the **ARPAnet**. Collaborative AI research among universities became heavily dependent on this network, and the notion of electronic messaging among researchers across the various sites evolved into the email that we take for granted today. Similarly, the ARPAnet, and its packet switching technology, were eventually taken over by the National Science Foundation (NSF) and,

---

[7] See https://en.wikipedia.org/wiki/Douglas_Engelbart. (accessed August 13, 2022). SRI became an independent entity outside of Stanford University and is known today simply as SRI International.

[8] https://www.sri.com/hoi/shakey-the-robot/. (accessed August 13, 2022).

[9] Also often called **DARPA**, for Defense Advanced Research Projects Agency.

in turn, became a coordinated independent entity that is today known as the Internet.

AI Meets Medicine and Biology: The 1960s and 1970s

As AI was developing as a research discipline, it is not surprising that some of the challenging problems that attracted investigators were drawn from biomedical science. An early example from 1965 was MIT work by Joseph Weizenbaum who was exploring **chatbot** technology (conversational natural language processing and response generation; see Chap. 9). He developed a program known as "The Doctor", but more affectionately referred to as "Eliza", which attempted to provide psychiatric assessments of patients. The focus was on maintaining the conversation intelligently rather than actually reaching a psychiatric diagnosis. The program became a popular, easy-to-use "toy" at AI centers since it was available for conversations over the ARPAnet, and it did respond in ways that suggested, at some level, that it understood what the user was saying. A few years later, at Stanford, a psychiatrist on the medical school faculty, Ken Colby, worked with AI researchers to develop a conversational program, known as "Parry", that would simulate the behavior of a patient with paranoid schizophrenia. He undertook the work largely for educational purposes, and his students and residents enjoyed "interviewing" the program to learn about its thought disorder and to try to keep the "patient" from shutting down and refusing to communicate further. Of course, as Parry became known in the AI community, it was inevitable that people would begin to wonder how Eliza would handle a therapeutic session with Parry. Accordingly, in 1972, an ARPAnet link was created between Eliza at MIT (Cambridge, MA) and Parry at Stanford (Palo Alto, CA). Without human intervention, the two programs had a conversation,[10] and this somewhat hysterical match-up has become part of AI lore [12].

Emergence of AIM Research at Stanford University

A more serious and ground-breaking AI research effort in biomedicine was the Dendral Project at Stanford University. It began as an effort developed by a remarkable scientist, Joshua Lederberg, who had been attracted to Stanford as founding chair of their Department of Genetics in the late 1950s. He arrived shortly after receiving the Nobel Prize in Physiology or Medicine (at age 33!) for his ground-breaking work, at the University of Wisconsin, on genetic transfer between bacteria. Then, in the mid-1960s, a young researcher, Edward Feigenbaum, joined the faculty in Stanford's nascent computer science department, arriving from UC Berkeley

---

[10] See https://tools.ietf.org/html/rfc439 for a transcript of the interchange between the two programs. (accessed August 13, 2022).

after studying with Herbert Simon at Carnegie Tech (Carnegie Mellon University today). Lederberg and Feigenbaum teamed up with Carl Djerassi, an eminent professor in the Chemistry Department, who was an expert in organic and hormonal chemistry and who had been instrumental in the development of birth control pills a decade earlier.

Lederberg was himself an excellent programmer (in addition to his skills as a geneticist) who became fascinated with the challenge of determining organic compound structures from mass spectral data—a task mastered by very few organic chemists. He wondered if there might be a computational solution and felt that the first requirement was to consider all the possible structures consistent with a compound's chemical formula ($C^aH^bO^c$, where the superscripts indicate the number of carbon, hydrogen, and oxygen atoms in one molecule of the compound). As the number of atoms in a compound increases, the number of potential structures becomes very large. Lederberg developed an algorithmic approach, which he called the "dendritic algorithm,"[11] and wrote a program that could generate the entire exhaustive set of potential structures for any organic compound. Pruning that large space to define a couple of likely structures was guided by mass spectral analysis (**mass spectroscopy**) of the compound, and it was in this area that Djerassi had special expertise. With the addition of Feigenbaum and other computer scientists to the team, the Dendral Project thus sought to encode the rules used by organic chemists who knew how to interpret mass spectra in order to infer the small number of structures, from among all those generated by the dendritic algorithm, that were consistent with the spectral data. The focus on knowledge representation and the use of **production rules**, plus the capture and encoding of expertise, placed this early work solidly in the AI arena.

Another key contributor to this work in the early years was Bruce Buchanan,[12] a research scientist with computing expertise and formal training that included a PhD in Philosophy of Science. He stimulated and participated in efforts to view the Dendral work as research on **theory formation**. Although the system was initially based solely on rules acquired from Djerassi and other experts in interpretation of the mass spectra of organic compounds, Buchanan and others pursued the possibility that it might be possible to infer such rules from lots of examples of mass spectra and the corresponding compounds of known structure. This machine learning approach, which greatly enhanced the Dendral program's performance over time as new rules were added, became known as Meta-Dendral.

By the early 1970s, Dendral had become well known in computer science circles [13] and the biomedical focus had spawned methods that generalized for use in other domains—a phenomenon that was to occur many times in subsequent decades as biomedicine became a challenging real-world stimulus to novel approaches that were adopted broadly by AI researchers in areas beyond medicine. DENDRAL also

---

[11] The name was inspired by the expanding network of possible solutions that reminded him of a neuron's dendrites.

[12] See Buchanan's foreword to this volume.

spawned a dynamic research environment at Stanford, linking the school of medicine with the university's young computer science department. As other projects were developed that focused on capturing biomedical expertise in computer programs, Feigenbaum generalized the efforts in an overriding principle that had guided much of the work:

> The key empirical result of DENDRAL experiments became known as the knowledge-is-power hypothesis (later called the Knowledge Principle), stating that knowledge of the specific task domain in which the program is to do its problem solving was more important as a source of power for competent problem solving than the reasoning method employed.—Edward A. Feigenbaum, 1977 [14].

The process of capturing and encoding expert knowledge became known as **knowledge engineering.** See Chap. 4 for a focused discussion on knowledge-based systems, their subsequent evolution, and the current status of such work.

As DENDRAL grew and new projects were started at Stanford, it became clear that the computing facilities available for the research work were too limited. Furthermore, other medical AI projects were underway at a handful of other institutions and most researchers working on medical AI problems were feeling similar computational constraints. Lederberg accordingly submitted a successful proposal to the **Division of Research Resources (DRR)** at the **National Institutes of Health (NIH)**. He envisioned a major computing facility that would support medical AI research, not only at Stanford but at other universities around the US. The resulting shared resource was also granted one of the few remaining available connections to the ARPAnet—the first computer on the network that was not funded by the DOD. In this way the computer could be used by researchers anywhere in the country, using their own local connections to the ARPAnet to provide them with access to the computational power available at Stanford.[13] This shared computing resource, installed on the Stanford medical school campus in 1973, was known at the Stanford University Medical Experimental Computer for Artificial Intelligence in Medicine, more commonly referred to as **SUMEX-AIM**, or simply SUMEX. With grant renewals every 5 years, SUMEX served the national (and eventually the international) AI in Medicine community for 18 years.[14] With the departure from Stanford of Dr. Lederberg (who became President of Rockefeller University in New York City in the mid-1970s), Feigenbaum took over as Principal Investigator of SUMEX-AIM for several years.

---

[13] Since local area networking did not yet exist, most connections to the ARPAnet relied on dial-up modems with **acoustic couplers**. The network had local phone numbers for **terminal interface processors** (known as TIPs), scattered around the country, so investigators could generally access the network, and hence the computer at Stanford, with a local phone call.

[14] See "The Seeds of Artificial Intelligence. SUMEX-AIM." Published in 1980 by the Division of Resarch Resources at NIH. https://eric.ed.gov/?id=ED190109. (accessed August 13, 2022).

Three Influential AIM Research Projects from the 1970s

The notion of using computers to assist with medical diagnosis often traces its roots to a classic article that was published in *Science* in 1959 [15]. It was written by two NIH physician-scientists, one a dentist (Robert Ledley) and the other a radiologist (Lee Lusted). The paper laid out the nature of **Bayesian probability theory** and its relevance to medical diagnosis, arguing that computers could be programmed to assist with the Bayesian calculations and thus could serve as diagnostic aids. They acknowledged the challenges in deriving all the necessary probabilities and recognized the problem of conditional dependencies when applying Bayes' theorem for a real-world problem like medical diagnosis. However, their work stimulated a number of research projects that sought to use probability theory for diagnosis, with especially influential projects by Homer Warner and colleagues at the University of Utah [16] and by Timothy deDombal and his team at Leeds in the United Kingdom [17].

It was the challenges with statistical approaches, and their lack of congruence with the way in which human experts solved similar problems, that led scientists to consider whether AI methods might not be adapted for such clinical decision making problems. Three AIM research efforts from the 1970s are particularly well known and played key roles in the evolution of the field. Unlike DENDRAL, these projects were focused on clinical medicine, and two of them were created using the SUMEX-AIM resource. All three programs were envisioned as potential sources of consultative decision support for clinicians as they thought to diagnose and/or manage patients.

INTERNIST-1/QMR

One of the early SUMEX projects was developed over the ARPAnet from the University of Pittsburgh. There an esteemed physician leader, Dr. Jack Myers, had stepped down as Chair of Medicine and in the early 1970s became interested in sharing his clinical knowledge and experience in a novel way (rather than writing "yet another textbook"). Renowned as a master clinician and diagnostician, and a past President of the American College of Physicians and Chairman of the American Board of Internal Medicine, he collaborated with an MIT/Carnegie Tech-trained computer scientist, Harry E. Pople, Jr., PhD. Randolph A. Miller, then a second year Pitt medical student who had learned to program in machine language and a higher level language while in high school, joined the project in its second year. They worked together in an effort to create a program that would assist in the diagnosis of adult patients with problems whose diagnoses fell in the realm of internal medicine.

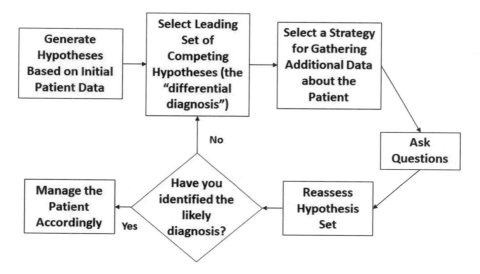

Fig. 2.1 The *hypothetico-deductive approach*, as applied to medical diagnosis. The Internist-1 program implemented these general notions in a program that tackled the diagnosis of essentially all diseases in internal medicine

The basic notion behind *INTERNIST-1*[15] was that it should be possible to simulate by computer the **hypothetico-deductive approach** that cognitive studies had shown were often used by expert clinicians as they attempted to diagnose challenging cases (Fig. 2.1) [18]. Myers invited medical students, including Miller and others, to spend medical school elective time conducting intensive analyses of the peer-reviewed literature on a disease topic of their choosing, which was then augmented by Myers' own experience. They thus characterized 650 disorders in internal medicine using 4500 possible patient descriptors. Miller took a sabbatical research year, working full time with Pople and Myers in 1974–75 to write the INTERNIST-1 Knowledge Base (KB) editor program.

Miller's programming enabled Pople's diagnostic algorithms to access and manipulate a KB that otherwise exceeded the computer system's available address space. The team developed a computational algorithm that used presenting history, symptoms, physical exam findings, and lab results from a patient to generate a set of diagnoses that could potentially explain the patient's problems. They also created a refinement process that selected a strategy and identified additional questions that would allow the program to distinguish between competing hypotheses and to generate new ones.

INTERNIST-1 could accurately diagnose many difficult cases. In addition, it could deal with multiple concurrent disorders in the same patient. It was ultimately tested with some of the most difficult diagnostic challenges in the clinical literature

---

[15] The community often referred to the program simply as *Internist*, although this simpler name was legally unavailable for ownership/copyright reasons.

(Clinical Pathological Conferences published in the *New England Journal of Medicine*) where it correctly diagnosed more of the cases than did the physicians who had actually cared for the patients [18].

While the evaluation of INTERNIST-1 showed the potential of the heuristic AI approach to assist human beings with diagnosis, it also uncovered a number of shortcomings that showed that the system was not suitable for widespread clinical use [19]. After Miller joined the Pitt faculty, he observed that INTERNIST-1 was of great interest to medical students and faculty clinicians. However, it was also clear that the system was impractical to use—especially because it required the user to take an hour or more to enter all information about the patient, and then to respond to queries from the program. Recognizing this, he decided that the most useful element of INTERNIST-1 was its knowledge base.

Beginning in 1983, he began working on a different approach to diagnostic assistance—one that recognized the human clinician-user was the most knowledgeable intelligence in the diagnostic consultation process. The doctor knew the patient far better than the computer system could. The new diagnostic assistant system, Quick Medical Reference (QMR), ran on the newly available personal computers. Miller felt that QMR should support the clinician's problem-solving as efficiently as possible. He worked with colleagues to develop QMR as a toolkit to assist clinicians with about a dozen specific diagnostic assistance tasks, which the user could select individually or chain together serially to address the dilemmas that had puzzled them. The user could invoke QMR quickly on a personal computer in the office. For example, it allowed questions such as "What is the differential diagnosis of finding x?" or "How can I best screen a patient for disease y?" QMR allowed the user to rank and influence the differential diagnosis produced, and to determine the mode for generating questions, in a way that had not been possible with INTERNIST-1. Eventually, over the course of a decade, QMR was marketed as a commercial product.

One lesson of this work, and other medical systems to be described shortly, was that consultative decision aids were not likely to be used if they did not integrate well into clinicians' existing workflow [19] (see also Chap. 17 for more discussion of this issue). It took the revolution in networking and electronic health records, which introduced new ways of accessing pertinent patient data, for such programs to be more realistically used, even though their early capabilities were impressive.

CASNET

Another center of excellence for research on medical AI in the 1970s was based at Rutgers University in New Brunswick, New Jersey. Their computer science department, chaired by Saul Amarel, had recruited a young faculty member, Casimir Kulikowski, who had applied his computer science expertise to medical problems during his training and early postdoctoral work. Amarel and Kulikowski successfully proposed a second computing resource for applied artificial intelligence in

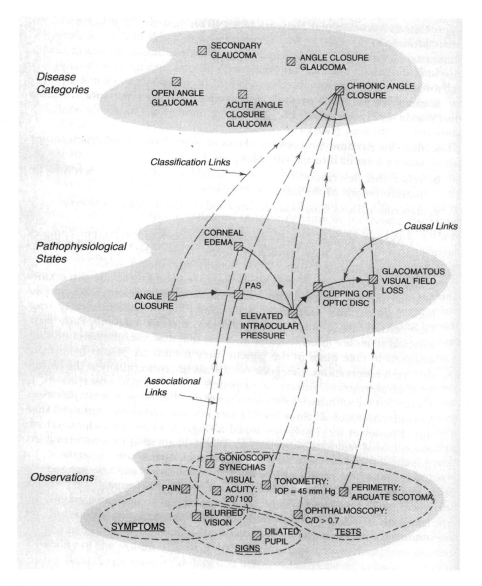

Fig. 2.2 CASNET's three-level description of a disease process. Note the *causal links* at the level of pathophysiological states. Observations (symptoms, signs, or tests) could be associated with either pathophysiological states or disease categories. (Reproduced with permission from C. Kulikowski and S. Weiss)

medicine. Like SUMEX, the Rutgers Resource was funded by the Division of Research Resources at NIH and was in time connected to the ARPAnet. Their initial major project involved a collaboration with Dr. Arin Safir, an ophthalmologist at Mt.

Fig. 2.3 An example of a MYCIN rule. Rules were encoded using the LISP programming language (at the top). Given the standardized approach to representing the knowledge, it was possible to write code to translate the rules into English (at the bottom). This provided transparency during interactions with clinical users

```
PREMISE:   ($AND  (SAME CNTXT GRAM GRAMPOS)

                  (SAME CNTXT MORPH COCCUS)

                  (SAME CNTXT CONFORM CLUMPS))

ACTION:    (CONCLUDE CNTXT IDENT STAPHYLOCOCCUS TALLY 700)
```

or (translated into English):

IF: 1) The gramstain of the organism is grampos

         2) The morphology of the organism is coccus

         3) The growth conformation of the organism is clumps

THEN: There is suggestive evidence (.7) that the identity of the

organism is staphylococcus.

Sinai Medical Center in New York City, who provided the necessary clinical expertise.

This system focused on modeling **causal reasoning** using a network-based representation of the pertinent domain knowledge. The program, known as CASNET (for *causal associational network*) assisted with the diagnosis of various forms of glaucoma. Their networked approach modeled the ability of expert clinicians to reason from observations about a patient to the delineation of existing physiological states (Fig. 2.2), which in turn helped to distinguish among potential diagnostic explanations for the findings. This important work was pursued with involvement of a talented PhD student, Shalom Weiss, who made portions of the project the focus of his doctoral dissertation [20].

MYCIN

This Stanford project began as doctoral research for a medical student who was also pursuing a PhD in what today would be called **biomedical informatics**. Edward Shortliffe had come to Stanford to study medicine in 1970—partly because of the school's flexibility (which would permit a medical student to pursue a simultaneous second degree in a computer-related discipline), but also because of the advanced biomedical computing environment that Lederberg and others had created. He quickly got to know AI researchers in the computer science department on the main campus, and especially those who were involved with the Dendral project. Guided by medical school faculty (Stanley Cohen, then Chief of Clinical Pharmacology and a genetics researcher,[16] and Stanton Axline, an infectious disease expert), Shortliffe built on the Dendral notion of encoding expert knowledge in production rules. His

---

[16] Cohen, who succeeded Lederberg as chair of genetics, briefly served as Principal Investigator of the SUMEX-AIM resource upon the Lederberg's departure for Rockefeller University. After a year, Feigenbaum took over that role until he was succeeded by Shortliffe.

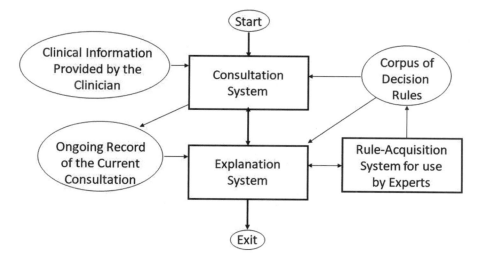

Fig. 2.4 This diagram provides an overview of the MYCIN system, identifying the three subsystems (rectangles), the corpus of decision rules, and the dynamic information that was generated during the consideration of a specific case. See text for details

principal computer science colleague was Bruce Buchanan. The idea was to develop a consultation program that would advise physicians on the selection of antimicrobial therapy for patients with severe infections. The resulting project was known as MYCIN, with Cohen serving as Shortliffe's dissertation advisor [21].

MYCIN used a collection of decision rules, acquired from Cohen, Axline, and others as the research group discussed actual cases taken from Stanford's wards. These rules were then encoded and stored in a growing collection (Fig. 2.3).

The rules were then kept separate from the actual program, which had three components (see rectangles in Fig. 2.4). The primary focus was the Consultation Program, which obtained patient data and offered advice, but also important was the Explanation Program, which could offer English-language explanations of why questions were being asked and why the program had offered its recommendations. The program itself knew how to handle a consultative interaction, but knew nothing about the domain of infectious diseases. All such knowledge was stored in the corpus of decision rules. A third subsystem, the Rule-Acquisition Program, was developed to allow experts to offer new rules or to edit existing ones. By running a challenging case through the Consultation Program, and using the Explanation Program to gain insight into why the program's performance might have been inappropriate for a given case, the expert could use the Rule-Acquisition Program to update the system's knowledge – entering new rules (for translation from English into LISP-coded versions) or editing existing ones. By re-running the case, the expert could see if MYCIN's advice had been suitably corrected.

MYCIN was formally evaluated in a blinded experiment that had infectious disease experts compare its performance with nine other prescribers who were

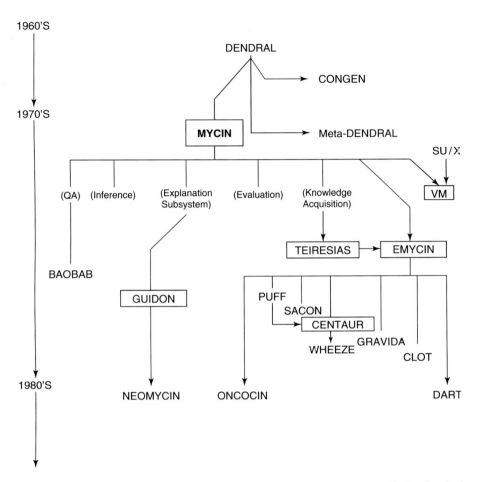

Fig. 2.5 Just as MYCIN drew inspiration from the earlier DENDRAL work, several other Stanford research projects built on the methods and concepts that MYCIN had introduced. This diagram shows many of these projects and their ancestry. Those projects depicted in rectangles were themselves the basis for computer science doctoral dissertations (VM: LM Fagan; TEIRESIAS: R Davis; EMYCIN: W van Melle; GUIDON: WJ Clancey; CENTAUR: J Aikins)

presented with the same ten cases [22]. The comparison group included the actual therapy given to the patient, Stanford infectious disease faculty members and a fellow, a medical resident, and a medical student. MYCIN was shown to perform at the top of the comparison group, as judged by the evaluators (who did not know which advice had been offered by the program).

The AI approach developed for MYCIN became known as a **rule-based expert system**. The architecture was attractive because the knowledge base was kept in rules that were separate from the program, offering the possibility that the system could provide advice in a totally different domain if the infectious disease rules were removed and a new set of rules was substituted. The program without the rules was termed "empty MYCIN" or "essential MYCIN"—generally simply referred to as EMYCIN [23]. This work provided further support for Feigenbaum's *knowledge is power* aphorism, previously mentioned. MYCIN also stimulated several other research projects in what became known as the Stanford Heuristic Programming Project, many of which were also focused on medical topics and were doctoral dissertations in computer science (Fig. 2.5). This diagram conveys the way in which Stanford's AIM science advanced over two decades, with each project introducing methods or concepts on which subsequent research could build. An important lesson is that AIM research is about more than building systems in the engineering sense. Equally important is its dependence on the scientific method, with experiments offering lessons that generalize and can feed back into the evolution of the field [24].

Cognitive Science and AIM

As the 1970s progressed, AIM researchers became aware of the synergy between their work to capture and convey clinical expertise and the work of researchers in educational psychology and cognitive science, many of whom were focused on medical problem solving. Since AIM researchers were seeking to encode clinical expertise and to produce systems that could reason using that knowledge, they were naturally drawn to work that studied clinicians as they solved problems. An esteemed physician at Yale University's medical school, Alvan Feinstein, had published an influential volume in 1967, *Clinical Judgment* [25]. Feinstein is commonly viewed as the founder of the field of clinical epidemiology, and the focus of his volume was on defining and teaching clinical thinking. The work inspired others to pursue related aspects of clinical expertise, and several groups tackled tasks in medical problem solving, using methods from psychology and cognitive science.

Particularly influential was a volume by Elstein, Shulman, and Sprafka, educational psychologists at Michigan State University [26]. They performed a variety of studies that sought to apply contemporary psychological theories and methods to address the complexity of problem solving in cases derived from real-life clinical settings. Their work influenced the thinking of AIM researchers, who were seeking to capture elements of medical reasoning, even if their programs were not formally modeling the workings of the human mind.

Meanwhile, at Tufts New England Medical Center in Boston, two nephrologists were becoming interested in the nature of medical problem solving and the role that computers might play in capturing or simulating such reasoning. William Schwartz had published a thoughtful piece in 1970 that anticipated the future role that computers might play in medicine and the impact that such changes might impose on clinical practice and even on the types of people who would be drawn to becoming a physician [27]. The second nephrologist, Jerome Kassirer,[17] had developed a collaboration with a computer science graduate student at MIT, Benjamin Kuipers, and they performed and published a number of experiments (further discussed in Chap. 5) that offered insights into clinical reasoning processes, including a classic paper on causal reasoning in medicine that appeared in 1984 (by which time Kuipers had joined the faculty at the University of Texas in Austin) [28].

The interest in expert reasoning in medicine, shared by Schwartz and Kassirer, also attracted a Tufts cardiologist, Stephen Pauker, and a computer scientist at MIT, Anthony Gorry. Pauker also knew how to program and this group sought to develop an experimental program that explicitly simulated the cognitive processes that they had documented in studies of expert physicians who were solving problems. This led to the development of the *Present Illness Program* (PIP - see also Chap. 4) which leveraged early cognitive science and AI and was arguably the first AIM research project to be published in a major clinical journal [29]. When Gorry departed MIT for Rice University, he was succeeded later in the decade by Peter Szolovits, himself a leader in AIM research and knowledge-based systems (see Chap. 4).

By the early 1980s there was pertinent related work underway at McGill University. Vimla Patel and Guy Groen were examining the relationship between comprehension of medical texts or descriptions with approaches to problem solving by individuals with varying levels of expertise [30]. This body of work, which extended throughout the next decade as well, provided an additional set of cognitive insights that informed the work of the AIM research community, while attracting the McGill group to become interested in how their work might influence the development of computational models of clinical expertise (see Chap. 5).

The work described briefly in this section laid the groundwork for subsequent work on expert reasoning and cognition that accounts for this book's emphasis on the interplay between AIM and cognitive science. These relationships were further solidified by the close interactions, and attendance at one another's meetings, between members of the AIM community and those in the Society for Medical Decision Making (SMDM).[18] The emergence of cognitive informatics as a specialty area within AIM research was built upon this early work and also on the growing recognition of the importance of cognitive issues in related areas of computer science, including computer-based education and human-computer interaction.

Reflecting on the 1970s

By the end of the decade, medical AI was having a significant impact on AI more generally. The top journal in the field, *Artificial Intelligence*, devoted an entire issue to AIM research [31], and the field of expert systems was being applied broadly in

---

[17]Years later Kassirer became the Editor-in-Chief of the *New England Journal of Medicine* (1992–2000).

[18]https://smdm.org/. (accessed August 13, 2022).

Fig. 2.6 The RX project was an early example of machine learning in the form of data mining under AI control. The goal was to use existing knowledge, plus real world data, to support the discovery of hypotheses that could in turn be formally explored using large amounts of data and statistical methods – thereby adding to current knowledge. For more details see https://www.bobblum.com/ESSAYS/COMPSCI/rx-project.html. (Figure reproduced with the permission of R.L. Blum)

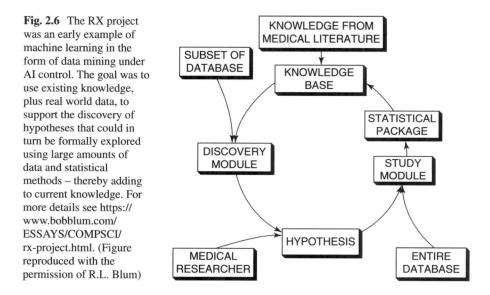

other areas of society. A community of medical AI researchers had come together to hold annual meetings (dubbed AIM Workshops) and to form new collaborations while embracing an increasing number of research projects. The first Symposium on Computer Applications in Medical Care (SCAMC), held in Arlington, VA in 1977,[19] had an entire session devoted to AIM research projects. AIM research was heavily cited in computer science research papers outside the field of medicine.

There was also important exploratory machine learning research in the medical arena, inspired in part by the Meta-Dendral work mentioned earlier. As clinical databases became available in specialized areas of medicine [32], it was natural to explore how computers might be able to learn, or discover new relationships. Blum pursued such work, proposing a cycle for discovery and clinical studies through the principled examination of such databases (Fig. 2.6) [33]. His RX program ultimately discovered and analyzed an association between prednisone and cholesterol that was published in a major clinical journal [34].

By the end of the 1970s, the AIM field was devoted to the notion that knowledge representation and use was the key to intelligent behavior by computer programs. As we describe in subsequent sections, the *knowledge is power* aphorism has been somewhat forgotten in today's AI research and application communities—arguably to their detriment.

---

[19] SCAMC went on to become the major US meeting in the field of biomedical informatics, merging with other organizations in 1989–1990 to create today's American Medical Informatics Association (AMIA), https://www.AMIA.org, (accessed August 13, 2022).

Evolution of AIM During the 1980s and 1990s

The next two decades were characterized by substantial evolution of AI and AIM, partly because of the remarkable changes in computing technology, but also because of the ups and downs of academic, industrial, and government interest in AI and its potential.

AI Spring and Summer Give Way to AI Winter

By the early 1980s there was rapidly growing interest in AI, medical applications, and especially in expert systems [35]. Companies began to recruit AI scientists and commercial expert systems were introduced to the marketplace or used for internal purposes [36]. Cover stories on AI and expert systems began to appear in major popular news magazines, often with prominent featuring of medical programs such as the ones described in the previous sections of this chapter. They tended to make wild predictions about the impact AI would soon be having on society, much of which ironically did not align well with what the system developers believed to be reasonable. However, the enthusiasm continued for several years and led, for example, to a major investment by the Japanese Ministry of International Trade and Industry which formed their *Fifth Generation Computer Project*[20] starting in 1982.

Early in the decade new companies, such as Teknowledge and Intellicorp, were also created specifically to commercialize expert systems. In parallel, hardware companies such as Symbolics, LISP Machines Inc., and Xerox Corporation introduced single-user machines that were designed to run the LISP programming language, to offer graphical user interfaces with mouse pointing devices, and to support the development of expert systems and other AI-related applications. Note that these machines appeared only shortly after the introduction of the first personal computers (e.g., the Apple II in the late 1970s followed by the first IBM PC and the Apple Macintosh a few years later). In parallel, the first commercial **local area networking** products were introduced (e.g., Ethernet from Xerox Corp and a competitor known as Wangnet), which had a profound effect on the ways in which computers and programs were designed to interact and share data.

The rapid change in the early 1980s continued throughout the decade. For example, it was not long until the first general-purpose workstations running the Unix operating system were introduced (e.g., by SUN Microsystems), and these rapidly made the notion of a LISP machine obsolete. The LISP machine market disintegrated and "Unix Boxes" (high-end workstations that were much more powerful than the existing personal computers) began to dominate in the AI research community.

---

[20] See https://en.wikipedia.org/wiki/Fifth_generation_computer. (accessed August 13, 2022).

Fig. 2.7 Graphic shows
the two periods often
called *AI Winter*, one at the
end of the 1970s (which
had little impact on AIM)
and the second in the late
1980s and early 1990s
(which did affect AIM
work for several years)

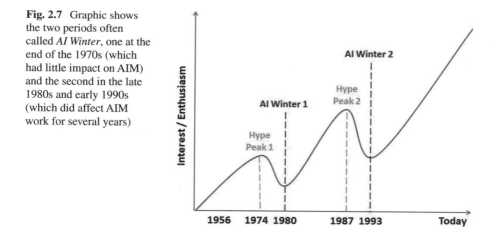

As the decade proceeded, the AI "luster" also began to fade, as highly touted systems tended to fail to live up to their expectations. Companies often found that the systems were expensive to maintain and difficult to update. They generally had no machine learning component, so maintenance was crucial in order to incorporate new knowledge into them. Performance was accordingly viewed as "brittle".

In the early 1980s ARPA had again begun to fund its support of general AI research, with an emphasis on knowledge-based systems—no doubt encouraged to do so by the major Japanese investment in their own project in the area. ARPA had lowered its enthusiasm for AI research in the mid- to late-1970s, even as the AIM activities were taking off. But AIM researchers were not supported by DARPA but rather by NIH or, in a few cases, by the National Science Foundation (NSF), and their work and impact had continued apace as described previously. Support for AIM research also continued during the 1980s, while ARPA was ramping up its own support for AI generally. However, as the decade came to an end, the AI community faced a clear diminution in the enthusiasm that had been strong only a few years earlier. Thus, there was again a dip in funding support for AI as the 1990s began, and some of this affected the AIM research community as well.

The dips in support for AI, and in belief for its potential, occurred in the late 1970s and again in the period between 1987 and 1993. These two drops in funding and interest have been called **AI Winter** #1 and #2[21] (see Fig. 2.7). During these periods it became unhelpful for companies or researchers to emphasize that they were working on AI problems. It was hard to attract interest from collaborators or funding agencies at a time when AI was viewed as having been oversold and having failed to demonstrate the utility that had been promised. By the early 1990s, those working in AI areas, including AIM, often sought new terms for what they were

---

[21] See https://en.wikipedia.org/wiki/AI_winter. (accessed August 13, 2022).

doing, hoping they would avoid the taint of the AI label. For example, work on knowledge base and terminology development often fell under the term **ontology** research,[22] and some types of machine learning research were often called **knowledge discovery in databases (KDD)**.[23]

As is shown in Fig. 2.7, there has been no downturn in enthusiasm for AI and its promise for almost 30 years. Those who lived through the early AI winters often wonder if the extreme enthusiasm for AI today, with remarkable investment in almost all areas of science (and medicine/health), is a harbinger of what could become a third period of disenchantment. However, most observers feel that the field has greatly matured and that current approaches are better matched to the state of computing and communications technology than was possible when earlier research, and commercial experiments, were being undertaken. As you read this book, you should develop your own sense of whether today's enthusiasm is well matched to the reality of what is happening, especially in AIM, and whether we can be optimistic about ongoing progress and impact. We return to this topic in Chaps. 19 and 20.

AIM Deals with the Tumult of the 80s and 90s

The expert systems fervor in the 1980s, which had been driven in part by medical AI projects that offered new methods and models for analyzing data and offering advice, put the AIM community in a highly visible position. AI in Medicine had become a worldwide phenomenon, with some medical focus in Japan during the Fifth Generation Computer Project. The major new source of AIM research energy, however, was in Europe, where a medical AI community began to coalesce. The first European meeting that focused on AIM (1985) was organized by Ovo de Lotto and Mario Stefanelli as a 2-day conference in Pavia, Italy. The meeting's success led to the decision to hold such meetings biannually under the name *Artificial Intelligence in Medicine Europe* (AIME). They quickly attracted an audience from the US and other parts of the world, so eventually the meeting name was adjusted to be simply *Artificial Intelligence in MEdicine*, continuing the AIME acronym.[24]

A retrospective paper analyzing three decades of trends in the content of AIME meetings, published in 2015, provides some instructive insights on how the field evolved over that time [37]. At the first meeting in 1985, essentially all the papers dealt with knowledge-based systems and knowledge engineering, reflecting the expert systems phenomenon. However, the number of papers in those categories

---

[22] See https://en.wikipedia.org/wiki/Ontology_(information_science). (accessed August 13, 2022).

[23] See   https://www.techopedia.com/definition/25827/knowledge-discovery-in-databases-kdd. (accessed August 13, 2022).

[24] The first meeting hosted outside of Europe (by the University of Minnesota) was held in 2020, although it needed to be held virtually due to the COVID-19 pandemic that prevented most travel to conferences.

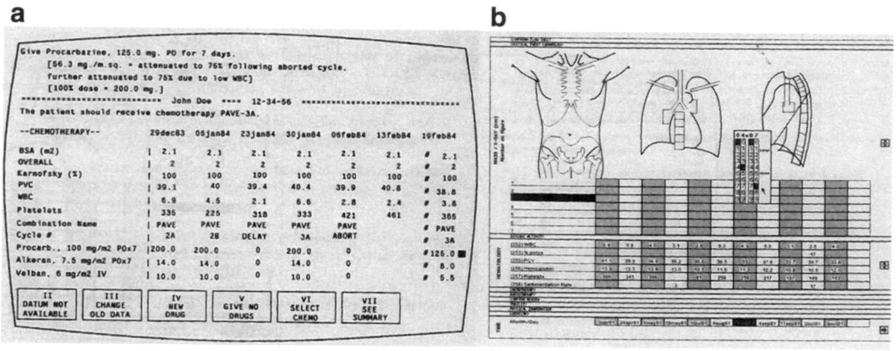

a   **b**

Fig. 2.8 The original ONCOCIN interface used a simple ASCII terminal and all interaction was through a computer keyboard (**a**). Within a few years, with reimplementation on a LISP machine, the program offered a greatly improved interface to clinician users (**b**)

decreased substantially over time while major new areas of emphasis were ontologies and terminologies, **temporal reasoning**, natural language processing (see Chap. 7), guidelines/protocols (see Chap. 10), management of uncertainty, and image/signal processing (see Chap. 12). The largest increase, which began slowly in the 1990s, was in the area of machine learning. By 2013 it had surpassed knowledge engineering as the most dominant topic at the meetings when measured cumulatively over three decades. This is not surprising given the AI emphasis on machine learning that today makes it the most active subfield of the discipline (see Chap. 6).

By the end of the 1980s, there was consensus that the AIM field was so active and productive that it warranted its own journal. *Artificial Intelligence in Medicine* was first published in 1989 with Kazem Sadegh-Zadeh, from the University of Münster in Germany, serving as founding editor [38]. This journal, published by Elsevier, is a major source of current research results in the field to this day. Several other peer-reviewed journals also publish AIM methodologic research papers,[25] and the more applied work has appeared in a variety of clinical, public health, and general science journals.

The rapid evolution in networking, hardware capabilities, and computing power during the 1980s also had a major influence on AIM research and capabilities during that decade. As an example, consider the ONCOCIN program, which was developed to apply knowledge-based methods to provide advice to oncologists caring for patients enrolled in cancer chemotherapy clinical trials [39]. The program was initially conceived to run on an computer terminal attached to a mainframe computer running a LISP programming environment (Fig. 2.8a). The terminal could display

---

[25] Examples include the *Journal of the American Medical Informatics Association* (JAMIA, Oxford University Press), *Journal of Biomedical Informatics* (JBI, Elsevier), and *Intelligence-Based Medicine* (Elsevier).

Table 2.1 Some Questions Asked by AIM Researchers in an Online Discussion Forum - 1991

Question	Brief response (details in ref. [39])
1. Are AIM systems intended to address user needs?	AIM research is driven by desire to develop tools that address clinical needs, but like all basic research, there can be a long trajectory before reaching those goals
2. Has AIM research contributed to AI? To cognitive psychology? To clinical medicine?	Basic methodological innovation is often required, even when working on applied goals. There is ample evidence that AI, computer science, and cognitive psychology have all been affected by AIM research. Contributing to clinical medicine remains a future goal, although the work has already stimulated much discussion in the clinical world
3. Is AIM part of information science, computer science, AI, engineering, or biomedicine?	Created at the intersection of all these fields, AIM is a key component of the field of biomedical informatics (BMI), which itself merges those disciplines
4. Are AIM researchers adequately trained? To what extent is there a problem with inbreeding?	Daunting as it may be to study broadly the many fields that come together in BMI and AIM, it has been the lack of expertise *at that intersection* which has accounted for many of the problems in developing and implementing computer-based systems for biomedicine. Hence training in BMI is optimal. Inbreeding will be less of an issue as more BMI training programs are introduced
5. Why is it so difficult for AIM systems to be tested in clinical settings with regard to process or outcome of clinical care?	This question reveals unfamiliarity with the many AIM system evaluations that have been published. Most focus on the quality of decisions. Demonstrations of impact on the quality of care and patient outcome remain to be undertaken
6. Why isn't AIM research better funded?	All AI-related research funding has suffered during the downturn in interest in AI. But it will rebound as we continue to demonstrate the value and innovation in what we do
7. Why have AIM systems been so difficult to transport from site to site successfully?	With the demise of the "Greek Oracle" (consultation model) [19], integration with local information systems has become the crucial delivery mechanism. In the lack of standards or facile access to such systems, it is very hard to move a developed system to a new integrated environment

only ASCII characters[26] and all interactions were by computer keyboard. Within a few years, with the introduction of Xerox LISP machines that were self-contained for single users and included both a mouse pointing device and high quality graphical capabilities, ONCOCIN was ported to a LISP device that provided a greatly improved interface that was intuitive for clinicians to use (Fig. 2.8b).

The democratization of the Internet, which occurred during the late 1980s and early 1990s (with the commercialization of its management and creation of the domain system), created opportunities for collaboration at a distance as well as the

---

[26] American Standard Code for Information Interchange (ASCII), is a character encoding standard for electronic communication. ASCII codes represent text in computers, telecommunications equipment, and other devices.

emergence of communities with shared interests. At a time when AI Winter was affecting the AIM research community, it is not surprising that forums for sharing opinions, asking questions, and providing pointers to information of interest would emerge. One such list, simply called *ai-medicine@stanford.edu*, had been created in advance of the AIME meeting held in Maastricht, The Netherlands in August 1991. A keynote presentation at that meeting assessed a variety of soul-searching questions that AIM researchers had been asking one another on the list server. Later published in the *AI in Medicine* journal, the paper looked at AI in Medicine's "adolescence" and anticipated its future directions [40]. Table 2.1 summarizes seven key questions and briefly provides the response from the article, although interested readers should peruse the full paper. Many of the questions (and answers) are still relevant today, some 30 years later. Fifteen years after the Maastricht meeting, the AIME meeting, held in Amsterdam in 2007, provided a panel that reassessed the questions and answers from 1991, while adding thoughts about how the field had evolved in the intervening years [41].

As AIM's first four decades came to an end (with the century), work on advanced systems was continuing apace, with improved funding and enthusiasm. With growing implementation of electronic health records (EHRs) and creation of digital imaging databases, coupled with the general availability of enhanced computational power, machine learning (ML) research was gaining in interest and impact. The ML revolution was on the horizon and today has been a dominant element in AI in general and in AIM. In the next section, we briefly examine the two decades that led to the present.

The Last 20 Years: Both AI and AIM Come of Age

The early 2000s were dominated by the completion of the human genome project and the associated rise of interest in **bioinformatics**, while the adoption of EHRs continued silently in the background at a slow pace. Several techniques in supervised machine learning were first applied to large biomedical datasets in the context of **genomics** and bioinformatics work [42, 43].

Meanwhile, in computer science, there were two major developments underway: (1) the availability of commodity **graphical processing units** (GPUs),[27] beginning in about 2001, for efficiently manipulating image data–which at their core comprise an array of numbers, and (2) the availability of large, labeled datasets (such as the introduction of ImageNet[28] in 2010) to support efforts to learn increasingly complex classifiers via **supervised machine learning**. The availability of ImageNet and the recognition that GPUs could be as flexible as CPUs (but orders of magnitude faster in array operations) led to accelerated progress in image recognition—partly due to

---

[27] https://en.wikipedia.org/wiki/GeForce_3_series. (accessed August 13, 2022).

[28] https://en.wikipedia.org/wiki/ImageNet#History_of_the_database. (accessed August 13, 2022).

the creation of annual contests using shared datasets.[29] The computing ability offered by GPUs accelerated the adoption of artificial neural networks (which, as was mentioned earlier in this chapter, had been explored since the 1960s, initially inspired by the concept of perceptrons). Ideas put forward by Geoffrey Hinton, Yann LeCun, and Yoshua Bengio for deep neural networks [44] became widely adopted beginning in 2006 (earning the trio the 2018 ACM A.M. Turing Award[30]). A landmark was reached in 2012, when a deep convolutional neural network called AlexNet achieved a 16% error rate in the ImageNet challenge (the previous best performance had hovered at around 25%). That same year, Andrew Ng and Jeff Dean (both at Google) demonstrated the feasibility of **unsupervised machine learning** (see Chap. 6) by training a computer to recognize over 20,000 object categories, such as cat faces and human faces, without having to label images as containing a face or a cat [45].

The developments in computer science percolated to medicine, initially in the form of image analysis advances in radiology and pathology. For a few years expert systems (and knowledge-based approaches in general) took a back seat given the challenges in acquisition of patient data in electronic form to enable the machine learning approaches. Adoption of electronic medical records regained momentum after the passage of the Health Information Technology for Economics and Clinical Health (**HITECH**) Act in 2009. By 2012 the powerful compute capabilities (in the form of **cloud computing**) were readily accessible for a nominal fee; machine learning using neural networks had proved its worth in image, text and speech processing; and patient data in electronic form were available in large amounts–leading to a renewed enthusiasm about the potential of AI in Medicine.

As a result, the application of supervised machine learning to medical datasets became commonplace, leading to rapid advances in learning classifiers using large amounts of labeled data. Computers approximated human ability in reading retinal images [46], X-rays [47], histopathology slides [48], and the entire medical record to provide diagnostic as well as prognostic outputs [49]. However, as mentioned earlier, in the hype around "deep learning" the *knowledge is power* aphorism was often forgotten and, on occasion, re-discovered [50].

It is too soon to tell if this third AIM wave will deliver on the hype or lead to another, and potentially more severe, AI winter (Fig. 2.7). However, old concerns around explainability and trustworthiness of AI systems in medicine [51] are again being actively discussed (see Chaps. 8 and 18), with a keen focus on prevention of bias and ensuring fairness in their use in medical decision making [52, 53].

Given today's massive amount of activity in the field, there are several ongoing debates. For example, it is unclear if the unstructured content from clinical notes holds much value in improving diagnostic or prognostic systems given the high prevalence of copy-and-pasting, use of templates, and pressures to over-document

---

[29] https://www.image-net.org/challenges/LSVRC/. (accessed August 13, 2022).

[30] Often called the "Nobel Prize in Computer Science". See https://awards.acm.org/about/2018-turing. (accessed August 13, 2022).

in light of billing concerns (see Chaps. 10 and 11). As another example, there is increasing tension between the need to share data for training AI systems and the desire to ensure patient privacy (see Chap. 18). Once considered a forward-thinking piece of legislation, the **Health Insurance Portability and Accountability Act (HIPAA)** from 1996 is increasingly considered a hindrance to building AI systems[31] while also being inadequate to protect patient privacy [54].

While the media hype around AI in medicine continues, there are several exciting possibilities to integrate the advances from the pre-2000s with recent developments. A particularly noteworthy direction is on combining symbolic computing with deep neural networks [44] (see Chap. 6). As Bengio, Lecun and Hinton note, it was a surprise that the simple approach (creating networks of relatively simple, nonlinear neurons that learn by adjusting the strengths of their connections) proved so effective when applied to large training sets using huge amounts of computation (thanks to GPUs!). It turned out that a key ingredient was the depth of the networks; shallow networks did not work as well, but until the last decade or so we lacked the computational power to work with neural networks that were "deep". In outlining the promising future directions for AI research, these authors reflect in their Turing lecture [43] on the role that the symbolic AI research from the twentieth century might play in guiding how we structure and train neural nets so they can capture underlying causal properties of the world. In the same vein, we encourage the reader to reflect again on the rich history of symbolic reasoning systems built by AIM researchers in the twentieth century (as presented earlier in this chapter and recapitulated in some detail in Chap. 4). It is exciting to consider how that earlier work might be complementary to the machine learning developments in the last 20 years. As we suggested in Chap. 1 and earlier in this chapter, future work may demonstrate that combining the two paradigms, with a better focus on the role of cognitive science in designing ML systems (see Chaps. 5, 6 and 20), might catalyze rapid progress in the core diagnostic and prognostic tasks of AI in Medicine.

Today's cutting edge research will be tomorrow's history. The following chapters provide a glimpse of how current research and practice may evolve as both methods and computational capabilities continue to advance.

Questions for Discussion

- How would you characterize the notion of "intelligence", first as a characteristic of human beings (or other organisms) and second as a feature of modern computing? How do those characterizations diverge from one another? In what sense are devices that you use every day "intelligent".
- What has been the role of communications technology in advancing both artificial intelligence research and its applications in biomedicine?
- Given the explosive interest in expert systems, including their potential use in biomedicine, to what do you attribute their failure to meet early expectations and

---

[31] https://hai.stanford.edu/news/de-identifying-medical-patient-data-doesnt-protect-our-privacy. (accessed August 13, 2022).

the emergence of the AI Winter of 1987–1993? Consider inherent characteristics of the approach as well as the then-current communications and computational technologies.

- What accounts for the slow progress in machine learning (despite some impressive early examples) until the last two decades?
- Do we need a resurgence of expertise in the area of knowledge engineering for the development of medical AI systems? Why or why not?
- What uses might unsupervised learning have in medicine?
- How might prior medical knowledge, codified in knowledge structures such as ontologies, be provided to deep neural networks to improve their performance?
- What are the principal barriers that you envision in the ongoing effort to develop, test, and implement medical AI systems that interact directly with clinicians? With patients?

Further Reading

Dyson G. Turing's Cathedral: The Origins of the Digital Universe. New York: Vintage Books, 2012.

- A historical description of scientific innovation, told in the context of work by a team of young mathematicians and engineers, led by John von Neumann at Princeton's Institute for Advanced Study, who applied the ideas of Alan Turing to develop the fastest electronic computer of its era. That work also introduced the concept of RAM (random access memory) that we still use in most computers today. See also Alice Rawsthorn's book review, "Genius and Tragedy at Dawn of Computer Age" (New York Times, March 25, 2012).

Simon HA. The Sciences of the Artificial (3rd edition). Cambridge, MA: MIT Press, 1996.

- Originally published in 1968, this is a classic volume by a Nobel Laureate (Economics) who was also an early luminary in the field of AI. His assessment of AI includes topics that include not only his thoughts as a cognitive psychologist, but also analyses of the organization of complexity, the science of design, chaos, adaptive sysstems, and genetic algorithms.

Clancey WJ, Shortliffe EH. Readings in Medical Artificial Intelligence: The First Decade. Reading, MA: Addison-Wesley, 1984.

- This book is a compendium of classic papers describing the first generation of AIM systems, including MYCIN, CASNET and INTERNIST-1. It provides a detailed account of the methods underlying the development of these systems, including methods for the elicitation of expert knowledge and probabilistic inference procedures.

Shortliffe EH. Artificial intelligence in medicine: Weighing the accomplishments, hype, and promise. *IMIA Yearbook of Medical Informatics* 2019;28(01):257–62, (https://doi.org/10.1055/s-0039-1677891).

- This paper can be considered as the third in a series that includes refs. [40, 41] in that it describes the state of the field approaching the year 2020. The paper provides a historically-informed perspective on recent developments in machine learning methodology, takes stock of achievements to date and considers challenges that remain for clinically impactful deployment of AIM systems.

Szolovits P. (ed.) (1982). Artificial Intelligence in Medicine. (AAAS Selected Symposium). Boulder, CO: Westview Press. (https://www.google.com/books/edition/Artificial_Intelligence_In_Medicine/8tmiDwAAQBAJ)

- This book is an edited volume, published originally by the American Association for the Advancement of Science (AAAS), with chapters summarizing much of the medical AI research of the 1970s. It includes an especially important paper by Harry Pople describing the evolution of the INTERNIST-1 system.

Bengio Y, Lecun Y, Hinton G. Deep Learning for AI. Communications of the ACM 2021;64(7):58–65 (https://doi.org/10.1145/3448250).

- Yoshua Bengio, Yann LeCun, and Geoffrey Hinton are recipients of the 2018 ACM A.M. Turing Award for breakthroughs that have made deep neural networks a critical component of computing. This commentary describes their reflections on the progress to date in building deep neural networks and their thoughts on the future of deep learning, including the role of symbolic AI.

References

1. Whitehead AN, Russell B. Principia Mathematica. 2nd ed. Andesite Press; 2015, Originally published in 1910.
2. McCulloch WS, Pitts W. A logical calculus of the ideas immanent in nervous activity. Bull Math Biophys. 1943;5:115–33. https://link.springer.com/article/10.1007/BF02478259
3. Post EL. Formal reductions of the general combinatorial decision problem. Am J Math. 1943;65(2):197–215. https://doi.org/10.2307/2371809.
4. Polya G. How to solve it: a new aspect of mathematical method. Princeton, NJ: Princeton University Press; 2015, Originally published in 1945.
5. Bush V. As we may think. The Atlantic, July 1945. https://www.theatlantic.com/magazine/archive/1945/07/as-we-may-think/303881/.
6. Turing AM. Computing machinery and intelligence. Mind. 1950;LIX(236):433–60. https://doi.org/10.1093/mind/LIX.236.433.
7. Shannon CE. Programming a computer for playing chess. Computer Chess Compendium. 1943:2–13. https://doi.org/10.1007/978-1-4757-1968-0_1.
8. Rosenblatt F. The perceptron: a probabilistic model for information storage and organization in the brain. Psychol Rev. 1958;65(6):386–408. https://doi.org/10.1037/h0042519.
9. Samuel AL. Some studies in machine learning using the game of checkers. IBM J Res Dev. 1959;44:206–26. https://ieeexplore.ieee.org/document/5389202
10. Minsky M. Semantic information processing. Cambridge, MA: MIT Press; 1960.
11. Minsky M, Papert SA. Perceptrons: an introduction to computation geometry. Cambridge, MA: MIT Press; 1987, Originally published in 1969.
12. Garber M. When PARRY met ELIZA: a ridiculous chatbot conversation from 1972. The Atlantic, June 9, 2014. https://www.theatlantic.com/technology/archive/2014/06/when-parry-met-eliza-a-ridiculous-chatbot-conversation-from-1972/372428/.

13. Lindsay RK, Buchanan BG, Feigenbaum EA, Lederberg J. Applications of artificial intelligence for organic chemistry: the DENDRAL project. New York: McGraw-Hill (advanced computer science series); 1980. https://collections.nlm.nih.gov/catalog/nlm:nlmuid-10158490 6X7379-doc

14. Feigenbaum EA. The art of artificial intelligence: themes and case studies of knowledge engineering. Proceedings of the fifth international joint conference on artificial intelligence, Cambridge, MA; 1977. https://www.ijcai.org/proceedings/1977-2.

15. Ledley RS, Lusted LB. Reasoning foundations of medical diagnosis: probability, logic, and medical diagnosis. Science. 1959;130(3380):892–930. https://doi.org/10.1126/science.130.3366.9.

16. Warner HR, Toronto AF, Veasy L. Experience with Bayes' theorem for computer diagnosis of congenital heart disease. Ann N Y Acad Sci. 1964;115:558–67. https://doi.org/10.1111/j.1749-6632.1964.tb50648.x.

17. de Dombal FT, Leaper DJ, Staniland JR, McCann AP, Horrocks JC. Computer-aided diagnosis of acute abdominal pain. Br Med J. 1972;1:376–80. https://doi.org/10.1136/bmj.2.5804.9.

18. Miller R, Pople H, Myers J. INTERNIST-1: an experimental computer-based diagnostic consultant for general internal medicine. N Engl J Med. 1982;307:468–76. https://doi.org/10.1056/nejm198208193070803.

19. Miller RA, Masarie FE. The demise of the "Greek Oracle" model for medical diagnostic systems. Methods Inf Med. 1990;29(1):1–2. https://doi.org/10.1055/s-0038-1634767.

20. Weiss SM, Kulikowski CA, Amarel S, Safir A. A model-based method for computer-aided medical decision-making. Artif Intell. 1978;11:145–72. https://doi.org/10.1016/0004-3702(78)90015-2.

21. Shortliffe EH. Computer-based medical consultations systems: MYCIN. New York: American Elsevier; 1976.

22. Yu VL, Fagan LM, Wraith SM, Clancey WJ, Scott AC, Hannigan J, Blum RL, Buchanan BG, Cohen SN. Antimicrobial selection by a computer: a blinded evaluation by infectious disease experts. JAMA. 1979;242:1279–82. https://doi.org/10.1001/jama.1979.03300120033020.

23. van Melle W. A domain-independent system that aids in constructing knowledge-based consultation programs. PhD dissertation, Computer Science Department, Stanford University, 1980. Published as van Melle W, System aids in constructing consultation programs. Ann Arbor, MI: UMI Research Press; 1981.

24. Buchanan BG, Shortliffe EH. Rule-based expert systems: the MYCIN experiments of the Stanford heuristic programming project. Reading, MA: Addison-Wesley; 1984.

25. Feinstein AR. Clinical judgment. Malabar, FL: Krieger Publishing Co.; 1967.

26. Elstein AS, Shulman LS, Sprafka SA. Medical problem solving: an analysis of clinical reasoning. Cambridge, MA: Harvard University Press; 1978.

27. Schwartz WB. Medicine and the computer: the promise and problems of change. N Eng J Med. 1970;283(23):1257–64. https://doi.org/10.1056/nejm197012032832305.

28. Kuipers BJ, Kassirer JP. Causal reasoning in medicine: analysis of a protocol. Cogn Sci. 1984;8:363–85. https://doi.org/10.1016/S0364-0213(84)80007-5.

29. Pauker SG, Gorry GA, Kassirer JP, Schwartz WB. Towards the simulation of clinical cognition: taking a present illness by computer. Am J Med. 1976;60(7):981–96. https://doi.org/10.1016/0002-9343(76)90570-2.

30. Patel VL, Groen GJ. Knowledge-based solution strategies in medical reasoning. Cogn Sci. 1986;10:91–116. https://doi.org/10.1207/s15516709cog1001_4.

31. Sridharan NS. Guest editorial: special issue on artificial intelligence in biomedicine. Artif Intell. 1978;11(1–2):1–4. https://doi.org/10.1007/s13755-017-0040-y.

32. Fries JF. The chronic disease databank: first principles to future directions. J Med Philos. 1984;9:161–80. https://doi.org/10.1093/jmp/9.2.161.

33. Blum RL. Discovery and representation of causal relationships from a large time-oriented clinical database: the RX project. In: Lecture notes in medical informatics, vol. 19. Berlin: Springer; 1982. https://doi.org/10.1007/978-3-642-93235-9_1.

34. Blum RL. Computer-assisted design of studies using routine clinical data: analyzing the association of prednisone and cholesterol. Ann Intern Med. 1986;104(6):858–68. https://doi.org/10.7326/0003-4819-104-6-858.

35. Hayes-Roth R, Waterman DA, Lenat DB. Building expert systems. Reading, MA: Addison-Wesley; 1983.

36. Feigenbaum EA, McCorduck P, Nii HP. The rise of the expert company: how visionary companies are using artificial intelligence to achieve higher productivity and profits. New York: Times Books; 1988.

37. Peek N, Combi C, Marin R, Bellazzi R. Thirty years of artificial intelligence in medicine (AIME) conferences: a review of research themes. Artif Intell Med. 2015;65:61–73. https://doi.org/10.1016/j.artmed.2015.07.003.

38. Sadegh-Zadeh K. Machine over mind (editorial). Artif Intell Med. 1989;1:3–10. https://doi.org/10.1016/0933-3657(89)90012-2.

39. Hickam DH, Shortliffe EH, Bischoff MB, Scott AC, Jacobs CD. A study of the treatment advice of a computer-based cancer chemotherapy protocol advisor. Ann Intern Med. 1985;103:928–36.

40. Shortliffe EH. The adolescence of AI in medicine: will the field come of age in the 90s? Artif Intell Med. 1993;5:93–106. https://doi.org/10.1016/j.artmed.2008.07.017.

41. Patel VL, Shortliffe EH, Stefanelli M, Szolovits P, Berthold MR, Bellazzi R, Abu-Hanna A. The coming of age of artificial intelligence in medicine. Artif Intell Med. 2009;46:5–17.

42. Ding CHQ, Dubchak I. Multi-class protein fold recognition using support vector machines and neural networks. Bioinformatics. 2001;17(4):349–58. https://doi.org/10.1093/bioinformatics/17.4.349.

43. Furey TS, Cristianini N, et al. Support vector machine classification and validation of cancer tissue samples using microarray expression data. Bioinformatics. 2000;16(10):906–14. https://doi.org/10.1093/bioinformatics/16.10.906.

44. Bengio Y, Lecun Y, Hinton G. Deep learning for AI. Commun ACM. 2021;64(7):58–65. https://doi.org/10.1145/3448250.

45. Quoc VL, Ranzato MA, et al. Building high-level features using large scale unsupervised learning. *arXiv* 2012;1112.6209v5. https://arxiv.org/abs/1112.6209.

46. Gulshan V, Peng L, et al. Development and validation of a deep learning algorithm for detection of diabetic retinopathy in retinal fundus photographs. JAMA. 2016;316(22):2401–10. https://doi.org/10.1001/jama.2016.17216.

47. Irvin J, Rajpurkar P, et al. CheXpert: a large chest radiograph dataset with uncertainty labels and expert comparison. Proc AAAI Conf Artif Intell. 2019;33:590–7. https://doi.org/10.1609/AAAI.V33I01.3301590.

48. Komura D, Ishikawa S. Machine learning methods for histopathological image analysis. Comput Struct Biotechnol J. 2018;16:34–42. https://doi.org/10.1016/j.csbj.2018.01.001.

49. Rajkomar A, Oren E, et al. Scalable and accurate deep learning with electronic health records. NPJ Digit Med. 2018;1:18. https://doi.org/10.1038/s41746-018-0029-1.

50. Nestor, B, McDermott MBA, et al. Proceedings of the 4th machine learning for healthcare conference, PMLR. 2019;106:381–405. https://proceedings.mlr.press/v106/nestor19a.html.

51. Markus AF, Iors JA, Rijnbeek PR. The role of explainability in creating trustworthy artificial intelligence for health care: a comprehensive survey of the terminology, design choices, and evaluation strategies. J Biomed Info. 2021;113:103655. https://doi.org/10.1016/j.jbi.2020.103655.

52. Char DS, Shah NH, Magnus D. Implementing machine learning in health care: addressing ethical challenges. N Engl J Med. 2018;378:981–3. https://doi.org/10.1056/NEJMp1714229.

53. McCradden MD, Joshi S, et al. Ethical limitations of algorithmic farness solutions in health care machine learning. Lancet Digital Health. 2020;2(5):E221–3. https://doi.org/10.1016/S2589-7500(20)30065-0.

54. Mandl KD, Perakslis ED. HIPAA and the leak of "deidentified" EHR data. N Engl J Med. 2021;384:2171–3. https://doi.org/10.1056/NEJMp2102616.

Chapter 3
Data and Computation: A Contemporary Landscape

Ida Sim and Marina Sirota

After reading this chapter, you should know the answers to these questions:
- What type of data can be leveraged for medical research and care?
- How do we know and learn about the world through data and computation?
- What computational infrastructures currently exist to support research discovery and clinical care?
- What are artificial intelligence and machine learning and how are they related?
- What types of knowledge representation exist?
- What are open challenges in the field moving forward?

Understanding the World Through Data and Computation

Data has been called the "new oil" [1] or likened to "sunlight" [2] in its ubiquity and importance. Yet no one goes to medical school to learn data; one goes to medical school to learn what's needed to diagnose, treat, and care for people. What then is the role of data in biomedicine? Ackoff [3] is often credited with positing the data-information-knowledge continuum, in which data are raw observations, information is data in context, and knowledge is an understanding about the world that is useful for explaining, predicting, and guiding future action. Knowledge—what we learn in medical school—may be explicit and codifiable (e.g., guidelines, textbooks), tacit and not codifiable (e.g., expertise, heuristics), or process knowledge (e.g., how to

I. Sim (✉) · M. Sirota
University of California San Francisco, San Francisco, CA, USA
e-mail: ida.sim@ucsf.edu; marina.sirota@ucsf.edu

© The Author(s), under exclusive license to Springer Nature Switzerland AG 2022
T. A. Cohen et al. (eds.), *Intelligent Systems in Medicine and Health*, Cognitive Informatics in Biomedicine and Healthcare,
https://doi.org/10.1007/978-3-031-09108-7_3

remove a gallbladder). Here is a clinical example. An observation that a patient's Hemoglobin A1c (**HbA1c**) is 8.2% is data; that this HbA1c of 8.2% is above the normal range is information, i.e., data in context; that a high HbA1c is associated with increased risk of adverse cardiovascular outcomes is knowledge. Knowledge is used, along with data and information about specific patients or populations, to guide actions in clinical care and population health respectively.

In recent years, machine learning and other computational approaches have powered a new path to transforming data into knowledge. But of course, biomedicine had been generating knowledge from data well before the modern era of computing. The dominant epistemology of clinical medicine—"the investigation of what distinguishes justified belief from opinion" [4]—became increasingly grounded in the scientific method starting at the turn of the twentieth century, progressed as a result of the 1910 Flexner Report [5] to formalized teaching of physiology and biochemistry in medical school (See Chap. 16), and culminated with the tenets of evidence-based medicine (EBM) as described by Guyatt and others in 1992 [6]. EBM is marked by scrupulous attention to experimental sources of bias that may cloud attempts to distinguish "justified belief from opinion." The randomized controlled trial (RCT), which controls for both known and unknown confounders through randomization, was held up as the gold standard for resolving questions of causation, sitting atop the evidence hierarchy save for the aggregation of RCTs in meta-analysis (Fig. 3.1).

However, this classical formulation of EBM addresses only questions of causation (does X cause Y). RCTs are not an appropriate study design for other types of questions central to clinical care [7], including description of **natural history** (what happens to people with Stage 5 lung cancer), **classification** (does this

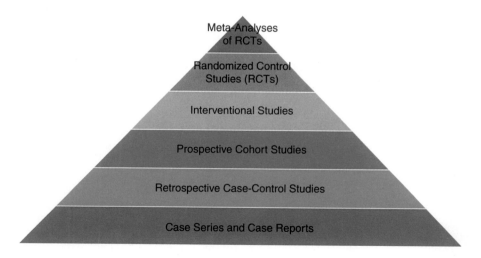

Fig. 3.1 Hierarchy of evidence according to evidence-based medicine

patient belong in (i.e., is classifiable into) the group of patients with Type 2 diabetes), **prediction** (how long will this patient with Stage 5 cancer live), and **explanation** (how does a high HbA1C result in elevated cardiovascular risk). An expanded version of EBM now addresses these other epistemological tasks using other study designs such as case control studies, prospective cohort studies, and prognostic rules [8].

Evidence : data + "study" design + analysis

Evidence is generated from data collected according to some study protocol (e.g., for an RCT, cohort study, or systematic review) and analyzed through biostatistical methods (e.g., intention-to-treat analysis for RCTs). The analyses generate findings which are used to support claims of knowledge (e.g., dexamethasone reduces 28-day mortality in some hospitalized patients with COVID-19 [9]). A particular claim of knowledge is justified beyond simple belief based on the evidentiary strength of the study design and analytic method. The claim that dexamethasone is efficacious for COVID-19 as supported by a well-conducted RCT can be contrasted with a belief in some circles of hydroxychloroquine's efficacy.

The contemporary landscape of biomedical epistemology is in tension and flux. While much of clinical research is still firmly embedded in traditional EBM approaches to generating evidence and knowledge, new computational approaches analyze vast amounts of data using "study designs" or algorithms that are wholly different from how clinical researchers and clinicians have been taught to know the world. Logistic regression and various machine learning algorithms are both analytic methods applied to data to generate evidence for claims of knowledge. These two ways of knowing [10]—EBM and data science—are complementary and can both be advanced with contemporary computational capabilities. This chapter reviews the foundations of data and computation as an underpinning to the following chapters.

Types of Data Relevant to Biomedicine

There are many broad classes of data relevant to biomedicine and healthcare, including Electronic Health Records (EHR), -omics, imaging, mobile and social media, environmental, public health, and clinical research data. The EHR captures patient information including demographics, diagnosis codes, lab test results, medications, allergies, and clinical notes generated from the provision of health care. While these data are originally collected for clinical and reimbursement purposes, they provide an incredible opportunity to mine and apply machine learning techniques for predicting disease risk or understanding disease better. These data have been used widely to predict patient outcomes such as hospital readmission rate [11] or pregnancy outcomes [12]. Other clinical datasets include MIMIC-IV [13], a large, single-center database containing information relating to patients admitted to critical care units at a large tertiary care hospital. MIMIC is a rare example of a large clinical dataset available for use by the broader research community. There are efforts in clinical trials data sharing through repositories such as ImmPort [14] and Vivli [15]. Finally clinical imaging is another field with many opportunities to apply advanced machine learning and predictive modeling techniques for diagnostic purposes, as further described in Chap. 12.

Genomic and other molecular profiling technologies allow us to extract large amounts of data from patient samples, elucidating previously unknown factors involved in disease, such as drug targets or disease biomarkers. Much of the data from these types of experiments are publicly available. For instance, gene expression data are hosted in the Gene Expression Omnibus (GEO) [16] that as of July 2021, contains data on over 4.5 million samples and over 150,000 experiments. These data are very rich, capturing a number of different disease areas. With the technologies getting cheaper and more advanced, many of the transcriptomic studies now capture expression on a single cell level. dbGAP [17] and Short Read Archive (SRA) both house sequencing data with additional security for ensuring patient privacy. There are also disease-specific databases such as the Cancer Genome Atlas (TCGA) [18] that contains molecular measurements on more than 10,000 cancer samples and adjacent normal controls including transcriptomics, genetics, methylation and proteomics. The Preterm Birth Data Repository [19] is another example of a data repository, which as of July 2021 hosted over 45 molecular studies relating to pregnancy outcomes with a focus on preterm birth. A more in-depth description of applications of artificial intelligence to molecular measurements as part of the field of translational bioinformatics can be found in Chap. 14.

Clinical and molecular datasets can furthermore be enhanced by public health data such as The National Health and Nutrition Examination Survey (NHANES). NHANES is a program of studies designed to assess the health and nutritional status of adults and children in the United States and uniquely combines interviews and physical examinations. CalEnviroscreen [20] is a database that captures environmental exposures across the state of California. Birth and death records (e.g., OSHP [21]) have been used extensively for research purposes. For instance in our own work, we have integrated the environmental exposure data from the CalEnviroscreen together with birth records information in order to identify arsenic and nitrate as water contaminants that are associated with preterm birth [22]. Finally in the last several years, mobile/social media data such as actigraphy, Twitter, and smartwatch data has been used to improve disease diagnosis (e.g., of atrial fibrillation [23]), monitor symptoms [24], and drive health behavior change [25, 26]. Newer modalities of data acquisition including Ecological Momentary Assessments (EMAs) [27] that prompt users for their behaviors and experiences in real time in their natural environments are offering an unprecedented view into people's lived experience of health and disease.

The truth, however, is that there is no such thing as "health" and "non-health" data: all data can have implications for health. For example, individual-level data such as your online purchases, social media, geolocation, financial and criminal record data can be mined for predictors of health risk and health status. Environmental and population-level data such as block-level air pollution and noise [28], and voting patterns in your state [29], could be as predictive for health as traditional EHR data. The boundaries dividing health from general societal data and computing infrastructure are increasingly porous.

Knowing Through Computation

The explosive availability of Big Data—distinguished by high Velocity (speed of data generation), Volume, and Variety—enables new levels of data-driven reasoning, of which there are two major flavors. **Abductive reasoning** as originally coined by Pierce in 1955 [30] can be characterized as a cyclical process of *generating* possible explanations or a set of hypotheses that are able to account for the available data (see also the similar discussion of these concepts as they apply to human reasoning in Chap. 5). More recently, the term abductive reasoning has been expanded to the notion of "Inference to the Best Explanation" [31], by which a hypothesis or theory is arrived at that *best explains* the available data. Over time, clinical research using traditional statistics also endeavors to arrive at a "best explanation." A study postulates a hypothesis, data is collected and analyzed drawing on deep domain expertise, and the null hypothesis is accepted or rejected thus arriving at a provisional explanation of the observed data. Randomized controlled trials are a type of study design that controls for known and unknown confounders to strengthen a claim of causation, yielding a "best explanation" that can be contravened by other or subsequent trials. In computation, case-based reasoning is a classic example of abductive decision support systems, which are nowadays overshadowed by inductive machine learning approaches.

Inductive reasoning involves an inferential process from the observed data to account for the unobserved. It is a process of generating possible conclusions based on available data. The power of inductive reasoning lies in its ability to allow us to go beyond the limitations of our current evidence or knowledge to novel conclusions about the unknown. **Machine learning**—computer algorithms that find and apply patterns in (huge amounts of) data—is quintessential inductive reasoning. Subtypes include **classification, prediction, causal reasoning,** and **modeling** (Box 3.1).

Box 3.1 Examples of Inductive Reasoning

Classification: inferring which class an instance belongs to based on classes of observed instances. E.g., a diagnostic decision support system "classifies" a given patient to a "disease" based on the similarity of their symptoms to the symptoms of prior patients known to have that disease.

   Prediction: inferring a future state based on past data. E.g., a clinical decision support system predicts whether a patient will require hospitalization based on historical hospital admissions data.

   Causation: inferring whether X caused Y. E.g., a deep neural network running over a clinical data warehouse is used to discover whether Drug X causes a Side Effect Y.

   Modeling: simulating the components, relationships, and actions within a biomedical or health system to explain, explore, or predict E.g., a discrete event model of endocrine feedback for a disease.

The combination of Big Data and machine learning is fueling a transformation in computational reasoning. Coupled with advances in cloud, social, mobile and other technologies, a new frontier is opening up for what computers can do with and for humans in health and biomedicine.

Motivational Example

Now that we have an overview of biomedical data and computation, we present and deconstruct an example clinical case (Box 3.2) to illustrate high-level issues and challenges that will shape the near future of data and computation.

Box 3.2 Illustrative Case

Andre is a 47-year-old man with mild Type 2 diabetes. He was returning from a business trip overseas when he felt short of breath, out of sorts, and had occasional sharp chest pains. He signed onto a telehealth service offered through his employer. The telehealth service's chatbot interviewed Andre, using an avatar that was Hispanic, as Andre is. After an initial set of questions, the chatbot handed over the case to a human physician, who conducted a video consultation with Andre while reviewing his electronic health record data along with his respiratory rate, body temperature, oxygen saturation and other data from his smartwatch. The physician recommended that Andre get evaluated in person at the nearest Emergency Room (ER). Andre is getting worried. On his way to the ER, Andre asks Siri what he might have. Siri tells him scary diagnoses like pneumonia, and something called pulmonary embolism. Siri explains that pulmonary embolism is when a blood clot forms in a leg after prolonged sedentariness (like a long flight) and breaks off to the lungs causing chest pain and shortness of breath.

At the ER, Andre was first seen by a resident physician-in-training who ordered multiple tests including labwork, a chest x-ray, and a chest CT. Based on those data, a decision support system ran predictive models that resulted in a ranked list of differential diagnoses, with an intermediate probability for pulmonary embolism. The resident presented the case to Dr. Jackson, the attending ER physician. After reviewing the data and output, Dr. Jackson went to talk with Andre and examine him. She noticed crackles in the lungs, an S3, a prominent right-sided cardiac lift and elevated jugular venous pressure. On further questioning, Andre mentioned that he had had a "bad cold" about 1 month before and had been feeling unwell even before the business trip. Suspecting biventricular failure from viral myopericarditis, Dr. Jackson ordered an echocardiogram and admitted Andre.

Andre is fortunate to have convenient timely access to "virtual-first" care through his employer. 9% of Americans have no health insurance [32] at all while 43% are underinsured [33]. When health care moved onto virtual platforms during the SARS-CoV-2 pandemic, marginalized populations had reduced access to health care due to lack of technology and/or technology literacy [34], adding "digital determinants of health" to the causes of health inequities (Chaps. 13 and 18). As with general consumer technology, chatbot services are increasingly common in health. Chapter 9 reviews natural language processing (NLP) and other computational issues underlying dialog systems. Culturally concordant avatars, language, and user interactions are needed to establish belonging and trust with digital interactions for all peoples (Chap. 18). Central to this book on cognitive informatics is the importance of a smooth handoff between computational and human care: the decision to refer to Andre to the ER is one that should involve a human, who in this case was able to access and review Andre's EHR and wearable data to get a better view of his overall status. The ability to access such data in real time requires health data interoperability encompassing network computing, data standards, and sociotechnical data sharing mechanisms. Siri and the decision support system in the ER illustrate the exciting possibilities of automated reasoning. Early diagnostic systems dating from the 1970s include INTERNIST-1 and **MYCIN** (Chap. 2). Simpler systems, such as the Modified Early Warning System (MEWS) for scoring physiologic observations to predict sepsis [35], have been widely used in clinical practice, and have evolved to machine-learning based models with better performance (Chap. 10). Advances in image recognition have given rise to imaging decision support systems such as for detecting pulmonary embolism (Chap. 12).

Andre's case illustrates the importance of framing clinical decision support not as a solely computational task but as one of human/AI collaboration requiring a human-in-the-loop approach. The ER resident who first evaluated Andre likely had

premature closure [36] on the potential diagnosis of pulmonary embolism (PE) and collected data (e.g., chest CT) with PE in mind while not pursuing other potential diagnoses. When presented with this restricted set of data, the decision support system backs up the resident's diagnostic hunch. Dr. Jackson, the more senior physician, performs a more thorough history and exam with a broader differential in mind, and notes signs of biventricular failure that the resident missed. These findings increase her suspicion for viral myopericarditis, a diagnosis which becomes more likely with additional history that Andre has felt increasingly unwell since a viral syndrome 1 month ago. That the decision support system did not rank viral myopericarditis high on the potential list of diagnoses is less a failure of the diagnostic algorithm than a failure of the human component. Cognitive informatics emphasizes a balanced approach to how humans and machines work together. One could imagine circumventing the resident's premature diagnostic closure by instrumenting Andre's existence—surveilling his exposure to a virus 1 month ago, tracking his progressively worsening symptoms and elevated heart pressures, sensing his decreased gait speed and mobility—to diagnose his condition before he hit the ER. Aside from the technical challenges of achieving accurate diagnosis using such multi-modal time-varying data, the continuous collection of vast amounts of data from our daily lives presents a potentially grave cost in privacy. Data privacy is a core element of trust, as is, increasingly, transparency and fairness of the algorithms underlying computational decision support (Chap. 18). The remainder of this chapter discusses the main data and computational issues raised by Andre's use case.

Computational Landscape

There exists frequent confusion between **artificial intelligence (AI)** and **machine learning (ML)** and between ML and statistics. AI is the ability of a machine to perform tasks (and behave) like an intelligent being. AI encompasses a broad range of functions that lead a machine to "seem" intelligent, that we can break up into functions relating to data acquisition and processing, "thinking", and action in the real world. Data acquisition and processing include machine vision and image processing (e.g., detecting breast cancer in a mammogram, Chap. 12), speech recognition (e.g., dialog systems, Chap. 9), and NLP (e.g., extracting smoking status from EHR free text, Chap. 7). Thinking includes reasoning (as above), planning (e.g., surgical robot planning), and learning (Chaps. 5 and 6). Action in the real world includes image generation (e.g., embodied conversational agents, Chap. 9), speech generation (e.g., dialog systems, Chap. 9) and autonomous systems (e.g., robots that deliver meds).

As shown in Fig. 3.2, AI is a subset of computer science and ML is a subset of AI. Confusingly, ML also overlaps with statistics and data science. In fact, if ML is "computer algorithms that find and apply patterns in data," statistics does so too. Although ML typically is used on huge amounts of data, both ML and statistics are just alternative ways to understand and draw inferences out of data. Because ML

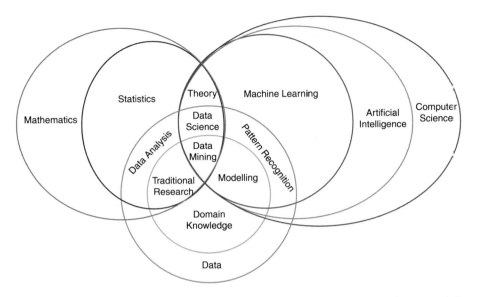

Fig. 3.2 Data Science Field/Term Diagram (adapted from Ryan J Urbanowicz, ryanurb@upenn.edu)

has commonalities with traditional analytics, ML is subject to the same pitfalls as traditional statistics, including bias, confounding, or inappropriate interpretation (Chap. 18). We can and should hold ML to the same expectations for scientific integrity as we do traditional analytics.

Knowledge Representation

Knowledge representation is the field of AI dedicated to representing information about the world in a form that a computer system can understand and use to solve complex tasks such as diagnosing a medical condition.

There are different approaches to data representation including symbolic, rule-based and graph-based formalisms. One of the most active areas of knowledge representation research are projects associated with the Semantic Web which seeks to add a layer of meaning on top of the internet. Rather than indexing web sites and pages via keywords, the Semantic Web creates large ontologies of concepts. An **ontology** is a set of concepts and categories in a subject area or domain that shows their properties and the relations between them. An example of an ontology in the biomedical domain is the Gene Ontology used to annotate genes.

A **rule-based** system has a knowledge base represented as a collection of "rules" that are typically expressed as "if-then" clauses. The set of rules forms the knowledge base that is applied to the current set of facts.

One of the earliest examples of such a system in the clinical domain was **MYCIN** [37], an early **backward chaining** expert system that used artificial intelligence to identify bacteria causing severe infections, such as bacteremia and meningitis, and to recommend antibiotics, with the dosage adjusted for a patient's body weight. Knowledge graphs are another method to model knowledge. A **knowledge graph** is a directed, labeled graph in which the labels have well-defined meanings. A directed labeled graph consists of nodes, edges (links), and labels. Anything can act as a node, for example genes, proteins, diagnoses. Edges between them can be relationships. This type of representation can be used for predicting and modeling different biological associations for instance drug-protein targets, gene-disease associations, protein-protein interactions, disease comorbidities. Knowledge-based systems are discussed in detail in Chap. 4 of this volume.

Machine Learning

Machine learning is a branch of artificial intelligence based on the idea that systems can learn from data, identify patterns and make decisions with minimal human intervention. Machine learning approaches which are in further detail described in Chap. 6 can be characterized into **supervised** and **unsupervised** approaches (Fig. 3.3). **Clustering** algorithms that aim to group objects with similar attributes using measures of distance or similarity. For instance, one can cluster patients based on their clinical profiles and identify subgroups of patients that might be similar to each other. Unsupervised algorithms, or those that do not rely on ground truth, include k-means, hierarchical clustering, and expectation-maximization clustering using Gaussian mixture models. Classification is a task of identifying which category an observation belongs to. Some examples include classifying an email to the "spam" or "non-spam" category, or in the biomedical domain, assigning a diagnosis to a given patient based on observed characteristics of the patient. **Classification** algorithms, which often rely on training data, include random forest, decision trees, naive bayes and others and are supervised, which means that there is some data that is used with existing labels. These concepts are further explored in Chap. 6.

Deep learning techniques deserve special mention due to the importance these methods are gaining currently. Deep learning methods rely on neural networks, which were first proposed in the 1940s, in which layers of neuron-like nodes mimic

Fig. 3.3 Types of Machine Learning (ML) Approaches

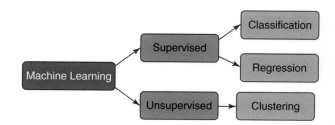

how human brains analyze information. The underlying mechanisms of trained neural networks can be hard to disentangle, and thus, they have mainly been applied within biomedicine for image recognition. However, the ability to train a neural network on massive amounts of data has raised special interest in applying them elsewhere in the field of biomedicine, although the interpretability of these approaches is often a challenge (Chap. 8). These methods have been applied extensively to image analysis [38] and have been recently extended to other types of data including EHR [39] and genetic data [40].

Data Integration to Better Understand Medicine: Multimodal, Multi-Scale Models

The wealth and availability of public genomic, transcriptomic and other types of molecular data together with rich clinical phenotyping and computational integrative methods provide a powerful opportunity to improve human health by refining the current knowledge about disease therapeutics and diagnostics. There are different types of integrative models that can be applied to bring together diverse data [41]. As presented by Richie et al., meta-dimensional analysis can be divided into three categories: (1) **Concatenation-based integration** involves combining data sets from different data types at the raw or processed data level before modelling and analysis; (2) **Transformation-based integration** involves performing mapping or data transformation of the underlying data sets before analysis, and the modelling approach is applied at the level of transformed matrices; and (3) **Model-based integration** is the process of performing analysis on each data type independently, followed by integration of the resultant models to generate knowledge about the trait of interest.

The ideal scenario is when the different types of data are collected on the same individuals. In this case both concatenation and transformation-based integration can be applied. In our prior work, we examined patient heterogeneity in a lupus cohort for which we had rich clinical as well as molecular measurements such as genotyping and methylation to identify several clinical clusters of SLE patients and molecular pathways associated with those clusters [42]. However, there are also situations when the data is not collected on the same individuals and therefore, we must use a model-based integration approach to bring the datasets together using phenotype as the common ground. For instance, if the goal is to identify genetic, transcriptomic and proteomic associations with a certain disease of interest, data sets could be extracted from the public domain, where DNA sequence data may be available on some of the patient samples, microarray data from a different subset of patient samples, and proteomic data on yet another subset of patient samples. Model-based integration would allow the independent analysis of each of the modalities, followed by an integration of the top models from each data set to identify integrative consensus models.

By integrating data across measurement modalities as well as by integrating molecular measures with rich clinical phenotyping we can get a bit closer to achieving precision medicine by improving diagnostics and therapeutics.

Distributed/Networked Computing

The modern world is a networked world including more recent technologies for computing such as cloud computing and graphical processing units (GPUs—more in Chap. 2), where both data and computation are distributed across time, space, and jurisdictions. A patient's EHR data may reside in several places: her current primary doctor's health system, the health systems of her previous care providers and of emergency visits, and third party telehealth companies for the occasional urgent care consult. Her genetic sequence, cancer genotype, and various wearable data such as Apple Watch or FitBit are likewise held and computed on in siloed and proprietary systems, each subject to access policies and terms of use that are often opaque to both the patient herself and to third parties. As messy as this all is, as discussed in the section on "Types of Data Relevant to Biomedicine", there is no such thing as "health" and "non-health" data. Because the value of data is in its aggregation, a challenge is how to bring together multiple sources of data for any given query to enable multiple types of computation.

In the traditional approach, data is brought to the query. That is, if a data requester wants to run a query, the requester obtains a copy of the data, installs it on his/her own machine and runs the query on the data that has been brought in. Because the data requester now holds a copy of the data, the original data holder has effectively lost control over its access. Moreover, if the datasets are very large, as is the case for many imaging, genomic, sensor, and real-world data studies, the data requester may not have sufficient storage and compute capacity. Thus, this approach is not compatible with any need for controlled access (which includes most cases of sharing patient data) nor for sharing large datasets.

The converse approach is bringing the query to the data. The data requester submits the query to the machine where the data resides, the query is run on that remote machine, and the results are returned back to the requester. Queries can, of course, be complex computations and analyses, not just simple search and retrieval queries. In this model, data holders retain control of the data and the requester does not ever have a copy of or control of the data.

Data Federation Models

This basic idea of bringing the query to the data can be implemented through different configurations of databases and query servers, each with their own benefits and challenges. In the simplest **Local Data Store** model, every data holder hosts its own data on its own server. External data requesters establish user accounts on that server under some access control model. The requester then has access to view the data and to analyze it, but not to download a copy of the data to the requester's own machine. However, this model is infeasible for widespread data sharing because data requesters wishing to query multiple databases must establish multiple user accounts and navigate multiple access policies and procedures and have no ability to combine data for aggregate analysis.

In the **One Single Centralized Datastore** model, data from multiple sources are aggregated into one "data warehouse." An example is the University of California's Health Data Warehouse that aggregates data from over 15 million patients seen at the five medical campuses of the University of California [43]. Another example is N3C, aggregating EHR data on 1.9 million COVID patients from 34 medical centers across the US into a single portal for secure data access and analysis [44]. This model benefits from economies of scale, and data requesters need to submit their queries to only one database under a uniform data access policy. However, this model still does not allow aggregation of data across data warehouses. The silo is just a bigger silo.

The **federated query model** combines the bring-the-query-to-the-data approach with federated databases. Databases are federated when independent geographically dispersed databases are networked in such a way that they can respond to queries as if all the data were in a single virtual database. Thus, data requesters can submit a query to a federated query service and have that query be routed to all databases participating in that federation. Data holders maintain full control of their data, and neither the data requester nor the query service provider ever has direct access to the data.

Federation technology has progressed substantially in recent years. An example is the R2D2 initiative with a federated network of 12 health systems comprising 202 hospitals contributing COVID-related EHR data on 45 million patients [45]. In contrast to the N3C approach described above, data never leave the 12 health systems, which act as nodes on the network making their patient data available in a common data model. Queries and computations are submitted via a centralized service that then federates computation such as averages, regressions, and machine learning models to individual nodes on the network.

Interoperability

Whenever data is brought together for query and computation, whether in the centralized warehouse or federated model, the data must be interoperable. **Interoperability** is the ability of computer systems or software to exchange *and make use of* information; it is not enough to send data that is unintelligible to the recipient. Interoperability therefore includes both syntactic and semantic interoperability, which are enabled by the use of data interoperability standards. **Syntactic interoperability** refers to the format and ordering of what is exchanged, analogous to the grammar of an English sentence for exchanging ideas between humans. Examples of primarily syntactic standards include data exchange standards such as

HTML and, in health care, HL7 FHIR and DICOM for representing data in transit. **Semantic interoperability** refers to the meaning of what is exchanged, analogous to the words and their dictionary meaning in an English sentence. Semantic standards in healthcare include common terminologies such as SNOMED and LOINC. One needs both syntactic and semantic standards to enable full interoperability. A sentence using English words and German grammar is not interoperable between humans (Box 3.3).

Box 3.3 Interoperability
Interoperability is the ability of computer systems or software to exchange and make use of information. **Syntactic interoperability** *refers to the format and ordering of what is exchanged.* **Semantic interoperability** *refers to the meaning of what is exchanged.*

Data that is to be aggregated also need to share a common data model at rest. The University of California Health Data Warehouse, N3C warehouse, and the R2D2 federated network all use the Observational Medical Outcomes Partnership Common Data Model (OMOP CDM) [46]. This model was designed for cross-institutional queries of EHR data for quality improvement and research purposes, and binds data to a mandatory clinical vocabulary (OMOP Standardized Vocabularies) [47] that is based on SNOMED, LOINC, RxNORM and others. Note the same OMOP data model and associated vocabularies can be used for centralized or federated approaches and is fit-for-purpose for a wide range of EHR data interoperability use cases. Common data models and data exchange protocols must be defined and agreed upon across all contributors to data sharing and adopted uniformly by each contributor or federation node.

Computational Aspects of Privacy

Chapter 18 reviews the broader issues of Ethics, including Privacy. To understand the computational aspects of privacy, we need to distinguish privacy and security. **Privacy** is a concept that applies to people, rather than documents, in which there is a presumed right to protect that individual from unauthorized divulging of personal data of any kind. **Security** is the process of protecting information from destruction or misuse, including both physical and computer-based mechanisms. Security falls under IT. Privacy is when you are assured and protected from a company holding your geolocation data selling it without your knowledge or approval. Security is when no hacker can get into that company's systems to access or corrupt your geolocation data. You can have 100% security and no privacy; if you have no security, you also have no privacy.

Privacy is best protected by a combination of technical and legal means. Technically, the objective is to minimize the risk that an adversary can associate or re-identify your personal data with you. However, there is no guarantee of absolute protection against re-identification. Data—EHR, geolocation, fitness data—can be subjected to **de-identification** or **anonymization** to increase privacy. De-identified data is data that has identifying personal data such as names and birthdates removed or perturbed in such a way as to be non-identifying (Chap. 18). Anonymized data has identifying personal data removed or perturbed and the key linking a data record to a particular person is destroyed such that the data becomes anonymous. In truth, with sufficient external data, de-identified and even anonymized data can be re-identified. Thus, legal mechanisms such as data use agreements (DUA) are needed to supplement technical privacy protection.

The challenges of privacy protection are magnified when data need to be aggregated. The more data there is about an individual, the greater the risk the data will uniquely match an individual leading to re-identification.

The risk is further magnified with federated data sharing. Mechanisms such as differential privacy [48] are used where queries are federated over perturbed data and the answers are then operated on to "subtract" out the perturbations to arrive at the real answer without increasing the risk of re-identification. Another approach is synthetic data [49], where a synthetic dataset is created that matches the distributional properties of the original data set. In this way, computations can occur on the synthetic dataset with some provable level of accuracy to the original dataset. The details of computation for privacy are outside the scope of this book but are closely tied to the ability to safely aggregate and reuse large amounts of data for machine learning. The point to know is that the "old" way of privacy protection under HIPAA "safe harbor" [50]—removing a specified list of 18 identifying data elements—is increasingly insufficient for modern-day data sharing and computation.

Trends and Future Challenges

Chapter 19 anticipates the future of AI in medicine and healthcare. Here, we review trends and open challenges affecting the general use of data and computation for biomedicine.

Ground Truth

The availability of extensive molecular and clinical data provides an incredible opportunity to apply predictive modeling and ML techniques to improve diagnostics and therapeutics. However, ML models need rich and accurate training data, including labelling of ground truth (e.g., which patients have the disease that the

ML is trying to predict). Many datasets, especially large public datasets, are poorly labelled and are also heterogeneous and not well annotated, making them difficult to aggregate and use for ML. Annotation and labelling are difficult and time-consuming tasks. For example, labelling clinical and imaging data with ground truth labels of diagnosis requires expert time and costs. The limited availability of labelled data can be somewhat overcome by the sheer amount of data, but this bottleneck is important to recognize. New semi-supervised approaches are emerging that rely on small amounts of labelled data to predict missing labels for larger datasets, but these approaches risk perpetuating and amplifying biases and mis-labelling in the smaller set. The availability of accurate and unbiased labelled training data for ML will be an ongoing challenge.

Open Science and Mechanisms for Open data

Scientific culture is increasingly embracing open approaches to data sharing and reuse, adhering to FAIR (Findable, Accessible, Interoperable, Reusable) principles [51]. **Findability** requires indexing and shared metadata and persistent Digital Object Identifiers (DOIs) such as from DataCite or other services that span disciplines. **Accessibility** brings up data rights, ownership, access policies, and fair (as in just) credit for data sharing—all of which are wide open issues. We discussed **Interoperability** above.

Reusability needs to be distinguished between reusability by humans or reusability by computers. Human reusability is a lower bar. Data and metadata need to be findable and sufficiently interpretable by humans to facilitate additional data cleaning, alignment, and harmonization to achieve the aggregation purpose. In contrast, automated reusability by computers requires much more stringent adherence to compatible syntactic and semantic standards for all the data. This upfront work is challenging for data mapping but also governance reasons. People need to decide on common data elements, which necessitate agreement on potentially controversial scientific issues. For example, the N3C Consortium agreed on specific definitions of variables that all sites have to map their data into [52]. N3C also had to address privacy concerns for human data, as data reusability must take place under fair and just conditions that limit the risk of re-identification. Thus, N3C also defined three levels of access to N3C data in their secure enclave: a limited data set that can only be accessed with IRB approval, a de-identified data set that can be accessed without IRB approval, and a synthetic data set that requires only an N3C account and DUA [53]. Perhaps because of the additional challenges of protecting privacy, the ethos of open science and open data has a stronger hold in the life sciences than in clinical research and care.

As data, information and knowledge are shared, re-purposed, combined, and distributed in a networked world, the **provenance** of each component must be auditable lest errors and biases become compounded to an extent that threatens the integrity of computed inferences and decision support. Infrastructures for managing metadata and provenance are currently woefully inadequate. The FHIR [54] and

Open mHealth [55] data exchange standards model provenance (e.g., who measured a blood pressure reading in the clinic, what sensor model did the sleep duration come from) but these attributes are not consistently captured or described. The need for detailed provenance is critical for scientific reproducibility and is especially important for longitudinal studies of data that may drift over time. For example, the NIH's 4-year RECOVER initiative to study Post-Acute Sequelae of SARS-CoV-2 (PASC, aka "long COVID") will be collecting real-world, survey, and sensor data whose definition, collection, and post-processing methods are likely to change as more is known about PASC. Without a clear trace of data transformations and other provenance, the scientific value of the consortium data will diminish over time. Provenance architectures, managing the risks of re-identification, and mechanisms for tracking and assigning data sharing credit are two major open challenges.

Data as a Public Good

The ultimate value of data and computation to society rests on the willingness of the intended users to accept the outputs. How we collect, describe, and share data and how we construct our computational systems can earn the trust of users—or not. As discussed in Chap. 18, trustworthiness must be designed into data and computation from the outset and cannot be left as an afterthought. Lack of trust is corrosive and impedes data fluidity and data aggregation, which decreases the overall value of computation by reducing the amount and representativeness of the underlying data.

One of the central pillars of trustworthiness involves protecting the privacy of individuals. In the United States, the Health Insurance Portability and Accountability Act (HIPAA) [50] governs health data privacy by regulating healthcare organizations ("covered entities") on when they can use and disclose individuals' health information. This approach implicitly sets healthcare organizations as the principal custodians of health data, thus giving such organizations outsize control (and responsibility) over the trust fabric for the use of computers in health care. The European Union, in contrast, takes a person-centered rather than an organization-centered approach. The General Data Protection Regulation (GDPR) [56] explicitly places the individual in control of the use and disclosure of their own data, and defines a more expansive framing of data protection to include not only privacy but also appropriately scoped data requests, transparency, and fairness. As demonstrated by the SARS-CoV-2 pandemic, however, data also serve as a public good to inform public policies, drive machine learning models, or demonstrate the efficacy of pharmaceutical and non-pharmaceutical interventions. While care must be taken to re-purpose data originally collected for individual care, a justice-based model for data sharing [57] is emerging that focuses on fostering public trust in uses of such data for the public good with attention to the needs of vulnerable populations and eliminating health disparities. Data sharing that prioritizes public interest as well as personal privacy promotes optimal data use for society. Over time, the technical architecture of data, data sharing, and computation will morph to drive and align with society's evolving relationship to data, with deep implications for the future of cognitive informatics.

Questions for Discussion

- What are some existing clinical data resources and standards that allow for data analysis and integration?
- What molecular databases exist now that can be leveraged for biomedical research?
- How can supervised and unsupervised machine learning approaches complement traditional evidence-based medicine approaches?
- What is data federation and in what ways can it be achieved?
- What kind of data can be integrated to impact clinical decision making and care?
- What are key considerations in ensuring trustworthy data and computation?

Further Reading

Ritchie MD, Holzinger ER, Li R, Pendergrass SA, Kim D. Methods of integrating data to uncover genotype-phenotype interactions. Nat Rev Genet. 2015 Feb;16 (2):85–97. doi: 10.1038/nrg3868. Epub 2015 Jan 13. PMID: 25582081.

- This is a comprehensive review paper on integrative approaches. The authors explore meta-dimensional and multi-staged analyses — in the context of better understanding the role of genetics and genomics in complex outcomes. However the aforementioned approaches can also be leveraged for integrating other types of data.

Sim I. Mobile Devices and Health. N Engl J Med 2019; 381:956–968.

- Comprehensive review of leveraging mobile devices in health. This article discusses sensors, digital biomarkers, digital therapeutics and diagnostics, and the integration of mobile health into frontline clinical care. It concludes with open questions on the ethics, validation, and regulation of mobile health and the prevailing market forces that are shaping the growth of this technology sector.

Straus S, Glasziou P, Richardson WS, Haynes RB. (2018) *Evidence-Based Medicine: How to Practice and Teach It.* Elsevier. ISBN: 9780702062964.

- A comprehensive description of evidence-based medicine geared towards practicing clinicians. It reviews EBM approaches for the major types of clinical questions (therapy, diagnosis and screening, prognosis) and includes tools and calculators for teaching and applying EBM in practice.

Pedro Larrañaga, Borja Calvo, Roberto Santana, Concha Bielza, Josu Galdiano, Iñaki Inza, José A. Lozano, Rubén Armañanzas, Guzmán Santafé, Aritz Pérez, Victor Robles, Machine learning in bioinformatics, *Briefings in Bioinformatics*, Volume 7, Issue 1, March 2006, Pages 86–112, https://doi.org/10.1093/bib/bbk007.

- This is a comprehensive review of machine learning in bioinformatics. The authors present a number of modelling methods, such as supervised classification, clustering and probabilistic graphical models for knowledge discovery, as well as deterministic and stochastic heuristics for optimization. They present applications in genomics, proteomics, systems biology, evolution and text mining however the methodology is applicable to other types of data including clinical.

Alyass, A., Turcotte, M. & Meyre, D. From big data analysis to personalized medicine for all: challenges and opportunities. BMC Med Genomics 8, 33 (2015). https://doi.org/10.1186/s12920-015-0108-y.

- While there are incredible opportunities with the recent advances in high throughput technologies allowing for leveraging and integrating large datasets to achieve more precise modeling of human disease, there are also challenges that need to be recognized. Several bottlenecks include generation of cost-effective high-throughput data; hybrid education and multidisciplinary teams; data storage and processing; data integration and interpretation; and individual and global economic relevance. This article discusses challenges and opportunities in personalized medicine using big data.

References

1. The world's most valuable resource is no longer oil, but data. The Economist [Internet]. 2017 May 6 [cited 2021 June 13]. https://www.economist.com/leaders/2017/05/06/the-worlds-most-valuable-resource-is-no-longer-oil-but-data.
2. Are data more like oil or sunlight? The Economist [Internet]. 2020 Feb 20 [cited 2021 June 13]. https://www.economist.com/special-report/2020/02/20/are-data-more-like-oil-or-sunlight.
3. Ackoff RL. From data to wisdom. J Appl Syst Anal. 1989;16:3–9.
4. EPISTEMOLOGY | Definition of EPISTEMOLOGY by Oxford Dictionary on Lexico.com also meaning of EPISTEMOLOGY [Internet]. Lexico Dictionaries | English. [cited 2021 June 13]. https://www.lexico.com/en/definition/epistemology.
5. Beck AH. STUDENTJAMA. The Flexner report and the standardization of American medical education. JAMA. 2004;291(17):2139–40.
6. Evidence-Based Medicine Working Group. Evidence-based medicine. A new approach to teaching the practice of medicine. JAMA. 1992;268(17):2420–5.
7. Clarke B, Gillies D, Illari P, Russo F, Williamson J. The evidence that evidence-based medicine omits. Prev Med. 2013;57(6):745–7.
8. Oxford Centre for Evidence-Based Medicine: Levels of Evidence (March 2009) — Centre for Evidence-Based Medicine (CEBM), University of Oxford [Internet]. [cited 2021 July 23]. https://www.cebm.ox.ac.uk/resources/levels-of-evidence/oxford-centre-for-evidence-based-medicine-levels-of-evidence-march-2009.
9. RECOVERY Collaborative Group, Horby P, Lim WS, Emberson JR, Mafham M, Bell JL, Linsell L, Staplin N, Brightling C, Ustianowski A, Elmahi E, Prudon B, Green C, Felton T, Chadwick D, Rege K, Fegan C, Chappell LC, Faust SN, Jaki T, Jeffery K, Montgomery A,

Rowan K, Juszczak E, Baillie JK, Haynes R, Landray MJ. Dexamethasone in hospitalized patients with Covid-19. N Engl J Med. 2021;384(8):693–704.

10. Sim I. Two ways of knowing: big data and evidence-based medicine. Ann Intern Med. 2016;164(8):562–3.

11. Rajkomar A, Oren E, Chen K, Dai AM, Hajaj N, Hardt M, et al. Scalable and accurate deep learning with electronic health records. NPJ Digit Med. 2018;1:18.

12. Abraham A, Le B, Kosti I, Straub P, Velez-Edwards DR, Davis LK, et al. Dense phenotyping from electronic health records enables machine-learning-based prediction of preterm birth. medRxiv. 2020;2020.07.15.20154864.

13. Johnson A, Bulgarelli L, Pollard T, Horng S, Celi LA, Mark R. MIMIC-IV (version 1.0). PhysioNet. 2021. https://doi.org/10.13026/s6n6-xd98.

14. Bhattacharya S, Andorf S, Gomes L, Dunn P, Schaefer H, Pontius J, et al. ImmPort: disseminating data to the public for the future of immunology. Immunol Res. 2014;58(2–3):234–9.

15. Vivli - Center for Global Clinical Research Data [Internet]. [cited 2021 July 22]. https://vivli.org/.

16. Clough E, Barrett T. The gene expression omnibus database. Methods Mol Biol. 2016;1418:93–110.

17. Mailman MD, Feolo M, Jin Y, Kimura M, Tryka K, Bagoutdinov R, et al. The NCBI dbGaP database of genotypes and phenotypes. Nat Genet. 2007;39(10):1181–6.

18. Tomczak K, Czerwińska P, Wiznerowicz M. The cancer genome atlas (TCGA): an immeasurable source of knowledge. Contemp Oncol (Pozn). 2015;19(1A):A68–77.

19. Sirota M, Thomas CG, Liu R, Zuhl M, Banerjee P, Wong RJ, et al. Enabling precision medicine in neonatology, an integrated repository for preterm birth research. Sci Data. 2018;5:180219.

20. Admin O. CalEnviroScreen [Internet]. OEHHA. 2014 [cited 2021 July 22]. https://oehha.ca.gov/calenviroscreen.

21. Office of Statewide Health Planning and Development [Internet]. OSHPD. [cited 2021 July 22]. https://oshpd.ca.gov/.

22. Wang A, Gerona RR, Schwartz JM, Lin T, Sirota M, Morello-Frosch R, et al. A suspect screening method for characterizing multiple chemical exposures among a demographically diverse population of pregnant women in San Francisco. Environ Health Perspect. 2018;126(7):077009.

23. Large-Scale Assessment of a Smartwatch to Identify Atrial Fibrillation - PubMed [Internet]. [cited 2021 July 20]. https://pubmed.ncbi.nlm.nih.gov/31722151/.

24. Wesley DB, Blumenthal J, Shah S, Littlejohn R, Pruitt Z, Dixit R, et al. A novel application of SMART on FHIR architecture for interoperable and scalable integration of patient-reported outcome data with electronic health records. J Am Med Inform Assoc. 2021;28(10):2220–5. https://doi.org/10.1093/jamia/ocab110.

25. Tong HL, Quiroz JC, Kocaballi AB, Fat SCM, Dao KP, Gehringer H, et al. Personalized mobile technologies for lifestyle behavior change: a systematic review, meta-analysis, and meta-regression. Prev Med. 2021;148:106532.

26. Milne-Ives M, Lam C, De Cock C, Van Velthoven MH, Meinert E. Mobile apps for health behavior change in physical activity, diet, drug and alcohol use, and mental health: systematic review. JMIR Mhealth Uhealth. 2020;8(3):e17046.

27. Shiffman S, Stone AA, Hufford MR. Ecological momentary assessment. Annu Rev Clin Psychol. 2008;4:1–32.

28. Catlett CE, Beckman PH, Sankaran R, Galvin KK. Array of things: a scientific research instrument in the public way: platform design and early lessons learned. In: Proceedings of the 2nd International Workshop on Science of Smart City Operations and Platforms Engineering - SCOPE '17. Pittsburgh, PA: ACM Press; 2017. http://dl.acm.org/citation.cfm?doid=3063386.3063771.

29. Neelon B, Mutiso F, Mueller NT, Pearce JL, Benjamin-Neelon SE. Associations between governor political affiliation and COVID-19 cases, deaths, and testing in the U.S. Am J Prev Med. 2021;61(1):115–9.

30. Peirce CS. In: Buchler J, editor. Philosophical writings of Peirce. New York: Dover; 1955.

31. Harman G. The inference to the best explanation. Philos Rev. 1965;74:88–95.
32. Bureau UC. Health Insurance Coverage in the United States: 2019 [Internet]. The United States Census Bureau. [cited 2021 July 22]. https://www.census.gov/library/publications/2020/demo/p60-271.html.
33. Health Coverage Affordability Crisis 2020 Biennial Survey | Commonwealth Fund [Internet]. [cited 2021 July 22]. https://www.commonwealthfund.org/publications/issue-briefs/2020/aug/looming-crisis-health-coverage-2020-biennial.
34. Sisodia RC, Rodriguez JA, Sequist TD. Digital disparities: lessons learned from a patient reported outcomes program during the COVID-19 pandemic. J Am Med Inform Assoc. 2021;28(10):2265–8. https://doi.org/10.1093/jamia/ocab138.
35. An early warning scoring system for detecting developing critical illness – ScienceOpen [Internet]. [cited 2021 July 22]. https://www.scienceopen.com/document?vid=28251d22-8476-40a6-916d-1a34796816e4.
36. McSherry D. Avoiding premature closure in sequential diagnosis. Artif Intell Med. 1997;10(3):269–83.
37. Shortliffe EH. Mycin: a knowledge-based computer program applied to infectious diseases. Proc Annu Symp Comput Appl Med Care. 1977;5:66–9.
38. Esteva A, Kuprel B, Novoa RA, Ko J, Swetter SM, Blau HM, et al. Dermatologist-level classification of skin cancer with deep neural networks. Nature. 2017;542(7639):115–8.
39. Miotto R, Li L, Kidd BA, Dudley JT. Deep patient: an unsupervised representation to predict the future of patients from the electronic health records. Sci Rep. 2016;6(1):26094.
40. Eraslan G, Avsec Ž, Gagneur J, Theis FJ. Deep learning: new computational modelling techniques for genomics. Nat Rev Genet. 2019;20(7):389–403.
41. Ritchie MD, Holzinger ER, Li R, Pendergrass SA, Kim D. Methods of integrating data to uncover genotype-phenotype interactions. Nat Rev Genet. 2015;16(2):85–97.
42. Lanata CM, Paranjpe I, Nititham J, Taylor KE, Gianfrancesco M, Paranjpe M, et al. A phenotypic and genomics approach in a multi-ethnic cohort to subtype systemic lupus erythematosus. Nat Commun. 2019;10(1):3902.
43. Center for Data-driven Insights and Innovations (CDI2) | UCOP [Internet]. [cited 2021 July 22]. https://www.ucop.edu/uc-health/functions/center-for-data-driven-insights-and-innovations-cdi2.html.
44. Bennett TD, Moffitt RA, Hajagos JG, Amor B, Anand A, Bissell MM, et al. The National COVID Cohort Collaborative: clinical characterization and early severity prediction. medRxiv. 2021;2021.01.12.21249511.
45. Kim J, Neumann L, Paul P, Day ME, Aratow M, Bell DS, et al. Privacy-protecting, reliable response data discovery using COVID-19 patient observations. J Am Med Inform Assoc. 2021;28(8):1765–76. https://doi.org/10.1093/jamia/ocab054.
46. Chapter 4 The common data model | The book of OHDSI [Internet]. [cited 2021 July 22]. https://ohdsi.github.io/TheBookOfOhdsi/.
47. Chapter 5 Standardized vocabularies | The book of OHDSI [Internet]. [cited 2021 July 22]. https://ohdsi.github.io/TheBookOfOhdsi/.
48. Dwork C, Roth A. The algorithmic foundations of differential privacy. Found trends®. Theor Comput Sci. 2014;9(3–4):211–407.
49. El Emam K, Mosquera L. Practical Synthetic Data Generation: Balancing Privacy and the Broad Availability of Data. Sebastopol, CA: O'Reilly Media, Inc; 2020.
50. Office for Civil Rights. Summary of the HIPAA privacy rule [Internet]. HHS.gov. 2008 [cited 2021 July 22]. https://www.hhs.gov/hipaa/for-professionals/privacy/laws-regulations/index.html.
51. Wilkinson MD, Dumontier M, IJJ A, Appleton G, Axton M, Baak A, et al. The FAIR Guiding Principles for scientific data management and stewardship. Sci Data. 2016;3(1):160018.
52. COVID-19 Clinical Data Warehouse Data Dictionary Based on OMOP Common Data Model Specifications Version 5.3. :22.

53. N3C data overview [Internet]. National Center for Advancing Translational Sciences. 2020 [cited 2021 July 22]. https://ncats.nih.gov/n3c/about/data-overview.
54. Overview - FHIR v4.0.1 [Internet]. [cited 2021 July 22]. https://www.hl7.org/fhir/overview.html.
55. Open mHealth [Internet]. GitHub. [cited 2021 Jul 22]. https://github.com/openmhealth.
56. EUR-Lex - 32016R0679 - EN - EUR-Lex [Internet]. [cited 2021 July 22]. https://eur-lex.europa.eu/eli/reg/2016/679/oj.
57. University of California. President's Ad Hoc Task Force on Health Data Governance [Internet]. 2018 [cited 2021 July 22]. https://www.ucop.edu/uc-health/reports-resources/health-data-governance-task-force-report.pdf.

Part II
Approaches

Chapter 4
Knowledge-Based Systems in Medicine

Peter Szolovits and Emily Alsentzer

After reading this chapter, you should know the answers to these questions:
- What were some of the early approaches to building human diagnostic expertise into computer programs?
- What representations supported different styles of inference using programs' knowledge?
- What are inductive biases and how can they be encoded into model architecture and training?
- What are some approaches for learning representations of graph-based data? How have these methods been applied in the biomedical domain?
- How can biomedical knowledge captured in unstructured text be leveraged in machine learning models?

What Is a Knowledge-Based System?

Maintaining or restoring health has, not surprisingly, been a goal of people even during the pre-scientific era. Human mental capacity seems very good at observing phenomena, generalizing from those observations, making consequent predictions of what is likely to happen, choosing actions that try to optimize those expected outcomes, and passing those acquired chunks of knowledge on to future generations so they may benefit from the accumulation of learning without having

P. Szolovits (✉) · E. Alsentzer
Massachusetts Institute of Technology, Cambridge, MA, USA
e-mail: psz@mit.edu; emilya@mit.edu

© The Author(s), under exclusive license to Springer Nature
Switzerland AG 2022
T. A. Cohen et al. (eds.), *Intelligent Systems in Medicine and Health*, Cognitive
Informatics in Biomedicine and Healthcare,
https://doi.org/10.1007/978-3-031-09108-7_4

to rediscover these individually. Traditional healers experimented with natural medications to treat symptoms, so ancient Egyptian records pass on the knowledge that digitalis (from the purple foxglove) helps to treat certain types of congestive sickness. Although in that era, there was apparently no understanding that the heart pumped blood (first formally noted by Harvey in 1628 [1]), the empirical correlation between treatment with foxglove and improvements in some patients became part of medical knowledge. In 1785, Withering recognized that digitalis affected the function of the heart, further characterized its therapeutic and toxic effects [2], and published a guide to its proper use that remained the state of the art until real pharmacokinetic models supplanted it in the middle of the twentieth century.

This short story illustrates some of the different kinds of knowledge that medicine has accumulated over the years. Often, it begins with an empirical correlation that holds up frequently enough to be clinically useful. Later, that association may become interpreted as due to some mechanism whose operation is understood at some level of detail. Later yet, we may develop a more quantitative understanding of just how a disease develops, what we may expect from its unchecked development (*prognosis*), how it generates the signs and symptoms associated with it (*diagnosis*), and how it responds to therapeutic interventions (*treatment*). This evolution of understanding enables more and more sophisticated uses of such knowledge to improve medical care. Although we strive for a more mechanistic understanding of clinical phenomena in our research, we still do not understand the mechanisms of many diseases in detail, yet we accumulate useful knowledge of the above various sorts to help improve the lives of patients.

Knowledge-Based Systems (KBS) in health care build on such a tradition, and try to reproduce in computer programs the ways in which human practitioners think about and handle difficult medical cases. Most such efforts have not tried to supplant human clinicians, but have aimed to improve their decision making by providing an automated "second opinion", i.e., guidance on how to think about a clinical case, to interpret data available about the patient, and to choose appropriate further tests and treatments.

Many of the landmark KBS were developed in the latter half of the twentieth century and represented the earliest somewhat successful attempts to achieve such automation of medical advice [3, 4]. The knowledge leveraged by these systems was typically elicited through formal or informal interviews with human clinicians, often prompted by thinking through specific difficult clinical cases they had encountered, and through manual encoding of knowledge found in textbooks and journal articles. Although researchers recognized the potential value of learning from clinical databases, such electronic medical (or health) records (EHRs) existed only in a tiny set of leading academic-affiliated medical centers. Most records were kept exclusively on paper, so significant datasets were simply unavailable. Starting with the advent of Medicare and Medicaid in 1965, when the federal government took responsibility for paying for health care for the elderly and the poor, computerized records of such bills and payments began to be kept broadly, but contained only the data necessary for making payment decisions. For example, they may have recorded that a patient had a chest x-ray (a billable procedure), but not what was found on the x-ray, because the payment was the same, independent of resulting findings.

Only with the passage of the new funding for improving health care at the start of the Obama administration in 2009 did EHRs become widely adopted, through incentives under the HITECH Act[1] that subsidized hospitals, clinics and practices to install such systems. Today, most major academic medical centers have repositories of case records documenting the conditions of, and the care given to, millions of their patients, often going back in time for over a decade (or, in pre-2009 EHR systems, even longer). Regional, national and international repositories are far less common because of institutional concerns for patient confidentiality and each institution's desire to exploit their own data before sharing them. A few exceptions, such as the MIMIC [5] and Physionet [6] de-identified repositories from one Boston-area hospital and the eICU repository [7] donated from Philips' tele-ICU records have been available. Recently, however, large national repositories such as the UK Biobank [8], the US "All of Us" [9], "Million Vets" [10] and PCORI (Patient Centered Outcomes Research Institute)[2] datasets are becoming more easily available for researchers. Today machine learning systems offer methods underlying the exciting work enabled by such collections of data (see Chaps. 6, 10, and 11). This chapter also touches on machine learning, with the specific aim of studying how one can learn new knowledge and integrate it with what is already known. However, Chap. 6 provides a broad introduction to the topic.

How Is Knowledge Represented in a Computer?

Philosophers have debated the nature of knowledge for millennia, and we are unlikely to resolve that discussion here. However, it is helpful to ask what types of knowledge are useful in medicine and how one can represent such knowledge in the computer.

Davis et al., in 1993 [11], reviewed attempts to represent knowledge in artificial intelligence (AI) programs and noted five major characteristics of a knowledge representation. First, knowledge about anything other than formal objects (e.g.,

---

[1] "Health Information Technology for Economics and Clinical Health (HITECH) Act", part of the overall Recovery Act funding that tried to advance economic recovery from the 2008 recession. The subsidies depended on certification by the Office of the National Coordinator for Health Information Technology (ONC) that the purchased systems met "meaningful use" criteria.

[2] See https://www.pcori.org/. (accessed August 17, 2022).

mathematics) must be an imperfect surrogate for the thing represented. For example, no computer representation of "cancer" can encompass all its characteristics and associations. Second, a representation makes a set of **ontological** commitments— what real-world things can be represented in the computer? In a medical setting, for example, should we represent only biomedical entities, or should the representation also allow surrogates for a patient's social and economic environment, personal hopes and desires, degree of risk aversion, and the clinician's history of medical experience, past patients' outcomes, etc.? Third, a representation is tied to a fragmentary theory of intelligent reasoning. AI's roots are grounded in various traditions, including logic, psychology, biology, statistics and economics, each of which has inspired different styles of reasoning and has demanded different ways to represent underlying knowledge. The representation defines not only what inferences are possible, but also which are recommended. We discuss many of these below. Fourth, using a representation must be sufficiently efficient computationally to be practically useful. Fifth, a representation must serve as a medium of human expression, allowing people and the computer to communicate their knowledge to each other.

Rules: Inference Steps

From the logical tradition, rules have often been used to represent individual steps of inference. Such rules are usually written in the form of an implication,

$$LHS \rightarrow RHS$$

where the Left Hand Side (LHS) is a conjunction of conditions that, if true, justify asserting the conjunction of conditions in the Right Hand Side (RHS). If these conditions refer only to specific entities, then the rules are simple, such as in Fig. 4.1a.

a	**b**	**c**
Raining → Wet-Street	Raining → Wet-Street	∀x Human(x) → Mortal(x)
Raining	¬Wet-Street	Human(Socrates)
Wet-Street	¬Raining	Mortal(Socrates)

Fig. 4.1 Logical inference rules. In **sentential logic**, all statements and rules are about individual instances. Implications have a **left** and **right**-hand side separated by an arrow, and state that if the left hand side is true, then the right hand side is also. (**a**) Shows **modus ponens**, which derives a conclusion (Wet-Street) from its premises (that it is Raining, and that Raining implies Wet-Street). (**b**) Shows an example of **modus tollens**, where knowing the falsity of the right hand side (the street is not wet) contradicts the left (it must not be raining). (**c**) Shows an example of modus ponens, but now in **predicate logic**, which introduces variables (x) that may be bound to any individual (Socrates) and quantifiers **for all** (∀) and **there exists** (∃). In this case, the premises are that every human is mortal and that Socrates is human. Therefore, we may conclude that Socrates is mortal. The symbol → stands for implication, ¬ for negation, ∧ for and, and ∨ for or

It represents the knowledge that raining implies that the street will be wet and that it is raining, from which we may conclude that the street is wet. Figure 4.1b shows a deduction that proceeds in the opposite direction, so that based on the same implication between rain and the wet street, if the street is not wet, then it must not be raining.

This representation, called the **sentential logic**, is too limited for most uses because it cannot refer explicitly to generalizations. **Predicate logic** introduces variables into the notation and quantification over those variables, to extend the representational power of the language. Figure 4.1c uses an old chestnut, that if we know that all humans are mortal and Socrates is human, then he is mortal. To use such rules, we must do pattern matching to bind variables to specific entities. In addition to the universal quantifier ($\forall$), logic also provides an existential quantifier ($\exists$), as in

$$\exists x \, \text{Human}(x)$$

which says that there exists some human being (x).

Programming languages such as Prolog [12] and OPS5 [13] were created to implement such logical rules and to apply them efficiently to data structures that represent particular entities. OPS5 uses a collection of facts in its working memory and a set of implication rules to derive new facts from old via its rules. The facts may be structured, for example, to include various attributes, e.g., Socrates' age. The rules' LHS contain a logical combination of pattern matching specifications that allow them to match multiple specific facts, thus providing predicate logic facilities. The RHS can create new working set elements and delete or modify old ones. This method is called **forward chaining**, where the system works from known facts and rules to establish new facts. Such programming languages also introduced non-logical operations to help control their inferences and avoid infinite loops. For example, a rule in the sentential calculus that says that if A and B are both true, then "A and B" ($A \wedge B$) is also true, can "run away" because it can then produce $A \wedge (A \wedge B)$, $A \wedge A \wedge (A \wedge B)$, $A \wedge A \wedge A \wedge (A \wedge B)$, …, etc. Systems can include various rule ordering and other heuristics in order to prevent the automatic derivation of such useless inferences.

Prolog [12], by contrast, uses **backward chaining**, which traces back from a query (a fact pattern whose truth or matching entities are sought) by finding rules whose RHS can assert a fact that matches that query and then recursively uses each pattern in such rules' LHS as further queries. Because these query patterns typically contain variables, Prolog can, for example, find the entities that can be proven to have desired characteristics. Prolog uses Horn clauses, in which the RHS consists of only one element, and "negation as failure", where its inability to prove A allows it to assert ¬A. Although forward and backward-chaining seem quite distinct methods, forward-chaining systems can implement a backward-chaining style of reasoning by including explicit assertions about their goals among their facts.

The prime example of rule-based approaches in medicine was the MYCIN system [14], developed in the mid-1970s for diagnosis and treatment selection for bacteremia, later extended to meningitis. MYCIN's principal method was backward chaining from the goal of identifying significant organisms that needed to be treated (see Chap. 2). Given a (sub-)goal, it would find rules that could make an assertion satisfying that goal and then establish each of the LHS conditions in that rule as subgoals. Once those subgoals had been satisfied, it would assert the RHS with a computed certainty into its working memory. If no rule existed, then it would retrieve the matching fact from its working memory or just ask the user for the desired goal. In this way, its control structure essentially traced out a branching logic tree that dynamically collected the information that could help derive the overall goal. An example of one of MYCIN's rules, recognizing bacteroides as the organism in an infection, is shown in Chap. 2 (Fig. 2.3). A more heuristic (and less certain) rule suggesting other likely organisms in a patient receiving steroid treatments is shown in Fig. 4.2.

MYCIN's creators developed their own programming language in order to add several extensions to the basic rule-based framework. First, they wanted to represent uncertainty about both the rules implementing clinical knowledge and about the derived facts about the patient. Thus, each rule was associated with a **certainty factor** stating how strongly one should believe the conclusion of a rule, and the certainty of a derived fact was a combination of the certainties of the rule that derived it and of the facts matching the rule's LHS elements. Second, in MYCIN's domain, there was a natural organization of facts. Patients had possible sites of interest, each site had possible infections, each infection might have one or more cultures taken, each of which might grow out a particular organism, each of which might be treated with a particular drug. A **context mechanism** imposed this hierarchical organization on the variables in the rules so they did not need to state explicitly that, for example, if a rule contained variables for both a culture and an organism, the organism was grown from that culture. This simplified creation and interpretation of rules and allowed creation of an explanation mechanism unburdened by explaining such technical connections [16].

The therapy selection portion of MYCIN was implemented using methods other than backward chaining rules because its task was essentially a set covering that

RULE543

If:

      1) The infection which requires therapy is meningitis,
      2) Only circumstantial evidence is available for this case,
      3) The type of the infection is bacterial,
      4) The patient is receiving corticosteroids,

Then:

      There is evidence that the organisms which might be causing the infection are e.coli (.4), klebsiella-pneumoniae (.2), or pseudomonas-aeruginosa (.1)

Fig. 4.2 MYCIN's "steroids" rule. (From a paper describing MYCIN's explanation capabilities [15], used with permission)

chose a parsimonious combination of antibiotics to cover for all of the likely dangerous pathogens whose presence was concluded by the diagnostic portion of the program. MYCIN also included an interesting explanation facility, by which it was able to answer questions about how a fact about the patient was used in reaching its conclusions, whether and how various rules were used in analysis of a case, and even hypotheticals such as what facts would need to have been entered in order to reach a particular conclusion.

Yu et al. evaluated MYCIN's therapy recommendations against panels of Stanford infectious disease experts, who found that over 90% of the recommendations were acceptable [17]. The program identified (a) whether the patient had a significant infection, where agreement with the Stanford and national experts was an impressive 97%, (b) the identity of infecting organisms, with 77% agreement, and (c) the appropriate therapy, with 73% agreement. However, because the experts often disagreed among themselves, MYCIN's recommendations were still considered reasonable even in some cases where they did not match the majority recommendation of the experts. Interestingly, the Stanford and national panels at times disagreed about proper treatment for a case and thus about whether MYCIN's conclusions were appropriate, the program agreeing more often with the local experts, probably reflecting practice differences at different institutions. Another evaluation by Yu et al. that focused on meningitis cases showed slightly weaker results, but highlighted the frequent disagreements among human experts [18].

Patterns: Matching

Another highly influential knowledge representation tradition was to organize knowledge in terms of prototypes. Marvin Minsky named these constructs **frames**, which typically represented a core concept. They did so by specifying attributes of that object, default values for the attributes if they were not explicitly stated, restrictions on what values such attributes could take on, and procedures attached to the frame that could be run when a new attribute value was asserted or if an unknown attribute value was sought [19]. These procedures served a similar function to forward and backward chaining rules in rule-based systems.

The original motivation for frame representations was to address a difficult technical problem in reasoning about actions, which require some representation of *state* or *time*. Assertions in a logical formalism need to refer to object attributes in a specific state, say (robot1 holding block17 state5), representing that a (one-handed) robot, robot1, has the attribute holding, whose value is block17, in state5. If the robot then takes two steps forward and is thus in state6, we would not want to have to re-derive that it is still holding block17. Frame systems permitted such facts to persist across states unless the action that moved from one state to another explicitly altered an attribute.

In medical applications, the use of frames was mainly to represent prototypical situations. For example, a frame for a disease would have attributes that represented

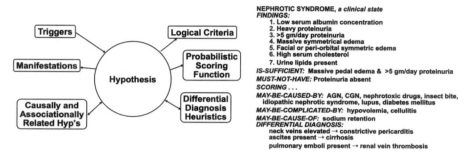

Fig. 4.3 Present Illness Program memory structure and an example of part of the frame for nephrotic syndrome

its typical signs, symptoms, predisposing factors, laboratory findings, drug or surgical treatments, etc.—often in the aggregate called *findings* or *manifestations*. These manifestations themselves were often represented as additional frames, so more details could be provided. For example, in the **Present Illness Program** [20], frames representing diseases and syndromes had a structure such as that shown in Fig. 4.3. Associated with each diagnostic hypothesis are its typical manifestation, some of which ("triggers") would serve to evoke the hypothesis if seen. The values of these attributes were typically also represented by frames; for example, the frame for edema (swelling) contained attributes for how long it had been present, whether it appeared for the first time, often or periodically, whether it exhibited a daily temporal pattern, whether it appeared red, etc. Links to other hypotheses could show ones that could either cause or be caused by this one, or that should be evoked when considering this one if specific differential manifestations were reported. The program's knowledge base, therefore, was a **semantic network** that tied together the representations of all the types of objects it represented. In addition, there were logical criteria by which a hypothesis could be definitively confirmed or excluded and a probabilistic scoring function that attempted to compute the hypothesis' probability given everything known so far about the patient and about linked diseases. Figure 4.3 shows (part of) the knowledge about nephrotic syndrome, as an example. This program focused on nephrology, representing details of 20 disease frames and another 50 frames for associated syndromes and clinical and physiologic states, which we might call phenotypes today.

This program operated by asking for a chief complaint—what brought the patient to the doctor—which was expected to evoke one or more disease hypotheses. Inspired by observation of how expert human diagnosticians pursued such cases (see discussion of the role of cognitive studies in Chap. 2 as well as Chap. 5), the program would then ask about additional prototypical findings expected for the evoked disorders. It could also use its scoring function to prioritize asking about findings relevant to the most likely diagnoses, use unexpected answers to evoke additional hypotheses and differentials, and eventually conclude the presence or absence of each of the evoked hypotheses based on logical criteria and the scoring function. Figure 4.4 shows the network of connections in the program's long-term

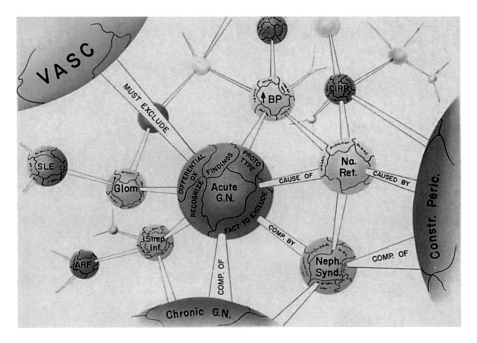

Fig. 4.4 The associative (long-term) memory. The associative memory consists of a rich collection of knowledge about diseases, signs, symptoms, pathologic states, "real-world" situations, etc. Each point of entry into the memory allows access to many related concepts through a variety of associative links shown as rods. Each rod is labeled to indicate the kind of association it represents. Note that the red spheres denote disease states, blue spheres denote clinical states (e.g., nephrotic syndrome) and yellow spheres denote physiologic states (e.g., sodium retention). Abbreviations used in this figure are *Acute G.N.* acute glomerulonephritis, *Chronic G.N.* chronic glomerulonephritis, *VASC* vasculitis, *CIRR* cirrhosis, *Constr. Peric.* constrictive pericarditis, *ARF* acute rheumatic fever, *Na Ret.* sodium retention, *SLE* systemic lupus erythematosus, ↑*BP* acute hypertension, *GLOM.* glomerulus, *Strep. inf.* streptococcal infection, *Neph. Synd.* nephrotic syndrome (Reproduced with permission from the original paper [20])

memory between these. Figure 4.5 shows a schematic of how new information evokes hypotheses by bringing nodes triggered by new facts into the short-term memory. Although the machinery of the program contained multiple methods, its fundamental approach to diagnosis was matching a patient's case to the prototypes described in its knowledge base. As in the case of MYCIN, the program's questioning behavior was dynamic, driven by its knowledge base and the previous answers it had been given.

The **INTERNIST-1** program [21], also originally developed in the 1970s (see Chap. 2), contained a vastly larger dataset of about 500 diagnoses and 3550 atomic manifestations, with 2600 two-way weighted links connecting each disease to its possible manifestations. Thus, diagnoses were represented by frames whose attributes included related manifestations, typically around 75 per diagnosis. The manifestations, unlike in the Present Illness Program described above, were simply atomic tokens that included in a cryptic way—e.g., "ALKALINE PHOSPHATASE

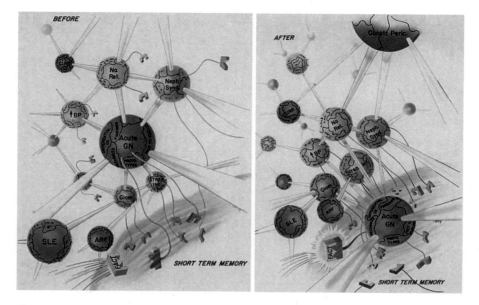

Fig. 4.5 Hypothesis generation. **BEFORE**: in the nascent condition (when there are no hypotheses in short-term memory), tentacles (daemons) from some frames in long-term memory extend into the short-term memory where each constantly searches for a matching fact. **AFTER**: the matching of fact and daemon causes the movement of the full frame (in the case, acute glomerulonephritis) into short-term memory. As a secondary effect, frames immediately adjacent to the activated frame move closer to short-term memory and are able to place additional daemons therein. Note that, to avoid complexity, the daemons on many of the frames are not shown. The abbreviations are the same as those used in Fig. 4.4. (Reproduced with permission from the original paper [20])

BLOOD INCREASED NOT OVER 2 TIMES NORMAL"—information that a frame representation might have explicitly given. One weight, the *frequency*, approximated the conditional likelihood of that manifestation occurring if a patient had the corresponding disease. The other, the *evoking strength*, indicated how strongly observing that manifestation should evoke consideration of that disease. Frequency was stated on a 1–5 scale, ranging from "occurs rarely" (1) to "in essentially all cases" (5). Evoking strength ranged from 0–5, meaning "nonspecific" (0) to "pathognomonic" (5). There has been much debate about how one might convert such numbers to probabilities [22] (also see the discussion of QMR-DT, below); generally, they are thought to be on a logarithmic scale. Additional links connected diagnoses to each other by causal and associational links, also using a small integer representation of likelihood, and each manifestation included an *importance* score stating how critical it was to include an explanation for it in the program's final conclusions (Table 4.1).

INTERNIST-1's main innovation, in addition to the estimated 15 man-years of physician effort to build its knowledge base, was a clever heuristic for forming possible multiple differentials in the diagnosis of a complex case. Given a set of

Table 4.1 INTERNIST-1's knowledge about alcoholic hepatitis. The first column of numbers is the evoking strength, a measure of the degree to which observing that manifestation should encourage consideration of the disease, on a scale of 0–5. The second is the frequency, an indication of how frequently that manifestation occurs in patients with the disease; its scale is 1–5, roughly logarithmic in probability. Most of this long table is omitted here to save space

Manifestations of alcoholic hepatitis	Evoking strength	Frequency
Age 16–25	0	1
Age 26–55	0	3
Age GTR than 55	0	2
Alcohol ingestion recent HX	2	4
Alcoholism chronic HX	2	4
Sex female	0	2
Sex male	0	4
Urine dark HX	1	3
Weight loss GTR than 10%	0	3
... 69 more rows for other manifestations		

manifestations stated to be present or absent, the program computed a score for each disease by taking into account the evoking strengths of associated manifestations, contributions from other diagnoses that had already been confirmed, penalizing for high-frequency manifestations that did not occur in the patient, etc. INTERNIST-1 would then form a differential around the highest-scoring diagnosis. Its clever technique was a heuristic that if another, lower-scoring disease could explain either the same or a subset of the observed manifestations of the top diagnosis, then it would be considered a competitor and would be part of the differential. However, if a lower-scoring disease explained manifestations not explained by the leading diagnosis, it was taken as evidence that perhaps the patient was suffering from multiple disorders. In that case, those lower-ranked diagnoses and the manifestations they explained were temporarily set aside. The program would then proceed to use a questioning strategy focused on just the formulated differential, driven by the size of the differential and numerical differences in the scores of the diagnoses in the differential. For example, if the leading diagnosis significantly outscored the others, a *confirm* strategy was used, to ask questions whose positive answers would most increase the score of that leader; if, on the other hand, the differential was very large, a *rule out* strategy would choose questions for which a negative answer would decrease the scores of less likely diagnoses so that they could drop from the differential. After concluding a diagnosis, a new differential would be formed around the remaining evoked diseases if their scores were sufficiently high. Thus, the program was able to diagnose complex cases in which the patient suffered from multiple disorders.

INTERNIST-1's ability to diagnose complex cases was developed using clinico-pathological conference cases from the New England Journal of Medicine and tested against other such cases not used during development [21]. Of 19 cases published in 1969 for which the program's knowledge base included all the diagnoses discussed in the Journal (out of 42 such cases that were published in the journal that

year), there were 43 major diagnoses (a little over two per case). The program identified 17 as definite and 8 more as tentative, failing to find 18 diagnoses. Although
this seems disappointing, a panel of Mass General clinicians missed 15 and even the
case discussants missed 8, showing that the program was doing a reasonably good
job on very complex cases.

The INTERNIST-1 algorithm was later reimplemented on the then new personal
computers as QMR (Quick Medical Reference), using the valuable knowledge base,
expanded to cover over 750 diagnoses and 5500 manifestations. It was subsequently
licensed to a company to try to create a commercial product, though that attempt did
not reach fruition except as an educational tool [23, 24]. Another program with
similar structure, DXPLAIN [25], was developed over many years at Massachusetts
General Hospital and has been widely used as a teaching tool in medical schools,
though not for active clinical decision support.

The task of identifying the right diagnoses in cases where two or more diseases
may be present is challenging and led to a number of subsequent approaches. One
of the INTERNIST-1 authors proposed a diagnostic system, Caduceus, that formalized and extended INTERNIST-1's differential diagnosis strategy to become a
search through a space of complex hypotheses, guided by additional knowledge
about anatomical and etiologic hierarchies and graphs representing chains of possible causality [26]. Mutual constraints from different hierarchies could combine
partial hypotheses to generate more coherent simple ones. For example, if a manifestation could be caused by a number of different diagnoses and if the program's
state "believes" (for other reasons) that a particular organ system is involved, then a
useful heuristic would be to combine those two partial hypotheses to say that the
intersection of the possible causes with the diseases of that organ system is likely,
by Occam's razor, to be a parsimonious explanation. Various search techniques
could then be used to explore different ways to combine evidence and partial
hypotheses into a unified whole. Unfortunately, the full knowledge base for this
proposed program was not constructed, though it remained an inspiring set of ideas
for subsequent efforts to view diagnostic reasoning as a search through a space of
hypotheses by decomposing complex cases heuristically into simpler individual
components [27].

Probabilistic Models[3]

Naive Bayes

Uncertainty lies at the heart of diagnostic reasoning. Some of the earliest diagnostic
efforts in the 1960s used **Naive Bayes** models to assess the impact of observations
about a patient, coupled with laboratory test results, to revise the probabilities of the

---

[3] This section assumes a basic understanding of probability theory and Bayes' Rule. A book such
as *Medical Decision Making* [28] provides appropriate background.

diseases that might be afflicting the patient. The programs typically assumed that the patient had exactly one disease and that all manifestations of that disease were **conditionally independent** of each other, depending only on what the actual disease was; it is in this sense that such models were termed *naive*. Programs built this way thus included an *a priori* probability distribution over the possible diseases and conditional probability distributions for each manifestation given each disease. This model is most appropriate for diagnosis of acute illnesses because newly presenting facts about a patient are likely to be caused by one rather than multiple diseases. It is not a good match to the diagnosis of a complex case such as the CPC cases used to test INTERNIST-1, where multiple diseases are typically simultaneously present. Such models were often applied appropriately to well-bounded problems. Examples include acute renal failure or congenital heart disease, where it was reasonable to use lab data to suggest which disease of a defined differential diagnosis was most likely.

A highly useful idea was added to allow such Naive Bayes models to optimize the order in which they asked about manifestations, to choose that question to ask that minimizes the expected **entropy** of the probability distribution resulting from asking that question. If a question has k possible answers, the program can use Bayes' Rule to compute the posterior probability distribution if it got each answer separately, then compute the entropy of that distribution, weight each entropy by the probability of getting that answer, and thus calculate the expected information gain from asking that question. The conditional independence of the manifestations allows this method to apply sequentially, optimizing its choice of questions dynamically based on previous answers, and thus often allows a program to ask for only a small fraction of all the possible manifestations known in the model and quickly to reach a probability distribution that indicates one disease as highly likely [29] (see Fig. 4.6).

Bayesian Networks

In cases where multiple diseases might be present, with several potentially making manifestations more likely, a number of projects adopted a bipartite network representation. In this, each disease has an *a priori* probability, independent of the others. Each finding depends on some subset of the diseases, but the findings are, as in INTERNIST-1, conditionally independent (See Fig. 4.7). This structure is a subset of more general Bayesian networks, directed acyclic graphical models that indicate the probabilistic dependencies among multiple nodes. In fact, the QMR-DT project [30, 31] reformulated the QMR database into just such a bipartite graph representation.

When a finding can be caused by multiple diseases, the conditional probability table for that finding has to have an entry for all possible combinations of the presence or absence of each causing disease. This is, of course, exponentially large and impractical for findings that may be caused by many diseases. Therefore, they adopted the **noisy-or assumption**, that a finding is absent only if none of its possible causes actually cause it. For a finding with just one possible disease cause, its probability is just the probability of the disease times the causal probability that the

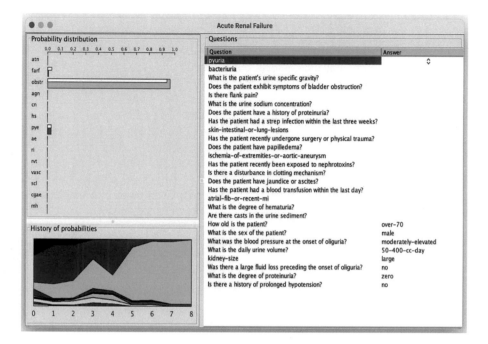

Fig. 4.6 A contemporary graphical user interface for a Naïve Bayes program for diagnosis of acute renal failure [29]. The bottom left panel shows the sequence of probability distributions after answering the questions as shown at the bottom of the right panel. Other possible but unanswered questions at the top of the right panel could be answered, but were considered less informative by the program's entropy minimization heuristic. The top left shows the current (in color) and the previous distributions. The case answers are as given in the example in the original paper, and lead to a diagnosis of a urinary tract obstruction

disease would cause the finding. For a finding with multiple possible causes, we calculate its probability in the way we compute the probability of the "or" of multiple events, namely one minus the product of the probabilities of each disease *not* causing the finding. If finding S could be caused by any of $D_1, D_2, \ldots, D_k$, then:

$$P(S|d_1,d_2,\ldots,d_k) = 1 - \left(1 - P(d_1)P(S|d_1)\right)$$
$$\left(1 - P(d_2)P(S|d_2)\right)$$
$$\ldots$$
$$\left(1 - P(d_k)P(S|d_k)\right),$$

where d_i is whether D_i is present or absent. This model also assumes that there is a "leak" term, namely that the finding might occur with some small probability even if all its causes are absent.

To build this model, they had to turn INTERNIST-1's frequency estimates into the causal probabilities and had to estimate prior probabilities for each disease. Also, because general solvers for Bayesian networks take time that is exponential in

Fig. 4.7 A bipartite Bayesian network showing four diseases and nine symptoms. The diseases may occur simultaneously, but are probabilistically independent of each other. The symptoms depend only on the diseases, and are conditionally independent of each other

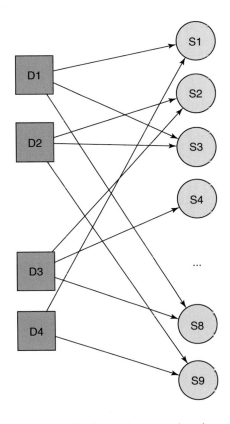

the number of undirected loops (i.e., multiple paths of influence), approximation methods had to be used to compute posterior probabilities of all the diseases given a set of observations of the findings.

In principle, one could combine the insights of QMR-DT with those of the Caduceus proposal so that a diagnostic program would formulate smaller differentials and use Bayesian methods to evaluate them. Such an idea was proposed in the Synopsis system [32], but not fully implemented.

Decision Analysis and Influence Diagrams

Medical practitioners have also used the **principle of rationality,** that the right action to take is the one with the best expected outcome. Often, this is done informally, but can also be formalized as the use of **decision analysis** [33] to assign numerical values to various outcomes and probabilities to the effects of various actions conditioned on what ails the patient. In simple cases, this can be represented by a **decision tree** containing *choice nodes* representing the choices facing the clinician leading to *chance nodes* representing the probabilistic outcomes of the chosen actions. At the leaves of such a decision tree are *value nodes*, showing the value of

that outcome. Given a decision tree, one can "fold back" the tree to assign values to
each of its nodes, starting with the specified outcomes. A simple example showing
a decision analysis for how to treat an elderly man with a gangrenous foot is shown
in Fig. 4.8, and an early example of a clinical application to coronary artery surgery
is also available [34]. Ascertaining probabilities is a difficult task because they
should reflect details of the case under consideration. Ascertaining values is even
harder because these should reflect the views of the patient—e.g., on a scale of 0
(death) to 1000 (full health), what is the value of living with an amputated leg? Such
judgments are hard to elicit and do not seem to remain stable as the situation evolves.
For long-term consequences of health decisions, the Quality-Adjusted Life Year
(QALY) is often used, adjusting the (expected) length of life for the presence of
disabling or morbid conditions. A review of its history, from the British viewpoint,
is presented in [35].

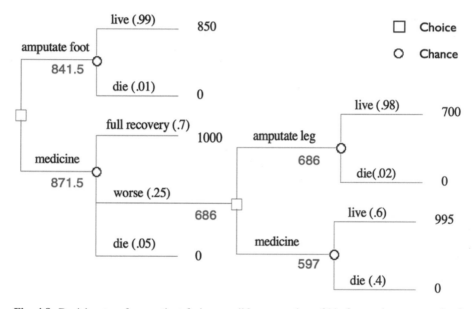

Fig. 4.8 Decision tree for a patient facing possible amputation of his foot or leg as a result of
gangrene. Squares represent decisions to be made, and circles the chance nodes that lead to different outcomes with different probabilities. The choices contemplated here are either to amputate the
patient's foot or to treat him medically. If the medical treatment fails and the gangrene gets worse,
then one can either amputate the whole leg or continue to treat medically. Each branch of the tree
terminates in a specific numeric value, in this case measured on a 0–1000 scale, where 0 represents
death, 1000 represents regained full health, and intermediate numbers the relative desirability of
different health states. For the example patient, life after having lost his foot to amputation is worth
850 points on this 1000-point scale, whereas life after having lost his whole leg is worth 700. The
example is a simplified version of one of the earliest clinical uses of decision analysis, on the clinical decision-making service at New England Medical Center. At each chance node, the expected
value (in red) is the sum of the products of the probability of each outcome times the expected
value of that outcome. At choice nodes, the expected value is the maximum of the values of the
choices, always assuming that the best choice will be chosen. (Figure is reproduced, with permission, from a review of probabilistic methods in medical decision support [36])

An **influence diagram** combines the idea of decision analysis with Bayesian network representations of the potentially more complex probabilistic relations among choices, chances and decisions. This provides a much more compact representation of complex decision problems and avoids having to specify the order of decisions, as in a decision tree [37]. Methods similar to those for solving Bayesian networks have been adapted to influence diagrams.

Reinforcement learning (RL) is a method of identifying an optimal decision policy to allow a decision maker to choose the best course of action under any modeled circumstance. In this method, an action is typically modeled to have an immediate reward (e.g., the patient's elevated heart rate decreases) and a long-term reward (e.g., the patient survives the hospital stay). In evaluating a potential action, one combines the immediate reward and then (in the manner of a decision tree or influence diagram) the discounted expected sequence of immediate and long-term rewards anticipated from the possible future states resulting from the action. Given a large database of past treatments of other patients, it is possible to estimate the relevant expected rewards, but not for actions that were rarely if ever taken in the past. It may thus be helpful sometimes to try a different, less explored therapy, in case one might discover a more successful approach. Of course, because medical actions affect real patients, this is often done only in simulation using retrospective data and strong independence assumptions rather than actually trying unproven ideas on patients. However, one can view a randomized clinical trial as a step in such an exploration strategy. The reinforcement learning approach has been gaining popularity as a way to exploit data on complex sequences of past decisions; a recent example explores optimal treatment for sepsis [38].

Causal Mechanisms: How Things Work

If we had a complete understanding of how the human body works, we could build mechanistic models that could predict its response to various conditions and treatments with precision. For most of medicine, we do not have such deep understanding, but there have been many attempts to build such models for at least parts of human (patho-)physiology. Perhaps the largest is Guyton's cardiovascular model [39], consisting of hundreds of differential equations connecting hundreds of variables representing concentrations, volumes and flows in the body, and hundreds of additional parameters that describe the strengths of interactions in the equations. In principle, one might "tune" such a model to the specific situation of an individual patient, i.e., measure all the variables and determine all the parameters, but many of these cannot be measured and in any case the effort required would be completely impractical. The Guyton-Coleman implementation of this model did lead to new insights into the relationship between cardiac output, blood pressure and control of sodium, among others, and NASA used the model to predict the effects of weightlessness on the circulatory system of astronauts as a safety check as they prepared for space travel [40]. The model continues to be developed in the twenty-first century, called Digital Human and expanding to about 5000 variables including renal, respiratory, endocrine, neural and metabolic physiology [41]. Much smaller lumped parameter models, such as CVSim [42], have also been built for teaching and research. Another early knowledge-based system for providing expert consultation on glaucoma used a causal model of the disease and its development combined with a **fuzzy logic** method of associating observables with pathophysiological states to determine the stage of advancement of the diseases [43].

Because the numerical relationships among many of the variables in such models are not known precisely, others have also pursued use of qualitative models that might represent, for example, that if the heart's contractility decreases, then so will cardiac output. This type of model is helpful for reasoning about the likely direction of changes induced by changes and interventions. Its downfall for clinical reasoning is that most systems in the body are controlled by feedback loops, so the correct differential equations add contributions from various components to compute outputs. However, in a qualitative representation that denotes changes only by their sign, we cannot in general tell the sign of a sum of a positive and a negative. The output is determined by their relative values, which are not provided in this qualitative formulation. In domains where quantitative data and models for at least some of the relationships are available, it is possible to build multi-level reasoning systems that analyze the situation qualitatively, but dive into quantitative details when such ambiguities arise. For example, the ABEL system used this approach for analysis of disorders of acid-base and electrolyte balance [44].

How Is Knowledge Acquired?

The systems described above each have their own ways of representing their rules of inference, patterns of disease/finding associations, probabilistic relationships, etc. They also have corresponding specialized tools to ease entering such data into their knowledge bases. More recently, two main approaches have taken hold for eliciting knowledge to use in KBS. One is based on a taxonomic organization of concepts into **ontologies** that describe each concept in terms of its super- and sub-categories and its attributes and constraints on them, adopting a frame-like view of the representation task. Information about super-categories is typically inherited by sub-categories and instances, making the expression of knowledge efficient. Classification and inheritance are the main inferences supported by such systems, and the constraints on attributes are typically limited in expressive power in order to stay away from the possibility of highly inefficient (or even incomplete) inference systems that would be needed for more powerful constraints. The other main approach is the construction of **knowledge graphs**, which can be constructed manually or via unsupervised methods that exploit the co-occurrence of terms in sentences, paragraphs, or articles.

Ontologies and Their Tools

One very popular tool for ontology construction is Protégé [45]. To create an ontology of a new domain, Protégé encourages the user to define a hierarchy of concepts (called classes) in the domain and allows specification of defaults and constraints on properties of the classes, including whether the property should be a simple value or another class, how many values or classes the property may include, etc. When a subclass is defined, it can simply be defined as a subclass of an existing class or it can be defined as containing instances of the superclass with specific properties. For example, bacteria may be a subclass of pathogens, but we do not know how to specify properties that invariably distinguish bacteria from other categories of pathogens. By contrast, we can say that a heart disease is a disease whose locus is in the heart, which allows the system to classify a disease as a heart disease even if it was not defined that way. Figure 4.9 shows part of the gene ontology from the

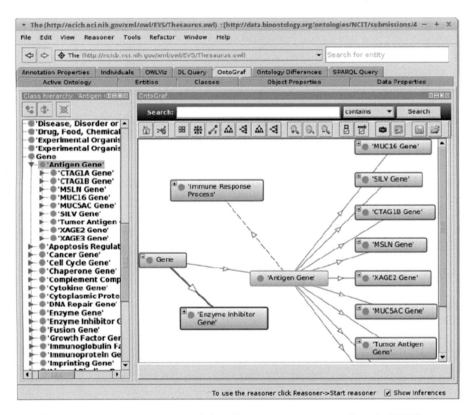

Fig. 4.9 The Protégé system, showing relationships among gene concepts from the NCI Thesaurus. (Figure is reproduced, with permission, from the original paper [45])

NCI Thesaurus.[4] The definitions of such properties are made in a description logic, and there is a tradeoff between the expressiveness of that logic and the computational tractability of doing inference with it [46]. One very important use of ontologies is to integrate the concepts used in different clinical systems. The Galen approach, using the GRAIL description logic, was an important early use of this technology [47].

An alternative approach was pioneered by the U.S. National Library of Medicine through the **Unified Medical Language Systems (UMLS)**, which created a Metathesaurus instead of trying to build a comprehensive ontology.[5] The Metathesaurus combines concepts and taxonomic and other relationships from (as of 2021) over 200 different terminological systems [48]. Machine and manual curation has assured that the nearly 13 million terms from 25 languages (though mostly English) map to over 4.4 million concepts, to help coordinate information among the terminologies. Reliably mapping many terms to a single concept is a major aid to clinical natural language processing, by noting that, for example, "acute myocardial infarct", "AMI" and "heart attack" represent the same concept. The UMLS also provides some linguistic tools for tasks such as lemmatization (identifying the root words of inflected words; e.g., "run" from "running") and assigns a semantic category to each concept from among a set of 189 such categories, which provides a low-resolution ontology of objects and relations. However, because the content of UMLS comes from many separately developed databases, taxonomic inconsistencies do arise, and relations other than the taxonomies are often sparse.

Manual curation of large knowledge bases is phenomenally costly and subject to gaps because it is difficult for people to think of everything needed. For example, the CYC knowledge base[6] has been under development for over 30 years, and among many applications are some in healthcare. CYC represents its knowledge in a logical form and contains 10,000 predicates over millions of concepts, encoding 25 million assertions in a higher-order logic that allows quantification not only over variables but also over sets and relations. It also includes a number of specialized inference engines to draw new conclusions from its store of knowledge. Nevertheless, it is difficult to determine just what the system knows or is able to infer.

Knowledge in the Era of Machine Learning

The advent of machine learning and deep learning methods has resulted in a shift in thinking regarding how knowledge is acquired, represented, and leveraged in biomedical models. Whereas knowledge-based systems of the twentieth century often involve probabilistic or causal reasoning over explicit knowledge, machine learning

---

[4] See https://ncithesaurus.nci.nih.gov/ncitbrowser. (accessed August 17, 2022).

[5] See https://www.nlm.nih.gov/research/umls. (accessed August 17, 2022).

[6] See https://cyc.com. (accessed August 17, 2022).

methods today are designed to implicitly learn patterns from copious amounts of data. This shift has been accelerated by the recent successes of deep learning methods (see Chap. 6). Extensive feature engineering of input data using domain knowledge is being replaced by methods that leverage an "end-to-end" design philosophy to automatically learn representations of the input data that are useful for prediction.

This transition has spurred a debate within the community as to the amount of structure and innate priors that should be incorporated into machine learning models—a debate with roots in philosophy that dates back to Plato, John Locke, and David Hume. On one side are what Judea Pearl terms the "radical empiricists", individuals who believe that knowledge comes from interaction with the environment and can be learned via analyzing large amounts of observed data [49]. Radical empiricists argue for flexible models with minimal a priori representational design assumptions. On the other side are "nativists" who believe that built-in machinery is necessary for generalized learning and argue for incorporating structural priors into models such as through symbolic or causal reasoning. In reality, this is a spectrum, and many current approaches fall in the middle of these two camps. The development of approaches that marry deep learning and structured methods is an active area of research.

The rest of this section provides an overview of the spectrum of approaches for representing and leveraging knowledge in modern machine learning models. The section focuses on graph and text based models that explicitly leverage biomedical domain knowledge and discuss the use of biomedical expert systems to train more sophisticated machine learning models. The reader may want to refer to Chap. 6 for an introduction to machine learning and to Chap. 7 for a discussion of natural language processing. The following discussion may be more useful if you first familiarize yourself with some of those basics.

Incorporating Knowledge into Machine Learning Models

While there are debates about the amount of innate machinery required for artificial intelligence, all machine learning methods are guided by human knowledge in their design. This can occur *implicitly* through the choice of model architecture and loss function or the selection and augmentation of the training data. It may also occur more *explicitly* by incorporating structured knowledge via knowledge graphs or by retrieving relevant text data (Fig. 4.10).

The choice of model architecture and loss function can encode useful **inductive biases** that enable more robust machine learning methods. Inductive biases can be any design decision that provides a basis for choosing one generalization over another [50]. For example, standard layers in neural networks incorporate invariances into the architecture that induce representational biases. Layers in **convolutional neural networks** (CNNs) exhibit equivariance and invariance to translation. Translation equivariance, which is achieved by weight sharing, means

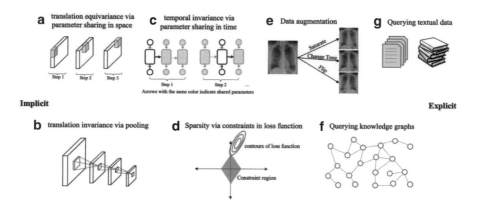

Fig. 4.10 Incorporating knowledge into machine learning models can occur implicitly through choice of model architecture (**a–c**) or loss function (**d**), through data augmentation (**e**), or explicitly by querying external knowledge sources such as knowledge graphs or textual data (**f, g**)

that changes in the input image result in similar changes in the output,[7] and translation invariance, which occurs due to pooling operations, means that small local translations do not necessarily change the pooled output values. These are both natural priors for image data where the representation of an object should not necessarily depend on its precise location in the larger image (Fig. 4.10a, b). Similarly, the sequential processing in recurrent layers found in **recurrent neural networks** (RNNs) impose notions of temporal invariance, which is particularly useful for processing time-series data and natural language that is read from start to end (Fig. 4.10c). Occam's razor—that the simplest solution is generally best—is often implemented by considering the complexity of a learned model, usually as a function of all its weights, as a cost that penalizes more complex models and encourages sparsity (Fig. 4.10d). These inductive biases are essential for developing robust machine learning models that can generalize beyond their training data and perform better in limited data regimes and under data distribution shifts. For example, the spatial translational equivariance of convolutional layers allows CNNs to recognize images with translated pixels without needing to augment the training data with many shifted images.

The process of selecting and annotating training data also injects human biases into the model development process. Perhaps most explicitly, **data augmentation** is the process of augmenting the training dataset with transformations of the input data with the goal of inducing the model to be invariant to the transformation. For example, transformations that rotate, flip, or randomly crop images are frequently used in model development for radiology images (see Chap. 12). Procedures for quickly annotating data also serve to inject human biases. For example, **data programming** allows domain experts to specify labeling functions that heuristically

---

[7] More precisely, a function f(x) is equivariant to a function g if $f(g(x)) = g(f(x))$.

and noisily label subsets of the data, which can later be combined and denoised to generate a training dataset [51]. Active learning methods select new data points for annotation by domain experts—for example, chest x-rays close to the model decision boundary might be sent to radiologists for annotation. Both of these approaches allow for implicitly incorporating experts' domain knowledge through efficient annotation of training data. Finally, the choice of input data sources, features, and labels can serve to bias model development. For instance, model developers make assumptions regarding which features may be worth collecting for training. These choices can have negative consequences for fairness when the training data skews towards majority populations or when the labels are biased proxies of the true outcome of interest [52]. See also Chap. 18 for discussion of resulting ethical issues.

There are an increasing number of efforts to leverage human knowledge more explicitly in machine learning models. Such approaches are diverse, including Bayesian neural networks, neural Turing machines, and machine learning for causal inference, among others. The remainder of the section focuses on two broad categories of models that query external information found in knowledge graphs and text. These approaches borrow from the long tradition of leveraging knowledge bases in expert systems, and their goal is to incorporate the strengths of such systems into modern machine learning frameworks.

Graph-Based Models

As noted in section "Ontologies and Their Tools", the biomedical informatics community has devoted significant time and resources into developing curated graphs of biomedical knowledge for diagnoses, labs, medications, drugs, and genes. The abundance of structured biomedical knowledge graphs has encouraged extensive research on leveraging graphs for tackling challenging biomedical machine learning problems.

Graph Representation Learning

A core challenge of leveraging graphs in machine learning is graph **representation learning**, i.e., learning an encoding of the graph that can capture the relevant structural and positional information. A graph is a structure consisting of a set of nodes and the set of directed or undirected edges that connect the nodes. Traditional machine learning approaches for representing graphs often use hand-engineered summary statistics [53] or kernel functions [54] to measure graph structure. For example, a node can be represented by its degree—i.e., the number of edges connected to the node, by its centrality within the graph, or by the number of motifs (e.g., triangles) within the node's local neighborhood. More recent approaches use data-driven techniques to learn **embeddings**, or low-dimensional vector representations that can encode graph structure. We outline four broad approaches for learning

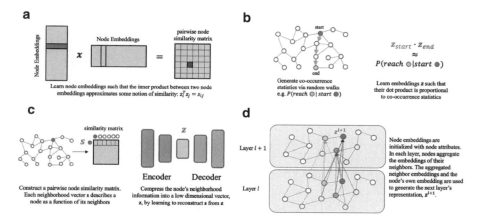

Fig. 4.11 Approaches for node representation learning include (**a**) matrix factorization, (**b**) random walk-based methods, (**c**) autoencoders, and (**d**) graph neural networks (GNNs). Every approach produces a low dimensional embedding for each node in the graph. These methods can be extended to learn embeddings for edges, subgraphs, or graphs

node embeddings, all of which can be extended to learn edge, subgraph, or graph embeddings (Fig. 4.11).

- **Matrix factorization** methods leverage techniques for dimensionality reduction to learn node embeddings. The goal is to learn embeddings for each node in the graph such that the similarity between two nodes' embeddings (e.g., the inner product between two embeddings) approximates some user-defined measure of node similarity. Methods largely differ in how they define their deterministic notion of pairwise node similarity; in its simplest form, the pairwise node similarity can be defined by the graph's **adjacency matrix**—a matrix that indicates which nodes are connected by edges in the graph.
- **Random walk** methods leverage stochastic measures of node similarity to learn node embeddings. The key idea is that nodes that co-occur on short random walks over the graph should have similar node embeddings.
- **Autoencoder** methods leverage neural networks to learn a compressed representation of each node's neighborhood by enforcing a bottleneck within the network. The models are trained in an unsupervised manner to compress the node information into a low dimensional vector and reconstruct the original input from the compressed representation.
- **Graph neural network** *(GNN)* methods generate node embeddings by aggregating information from each node's local neighborhood within the graph. More concretely, each layer of the GNN consists of three stages: *message, aggregate,* and *update*. Messages are sent from each neighbor in the node's neighborhood, aggregated, and used to update the node's previous representation. This message-passing scheme occurs in each layer of the neural network, and as the process repeats, the generated node representations contain additional information from nodes further away in the graph.

Graph neural network methods have largely replaced traditional methods for graph representation learning. These methods have several notable benefits. Unlike prior approaches, the GNN framework allows for the incorporation of node-specific features by initializing the hidden representation of each node with the desired features. For example, protein nodes in a protein-protein interaction network could be initialized with their gene expression data or disease nodes in a disease ontology such as the International Classification of Diseases (ICD) could be initialized with a textual description of the disease. Perhaps most importantly, graph neural networks can be inductive, that is they can operate over nodes that are unseen during training. This property allows for generalization of these methods to new nodes at test time.

While a thorough review of machine learning methods for graphs is outside the scope of this book, we refer the interested reader to a review [55], which includes a more thorough treatment of traditional and modern neural methods for graph representation learning.

Biomedical Applications of Graph Machine Learning

Graph machine learning methods have been applied to diverse biomedical application areas including predicting therapeutic applications of drug molecules, identifying protein interactions, and performing disease diagnosis [56]. Such approaches generally take two forms: graph-based applications, which are concerned with predicting properties of nodes, edges, subgraphs, or entire graphs, and **cross-modal applications**, which leverage graph representations as input to larger models for downstream tasks that may be independent of the original graph (Fig. 4.12).

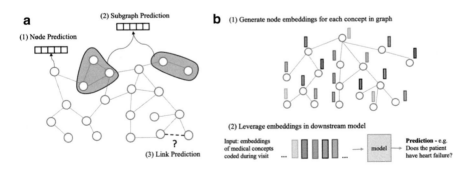

Fig. 4.12 (**a**) Graph-based applications involve predicting properties of nodes, edges, subgraphs, or entire graphs. Node prediction tasks compute values for each node in the graph, subgraph prediction tasks compute values for subsets of nodes in the graph, and link prediction tasks involve prediction of whether an edge exists between two nodes in a graph. (**b**) Cross-modal applications indirectly use graph-structured data for downstream tasks. Graphs are used to learn richer representations of the concepts. These concept embeddings are then leveraged in downstream tasks that do not necessarily relate to the original graph (e.g., heart failure prediction). The concept embeddings can either be pretrained or learned in an end-to-end manner on the downstream task

Biomedical graph-based applications largely focus on pharmaceutical and multi-omic applications. While there are some node prediction tasks, including protein function prediction [57, 58] and semantic type classification of medical terms [59], link prediction and graph classification tasks are more common. Tasks that predict the relationship between two entities can be formulated as a link prediction task in a biological network. For example, Zitnik et al. identify side-effects occurring with drug combinations by framing the problem as a multi-relational link prediction task on a graph containing protein-protein, drug-protein, and drug-drug interactions [60]. The link prediction framework has also been applied to identify protein-protein interactions [61], to detect miRNA-disease associations [62], to predict gene-disease associations [63], to identify disease candidates for established drugs [64] to predict molecular targets for drugs [65], and to perform knowledge graph completion of missing edges [66]. Finally, graph-level tasks largely focus on drug discovery; methods learn to encode small molecules, chemical reactions, and macromolecules for molecular property prediction [67], protein structure prediction [68], molecular dynamics applications [69], or for de novo molecule design [70]. Subgraph classification tasks are less common; one paper frames disease diagnosis as a subgraph classification task by representing each patient as a subgraph of medical codes in a larger graph containing phenotype-phenotype, phenotype-gene, and gene-gene relations [71].

Graph representation methods are increasingly being leveraged to generate embeddings of biomedical concepts that can be used in downstream cross-modal applications. Biomedical graphs are used to learn richer representations of the concepts based on the ontology structure, but the downstream tasks do not necessarily involve predicting properties of the graph itself. For example, GRAM (Graph-based Attention Model) incorporates the Clinical Classification Software (CCS) diagnosis ontology into a model for diagnosis prediction [72]. GRAM initializes the medical concept embeddings by employing GloVe, a method for generating embeddings based on co-occurrences within each visit [73]. Concepts are represented as a combination of the embeddings of their ancestors in the ontology via an **attention** mechanism. Similarly, Shang et al. use GNNs to encode ICD-9 diagnosis codes and ATC medication codes [74]. These embeddings are input into a BERT model (see Chap. 7) to generate representations of electronic health record (EHR) data for a single patient visit for medication recommendation.

Graph-derived embeddings can also be used to supplement text representations. A recent trend in clinical natural language processing (NLP) involves using relational information between entities in a knowledge graph to incorporate domain knowledge into NLP models. For example, umlsBERT extends BERT by enriching input embeddings with UMLS-derived semantic group embeddings and performing multi-label classification to encourage umlsBERT to identify all words associated with the same UMLS concept [75]. MacAveney et al. incorporate medical domain knowledge into its model for summarization of radiology reports by linking entities in the radiology reports with the UMLS ontology and generating an "ontology aware" encoding of the radiology report based on the linked entities [76].

Text-Based Models

While graphs provide useful sources of structured biomedical knowledge, existing knowledge graphs are limited in their completeness and breadth. Much of our biomedical knowledge is instead captured in unstructured text in journal articles, textbooks, and website pages. While the text can be used to construct structured knowledge graphs, thereby enabling the use of GNNs and other graph methods, a review of such methods is outside the scope of this chapter. We instead focus on methods that directly retrieve unstructured text for use in machine learning models. Rather than rely on knowledge implicitly stored as parameters in the model [77], such methods explicitly expose the role of world knowledge by asking the model to decide what knowledge to retrieve and use for the prediction. These retrieval-based models are commonly used for knowledge intensive tasks, such as fact verification and **open domain question answering**. Unlike traditional reading comprehension, in open domain question answering, the model does not receive a text document known to contain the answer and instead must identify and retrieve the necessary supporting information from a large corpus of documents. Most approaches consist of a separate *retriever*, which selects the necessary information, and a *reader*, which incorporates the retrieved information to make a final prediction. Traditionally, the retriever uses classical information retrieval methods and the reader employs neural networks. However, more recent approaches now include a retriever implemented with neural network methods, allowing the retriever and reader to be trained jointly end-to-end via backpropagation [78–80].

Retrieval-based methods have been leveraged in the biomedical domain for question answering. While many existing biomedical question answering datasets, such as emrQA and PubmedQA [81, 82], are closed-domain, i.e., they provide a single document containing the solution, there are some open-domain question-answering tasks that require methods to retrieve relevant knowledge. Epic-QA tasks models to answer questions about COVID-19 based on a large corpus of scientific and government articles [83]. The BioASQ workshop, which has been running since 2013, hosts a series of biomedical question-answering challenges that include open domain question answering over Pubmed articles [84]. Finally, several models leverage retrieval-based approaches to solve medical licensing exam questions—multiple-choice questions that can require extensive reasoning over external knowledge sources [85, 86].

Leveraging Expert Systems to Train Models

We conclude this chapter by briefly discussing approaches for injecting the knowledge from expert systems into machine learning models. The core idea of this approach is to transfer the knowledge from the more cumbersome, but domain knowledge-rich teacher model to a student model that has potential to generalize beyond the rules-based system. Such **knowledge distillation** approaches are starting to be used in the biomedical domain. For example, Ravuri et al. use the expert system QMR to generate synthetic training data, which is leveraged to train a deep learning model for disease diagnosis [87]. This approach yielded a more robust model that allows for incremental updating of the model with new diseases or symptoms. Similarly, McDermott et al. and Smit et al. developed BERT-based models to approximate CheXpert, a rules-based radiology report labeler and find that the BERT-based model actually has a tendency to correct errors in the original CheXpert labels [88, 89]. Finally Kodialam et al., reverse the traditional knowledge distillation framework by initializing their deep learning model to mimic a performant linear model in a technique they term reverse distillation [90]. All of these approaches are similar in their goal to transfer domain knowledge or other innate priors to the student model.

The older expert systems approaches have the benefit that their reasoning can be explained in relatively easy human-understandable terms. A chain of rule inferences can be shown as the basis for a conclusion, or the correspondence between a disease pattern and the facts observed about a patient can explain why that disease is a plausible diagnosis. By contrast, complex neural network-based systems seem inscrutable; the "answer" is a result of a vast number of arithmetic computations that, individually, have no obvious correspondence to the logic of the domain. Therefore, there are many attempts to develop means to provide explanations or justifications for the answers produced by neural network models. (See Chap. 8.) Especially in highly consequential domains, such as health care, demanding such transparency is highly justified. One promising approach is enabled by building a high-performance neural model starting with an explainable expert system, such as the ones mentioned in the previous paragraph, so a conclusion might be approximately justified by explaining how the expert system could have reached the conclusion actually derived by the neural model.

Looking Forward

We have reviewed various methods that have been developed to apply human knowledge to biomedical decision making tasks and to augment that knowledge by learning from the vast case repository of clinical experience that is now being captured in databases. The initial enthusiasm among some to imagine a world in which all knowledge can be rediscovered by applying machine learning (especially deep neural networks of various architectures) to heterogeneous clinical data has faded somewhat with experience. Unlike models based on explicit expressions of knowledge, such ML models are often inscrutable. Although they tend to work very well on average, they may fail catastrophically and unpredictably in some cases. And as clinical practice changes, patients age, and new diseases rise to prominence, models trained on historical data may become more and more inaccurate.

The central challenge in knowledge-based systems in medicine is to develop new means of integrating knowledge that derives from many different sources: causal understanding of the biochemical, genetic and pathophysiologic mechanisms involved in disease, the empirical observational data arising from clinical records, and the occasional clinical trials that test specific interventions. These learned models will need to account properly for the evolution of each patient's state over time and the uncertainties about both observations and conclusions, thus needing connections to research on knowledge representation.

These are significant challenges. However, the aging of our population and thus the increase in chronic diseases, the growth in data collection, and the inexhaustible demand of people for improved health care provide outstanding opportunities for exciting research and important applications.

Questions for Discussion

- Think about some of your own expertise. Which forms of knowledge representation might be most appropriate to express it?
- How important is uncertainty in the domains you are interested in? How do you think knowledge in those domains can support inference about the likelihood of particular events and conditions?
- How would you best explain the recommendations of a decision support system? Would that explanation necessarily mirror the way in which it derived that recommendation?
- Consider the problem of predicting the causal gene of patients with suspected Mendelian genetic disorders. Each patient is represented by a set of phenotypes (symptoms) and a list of candidate genes. What inductive biases or assumptions might you want to incorporate into your diagnosis model?
- Incorporating knowledge graphs into machine learning models has the potential to improve model performance and generalizability, but the utility of these hybrid models is still an open research question. How would you design an experiment to measure the usefulness of incorporating knowledge graphs into models versus simply adding more training data? What are the pros and cons of each approach?

Further Reading

Szolovits P, Pauker SG. Categorical and probabilistic reasoning in medical diagnosis. Artif Intell. 1978;11(1–2):115–44. https://doi.org/10.1016/0004-3702(78)90014-0.

- This paper reviews early approaches to capturing human-like reasoning about clinical tasks, emphasizing the need to be able to deal with multiple disorders and uncertainty.

Szolovits P. Artificial intelligence in medicine. Westview Press; 1982. Re-published by Routledge; 2019.

- A presentation of the first generation of AI systems for medical reasoning, with lessons even for today's world.

Battaglia PW, Hamrick JB, Bapst V, Sanchez-Gonzalez A, Zambaldi V, Malinowski M, et al. Relational inductive biases, deep learning, and graph networks. ArXiv180601261 Cs Stat. 2018. http://arxiv.org/abs/1806.01261.

• This article discusses the many types of inductive biases that can be incorporated into neural networks and provides an introduction to graph neural networks.

Hamilton WL. Graph representation learning. Synth Lect Artif Intell Mach Learn. 14(3):1–159. https://www.cs.mcgill.ca/~wlh/grl_book/.

• This textbook provides an introduction to graph representation learning, including methods for embedding graph data, graph neural networks, and deep generative models of graphs.

Li MM, Huang K, Zitnik M. Representation learning for networks in biology and medicine: advancements, challenges, and opportunities. ArXiv210404883 Cs Q-Bio. 2021; Available from http://arxiv.org/abs/2104.04883.

• This review article introduces approaches for graph representation learning and describes their applications to the biomedical domain.

References

1. Ribatti D. William Harvey and the discovery of the circulation of the blood. J Angiogenesis Res. 2009;1(1):3.
2. Bessen HA. Therapeutic and toxic effects of digitalis: William Withering, 1785. J Emerg Med. 1986;4(3):243–8.
3. Szolovits P. Artificial intelligence in medicine, vol. 51. Boulder, CO: Westview Press; 1982. https://groups.csail.mit.edu/medg/people/psz/ftp/AIM82/.
4. Clancey WJ, Shortliffe EH. Readings in medical artificial intelligence. Reading, MA: Addison-Wesley; 1984. http://www.shortliffe.net/Clancey-Shortliffe-1984/Readings%20Book.htm.
5. Johnson AEW, Pollard TJ, Shen L, Lehman L-w H, Feng M, Ghaseemi M, et al. MIMIC-III, a freely accessible critical care database. Sci Data. 2016;3:160035. https://www.nature.com/articles/sdata201635/.
6. Moody GB, Mark RG, Goldberger AL. PhysioNet: a web-based resource for the study of physiologic signals. IEEE Eng Med Biol Mag. 2001;20(3):70–5.
7. Pollard TJ, Johnson AEW, Raffa JD, Celi LA, Mark RG, Badawi O. The eICU Collaborative Research Database, a freely available multi-center database for critical care research. Sci Data. 2018;5(1):180178.
8. Bycroft C, Freeman C, Petkova D, Band G, Elliott LT, Sharp K, et al. The UK Biobank resource with deep phenotyping and genomic data. Nature. 2018;562(7726):203–9.
9. The "All of Us" Research Program. N Engl J Med. 2019;381(7):668–676.
10. Gaziano JM, Concato J, Brophy M, Fiore L, Pyarajan S, Breeling J, et al. Million Veteran Program: a mega-biobank to study genetic influences on health and disease. J Clin Epidemiol. 2016;70:214–23.
11. Davis R, Shrobe H, Szolovits P. What is a knowledge representation? AI Mag. 1993;14(1):17.
12. Kowalski RA. The early years of logic programming. Commun ACM. 1988;31(1):38–43.
13. Forgy CL. OPS 5 user's manual. Carnegie-Mellon University; 1981 p. 57. https://kilthub.cmu.edu/articles/journal_contribution/OPS5_user_s_manual/6608090/1.

14. Shortliffe EH. Computer-based medical consultations: MYCIN. New York: Elsevier; 1976. http://www.shortliffe.net/Shortliffe-1976/MYCIN%20thesis%20Book.htm.
15. Clancey WJ. The epistemology of a rule-based expert system—a framework for explanation. Artif Intell. 1983;20(3):215–51.
16. Shortliffe EH, Davis R, Axline SG, Buchanan BG, Green CC, Cohen SN. Computer-based consultations in clinical therapeutics: explanation and rule acquisition capabilities of the MYCIN system. Comput Biomed Res. 1975;8(4):303–20.
17. Yu VL, Buchanan BG, Shortliffe EH, Wraith SM, Davis R, Scott AC, et al. Evaluating the performance of a computer-based consultant. Comput Programs Biomed. 1979;9(1):95–102.
18. Yu VL, Fagan LM, Wraith SM, Clancey WJ, Scott AC, Hannigan J, et al. Antimicrobial selection by a computer. A blinded evaluation by infectious diseases experts. JAMA. 1979;242(12):1279–82.
19. Minsky M. A framework for representing knowledge. MIT-AI Laboratory; 1974. https://courses.media.mit.edu/2004spring/mas966/Minsky%201974%20Framework%20for%20knowledge.pdf.
20. Pauker SG, Gorry GA, Kassirer JP, Schwartz WB. Towards the simulation of clinical cognition. Taking a present illness by computer. Am J Med. 1976;60(7):981–96.
21. Miller RA, Pople HE, Myers JD. INTERNIST-I, an experimental computer-based diagnostic consultant for general internal medicine. N Engl J Med. 1982;307(8):468–76.
22. Lasko TA, Feldman MJ, Barnett GO. DXplain evoking strength—clinician interpretation and consistency. Proc AMIA Symp. 2002;1073.
23. Miller R, Masarie FE, Myers JD. Quick medical reference (QMR) for diagnostic assistance. MD Comput. 1986;3(5):34–48.
24. Miller RA, Masarie FE. Use of the Quick Medical Reference (QMR) program as a tool for medical education. Methods Inf Med. 1989;28(4):340–5.
25. Hupp JA, Cimino JJ, Hoffer EP, Lowe HJ, Barnett GO. DXplain—a computer-based diagnostic knowledge base. In: Proc MEDINFO; 1986. p. 117–21.
26. Pople HE Jr. Heuristic methods for imposing structure on ill-structured problems: the structuring of medical diagnostics. In: Szolovits P, editor. Artificial intelligence in medicine. AAAS symposium series, vol. 51. Boulder, CO: Westview Press; 1982. http://groups.csail.mit.edu/medg/people/psz/ftp/AIM82/ch5.html.
27. Wu TD. A problem decomposition method for efficient diagnosis and interpretation of multiple disorders. Comput Methods Programs Biomed. 1991;35(4):239–50.
28. Sox HC, Blatt MA, Marton KI, Higgins MC. Medical decision making. Philadelphia: ACP Press; 2007.
29. Gorry GA, Kassirer JP, Essig A, Schwartz WB. Decision analysis as the basis for computer-aided management of acute renal failure. Am J Med. 1973;55(3):473–84.
30. Middleton B, Shwe MA, Heckerman DE, Henrion M, Horvitz EJ, Lehmann HP, et al. Probabilistic diagnosis using a reformulation of the INTERNIST-1/QMR knowledge base. II. Evaluation of diagnostic performance. Methods Inf Med. 1991;30(4):256–67.
31. Shwe MA, Middleton B, Heckerman DE, Henrion M, Horvitz EJ, Lehmann HP, et al. Probabilistic diagnosis using a reformulation of the INTERNIST-1/QMR knowledge base. I. The probabilistic model and inference algorithms. Methods Inf Med. 1991;30(4):241–55.
32. Wu TD. A decompositional approach to the diagnosis of multiple disorders (PhD Thesis). Cambridge, MA: MIT; 1982. http://groups.csail.mit.edu/medg/ftp/twu/twu-thesis-v0.9.pdf.
33. Raiffa H. Decision analysis: introductory lectures on choices under uncertainty. ISBN: 9780070525795: Amazon.com: Books. Random House; 1968.
34. Pauker SG. Coronary artery surgery: the use of decision analysis. Ann Intern Med. 1976;85(1):8–18.
35. MacKillop E, Sheard S. Quantifying life: understanding the history of quality-adjusted life-years (QALYs). Soc Sci Med. 2018;211:359–66.
36. Szolovits P. Uncertainty and decisions in medical informatics. Methods Inf Med. 1995;34(1/2):111–21.

37. Howard RA, Matheson JE. Influence diagrams. Decis Anal. 2005;2(3):127–43.
38. Komorowski M, Celi LA, Badawi O, Gordon AC, Faisal AA. The Artificial Intelligence Clinician learns optimal treatment strategies for sepsis in intensive care. Nat Med. 2018;24(11):1716.
39. Guyton AC, Coleman TG, Granger HJ. Circulation: overall regulation. Annu Rev Physiol. 1972;34(1):13–44.
40. Montani J-P, Vliet BNV. Understanding the contribution of Guyton's large circulatory model to long-term control of arterial pressure. Exp Physiol. 2009;94(4):382–8.
41. Hester RL, Summers R, Ilescu R, Esters J, Coleman T. DigitalHuman (DH): an integrative mathematical model of human physiology. 6.
42. Heldt T, Mukkamala R, Moody GB, Mark RG. CVSim: an open-source cardiovascular simulator for teaching and research. Open Pacing Electrophysiol Ther J. 2010;3:45–54.
43. Weiss S, Kulikowski CA, Safir A. Glaucoma consultation by computer. Comput Biol Med. 1978;8(1):25–40.
44. Patil R, Szolovits P, Schwartz WB. Modeling knowledge of the patient in acid-base and electrolyte disorders. In: Szolovits P, editor. Artificial intelligence in medicine. Boulder, CO: Westview Press; 1982. http://groups.csail.mit.edu/medg/people/psz/ftp/AIM82/ch6.html.
45. Musen MA. The Protégé project: a look back and a look forward. AI Matters. 2015;1(4):4–12.
46. Levesque HJ, Brachman RJ. Expressiveness and tractability in knowledge representation and reasoning. Comput Intell. 1987;3(1):78–93.
47. Rector AL, Horrocks IR. Experience building a large, re-usable medical ontology using a description logic with transitivity and concept inclusions. In: AAAI conference on artificial intelligence; 1997. AAAI Technical Report SS-97-06:8.
48. Bodenreider O. The Unified Medical Language System (UMLS): integrating biomedical terminology. Nucleic Acids Res. 2004;32(Suppl_1):D267–70.
49. Pearl J. Radical empiricism and machine learning research. J Causal Inference. 2021;9(1):78–82.
50. Mitchell TM. The need for biases in learning generalizations. New Jersey: Department of Computer Science, Laboratory for Computer Science Research, Rutgers Univ; 1980. http://www.cs.cmu.edu/~tom/pubs/NeedForBias_1980.pdf.
51. Ratner A, Sa CD, Wu S, Selsam D, Ré C. Data programming: creating large training sets, quickly. In: Proceedings of the 30th international conference on neural information processing systems (NIPS'16). Red Hook, NY: Curran Associates Inc.; 2016. p. 3574–82.
52. Obermeyer Z, Powers B, Vogeli C, Mullainathan S. Dissecting racial bias in an algorithm used to manage the health of populations. Science. 2019;366(6464):447–53.
53. Henderson K, Gallagher B, Li L, Akoglu L, Eliassi-Rad T, Tong H, et al. It's who you know: graph mining using recursive structural features. In: Proceedings of the 17th ACM SIGKDD international conference on knowledge discovery and data mining (KDD '11). New York: Association for Computing Machinery; 2011. p. 663–71. https://doi.org/10.1145/2020408.2020512.
54. Vishwanathan SVN, Schraudolph NN, Kondor R, Borgwardt KM. Graph kernels. J Mach Learn Res. 2010;11(40):1201–42.
55. Hamilton WL. Graph representation learning. Synth Lect Artif Intell Mach Learn. 2020;14(3):1–159.
56. Li MM, Huang K, Zitnik M. Graph representation learning in biomedicine. arXiv:210404883 [cs, q-bio] 2021. http://arxiv.org/abs/2104.04883.
57. Kulmanov M, Khan MA, Hoehndorf R, Wren J. DeepGO: predicting protein functions from sequence and interactions using a deep ontology-aware classifier. Bioinformatics. 2018;34(4):660–8.
58. Zitnik M, Leskovec J. Predicting multicellular function through multi-layer tissue networks. Bioinformatics. 2017;33(14):i190–8.
59. Yue X, Wang Z, Huang J, Parthasarathy S, Moosavinasab S, Huang Y, et al. Graph embedding on biomedical networks: methods, applications and evaluations. Bioinformatics. 2020;36(4):1241–51.
60. Zitnik M, Agrawal M, Leskovec J. Modeling polypharmacy side effects with graph convolutional networks. Bioinformatics. 2018;34(13):i457–66.

61. Kovács IA, Luck K, Spirohn K, Wang Y, Pollis C, Schlabach S, et al. Network-based prediction of protein interactions. Nat Commun. 2019;10(1):1240.
62. Ji B-Y, You Z-H, Cheng L, Zhou J-R, Alghazzawi D, Li L-P. Predicting miRNA-disease association from heterogeneous information network with GraRep embedding model. Sci Rep. 2020;10(1):6658.
63. Luo P, Li Y, Tian L-P, Wu F-X. Enhancing the prediction of disease–gene associations with multimodal deep learning. Bioinformatics. 2019;35(19):3735–42.
64. Zhang R, Hristovski D, Schutte D, Kastrin A, Fiszman M, Kilicoglu H. Drug repurposing for COVID-19 via knowledge graph completion. J Biomed Inform. 2021;115:103696.
65. Lu Y, Guo Y, Korhonen A. Link prediction in drug-target interactions network using similarity indices. BMC Bioinformatics. 2017;18(1):39.
66. Ebeid IA, Hassan M, Wanyan T, Roper J, Seal A, Ding Y. Biomedical knowledge graph refinement and completion using graph representation learning and top-K similarity measure. In: Toeppe K, Yan H, Chu SKW, editors. Diversity, divergence, dialogue. Cham: Springer; 2021. p. 112–23.
67. Wu Z, Ramsundar B, Feinberg EN, Gomes J, Geniesse C, Pappu AS, et al. MoleculeNet: a benchmark for molecular machine learning. Chem Sci. 2017;9(2):513–30. https://doi.org/10.1039/c7sc02664a.
68. Jumper J, Evans R, Pritzel A, Green T, Figurnov M, Ronneberger O, et al. Highly accurate protein structure prediction with AlphaFold. Nature. 2021;596:583–9.
69. Park CW, Kornbluth M, Vandermause J, Wolverton C, Kozinsky B, Mailoa JP. Accurate and scalable graph neural network force field and molecular dynamics with direct force architecture. npj Comput Mater. 2021;7(1):1–9.
70. Xiong J, Xiong Z, Chen K, Jiang H, Zheng M. Graph neural networks for automated de novo drug design. Drug Discov Today. 2021;26(6):1382–93.
71. Alsentzer E, Finlayson S, Li M, Zitnik M. Subgraph neural networks. Adv Neural Inf Process Syst. 2020;33:8017–29.
72. Choi E, Bahadori MT, Song L, Stewart WF, Sun J. GRAM: graph-based attention model for healthcare representation learning. In: Proceedings of the 23rd ACM SIGKDD international conference on knowledge discovery and data mining (KDD '17). New York: Association for Computing Machinery; 2017. p. 787–95. https://doi.org/10.1145/3097983.3098126.
73. Pennington J, Socher R, Manning C. GloVe: global vectors for word representation. In: Proceedings of the 2014 conference on empirical methods in natural language processing (EMNLP). Doha: Association for Computational Linguistics; 2014. p. 1532–43. https://aclanthology.org/D14-1162.
74. Shang J, Ma T, Xiao C, Sun J. Pre-training of graph augmented transformers for medication recommendation. In: Proceedings of the twenty-eighth international joint conference on artificial intelligence. Macao: International Joint Conferences on Artificial Intelligence Organization; 2019. p. 5953–9. https://www.ijcai.org/proceedings/2019/825.
75. Michalopoulos G, Wang Y, Kaka H, Chen H, Wong A. UmlsBERT: clinical domain knowledge augmentation of contextual embeddings using the unified medical language system Metathesaurus. In: Proceedings of the 2021 conference of the North American Chapter of the Association for Computational Linguistics: human language technologies. Online: Association for Computational Linguistics; 2021. p. 1744–53. https://aclanthology.org/2021.naacl-main.139.
76. MacAvaney S, Sotudeh S, Cohan A, Goharian N, Talati I, Filice R. Ontology-aware clinical abstractive summarization. In: Proceedings of the 42nd international ACM SIGIR conference on research and development in information retrieval. https://dl.acm.org/doi/10.1145/3331184.3331319.
77. Petroni F, Rocktäschel T, Riedel S, Lewis P, Bakhtin A, Wu Y, et al. Language models as knowledge bases? In: Proceedings of the 2019 conference on empirical methods in natural language processing and the 9th international joint conference on natural language processing (EMNLP-IJCNLP). Hong Kong: Association for Computational Linguistics; 2019. p. 2463–73. https://aclanthology.org/D19-1250.

78. Lewis P, Perez E, Piktus A, Petroni F, Karpukhin V, Goyal N, et al. Retrieval-augmented generation for knowledge-intensive NLP tasks. Adv Neural Inf Process Syst. 2020;33:9459–74.
79. Lee K, Chang M-W, Toutanova K. Latent retrieval for weakly supervised open domain question answering. In: Proceedings of the 57th annual meeting of the Association for Computational Linguistics. Florence: Association for Computational Linguistics; 2019. p. 6086–96. https://aclanthology.org/P19-1612.
80. Guu K, Lee K, Tung Z, Pasupat P, Chang M-W. REALM: retrieval-augmented language model pre-training. arXiv:200208909 [cs]. 2020. http://arxiv.org/abs/2002.08909.
81. Pampari A, Raghavan P, Liang J, Peng J. emrQA: a large corpus for question answering on electronic medical records. In: Proceedings of the 2018 conference on empirical methods in natural language processing. Brussels: Association for Computational Linguistics; 2018. p. 2357–68. https://aclanthology.org/D18-1258.
82. Jin Q, Dhingra B, Liu Z, Cohen W, Lu X. PubMedQA: a dataset for biomedical research question answering. In: Proceedings of the 2019 conference on empirical methods in natural language processing and the 9th international joint conference on natural language processing (EMNLP-IJCNLP). Hong Kong: Association for Computational Linguistics; 2019. p. 2567–77. https://aclanthology.org/D19-1259.
83. Goodwin T, Demner-Fushman D, Lu Wang L, Lo K, Hersh W, Dang H, et al. Epidemic question answering. Epidemic Question Answering: TAC; 2020. https://bionlp.nlm.nih.gov/epic_qa/#objective.
84. Tsatsaronis G, Balikas G, Malakasiotis P, Partalas I, Zschunke M, Alvers MR, et al. An overview of the BIOASQ large-scale biomedical semantic indexing and question answering competition. BMC Bioinformatics. 2015;16(1):138.
85. Zhang X, Wu J, He Z, Liu X, Su Y. Medical exam question answering with large-scale reading comprehension. In: Proceedings of the thirty-second aaai conference on artificial intelligence and thirtieth innovative applications of artificial intelligence Conference and Eighth AAAI Symposium on Educational Advances in Artificial Intelligence. New Orleans, Louisiana, USA: AAAI Press; 2018. p. 5706–13.
86. Ha LA, Yaneva V. Automatic Question Answering for Medical MCQs: Can It go Further than Information Retrieval? In: Proceedings of the International Conference on Recent Advances in Natural Language Processing (RANLP 2019). Varna, Bulgaria: INCOMA Ltd.; 2019. p. 418–22. Available from: https://aclanthology.org/R19-1049.
87. Ravuri M, Kannan A, Tso GJ, Amatriain X. Learning from the experts: from expert systems to machine-learned diagnosis models. In: Machine learning for healthcare conference. PMLR; 2018. p. 227–43. http://proceedings.mlr.press/v85/ravuri18a.html.
88. McDermott MBA, Hsu TMH, Weng W-H, Ghassemi M, Szolovits P. CheXpert++: approximating the CheXpert labeler for speed, differentiability, and probabilistic output. In: Machine learning for healthcare conference. PMLR; 2020. p. 913–27. http://proceedings.mlr.press/v126/mcdermott20a.html.
89. Smit A, Jain S, Rajpurkar P, Pareek A, Ng A, Lungren M. CheXbert: combining automatic labelers and expert annotations for accurate radiology report labeling using BERT. In: Proceedings of the 2020 conference on empirical methods in natural language processing (EMNLP). Online: Association for Computational Linguistics; 2020. p. 1500–19. https://aclanthology.org/2020.emnlp-main.117.
90. Kodialam R, Boiarsky R, Lim J, Sai A, Dixit N, Sontag D. Deep contextual clinical prediction with reverse distillation. Proc AAAI Conf Artif Intell. 2021;35(1):249–58.

Chapter 5
Clinical Cognition and AI: From Emulation to Symbiosis

Vimla L. Patel and Trevor A. Cohen

After reading this chapter, you should know the answers to these questions:
- How do contemporary AI systems differ from expert human decision makers?
- Why is understanding clinical cognition critical for the future of sustainable AI?
- What constraints on human decision making suggest a complementary role for AI in clinical decision making?
- How might AI enhance the safety of clinical practice?

Augmenting Human Expertise: Motivating Examples

One of the more controversial claims about AI systems in medicine is that they have the potential to replace the role of the physician, especially in perceptual domains such as radiology and pathology, in which interpretation of images is a prominent component of physician work. While it is natural that practitioners with a focus on image interpretation would consider the implications of current AI technologies for the professional viability of their fields (see, for example [1]), a strong counterargument to this claim is that these technologies may play a complementary role in the field and allow radiologists (and pathologists) to focus on assessment and

V. L. Patel (✉)
New York Academy of Medicine, New York, NY, USA
e-mail: vpatel@nyam.org

T. A. Cohen
University of Washington, Seattle, WA, USA
e-mail: cohenta@uw.edu

© The Author(s), under exclusive license to Springer Nature
Switzerland AG 2022
T. A. Cohen et al. (eds.), *Intelligent Systems in Medicine and Health*, Cognitive
Informatics in Biomedicine and Healthcare,
https://doi.org/10.1007/978-3-031-09108-7_5

communication of AI-based image interpretations, and the positioning of these interpretations within a broader diagnostic workflow [2]. Alternatively, and in line with the main motivating argument for the current chapter, it has been proposed that physicians and AI systems might play a complementary role in diagnosis itself [1, 3, 4], though less attention has been paid to several other crucial areas of a clinician's task.

This chapter considers the proposal of complementary physician/AI systems from a **cognitive informatics** perspective, focusing on the strengths and weaknesses of the information processing systems concerned. Before proceeding to address these issues, the section below presents some examples from the published literature of systems that establish a case for the utility of human-machine collaboration in order to augment human abilities.

The burgeoning literature on AI-based diagnostic systems in radiology is replete with examples of hybrid human/AI systems outperforming either component taken alone in diagnostic tasks. For example, Lakhani and Sundaram report results from a combined human/AI workflow in which a board-certified cardiothoracic radiologist was enlisted to resolve disagreements between two convolutional network architectures trained to identify pulmonary tuberculosis in chest radiographs [5]. This arbitration process improved ensemble model specificity from 94.7% to 100% without loss in sensitivity, with the radiologist reviewing only those 13 of 150 test cases in which disagreement between models occurred. Patel and colleagues report results from a workflow in which images with low-confidence predictions for the presence or absence of pneumonia from a convolutional network were reconsidered by groups of radiologists in concert [6]. Probabilistic estimates from these experts were then used as an alternative to the model's original predictions, resulting in an approximately 10% improvement in accuracy over that obtained with deep learning alone.

In both cases, the combined human/AI system also outperformed its human component, an individual radiologist in the tuberculosis study, and a group of radiologists in the pneumonia study. Another common finding of interest is that the predominant mode of improvement with human oversight is an improvement in specificity. That is to say, the AI models alone tended toward overdiagnosis, which supports a pragmatic argument for the judicious use of human expertise to reduce false positive diagnoses in those cases in which uncertainty is identified either through disagreement between models, or through low-probability predictions from a single model.

Similar findings have been observed in dermatology diagnosis. Combined human/AI systems outperformed their independent components [7], with a 2.5% increase in specificity when enforcing the same level of sensitivity. Notably, some work in this area has also investigated the role of representation—advantages in performance for the human-computer collective were observed to be contingent upon the granularity (probabilities of differential diagnoses vs. global risk of malignancy) and cognitive demand of the representation used to convey predictions to physicians [8]. These results illustrate the need to consider the constraints on human information processing when attempting to integrate AI into clinical decision making processes. While these results concern perceptual domains of medicine, it has also been argued that AI can play a complementary role in verbal domains by supporting the aggregation and synthesis of information required to reach a diagnostic conclusion [3].

These sorts of pragmatic motivating arguments for the consideration of human cognition are very different from those that motivated considerations of human information processing earlier in the development of AIM. With early systems, there was a desire to develop models that emulated procedures characteristic of human intelligence, with two early systems (INTERNIST-1 [9] and the Present Illness Program [10]) deliberately designed to model the generation and testing of a set of diagnostic hypotheses that cognitive studies had suggested were characteristic of the behavior of medical experts [11].

The section that follows considers the intersection among cognitive science, clinical cognition and AI, from earlier studies to current work, with a focus on the shared roots of these fields and the need for AI development to consider human cognition.

Cognitive Science and Clinical Cognition

Cognitive science, or the science of cognition, includes numerous subfields of psychology, philosophy, linguistics, cognitive anthropology, neuroscience and computer science. Basic research in cognitive science uses theories and methods from a combination of these domains to investigate problems, including clinical problems. For example, a program of research has used theories and methods from cognitive science to investigate clinical cognition and medical decision making (for examples see: [12–14]). Table 5.1, illustrates how research in basic cognitive sciences is related to our understanding of clinical cognition.

Similarly, our understanding of the reasoning processes and knowledge associated with diagnostic and patient management provides a basis for influencing the development of medical AI and decision support systems. For example, research in characterizations of expert and novice clinical knowledge organization in human memory can be used in creating representations of such knowledge in clinical AI systems. Table 5.2 shows the corresponding relationships between medical cognition and research in AI. The science of cognition provides the foundation needed to drive AI-based decision-support systems that can augment human behavior.

Research in clinical cognition draws on the theories, and methods developed in basic cognitive science, and contributes to applications in biomedical informatics in a number of ways. We are beginning to see a greater awareness of the concept of clinical cognition and its relationship to clinical support systems. A recent literature

Table 5.1 Correspondences between cognitive science and medical cognition

Cognitive science	Medical cognition
Knowledge organization and human memory	Organization of clinical and basic science knowledge
Problem solving, heuristics/reasoning strategies	Medical problem solving and decision making
Perception/attention	Interpretation of radiologic and other visual data
Diagrammatic reasoning	Perceptual processing of patient data displays
Text comprehension	Learning from medical texts
Dialog analysis	Medical discourse analysis
Distributed cognition	Collaborative practice in health care
Coordination of theory and evidence	Diagnostic and therapeutic reasoning
Natural intelligence	Expertise in clinical practice

Table 5.2 Correspondences between medical cognition and research in AI

Medical cognition	Medical AI
Organization of clinical basic science knowledge	Development and use of medical knowledge bases in intelligent systems
Medical problem solving and decision making	Medical artificial intelligence/decision support systems
Radiologic and dermatologic diagnosis	Visual data analytics/machine learning
Perceptual processing of patient data displays	Biomedical information visualization
Learning from medical texts/medical discourse analysis	Natural language processing
Collaborative practice in health care	Technology-supported collaborative environments
Diagnostic and therapeutic reasoning	Clinical support systems
Natural intelligence in clinical practice	Interactive environments for collaborative problem solving

evaluation from a biomedical informatics journal identified 57 articles that were related to cognitive informatics [15]. The topics of these articles ranged from characterizing the limits of clinician problem-solving and reasoning behavior and characterization of distributed clinical teams, to developing cognitively plausible interventions for supporting clinician activities. The reader is referred to Chap. 4 in Shortliffe and Cimino's textbook of Biomedical Informatics for comprehensive coverage of this topic [16].

Symbolic Representations of Clinical Information

Much of the research in late 1980s and 90s, such as the research in Patel's laboratory, fell into the **symbolic** tradition, and dealt with models of diagnostic reasoning. The theoretical foundation of cognitive modeling is the idea that cognition is a kind of computation (where computation involves the manipulation of symbols). The claim is that what the mind does, in part, is to perform cognitive tasks by mental computing. This computational theory of mind provides the fundamental underpinning for most contemporary theories of cognitive science. The basic premise is that much of human cognition can be characterized as a series of computations on mental representations. In medical cognition, **mental representations** are internal states that reflect a clinician's hypothesis about a patient's condition. For example, noticing an abnormal enlargement of the neck region, which prompts the clinician to elicit further inferences about the patient's underlying condition (such as family history of a thyroid condition), may influence the physician's information-gathering strategies and contribute to an evolving problem representation.

In artificial intelligence, symbolic AI is an approach to AI based on the manipulation of knowledge represented in language-like (symbolic) structures in which all relevant semantics (meaning) is explicit in the syntax (formal structure). This also provids a framework for the study of human cognition as the manipulation of symbolic structures. It involves the explicit embedding of human knowledge and behavior rules into computer programs. This type of research in early decades has in recent years been superseded by connectionist AI (neural networks), though in cognitive science both symbolic and connectionist approaches have had periods of historical predominance [17]. All the steps in symbolic AI are based on human-readable representations of the problem that use formal logic. This reasoning process can be easily understood, and a symbolic AI program can therefore explain why a certain conclusion is reached, including the reasoning steps. An explanation that is understandable to human beings helps create a shared meaning of the reasoning process underlying clinical problem-solving, which is an important step in building trust (see Chap. 18).

As the investigations moved from laboratory conditions to realistic clinical environments, it became evident that cognitive factors alone did not account for all the variance in clinicians' performance. Besides cognition, other differences were found to influence decision making, due to socio-cultural, organizational and technological factors. This alerted researchers in their early work to consider the situated nature of the clinical environment in addition to human cognition [18, 19].

Clinical Text Understanding

Early research in language understating lead to development of an influential method of analyzing the process of text understanding or **text comprehension,** based on the assumption that text can be described at multiple levels, from surface codes (e.g., words and syntax) to a deeper level of semantics (meaning) [20, 21]. **Comprehension** refers to cognitive processes associated with understanding or deriving meaning from written text, conversation, or other informational resources. It involves the processes that people use when trying to make sense of a piece of text, such as a sentence, or a verbal utterance, such as verbal exchanges during a conversation. This work influenced the studies of medical text understanding by physicians at various levels of expertise, where formal methods of natural language representations, such as propositional and semantic representations were used.

Propositions are a form of natural language representation that captures the essence of an idea (i.e., semantics) or concept without explicit reference to linguistic content. Propositional representations constitute an important construct in theories of comprehension. Propositional knowledge can be expressed using a predicate calculus formalism or as a semantic network.

The formalism is informed by an elaborate propositional language [22]. Patel and Frederiksen [23] and Patel and Groen [24] introduced the use of propositional analysis as a method of natural language representation in the clinical domain. The method provided the means to characterize the information clinicians and medical students understood from reading a text, based on their summaries or explanations of the patient problems. Figure 5.1 presents a schematic representation of natural language analysis of clinical text, using a propositional representation representing a **text-based** model and its relationship to semantic and conceptual level analysis, representing a **situational** model [25].

These studies have shown that individuals at different levels of expertise represent clinical text differently [26–29]. This means that these various representations

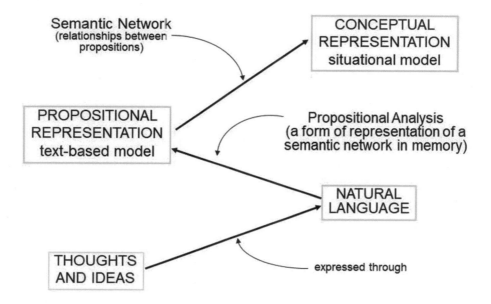

Fig. 5.1 Schematic representation of text (propositions with text-based model) using propositional analysis and its relationship to semantic structure and higher-level conceptual representation (situational model)

will lead to different interpretations of a patient's problem, leading to inconsistent diagnostic decisions. The details of the results show that expert physicians (Board certified in their domain of expertise), are able to separate relevant clinical information that can be used to inform the diagnostic decision-making process, from information that is not pertinent to this process. Non-experts remember considerably more information, but much of this is usually not relevant to the diagnostic decision at hand [26, 27]. Theories and methods of text comprehension have been widely used in the study of medical cognition and have been instrumental in characterizing the process of guideline development and interpretation (for examples see [30]).

Medical expertise is one of those areas of research where the importance of comprehension processes has been demonstrated [24]. Medical problem solving depends on understanding the problem because problem interpretation and analysis in medicine requires construction of appropriate clusters of information in long-term memory that match the current patient presentation. The construction-integration model was developed to account for the process of text comprehension [31, 32]. This model consists of a hybrid symbolic/connectionist architecture developed by Kintsch to account for the process of text comprehension. A model of diagnostic problem solving based on the construction-integration theory involves an interaction between the textbase and the long-term memory store, from which a situation model (Refer to Fig. 5.1) is derived through the cyclical process of construction and integration. A detailed account of how the construction-integration theory is used to explain some important aspects of expertise in medicine is given elsewhere [33]. The authors present a series of studies which serve as evidence for the validity of the construction-integration theory in accounting for the construction of schema during real-time diagnostic reasoning.

The study of medical cognition has been summarized in a series of articles [12, 34] and edited volumes (e.g., [35]). In more recent times, medical cognition is discussed in the context of informatics, generating a new field of investigation, cognitive informatics (for example, [13–15, 36]). Furthermore, foundations of cognition play a significant role in investigations of human computer interaction (HCI), including human factors and patient safety [37].

Clinical Cognition, Reasoning and the Evolution of AI

AI in medicine and medical cognition mutually influenced each other in several ways, including providing a basis for developing formal models of competence in problem-solving tasks. It is not necessary to replicate literally the human mind in order to exhibit intelligent behavior, and besides this may not always be desirable since human beings are error prone. However, in areas such as natural language understanding, commonsense reasoning and the ability to generalize effectively from small numbers of examples, human beings are still far superior to the best contemporary AI systems. Learning the mechanisms underlying these human abilities could lead to advances in AI. Using techniques and insights drawn from cognitive psychology, more robust and comprehensive AI systems could be built, resulting in models motivated not only by mathematics and a desire to optimize performance, but also by learning from the strengths of human psychology.

Early studies in linking clinical cognition to intelligent systems in medicine began with Anthony Gorry's series of studies in the 70s, comparing a computational model of medical problem solving with the actual problem-solving behavior of physicians [38]. Drawing on this work, others [10] developed a clinical program, where they were guided by the nature and organization of expert knowledge—which was a central concern to both developers of clinical expert systems and researchers in clinical cognition. Medical expert consultation systems, such as INTERNIST-1 [9] and MYCIN [39], introduced ideas about knowledge-based reasoning strategies across a range of cognitive tasks. MYCIN, in particular, had a substantial influence on studies in clinical cognition (see Chap. 2).

A landmark publication that significantly influenced clinical cognition is Newell and Simon's *Human Problem Solving* [40], relating human problem solving to research in artificial intelligence. It described a theoretical framework, extended a language for the study of cognition, and introduced protocol-analytic methods [41] that have become prevalent and dominant methods in investigations of high-level cognition, including the use of this framework for knowledge elicitation techniques in the development decision support systems. This work provided a foundation for the formal investigation of symbolic-information processing (problem solving) approaches.

Protocol analysis is among the most commonly used methods. It refers to a class of techniques for representing verbal **think-aloud protocols**, which are the most common source of data used in studies of problem solving. In these studies, subjects are instructed to verbalize their thoughts as they perform an experimental task. Ericsson and Simon [41] specify the conditions under which verbal reports are acceptable as legitimate data. Data collected during **retrospective think-aloud** protocols, where the subject has had the opportunity to reconstruct the information in memory (with potential for memory distortion), are considered suspect. Think-aloud protocols recorded while collecting observational data in context, provide rich data for the characterization of cognitive processes. In studies of expertise, Patel and colleagues used the think-aloud paradigm to generate sparse data, showing that the use of specific probes could constrain data collection, where subjects were asked to provide explanations for a patient's pathophysiological condition.

Bridging Cognition to Medical Reasoning

The study of expertise is one of the principal paradigms in problem-solving research, which has been documented in a number of volumes in the literature [42–45]. Comparing experts to novices provides us with the opportunity to explore the aspects of performance that undergo change and result in increased problem-solving skill. A goal of this approach has been to characterize expert performance in terms of the knowledge and cognitive processes used in comprehension, problem solving, and decision making, using carefully developed laboratory tasks [46].

The origin of medical problem-solving research on medical thinking is associated with the seminal work of Elstein and colleagues, who studied the problem-solving processes of physicians by drawing on then-contemporary methods and theories of cognition, based on psychology [11]. Their highly publicized research findings led to an elaborated model of **hypothetico-deductive reasoning**, which proposed that physicians reasoned by first generating and then testing a set of hypotheses to account for clinical data (i.e., reasoning from hypothesis to data). This model of problem-solving has had a substantial influence on studies of medical education. These authors were the first to use experimental methods and psychological theories to investigate problem solving in medicine. Patel and colleagues studied the knowledge-based solution strategies of expert cardiologists as evidenced by their **pathophysiological explanations** of a complex clinical problem [24]. The results indicated that expert physicians who accurately diagnosed the problem, employed a **forward (data-driven) reasoning** strategy—using patient data to lead toward a complete diagnosis (i.e., reasoning from data to hypothesis). This contrasts with subjects who misdiagnosed or partially diagnosed the patient problem. They tended to use a **backward or hypothesis-driven reasoning** strategy. Figure 5.2 shows a diagrammatic representation of data-driven reasoning. From the presence of puncture wound mark on the arm to a young unemployed male, (clinical findings on the *left side of figure*), the physician reasons forward to conclude the diagnosis of infection (*right side of the figure*). Figure 5.3 shows a representation of hypothesis-driven reasoning. When making the diagnosis of myxedema, the physician explains an inconsistent finding of respiratory failure to be the result of a hypometabolic state of the patient.

Although expert clinicians, in their own domain of expertise, typically use data-driven reasoning or general heuristics during clinical tasks, this type of reasoning sometimes breaks down, and the physician must resort to hypothesis-driven

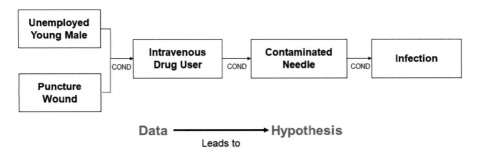

Fig. 5.2 A diagrammatic representation of data-driven reasoning when an unemployed young male presents with fever and a puncture wound mark on the arm. Presenting signs and symptoms through data-driven inferences, indicated likelihood of this patient being an intravenous drug user, with possible use of a contaminated needle, leading to infection. *COND* refers to a conditional relation, based on propositional analysis. Arrows indicate directionality

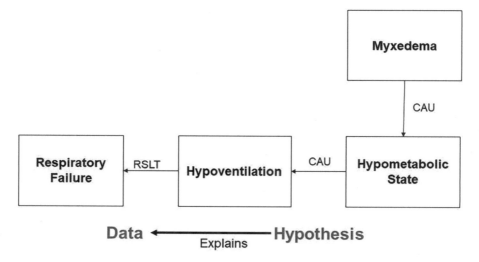

Fig. 5.3 A diagrammatic representation of hypothesis-driven reasoning. An anomalous finding of respiratory failure, which is inconsistent with the main diagnosis (myxedema), is accounted for as a result of a hypometabolic state of the patient, in a backward-directed inference. *CAU* indicates a causal relation, and *RSLT* identifies a resultive relation in propositional analysis. Arrows indicate directionality

reasoning. In everyday practice, both types of reasoning are used. Forward directed reasoning was found to be the hallmark of expertise, as shown in other knowledge-based domains, such as physics [47]. Although data-driven reasoning is highly efficient, it is often error-prone in the absence of adequate domain knowledge, since there are no built-in checks on the legitimacy of the inferences that a person makes. In contrast, hypothesis-driven reasoning is slower and may make heavy demands on working memory, because one must keep track of goals and hypotheses. It is, therefore, most likely to be used when there is uncertainty, domain knowledge is inadequate, or the problem is complex. This type of reasoning is not used in regular time-constrained practice because details interfere with the utility of efficient decision making. Other chapters in the book discuss the concepts of forward and backward chaining in systems (Chaps. 3 and 4). It should be noted that forward reasoning by expert systems consists of straightforward chaining of rules, whereas the forward reasoning of human experts invariably has missing steps in the inferencing process [28]. This indicates that forward reasoning may be generated by a process considerably more complex than the simple chaining of rules.

Hypothesis-driven reasoning is usually exemplary of a *weak method* of problem solving in the sense that is used in the absence of relevant prior knowledge and when there is uncertainty about a problem solution. In problem-solving terms, strong methods engage knowledge, whereas weak methods refer to general strategies that do not. Weak does not necessarily imply ineffectual in this context. Furthermore, hypothesis-driven reasoning may be more conducive to the novice learning experience in that it can guide the organization of knowledge [48]. Causal reasoning as part of the backward reasoning is an indispensable part of human thought, and it has been argued that formalizing it is a prerequisite to achieving human-level machine intelligence [49]. These types of reasoning relate to Kahneman's "fast" and "slow", models of reasoning [50], where the author proposes two types of reasoning corresponding to two different components of the human brain. There are identified as **System 1** and **System2**. System 1 processes information fast, but is slow to learn, since it learns through experience—often through sensory perception and pattern matching strategies—and it is error prone. System 2 processes information slowly, but is fast to learn. It learns from theory through explanatory processes with a logical inference engine, and is relatively reliable because it has built in error checks. This process is effortful and is triggered under uncertain conditions. The characterization of the two systems is not unlike the forward and backward reasoning in medical decision making developed by Patel and Groen and described above. The authors showed a formal relationship between comprehension and problem solving [51] in clinical medicine. The recognition of the relationship between the cognitive studies in clinical comprehension and problem solving, and AI dates back at least to 1991, when the two keynote presentations at the *Artificial Intelligence-Europe* meeting in Maastricht, Netherlands discussed the two topics and their synergies [28, 52]. These relationships show that collaboration among cognitive science, AI and neuroscience can produce an understanding of the mechanisms in the brain that generate human cognition. Thus, it is important to build AI systems with the ability to understand, think, reason and learn flexibly and rapidly, which will require deeper understanding of how the human mind functions as we do our tasks.

Models of Medical Reasoning

It is generally accepted there are two basic forms of reasoning: **deductive reasoning**, which in medicine consists of deriving a diagnosis (conclusion) from diagnostic category or a pathophysiological process (hypothesis). The other form is **inductive reasoning**, which consists of generating a diagnosis (conclusion), from patient data. However, reasoning in the "real world" does not fit neatly into any of these basic reasoning types. A third form of reasoning was identified as best capturing the generation of clinical hypotheses, where deduction and induction are intermixed. This is termed **abductive reasoning** [53], which is based in philosophy and is illustrated by the clinician generating a plausible explanatory hypothesis through a process of heuristic rule utilization (see for example, [54]).

Abductive reasoning is thought of as a cyclical process of generating possible explanations (i.e., identification of a set of hypotheses that are able to account for the clinical case on the basis of the available data) from a set of data and testing those explanations (i.e., evaluation of each generated hypothesis on the basis of its expected consequences) for the abnormal state of the patient at hand [11, 55–57]. Abductive reasoning is a data-driven process and dependent on domain knowledge. Within this generic framework, various models of diagnostic reasoning may be constructed. Following Patel and Ramoni [58], we can distinguish between two major models of diagnostic reasoning: **heuristic classification** [59] and **cover and differentiate** [60]. However, these models can be seen as special cases of a more general model: the **select and test** model [57], where the processes of hypothesis generation and testing can be characterized in terms of four types of processes: abstraction, abduction, deduction, and induction.

During **abstraction,** pieces of data in the data set are selected according to their relevance for the problem solution and chunked in **schemas** representing an abstract description of the problem at hand (e.g., abstracting that an adult male with hemoglobin concentration less than 14 g/dL is an anemic patient). Following this, hypotheses that could account for the current situation are related through a process of *abduction*, characterized by a "backward flow" of directed inferences. This model of reasoning can be used to explain the medical diagnostic process. Expert clinicians are selective in the data they collect (**abstraction**), focusing only on the data that are relevant to the generated hypotheses, while ignoring other less-relevant data [24, 27]. Successful clinicians focus on the fewest pieces of data and are better able to integrate these pieces of data into a coherent explanation for the problems [61]. Typically, physicians generate a small set of hypotheses very early in the case (**abduction**), as soon as the first pieces of data become available, as was first shown by Elstein's group [11], and later corroborated by other researchers (For example, [62, 63]). Physicians sometimes make use of the hypothetico-deductive process (**deduction**), which involves four stages: cue acquisition, hypothesis generation, cue interpretation, and hypothesis evaluation [11]. The reader is referred to the comprehensive summary of the research in clinical reasoning provided by Patel and colleagues in a recent book chapter [34]. The complex nature of clinical reasoning and decision making illustrates why is it so difficult to develop intelligent systems that can behave like human beings.

Knowledge Organization, Expert Perception and Memory

The discussion so far has focused more on expertise and the processes of diagnostic reasoning. Research has also revealed differences in knowledge representation with levels of expertise. A recurring finding from studies of expertise is that experts represent knowledge at a higher level of abstraction than their less experienced counterparts [64]. For example, Norman and colleagues investigated the ability of clinicians of different levels of dermatology expertise to make clinical diagnoses based on images presented as slides. Experts were more accurate in their diagnoses, and also exhibited a tendency to categorize slides at higher levels of abstraction. A similar finding was found in the study of expertise in radiology: less experienced subjects focused on surface anatomical features, while experienced radiologists developed deeper, more principled problem representations [65]. While this was not unexpected in *visual* domains of medicine, Patel and her colleagues identified an analogous difference in levels of abstraction in *verbal* problem solving, with expert physicians tending to represent case information from written scenarios at a higher level of abstraction than novice physicians [33]. Specifically, experts are distinguished by their emphasis on the *facet* level [66], which represents intermediate solutions to diagnostic problems. An example might be the cluster of symptoms associated with congestive cardiac failure—once these are recognized a specific *diagnosis* that explains the cause of the congestive cardiac failure can be sought. For experts, these facet-level pre-diagnostic hypotheses serve as intermediate steps in a diagnostic process, narrowing down the space of possible solutions to mediate effective problem solving. In addition, the aggregation of information into larger, meaningful units allows expert problem solvers to represent complicated cases within the laboratory-determined constraints on working memory capacity (famously, 7+-2 units of information) [67]. Such patterns of knowledge organization have immediate implications for the design of AIM systems. Adler-Milstein and her colleagues use the analogy of "wayfinding" to describe the use of AI to support the process of diagnosis by gathering, organizing and prioritizing information that is germane to the solution of a diagnostic problem [3]. How then, should the information be organized once gathered? The section on "AI, Machine Learning, and Human Cognition" considers how what is known about clinical knowledge organization and decision making might be used to guide this process.

Understanding Clinical Practice for AI Systems

The Role of Distributed Cognition

The work discussed in previous sections has focused on the cognitive processes of individual decision makers, often captured in laboratory experiments. However, toward the turn of the twenty-first century, a new paradigm of cognitive research emerged, known as **distributed cognition** [68]. Distributed cognition broadens the focus of cognitive research, moving from the study of individuals in laboratory settings to the study of groups of individuals at work in naturalistic environments. For example, Hutchins, a seminal figure in the field, conducted his influential work on navigation aboard naval vessels at sea [68]. A pragmatic advantage of this approach to research is that while representations in the mind (**internal representations**) cannot be observed directly, representations that occur in the work environment (**external representations**) can be recorded and studied. A famous example of an external representation concerns the "speed bug", a positionable plastic pointer that slides around the edge of the speedometer and can be used to demarcate appropriate landing speeds once these have been retrieved from a reference book [69]. This example is illustrative of a fundamental idea in distributed cognition: that an individual (or team of individuals) in a work environment constitute a composite cognitive system—a symbol processing system—with greater functionality than any of its individual components. From this perspective, the reference book of acceptable speeds is part of the long-term memory of the system, and the speed bug—a **cognitive artifact**—is part of its working memory [69]. In previous research, a significant paradigm shift was seen from a focus on individual cognition to collaborative and distributed cognition in healthcare. A special issue of the journal *AI in Medicine* included five original articles by prominent scholars that present complementary approaches to collaboration and distributed cognition in health and medicine, emphasizing situations where collaboration is between human and computer or facilitated by computers [70]. On account of the prominent role of cognitive artifacts such as whiteboards and different sorts of clinical notes in clinical practice, distributed cognition has proved to be an informative way to characterize such settings [71, 72], and identify opportunities to design tools that support their cognitive work [73].

As an illustrative example, Cohen and his colleagues used the distributed cognition paradigm to characterize the distribution of cognitive work in a psychiatry emergency department [71]. The work revealed ways in which cognition was distributed across teams and cognitive artifacts (such as written notes, see Fig. 5.4), and also over time, with these cognitive artifacts serving as bridges to maintain the continuity of cognitive tasks despite frequent staffing changes.

Considering a clinical environment from this perspective can lead to a more holistic picture of the ways in which AI technologies can offer support than the prevailing approaches of automated diagnostic decision making or prediction of adverse outcomes, including support for such cognitive tasks as information search, aggregation and synthesis [74].

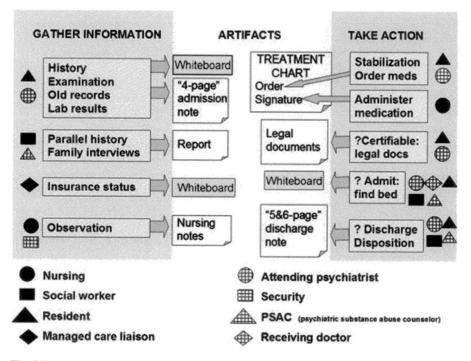

Fig. 5.4 Distribution of cognitive tasks in a psychiatric emergency department. The tasks, broadly categorized into information gathering tasks, and those involving actions taken on the basis of this information, are supported by a range of cognitive artifacts such as specific document types and the departmental whiteboard. Both the internal (mental) representations of the staff members and the external physical representations on these artifacts support the cognitive work required

AI, Machine Learning, and Human Cognition

The AI of today is a natural evolution of what we have seen over recent decades. For example, the deep neural networks currently used to classify images in radiology and other medical domains originated in the twentieth century [75, 76]. The changes, the reasons we are seeing AI in every aspect of life, appear to be less about AI advancement itself than they are about data generation and our current ability to leverage advanced computational power. However, there are certain barriers to the rapid growth of AI that are unlikely to be overcome by data and computational power alone. These barriers demonstrate that the path to the advancement of AI can be tricky and challenging. Present AI systems do not have a deep understanding— an understanding that integrates new observations with prior structured knowledge—but, rather, a shallow intelligence, that is the ability to emulate and, in the context of constrained tasks, sometimes even to improve upon some human pattern recognition and perception abilities. One cannot deny that there is intelligence in AI systems, but it does not follow the same rules as humans do.

The major goal of AI is to push forward the frontier of machine intelligence. Before going any further, it may be important to introduce a few terms. Machine learning and **deep learning** are two subsets of artificial intelligence which have garnered a lot of attention over the past few years. Many machine learning applications aim to allow computers to analyze and act with less human intervention by learning from training data. Deep learning—itself a type of machine learning— aims to support analyses that use multilayered structures inspired by the neural connectivity of the human brain (see Chap. 6). While many other machine learning methods require less training data and computing power than deep learning, deep learning methods typically need less human intervention because they have the capacity to learn useful representations of incoming data by themselves, obviating the need for these to be engineered manually. Deep learning can be viewed as a statistical technique for recognizing patterns in sample data, using neural networks with multiple layers, where there is an attempt at imitating (albeit superficially) the structure and function of neural networks in the human brain. An important advantage of deep neural networks is that they are able to learn useful representations while training. For example, in image processing a deep learning model may propagate data through different layers of the network, with each layer successively learning to recognize higher level image features that collectively suggest a label, as learned from training data. This is similar in some ways to how expert problem solvers work—using abstraction to relate their observations to previously learned hierarchies of concepts and relations in order to find an answer. However, there are important differences between these processes.

Consider the case of text comprehension. Human beings, as they process texts, frequently derive a wide range of inferences, as explained earlier. Deep learning currently struggles with open-ended inference based on real-world knowledge at the level of human accuracy [77]. Furthermore, human reasoners have the capability to explain the sequences of inferences that drive their decision making processes.

However, the propagation of representations from layer to layer of a deep neural networks, en route to a prediction, defies explanation in human terms. This transparency issue is a fundamental concern when using deep learning for problem domains like medical diagnosis, where clinicians need to understand how a given system made a decision. Problems that have to do with commonsense reasoning are usually outside the scope of deep learning. Human beings solve even simple problems by integrating knowledge across vastly disparate sources. In medicine these may include observational data, knowledge of clinical science, laboratory data and so forth. This is not true for the majority of deep learning models, which learn complex statistical correlations among input and output features, but with no inherent representation of causality or associated domain knowledge. We need to reach human-level cognitive flexibility if we are to see AI models reach human-like performance. These issues are well addressed in recent scholarly literature [77–79]. However, such flexible human-like performance is not a prerequisite to improving healthcare with AI. Contemporary AI methods can already perform constrained tasks with human-like accuracy, and have other capabilities—such as the ability to process large amounts of data quicky—that can be leveraged to support human decision makers.

Reinforcing the Human Component

Artificial intelligence is poised to transform the healthcare industry. By developing new data analytics, intelligent clinical systems can analyze large and varied data sets, and clinicians can easily access the information they need to deliver care to their patients. AI and **augmented intelligence** have similar goals but differ in the way of achieving them. Augmented intelligence is like AI in that both fields use machine learning to enhance performance. However, instead of replacing human intelligence, augmented intelligence aims to use AI methods to build upon it in an assistive role. This change in emphasis has broad implications. Technologies mediate human performance, and influence the way people behave as they interact with them. This goes beyond merely supporting, enhancing or expediting performance. Tools, and artifacts not only enhance people's ability to perform tasks but also change the way in which they do so. The following sections provide some examples of how AI systems can be used to augment human cognition in medicine.

Augmenting Clinical Comprehension

One approach to leveraging what is known about medical cognition to inform the design of AIM systems involves using approaches that deliberately emulate the knowledge organization of expert clinicians. As an illustrative example, Fig. 5.5 shows one of four views of a narrative text discharge summary (from a fictional

PSYCHOSIS	MOOD	SUBSTANCE	DANGER
• with Psychotic Features Schizoaffective Disorder PTSD	• past diagnoses including Bipolar Disorder	• against the wall and abusing opiate analgesics	• to kill herself by cutting her wrists
• about her agitation she claimed "the voices made me do it."	• from depression and having flashbacks	• and alcohol	• to a past sexual assault

PSYCHOSIS

HISTORY OF PRESENT ILLNESS:

1. with Psychotic Features Schizoaffective Disorder PTSD
2. about her agitation she claimed "the voices made me do it."
3. to take Risperdal but continued to endorse command AH
4. for safety saying "I don't know what the voices might make me do."

PAST PSYCHIATRIC HISTORY:

1. of paranoid ideation and command AH
2. on Haldol Zyprexa Risperdal Prozac Paxil Depakote

The patient has had a number of past diagnoses including Bipolar Disorder **with Psychotic Features Schizoaffective Disorder PTSD** and Borderline Personality Disorder

The patient had brought herself into the CPMC ER on March 2, 2002 with the chief complaint of hearing a voice commanding her to kill herself by cutting her wrists

She also stated at that time that she was suffering from depression and having flashbacks to a past sexual assault

She endorsed racing thoughts but denied change in energy sleep appetite and concentration

She denied SI or HI

She cites current stressors as her son not doing well in school and fights she has been having with her boyfriend

In the ER the patient was mostly calm and cooperative with the medical staff but became irritable and challenging with the security officers when asked to comply with their requests

When confronted **about her agitation she claimed "the voices made me do it."**

She agreed **to take Risperdal but continued to endorse command AH**

The staff felt that the patient may be malingering but she could not contract **for safety saying " I don't know what the voices might make me do "**

PAST PSYCHIATRIC HISTORY

Her physical exam and laboratory-test results were within normal limits except for a cardiac murmur

Her BAL was 0 and her UTOX was negative

The patient has a history of numerous psychiatric admissions since the age of 22 for complaints **of paranoid ideation and command AH** in the context of feeling depressed or "hyper."

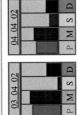

03 04 02	04 04 02
P M S D	P M S D

Fig. 5.5 View of a psychiatry discharge summary emphasizing psychosis-related elements. The summary was adapted from a text-based narrative developed in prior research, based on a case example from a textbook [80, 81]

patient encounter developed for research purposes) provided by a system that combines supervised machine learning with semantic word vector representations to draw connections between phrases in text and the diagnostically and prognostically important facet-level constructs of psychosis, mood, substance abuse and dangerousness [82, 83]. The figure shows a view that emphasizes phrases related to psychosis, such as those mentioning auditory hallucinations or paranoid ideation (as well as phrases mentioning antipsychotic medications such as Risperdal). Relevant phrases are also presented in the top and rightmost panels, and both these phrases and the four facets in the top panel serve as links to accommodate navigation, and switch perspective to emphasize the facet concerned. The interface also provides a graphical summary (bottom panel) of *other* narrative text records that indicates the extent to which content from each facet is represented, to facilitate exploration of historical narratives at a conceptual level that is conducive to problem solving. Evaluation of the interpretation of two case scenarios by 16 psychiatry residents revealed that the interface supported clustering of case-relevant information, with more detailed case recollection and better diagnostic accuracy in the more complex of the two scenarios when the interface was used [84]. In addition, residents using the interface better attended to clinically relevant elements of the case that had been neglected by non-expert participants in previous work [80], including important indicators of potential dangerousness to self and others. Qualitative evaluation of verbal think-aloud protocols captured during the process of exploring the cases using the interface revealed patterns of navigation used by residents to explore hypotheses at the facet level. These studies demonstrate the potential for AI to augment human decision making by simulating expert knowledge organization to reveal patterns in clinical data, rather than making decisions or predictions directly. From a distributed cognition perspective, the simulations of the knowledge and **retrieval structures**—structures that would typically support efficient decision making in the minds of the experts—are part of a larger cognitive system that includes residents, the interface and the AIM models that underlie it.

Supporting Specific Cognitive Tasks

The preceding section describes a system that was developed to support trainees (residents) by simulating knowledge organization and retrieval structures that are characteristic of expert medical cognition, and expertise in general. It is also possible to design systems to support the thought processes underlying a specific task, that have been characterized using cognitive methods. For example, Baxter and his colleagues describe the use of a **cognitive task analysis**—a systematic approach for collecting information about the mental processes underlying a particular task [85]—to inform the development of an expert system named FLORENCE to support decision making about ventilator settings in the context of neonatal respiratory distress [86]. This work involved a detailed characterization of the tasks, actors, communication events, documents and instruments in the neonatal intensive care unit concerned, resulting in a number of design implications for the system. These included practice recommendations for staff that identified contingencies in which the system's suggestions may be unreliable, the need for a distinctive alarm that would stand out from those already prevalent in the environment, and the incorporation of mnemonic devices already used by staff into the wording of the system's recommendations. These design implications were all informed by what had been learned about the cognitive capabilities of the team in the unit: their ability to recognize anomalous data that may lead to untrustworthy recommendations, the potential for their awareness of one alert to be drowned out by others, and the aids they use to remember procedural tasks developed to preemptively address potential causes of faulty readings that could mislead FLORENCE.

Mental Models of AI Systems

Interestingly, many of the design implications that emerged from the aforementioned cognitive task analysis concerned devising ways for human team members to recognize or preempt conditions under which an AIM system is likely to be incorrect. This requires having a mental model the system, akin to those shown to enhance learning to use devices in general [87]. Bansal and his colleagues provide empirical evidence that an accurate mental model of such conditions is fundamental to effective team performance in AI-advised decision making [88]. In these experiments, which were conducted with crowdsourced workers in the context of a simulated AI-advised task, better overall team performance was observed when using systems with error-prone conditions that were easier to understand because they depended upon fewer data features, and consistently led to a system error. The benefits of consistent model performance have also been shown in prior work by this group related to updating machine learning models, which was shown to have detrimental effects on overall team performance when it led to changes in decision-making on previously-observed examples [89]. These findings are also consistent with subsequent work showing that more accurate mental models of AI systems lead to better collaborative performance on word games [90]. Related work has investigated mediation of the development of accurate mental models of AI systems [91], and how such mental models are revised in response to surprising behavior [90]. While these findings mostly emerged from work outside the medical domain, they have clear implications for the development of AIM systems, and characterization of healthcare provider's mental models of AIM is an important area for future cognitive informatics research.

Conclusion

The influence of technology is not best measured quantitatively alone, since it is often qualitative in nature. The importance of cognitive factors that determine how human beings comprehend information, solve problems, and make decisions cannot be overstated. Investigations into the process of medical reasoning have been one such area where advances in cognitive science have made significant contributions to AI.

At the AI in Medicine conference in Amsterdam in 2009, researchers raised the question of whether we have forgotten about the role of the human mind as we perform our tasks in the evolution of AIM research [92]. This question is still salient today, perhaps more salient given that technological advances have surpassed our understanding of human behavior in such complex socio-technical environments. Today, a new question is whether we are getting the most out of our AIM inventions. It is time to reshape the current innovative technologies to serve human beings and augment our activities. In the clinical world, such augmented intelligence can provide clinicians with additional assistance they need to deliver a better quality of care for their patients.

Questions for Discussion

- Discuss, with examples, how the knowledge of cognitive science foundations can provide a better understanding of human-technology collaboration for developing contemporary AI systems for clinical practice. Can you think of principles of some of the component subfields of cognitive science that may also be valuable in such collaborative efforts?
- What are the ways to augment human intelligence for safer clinical practice, given what we know about current medical AI systems? Consider known limitations of human cognition, such as a propensity toward bias in diagnostic decision making and constraints on attentions span and working memory, how these limitations may manifest as vulnerabilities to medical error, and how AI methods may be used to preempt these patient safety concerns.
- Consider the potential and limitations of symbolic representation of knowledge in AI systems, and ways to circumvent these limitations with more contemporary approaches. Conversely, consider the limitations of contemporary deep learning models. How might the limitations of these approaches be addressed through incorporation of symbolic approaches, and vice versa?

Further Reading

Patel VL, Shortliffe EH, Stefanelli M, Szolovits P, Berthold MR, Bellazzi R, Abu-Hanna A. The coming of age of artificial intelligence in medicine. Artif Intell Med. 2009;46(1):5–17.

- The section on "Clinical Cognition, Reasoning and the Evolution of AI" of this paper argues for the importance of cognitive factors in the design of medical AI systems, and introduces many of the topics developed in this chapter.

Clark A. Natural-born cyborgs? International conference on cognitive technology. Berlin: Springer; 2001. p. 17–24.

- This book provides a readable introduction to the framework of distributed cognition, and its role in technology design.

Tschandl P, Rinner C, Apalla Z, Argenziano G, Codella N, Halpern A, Janda M, Lallas A, Longo C, Malvehy J, Paoli J, Puig S, Rosendahl C, Soyer HP, Zalaudek I,

Kittler H. Human–computer collaboration for skin cancer recognition. Nat Med. 2020;26(8):1229–34.

- This paper goes a step beyond establishing the benefits of the human-AI collaborative diagnosis in perceptual aspect of cognition, by investigating relationships between representation of AI output and diagnostic accuracy.

Patel VL, Kaufman DR. Cognitive science and biomedical informatics. In: Shortliffe EH, Cimino JJ, Chiang, M, editors. Biomedical informatics: computer applications in health care and biomedicine. 5th ed. Chap 4. New York: Springer; 2021.

- This chapter introduces cognitive research in healthcare and informatics, a discipline referred to as cognitive informatics. It presents the basic theoretical underpinnings of cognitive science with a focus on information-processing, natural language representation and distributed cognition frameworks.

References

1. Chan S, Siegel EL. Will machine learning end the viability of radiology as a thriving medical specialty? Br J Radiol. 2018;92(1094):20180416. https://doi.org/10.1259/bjr.20180416.
2. Jha S, Topol EJ. Adapting to artificial intelligence: radiologists and pathologists as information specialists. JAMA. 2016;316(22):2353–4. https://doi.org/10.1001/jama.2016.17438.
3. Adler-Milstein J, Chen JH, Dhaliwal G. Next-generation artificial intelligence for diagnosis: from predicting diagnostic labels to "wayfinding". JAMA. 2021;326(24):2467–8. https://doi.org/10.1001/jama.2021.22396.
4. Dreyer KJ, Geis JR. When machines think: radiology's next frontier. Radiology. 2017;285(3):713–8. https://doi.org/10.1148/radiol.2017171183.
5. Lakhani P, Sundaram B. Deep learning at chest radiography: automated classification of pulmonary tuberculosis by using convolutional neural networks. Radiology. 2017;284(2):574–82. https://doi.org/10.1148/radiol.2017162326.
6. Patel BN, Rosenberg L, Willcox G, Baltaxe D, Lyons M, Irvin J, Rajpurkar P, Amrhein T, Gupta R, Halabi S, Langlotz C, Lo E, Mammarappallil J, Mariano AJ, Riley G, Seekins J, Shen L, Zucker E, Lungren MP. Human–machine partnership with artificial intelligence for chest radiograph diagnosis. NPJ Digit Med. 2019;2(1):1–10. https://doi.org/10.1038/s41746-019-0189-7.
7. Hekler A, Utikal JS, Enk AH, Hauschild A, Weichenthal M, Maron RC, Berking C, Haferkamp S, Klode J, Schadendorf D, Schilling B, Holland-Letz T, Izar B, von Kalle C, Fröhling S, Brinker TJ, Schmitt L, Peitsch WK, Hoffmann F, et al. Superior skin cancer classification by the combination of human and artificial intelligence. Eur J Cancer. 2019;120:114–21. https://doi.org/10.1016/j.ejca.2019.07.019.
8. Tschandl P, Rinner C, Apalla Z, Argenziano G, Codella N, Halpern A, Janda M, Lallas A, Longo C, Malvehy J, Paoli J, Puig S, Rosendahl C, Soyer HP, Zalaudek I, Kittler H. Human–computer collaboration for skin cancer recognition. Nat Med. 2020;26(8):1229–34. https://doi.org/10.1038/s41591-020-0942-0.
9. Miller RA, Pople HE, Myers DJ. Internist-I, an experimental computer-based diagnostic for general internal medicine. In: Clancey WJ, Shortliffe EH, editors. Readings in medical artificial intelligence. Reading, MA: Addison-Wesley; 1984. p. 190–209.
10. Pauker SG, Gorry GA, Kassirer JP, Schwartz WB. Towards the simulation of clinical cognition: taking a present illness by computer. Am J Med. 1976;60(7):981–96. https://doi.org/10.1016/0002-9343(76)90570-2.

11. Elstein AS, Shulman LS, Sprafka SA. Medical problem solving: an analysis of clinical reasoning. Cambridge: Harvard University Press; 1978.
12. Patel VL, Arocha JF, Kaufman DR. Diagnostic reasoning and medical expertise. In: Medin DL, editor. The psychology of learning and motivation: advances in research and theory, vol. 31. San Diego: Academic Press, Inc.; 1994. p. 187–252.
13. Patel VL, Kaufman DR, Cohen T. Cognitive informatics in health and biomedicine: case studies on critical care, complexity and errors. London: Springer; 2014.
14. Patel VL, Kaufman D, Cohen T, editors. Cognitive informatics in health and biomedicine: case studies on critical care, complexity and errors with preface by Vimla L. Patel. London: Springer; 2014.
15. Patel VL, Kannampallil TG. Cognitive informatics in biomedicine and healthcare. J Biomed Inform. 2015;53:3–14.
16. Patel VL, Kaufman DR. Cognitive science and biomedical informatics. In: Shortliffe EH, Cimino JJ, Chiang M, editors. Biomedical informatics: computer applications in health care and biomedicine. 5th ed., Chap 4. New York: Springer; 2021.
17. Medler DA. A brief history of connectionism. Neural Comput Surveys. 1998;1:18–72.
18. Patel VL, Kaufman DR, Arocha JF. Steering through the murky waters of a scientific conflict: situated and symbolic models of clinical cognition. Artif Intell Med. 1995;7:413–38.
19. Patel VL, Kaufman DA, Arocha JF. Emerging paradigms of cognition and medical decision making. J Biomed Inform. 2002;35:52–75.
20. Kintsch W. Comprehension: a paradigm for cognition. Cambridge/New York: Cambridge University Press; 1998.
21. van Dijk TA, Kintsch W. Strategies of discourse comprehension. New York: Academic; 1983.
22. Frederiksen CH. Representing logical and semantic structure of knowledge acquired from discourse. Cogn Psychol. 1975;7(3):371–458.
23. Patel VL, Frederiksen CH. Cognitive processes in comprehension and knowledge acquisition by medical students and physicians. In: Schmidt HG, de Volder MC, editors. Tutorials in problem-based learning. Assen, Holland: van Gorcum; 1984. p. 143–57.
24. Patel VL, Groen GJ. Knowledge based solution strategies in medical reasoning. Cogn Sci. 1986;10(1):91–116.
25. Kintsch W. The representation of meaning in memory. Hillsdale, NJ: Lawrence Erlbaum Associates, Publishers. 1974.
26. Patel VL, Groen GJ. Developmental accounts of the transition from medical student to doctor: some problems and suggestions. Med Educ. 1991;25(6):527–35.
27. Patel VL, Groen GJ. The general and specific nature of medical expertise: a critical look. In: Ericsson KA, Smith J, editors. Toward a general theory of expertise: prospects and limits. New York: Cambridge University Press; 1991. p. 93–125.
28. Patel VL, Groen GJ. Real versus artificial expertise: the development of cognitive models of clinical reasoning. In: Stefanelli M, Hasman A, Fieschi M, Talmon J, editors. Lecture notes in medical informatics (44). Proceedings of the third conference on artificial intelligence in medicine. Berlin: Springer; 1991. p. 25–37.
29. Patel VL, Kaufman DR. Medical informatics and the science of cognition. J Am Med Inform Assoc JAMIA. 1998;5(6):493–502.
30. Peleg M, Gutnik LA, Snow V, Patel VL. Interpreting procedures from descriptive guidelines. J Biomed Inform. 2006;39:184–95.
31. Kintsch W. The role of knowledge in discourse comprehension: A construction integration model. Psychological Review. 1988;95:163–82.
32. Kintsch W, Welsch DW. The construction-integration model: a framework for studying memory for text. In: Hockley WE, Lewandowsky S, editors. Relating theory to data: essays on human memory in honor of Bennet Murdock. Hillsdale, NJ: Lawrence Erlbaum Associates; 1991. p. 367–85.
33. Arocha JF, Patel VL. Construction-integration theory and clinical reasoning. In: Weaver CA, Mannes S, Fletcher CR, editors. Discourse comprehension: essays in honor of Walter Kintsch; 1995. p. 359–81.

34. Patel VL, Kaufman DR, Kannampallil TG. Diagnostic reasoning and expertise in healthcare. In: Ward P, Schraagen JM, Gore J, Roth E, editors. The Oxford handbook of expertise: research & application. Oxford University Press; 2018.
35. Evans DA, Patel VL, editors. Cognitive science in medicine: biomedical modeling. Cambridge, MA: MIT Press; 1989.
36. Zheng K, Westbrook J, Kannampallil T, Patel VL, editors. Cognitive informatics: reengineering clinical workflow for more efficient and safer care. London: Springer; 2019.
37. Patel VL, Kaufman DR, Kannampallil TG. Diagnostic reasoning and decision making in the context of health information technology. In: Marrow D, editor. Reviews of human factors and ergonomics, vol. 8. Thousand Oaks, CA: Sage; 2013.
38. Gorry GA. Computer-assisted clinical decision-making. Methods Inf Med Suppl. 1973;7:215–30. PMID: 4617100.
39. Shortliffe EH. Computer-based medical consultations: MYCIN. New York: Elsevier; 1976.
40. Newell A, Simon HA. Human problem solving. Englewood Cliffs, NJ: Prentice-Hall. 1972.
41. Ericsson KA, Simon HA. Protocol analysis: verbal reports as data. Rev. ed. Cambridge, MA: MIT Press; 1993.
42. Ericsson KA. The road to excellence: the acquisition of expert performance in the arts and sciences sports and games. Mahwah: Lawrence Erlbaum Associates; 1996.
43. Ericsson KA. The Cambridge handbook of expertise and expert performance. Cambridge/New York: Cambridge University Press; 2006.
44. Ericsson KA, Smith J. Toward a general theory of expertise: prospects and limits. New York: Cambridge University Press; 1991.
45. Ericsson KA, Hoffman RR, Kozbelt A, Williams AM, editors. The Cambridge handbook of expertise and expert performance. Cambridge University Press; 2018.
46. Chi MTH, Glaser R. (1981). Categorization and representation of physics problems by experts and novices. Cognitive Science, 1981;5:121–52.
47. Larkin JH, McDermott J, Simon DP, Simon HA. Models of competence in solving physics problems. Cogn Sci. 1980;4(4):317–45. https://doi.org/10.1207/s15516709cog0404_1.
48. Patel VL, Evans DA, Kaufman DR. Reasoning strategies and use of biomedical knowledge by students. Med Educ. 1990;24:129–36.
49. Pearl J, Mackenzie D. The book of why: the new science of cause and effect. Basic Books; 2018.
50. Kahneman D. 35. Two selves. In: Thinking, fast and slow. New York: Farrar, Straus & Giroux; 2011.
51. Groen GJ, Patel VL. Relationship between comprehension and reasoning in medical expertise. In: Chi M, Glaser R, Farr M, editors. The nature of expertise. Hillsdale, NJ: Lawrence Erlbaum; 1988. p. 287–310.
52. Shortliffe EH. The adolescence of AI in medicine: will the field come of age in the 90s? Artificial Intelligence in Medicine 1993;5:93—106.
53. Peirce CS. Abduction and induction. In C. S. Peirce & J. Buchler (Eds.), Philosophical writings of Peirce. New York, NY: Dover; 1955a. pp. 150–6.
54. Magnani L. Abduction, reason, and science: processes of discovery and explanation. Dordrecht: Kluwer Academic; 2001.
55. Joseph GM, Patel VL. Domain knowledge and hypothesis generation in diagnostic reasoning. Med Decis Mak. 1990;10:31–46.
56. Kassirer JP. Diagnostic reasoning. Ann Intern Med. 1989;110:893–900.
57. Ramoni M, Stefanelli M, Magnani L, Barosi G. An epistemological framework for medical knowledge-based systems. IEEE Trans Syst Man Cybern. 1992;22(6):1361–75.
58. Patel VL, Ramoni MF. Cognitive models of directional inference in expert medical reasoning. In: Feltovich PJ, Ford KM, Hoffman RR, editors. Expertise in context: human and machine. Cambridge: The MIT Press; 1997. p. 67–99.
59. Clancey WJ. Heuristic classification. Artif Intell. 1985;27:289–350.
60. Eshelman L. MOLE: a knowledge acquisition tool for cover-and-differentiate systems. In: Marcus SC, editor. Automating knowledge acquistion for expert systems. Boston: Kluwer; 1988. p. 37–80.

61. Groves M, O'Rourke P, Alexander H. Clinical reasoning: the relative contribution of identification, interpretation and hypothesis errors to misdiagnosis. Med Teach. 2003;25(6):621–5. https://doi.org/10.1080/01421590310001605688. PMID: 15369910.
62. Feltovich PJ, Johnson PE, Moller JH, Swanson DB. The role and development of medical knowledge in diagnostic expertise. In: Clancey WJ, Shortliffe EH, editors. Readings in medical artificial intelligence: the first decade. Reading: Addison Wesley; 1984. p. 275–319.
63. Patel VL, Evans DA, Kaufman DR. Cognitive framework for doctor-patient interaction. In: Evans DA, Patel VL, editors. Cognitive science in medicine: biomedical modeling. Cambridge, MA: The MIT Press; 1989. p. 253–308.
64. Glaser R, Chi MTH, Farr MJ. The nature of expertise. Hillsdale, NJ: Lawrence Erlbaum Associates; 1988.
65. Lesgold A, Rubinson H, Feltovich P, Glaser R, Klopfer D, Wang Y. Expertise in a complex skill: diagnosing x-ray pictures. In: Chi MTH, Glaser R, Farr MJ, editors. The nature of expertise. Hillsdale: Lawrence Erlbaum Associates; 1988. p. 311–42.
66. Evans DA, Gadd CS. Managing coherence and context in medical problem-solving discourse. In: Evans DA, Patel VL, editors. Cognitive science in medicine: biomedical modeling. Cambridge, MA: MIT Press; 1989. p. 211–55.
67. Miller GA. The magic number seven plus or minus two: Some limits on our capacity for processing information. Psychological review. 1956;63:91–97.
68. Hutchins E. Cognition in the wild. Cambridge, MA: MIT Press; 1995.
69. Hutchins E. How a cockpit remembers its speeds. Cogn Sci. 1995;19:265–88.
70. Patel VL, editor. Distributed and collaborative cognition in health care: Implications for systems development. Special issue of Artificial Intelligence in Medicine. 1998;12(2).
71. Cohen T, Blatter B, Almeida C, Shortliffe E, Patel V. A cognitive blueprint of collaboration in context: distributed cognition in the psychiatric emergency department. Artif Intell Med. 2006;37:73–83.
72. Hazlehurst B, McMullen CK, Gorman PN. Distributed cognition in the heart room: how situation awareness arises from coordinated communications during cardiac surgery. J Biomed Inform. 2007;40:539–51.
73. Nemeth C, O'Connor M, Cook R, Wears R, Perry S. Crafting information technology solutions, not experiments, for the emergency department. Acad Emerg Med. 2004;11(11):1114–7. https://doi.org/10.1197/j.aem.2004.08.011.
74. Kannampallil TG, Franklin A, Mishra R, Almoosa KF, Cohen T, Patel VL. Understanding the nature of information seeking behavior in critical care: implications for the design of health information technology. Artif Intell Med. 2013;57(1):21–9. https://doi.org/10.1016/j.artmed.2012.10.002.
75. Fukushima K, Miyake S. Neocognitron: a self-organizing neural network model for a mechanism of visual pattern recognition. In: Competition and cooperation in neural nets. Berlin/Heidelberg: Springer; 1982. p. 267–85.
76. LeCun Y, Bottou L, Bengio Y, Haffner P. Gradient-based learning applied to document recognition. Proc IEEE. 1998;86(11):2278–324.
77. Marcus G. Deep learning: A critical appraisal. arXiv preprint arXiv:1801.00631. 2018.
78. Coiera E. The cognitive health system. Lancet. 2020;395(10222):463–66. https://doi.org/10.1016/S0140-6736(19)32987-3. Epub 2020 Jan 7. PMID: 31924402.
79. Kuang C. Can A.I. be taught to explain itself? The New York Times Magazine, Feature article. 2017. https://www.nytimes.com/2017/11/21/magazine/can-ai-be-taught-to-explain-itself.html.
80. Sharda P, Das AK, Cohen TA, Patel V. Customizing clinical narratives for the electronic medical record interface using cognitive methods. Int J Med Inform. 2006;75:346–68.
81. Spitzer RL, Gibbon ME, Skodol AE, Williams JBW. DSM-IV casebook: a learning companion to the diagnostic and statistical manual of mental disorders. 4th ed. American Psychiatric Association; 1994.
82. Cohen T. Augmenting expertise: toward computer-enhanced clinical comprehension. PhD dissertation. Columbia University; 2007.

83. Cohen T, Blatter B, Patel V. Simulating expert clinical comprehension: adapting latent seman- tic analysis to accurately extract clinical concepts from psychiatric narrative. J Biomed Inform. 2008;41(6):1070–87. https://doi.org/10.1016/j.jbi.2008.03.008.
84. Dalai VV, Khalid S, Gottipati D, Kannampallil T, John V, Blatter B, Patel VL, Cohen T. Evaluating the effects of cognitive support on psychiatric clinical comprehension. Artif Intell Med. 2014;62(2):91–104. https://doi.org/10.1016/j.artmed.2014.08.002.
85. Schraagen JM, Chipman SF, Shalin VL. Cognitive task analysis. Psychology Press; 2000.
86. Baxter GD, Monk AF, Tan K, Dear PRF, Newell SJ. Using cognitive task analysis to facilitate the integration of decision support systems into the neonatal intensive care unit. Artif Intell Med. 2005;35(3):243–57. https://doi.org/10.1016/j.artmed.2005.01.004.
87. Kieras DE, Bovair S. The role of a mental model in learning to operate a device. Cogn Sci. 1984;8(3):255–73. https://doi.org/10.1016/S0364-0213(84)80003-8.
88. Bansal G, Nushi B, Kamar E, Lasecki WS, Weld DS, Horvitz E. Beyond accuracy: the role of mental models in human-AI team performance. Proc AAAI Conf Hum Comput Crowdsourc. 2019;7:2–11.
89. Bansal G, Nushi B, Kamar E, Weld DS, Lasecki WS, Horvitz E. Updates in human-AI teams: understanding and addressing the performance/compatibility tradeoff. Proc AAAI Conf Artif Intell. 2019;33(01):2429–37. https://doi.org/10.1609/aaai.v33i01.33012429.
90. Gero KI, Ashktorab Z, Dugan C, Pan Q, Johnson J, Geyer W, Ruiz M, Miller S, Millen DR, Campbell M, Kumaravel S, Zhang W. Mental models of AI agents in a cooperative game setting. In: Proceedings of the 2020 CHI conference on human factors in computing systems. Association for Computing Machinery; 2020. p. 1–12. https://doi.org/10.1145/3313831.3376316.
91. Kulesza T, Stumpf S, Burnett M, Kwan I. Tell me more? The effects of mental model sound- ness on personalizing an intelligent agent. In: Proceedings of the SIGCHI conference on human factors in computing systems; 2012. p. 1–10. https://doi.org/10.1145/2207676.2207678.
92. Patel VL, Shortliffe EH, Stefanelli M, Szolovits P, Berthold MR, Bellazzi R, Abu-Hanna A. The coming of age of artificial intelligence in medicine. Artificial Intelligence in Medicine. 2009;46:5–17.

Chapter 6
Machine Learning Systems

Devika Subramanian and Trevor A. Cohen

After reading this chapter, you should be able to answer the following questions:

- What types of problems are suitable for machine learning?
- What are the steps in the design of a machine learning workflow for a clinical prediction problem?
- What are key techniques for transforming multi-modal clinical data into a form suitable for use in machine learning?
- What limitations in model-building arise from just using observational data? How does the use of prospective data mitigate some of these limitations?
- What are some examples of biases in observational data?
- What is feature engineering and when is it required?
- When is it appropriate to use an ensemble model instead of a single global model?
- What are the challenges in deploying machine learned models in clinical decision-making settings?

D. Subramanian (✉)
Rice University, Houston, TX, USA
e-mail: devika@rice.edu

T. A. Cohen
University of Washington, Seattle, WA, USA
e-mail: cohenta@uw.edu

© The Author(s), under exclusive license to Springer Nature
Switzerland AG 2022
T. A. Cohen et al. (eds.), *Intelligent Systems in Medicine and Health*, Cognitive
Informatics in Biomedicine and Healthcare,
https://doi.org/10.1007/978-3-031-09108-7_6

Identifying Problems Suited to Machine Learning

The exponential growth of a diverse set of digital health data sources (as described in Chap. 3) has opened new opportunities for data-driven modeling and decision-making in clinical medicine. These data sources including electronic health records (EHRs); large de-identified health datasets such as Medical Information Mart for Intensive Care (MIMIC) [1], which contains lab tests and time series of vital signs from Intensive Care Units (ICUs); the Cancer Genome Atlas (TCGA [2]), which includes imaging as well as proteomic and genomics data; and longitudinal, nationwide EHR datasets aggregated by companies such as Cerner. Machine learning is a critical enabling technology for analyzing and interpreting these massive data sources to support and improve clinical decision-making. Recent successes in machine learning have mainly focused on image-based predictive diagnostics: diabetic retinopathy [2], classification of skin cancer lesions [3], and identification of lymph node metastases in breast cancer [4] (see Chap. 12). Contemporary machine learning methods provide the means to go beyond these successes by exploiting the full range of data sources available today, including geno-type sequencing, proteomics and other -omics data, data from wearable devices such as continuous glucose monitors, from health apps on smartphones, and from patients' social media interactions (including text data). By integrating them with other classical data sources, physicians can leverage rich, time-indexed, multimodal representations of patients. Standardized frameworks such as the **Observational Medical Outcomes Partnership (OMOP** [5])[1] common data model for encoding disparate data types, make it possible to incorporate diverse data sources into a machine learning workflow.

There are two broad classes of problems that can be solved using machine learning: (1) *prediction problems* involving probabilistic estimation of a diagnosis, outcome of a therapy modality. risk of developing a disease, or disease progression from observational patient data; and (2) *probabilistic modeling* involving estimation of joint distributions of clinical variables from observational and interventional data, which can then be used to make "what-if" inferences to answer questions such as "will adding a specific therapeutic intervention reduce risk of hospital readmission?". **Supervised machine learning** models solve prediction problems. They learn mappings between predictor variables and outcome variables from paired associational training data that take the form (predictors, outcomes). A typical example might involve assigning a diagnostic label to a radiological image (predictors: pixels; outcomes: diagnoses). Training such models requires sets of predictors labeled with the outcomes of interest. **Unsupervised machine learning** models find patterns between a collection of clinically relevant variables, without the need for explicitly labeled data. Examples of patterns include finding phenotypic clusters and dimensionality reduction by inferring latent factors of variation among a large collection of variables.

The focus of the current chapter is on supervised machine learning models. This class of machine learning models currently predominates in AIM applications for tasks such as diagnosis assignment and outcome prediction. The discussion makes

---

[1] https://www.ohdsi.org/data-standardization/the-common-data-model/. (accessed August 19, 2022)

assumptions about the reader's knowledge of pertinent mathematics and notational conventions. Those who lack the requisite background may wish to focus on the conceptual aspects of the discussion rather than the mathematical details.[2]

There are unique technical challenges and opportunities that arise in defining solvable problems in the healthcare context. In setting up a prediction model, one needs to consider carefully the following: (1) *The prediction target*: what is to be predicted, (2) *Technical feasibility of prediction*: is it predictable at all, (3) *Economic feasibility of prediction*: is it worth predicting in the context of the clinical workflow, and (4) *Information source selection*: from what information sources can the prediction be made.

For example, consider the problem of determining the optimal time to insert a left ventricular assist device (LVAD—a surgically implanted artificial pump that assists the heart in circulating blood throughout the body) in a patient with chronic heart failure. The standard of care for LVAD insertion defines the optimal insertion time to be when the "pumping life" of the heart is estimated to be approximately 1 year. The prediction problem is then reduced to a mortality estimation problem—what is the probability of a patient's survival for 1 year given various clinical assessments of the heart's mechanical and electrical efficacy, coupled with a broad range of laboratory assessments on the condition of other vital organs. This prediction problem is solved routinely by expert cardiologists, so there is evidence that it is a solvable problem. Unfortunately, not all LVAD insertion decisions made by experts lead to optimal patient outcomes, which opens the possibility of machine learning analysis of this decision problem. The informational basis for prediction can initially be set to all the records reviewed by the expert cardiologist in making the LVAD insertion decision. Training data can be assembled from a retrospective study of EHR records containing all the relevant information (such as arterial blood pressure, EKG findings and ultrasound studies of cardiac function) together with the correct final go/no-go insertion decision. Note that the variable to predict is the *correct* decision, not necessarily the decision made by any individual doctor. The correct decision needs to be validated with information on the patient *after* the LVAD procedure, or by an expert committee. A predictive supervised machine learning model can extract probabilistic patterns to predict appropriate times for LVAD insertion from the curated dataset, in effect summarizing the experiences of the most successful expert cardiologists.

Defining outcome and predictor variables for a prediction problem can be tricky. One problem is that information about the outcome variable can be leaked through the predictors. Consider predicting diabetic ketoacidosis (DKA)[3] in a pediatric Type 1 diabetes[4] patient based on data gathered from the EHR, including demographic

---

[2] Introductory material on the pertinent mathematical details (e.g., probability theory, linear algebra, calculus) is provided in the suggested readings at the end of this chapter.

[3] DKA is a serious complication of diabetes resulting from the buildup of fatty acid byproducts called ketones in the bloodstream, with dangerous increases in blood acidity if untreated.

[4] Type 1 diabetes tends to arise first in children and requires treatment with insulin. The type of disease that arises in adults, who are often overweight, is Type 2 diabetes and can often be treated with medications rather than insulin.

information, lab tests, antibody titers, insulin dosing and modality. A supervised machine learning model built from retrospective patient data predicts that high values of beta-hydroxy-butyrate are predictive of DKA. Unfortunately, beta-hydroxy-butyrate is measured only for patients with DKA and is used in monitoring and management of that condition. By using beta-hydroxy-butyrate as a predictor, the answer has inadvertently been revealed to the algorithm.

Missing values in predictor variables pose a fresh set of challenges. Not all supervised learning methods can handle missing values. Those that cannot then drop data points, leading to models built on fewer samples, which may not be statistically robust. A further complication is the nature of missing data—was a measurement randomly omitted, or omitted for a specific cohort as in the beta-hydroxy-butyrate example above? Similarly, is there limited representation of specific demographic groups in the database, reflecting human biases in data collection that could yield large errors in prediction for that subgroup? Compensating for these biases in the construction of training data sets is essential for a successful machine learning project, and a detailed account of the origin of missing values in clinical data and methods to manage them is provided in Chap. 11.

The Machine Learning Workflow: Components of a Machine Learning Solution

This chapter seeks to introduce principles and mechanics of building data-driven predictive machine learning models for healthcare applications. At the heart of the process is the clinical question that needs answering, for it drives the selection of both the data and the machine learning model. Formulating clinical questions appropriate for data-driven machine learning analysis is still an art. One typically cycles through the steps shown in Box 6.1: specification of the clinical question, data source selection, data extraction and transformation, model specification and construction, model validation, and incorporation of the model into a clinical workflow.

Box 6.1 Steps in a Typical Workflow for Data-Driven Predictive Modeling in Healthcare
- **Step 0:** Specify the clinical question that needs to be answered
- **Step 1:** Identify data sources relevant to answering that question
- **Step 2:** Extract and transform raw data from the original sources into a form needed for analysis by specific machine learning (ML) algorithms
- **Step 3:** Select a suitable algorithm and build a model, ensuring appropriate choice of algorithm hyper-parameters
- **Step 4:** Validate model predictions; checking for robustness and going back to the earlier steps in the workflow, if warranted
- **Step 5:** Incorporate model into clinical workflow with a human-centered approach, and construct system-level impact assessments

Here is a specific example of a predictive modeling workflow.

- **The clinical question**: Is the risk of developing DKA in the next 3 months for a teenage, white, pediatric Type 1 diabetes patient with an HbA1c[5] increase of 1 point (from 7 to 8) over the last 3 months high enough to warrant an intervention? Which of the two following interventions is likely to be more successful—a social worker visit to ensure insulin compliance or an increase in insulin dosing?
- **The data sources**: Taking a data-driven perspective on this question would involve retrieving, from the EHR database, pertinent information on all Type 1 diabetes patients with similar demographic and clinical profiles, and examining the percentage of times interventions were applied, and their relative success, to recommend an evidence-based solution. While modern-day database tools allow easy retrieval of records from the EHR, the definitions of similar demographic and clinical profiles must be chosen carefully with an expert endocrinologist's help. For example, should gender be included in the demographic profile? Which lab tests are the most relevant to determine similarity in clinical profiles? Are there genetic markers available to risk-stratify patients? Predictive modeling is a collaboration between expert human beings and the machine, with the human expert providing nuanced decision criteria for cohort selection and the machine performing detailed analysis on expert-defined patient cohorts.
- **Data extraction and transformation**: Transforming raw clinical data into analysis-ready data sets can be challenging. This is primarily because the goal of data collection in hospitals is to support care and to manage costs and payments, and not necessarily to enable retrospective or predictive analyses. For structured fields, values may be missing or entered incorrectly. Further, approaches to handle time-series data sampled at different time scales are needed. There can also be wide variation in formats of unstructured data such as free text clinical notes. Since most machine learning algorithms take tabular data (two-dimensional arrays) or multi-dimensional arrays as input, data must be represented in these forms to be processed by these algorithms.
- **Model specification and construction**: In this example, the goal is to quantify the statistical association (if any) between risk of DKA in the next 3 months and the demographic and clinical profile of Type 1 diabetes patients. If there are enough patients in our analysis cohort, a supervised ML algorithm can be used to identify the probabilistic patterns that relate available predictors to DKA risk. In addition, it may be of value to know if there is a relationship between patient profiles and effectiveness of a specific type of intervention. Such associational queries can be easily answered using a range of supervised learning algorithms, which are covered in this chapter. Demographic and clinical data for pediatric

---

[5] HbA1c stands for Hemoglobin A1c, which reflects average blood sugar levels over the past 2–3 months.

Type 1 diabetes patients can be assembled from the EHR. These can be combined with patient data on interventions and their outcomes. From such a dataset, it is possible to build a simple logistic regression model to predict the probability of success of a specific intervention given a patient's profile. More sophisticated models to capture nonlinear interactions between predictors and outcomes, such as **gradient boosted decision trees**, can also be built if there are sufficient data to build them. Ultimately, an end-to-end machine learning pipeline (whose structure is dictated by the nature of the problem/data) is built and compared against a simple baseline model (such as a logistic regression). The pipeline is refined by evaluating whether it *overfits* or *underfits* the data (see section on "Bias and Variance"), and either reduce the number of parameters in the model or add more data (data augmentation) to support robust learning of model parameters.

- **Model validation**: Once a predictive model is constructed, there is a need to assess its performance on new (as yet unseen) data. In a retrospective study, a randomly selected portion of the available data (typically 20%), called the **test set**, is set aside and the remaining 80% is used to train the model. For classification problems, it is possible to use several performance measures. A detailed presentation of some widely-used performance metrics is provided in the next section on "Evaluating machine learning models: validation metrics". These metrics can be calculated over the set-aside test data to get an unbiased estimate of the performance of the trained model. With a prospective study, a new test set can be constructed by retrieving fresh data from the EHR to evaluate the performance of the model. A very important principle in model validation is to ensure that the *training and test sets are kept separate*—that is, the test set is not inadvertently used in the training process (for example, to select algorithm parameters). Model configuration may be accomplished with a held-out subset of the **training set** that is often referred to as a **validation set**. The test set estimates performance of the model on "unseen" data. The training set can be viewed as the analog of the "homework problem set" in human learning, and the test set serves as the "exam". Clearly, using problems identical to the homework in the exam provides an overoptimistic estimate of the model's (the student's) predictive performance. The choice of evaluation metric is also key and reflects priorities in the clinical use context—e.g., is it more important to avoid false negatives (failing to predict future DKA, leading to a missed opportunity of diagnosis) or to minimize false positives (incorrectly predicting future DKA, potentially leading to overtreatment).

- **Incorporation into clinical workflow and system-level assessment**: While having a predictive model with strong performance is a necessary component, it is unfortunately not all that is needed for clinical impact. One needs to determine where to inject the model's predictions in the workflow of a pediatric endocrinologist for maximal impact on patient outcomes. Human factor considerations play a critical role in the design of the user interface through which the model's decisions as well as its explanations are presented to the doctor (see Chap. 17). The final impact of the model can be estimated at the health system level with measures such as reduction in DKA admissions over a given time frame. While the discussion of validation here is focused on measures of accuracy, the reader is referred to Chap. 17 for a holistic account of evaluation that considers other important aspects such as system integration, usability, and eventual clinical outcomes.

Evaluating Machine Learning Models: Validation Metrics

A broad range of evaluation metrics are widely used to measure the performance of machine learning algorithms. While an exhaustive account of these metrics is not provided in this chapter, some of the most commonly applied ones are introduced, as well as some principles to consider when interpreting them. These metrics are introduced using the schematic representation of the results of a two-class classification system shown in Fig. 6.1.

Recall (Sensitivity) Recall measures the proportion of testing examples in the positive class that have been correctly identified by the model. This corresponds to the estimation of the *sensitivity* of a test in medicine (e.g., what proportion of cases of a disease in a population are detected by a laboratory test), and this term may be more familiar to a clinical audience. As is the case with some of the other metrics here, recall can be derived from the cells of a 2 × 2 table with cells corresponding to counts of correctly (true positive and true negative) and incorrectly (false positive

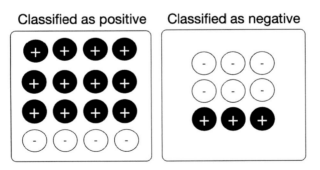

Fig. 6.1 Illustration of a possible output from a two-class classifier with an evaluation set of 25 examples, 15 of which are in the positive class (+), and 10 of which are in the negative class (−). Note that the classifier is imperfect, in that 4 members of the negative class have been classified as positive and 3 members of the positive class have been classified as negative

and false negative) classified examples. However, a straightforward way to think of recall is as the proportion of all the positive cases that were correctly identified by the model:

$$\frac{number\ of\ correctly\ classified\ positive\ examples}{total\ number\ of\ positive\ examples}$$

In the example in Fig. 6.1, recall would be estimated as 12/15 = 0.8.

Precision (Positive Predictive Value) It follows from the definition of recall that it is not affected by the number of negative examples that are incorrectly classified as positive cases (so-called false positives—the bottom row of the left panel in Fig. 6.1). However, it is also important to know what proportion of the ostensibly positive cases identified by a machine learning classifier were correctly identified. For example, a diagnostic system that falsely identifies many cases of a disease that then require extensive follow-up may do more harm than good, both at the individual and the societal level. Precision measures the proportion of a model's positive predictions that were true, and can be defined as:

$$\frac{number\ of\ correctly\ classified\ positive\ examples}{total\ number\ of\ classified\ positive\ examples}$$

Precision can be estimated from the leftmost panel of Fig. 6.1 as 12/16 = 0.75.

Precision corresponds to the *positive predictive value* of a clinical test—what proportion of people with a positive test truly have the condition it is intended to detect.

It is worth considering the trade-off between recall and precision. Given that machine learning classifiers often use a threshold (e.g., probability > 0.5) to assign discrete classes based on a probabilistic estimate, one might imagine simply setting this threshold to optimize for recall (by setting a low threshold such that most everything is classified as positive), or for precision (by setting a high threshold, such that the model only classifies examples it is very confident about as positive cases). In some circumstances, such as when the risk of missing a diagnosis is tolerable whereas the next step after automated detection is an invasive and expensive examination, precision may be more important than recall. In a screening scenario where it is desirable to detect most instances of a disease in the population, and a sequence of follow-up tests with greater precision is readily available, recall may be key. As such, the optimal performance characteristics of a machine learning model may vary depending upon how the predictions it makes will be used. Also, this trade-off suggests it may not be particularly meaningful to consider precision or recall in isolation.

The F-measure The F-measure evaluates performance by balancing precision against recall. With the most widely used variant of this measure, known as the F1

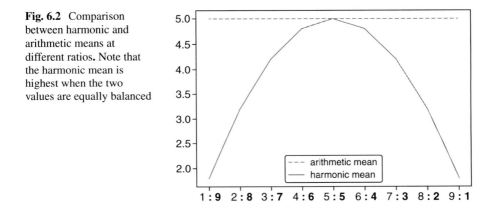

Fig. 6.2 Comparison between harmonic and arithmetic means at different ratios. Note that the harmonic mean is highest when the two values are equally balanced

measure, there is an equal balance between these two components. The F1 measure is the *harmonic mean*[6] between precision (p) and recall (r), which can be defined as follows:

$$F1(p,r) = \frac{2}{1/p + 1/r} = \frac{2}{(p+r)/pr} = \frac{2pr}{p+r}.$$

The implications for combining two metrics are that the harmonic mean rewards balanced combinations. The harmonic mean will be highest when p and r are relatively close together, and lowest when they are relatively far apart. Figure 6.2 illustrates that unlike the typically used arithmetic mean, the optimal harmonic mean of two values that sum to ten occurs when they are perfectly balanced. Likewise, the optimal F score will reflect a balance between precision and recall.

However, there may be tasks in which a perfect balance between precision and recall is not the optimal configuration. The F1 measure is the balanced form of the F-measure, which can be more generally formulated as follows:

$$F(p,r) = \frac{(1+\beta^2)pr}{\beta^2 p + r}$$

---

[6]The name 'harmonic' concerns the musical relationships that emerge from applying this mean to tonal frequencies. For example, the frequency of "middle C" is ~261.6 Hz, and that of the C above this ~523.3 Hz (about double). The harmonic mean of these frequencies is ~348.8 Hz, which is represented by "F" (albeit only approximately on evenly tempered keyboard instruments), the next point of harmonic progression when traversing the cycle of fourths.

The β parameter permits modification of the measure. For example, the F2 measure with $\beta = 2$ penalizes precision more heavily than recall, because the effects of precision on the denominator are multiplied by four, decreasing the overall score.

While the F measure effectively balances precision against recall (with the capability to shift emphasis), predictive models for classification generally produce a measure of confidence in their prediction—a *probability* that a test case falls into a particular category. Categories are assigned when this probability exceeds some threshold. Simply evaluating based on assigned categories discards information about the probabilistic estimates concerned. With a threshold of 0.5, a test case assigned a category-related probability of 0.6 and another assigned a probability of 0.9 would be treated identically when evaluating the model. However, it is often desirable to compare model performance across the full range of possible thresholds, without discarding these differences in a model's confidence in its predictions.

Measures Derived from Performance Curves This comparison can be accomplished by comparing the area under curves that measure performance characteristics of interest. Two widely used metrics of this nature are the area under the receiver operating characteristic curve (AUROC), and the area under the precision recall curve (AUPRC). Both of these metrics are estimated across a range of possible threshold values, effectively assessing model performance irrespective of the threshold chosen for category assignment.

The AUROC measures the area under a curve that is typically plotted as the sensitivity (recall) (y-axis) against the false positive rate—the proportion of all negative examples that have been misclassified as positive (x-axis).

In contrast the AUPRC measures the area under a curve that is typically plotted as the precision (y-axis) against the recall of a model (x-axis).

To illustrate these measures, consider a classification task with 10 positive test cases amongst 1000 in total.[7] Based on model output, the positive cases have been ranked among the 1000 cases, and the recall, precision, and false positive rate at the rank of each example is shown in Table 6.1.

Note in particular the *denominator* when calculating precision (number of predicted positives) and the false positive rate (number of negative examples). With precision, the denominator increases with recall. Moving down the ranked list of model predictions, each correctly classified positive example comes at the cost of many false positive results. On account of the class imbalance in the dataset these increases in the denominator result in substantial drops in precision with each positive example that is correctly classified. In contrast, the denominator of the false positive rate is constant, at 990—the number of negative examples. The false positive rate therefore increases gradually while working down the long list of negative examples.

---

[7]This presentation is inspired by Hersh's account of ranked retrieval evaluations [6].

Table 6.1 Performance characteristics of a hypothetical classifier

Rank	Recall	Precision (of predicted positives)	False positive rate (of 990 negative examples)
1	0.1 = 1/10	1.0 = 1/1 (all true positives)	0 (all true positives)
5	0.2 = 2/10	0.4 = 2/5	0.003 ≅ 3/990
15	0.3 = 3/10	0.2 = 3/15	0.012 ≅ 12/990
17	0.4 = 4/10	0.24 ≅ 4/17	0.013 ≅ 13/990
24	0.5 = 5/10	0.21 ≅ 5/24	0.019 ≅ 19/990
100	0.6 = 6/10	0.06 = 6/100	0.095 ≅ 94/990
191	0.7 = 7/10	0.04 ≅ 7/191	0.186 ≅ 184/990
300	0.8 = 8/10	0.03 ≅ 8/300	0.295 ≅ 292/990
488	0.9 = 9/10	0.02 ≅ 9/488	0.483 ≅ 479/990
1000	1.0 = 10/10	0.01 = 10/1000	1.0 = 990/990 (all false positives)

This disparity is illustrated in Fig. 6.3, in which the AUPRC and AUROC for these results are compared. In both cases the area under the curve is invariant to which value is assigned to the x-axis, and also the two graphs have a value in common—the model recall. Therefore, for illustrative purposes the assignment of axes for the AUPRC is reversed, such that recall occupies the x-axis in both graphs. To map between the graph and Table 6.1 move up the y axis (recall) while moving from top to bottom of the table. As the proportion of positive examples that are correctly classified increases, the corresponding part of the AUPRC (the area under the orange PR curve) drops precipitously as the PR curve moves rapidly leftward while the corresponding AUROC (the area under the blue ROC curve) rises gradually as the corresponding ROC curve moves slowly to the right.

Supervised Machine Learning

This section describes some of the key approaches and algorithms used in supervised machine learning. It is not intended to be an exhaustive account of these methods. More information can be found in one of the detailed and widely used textbooks of machine learning already available as resources, and several are suggested for further reading at the conclusion of this chapter. Rather, the goals in introducing these methods are first to familiarize the reader with standard nomenclature and notation used in machine learning, thereby eliminating a potential barrier to further exploration of related literature; and second to explain through illustration some fundamental concepts that relate to machine learning in general and must be understood before these methods can be applied in a principled manner. The key concepts that are developed during the course of the illustration of selected methods include the notion of a machine learning model with pliable parameters that can be fit to training data in order to make predictions; how training objectives can be configured to emphasize data points of greater predictive utility; and—of particular importance

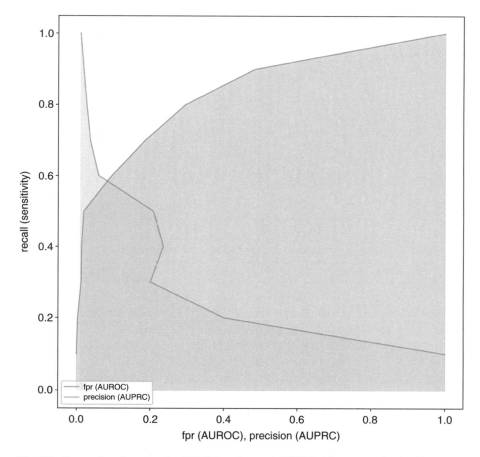

Fig. 6.3 Comparison between the AUROC and rotated AUPRC. The area under the blue curve shows the AUROC, and the area under the orange curve the AUPRC. The main contribution to the area under this orange curve occurs at low recall values (the bottom 20% of the y-axis)—precision drops precipitously as new positive examples are identified, because each of these carries the baggage of many negative examples in an imbalanced set. In contrast, the area under the blue AUROC curve continues to increase gradually throughout the full range of recall values, with larger changes to the false positive rate (fpr) delayed until around half of the positive examples have been identified

to supervised learning—the inherent trade-off between the ability of a model to conform to its training data and its ability to generalize to data outside of this training set. The general discussion offered is pertinent to applications in healthcare and biomedicine, as well as to other domains.

Machine learning is essentially an automated search for meaningful patterns in data. Traditional computational systems map inputs to outputs according to manually specified and programmed decision rules. In the clinical context, such systems are rigid and require frequent updates to accommodate changes in standard of care and/ or evolution of the understanding of disease. The promise of machine learning is the automatic inference of general decision rules from lots of specific examples of decision-making in a variety of contexts. It mirrors the residency phase of training of clinicians where clinically useful rules and patterns are learned directly by observation and integrated with those learned during didactic classroom learning. With retraining on suitable new data as they emerge, a machine learning system can adapt to new experiences and new examples without the need for explicit reprogramming.

The Structure of a Supervised Machine Learning Algorithm

In order to approach the topic of machine learning, it is necessary to become familiar with some notational conventions that are standard in the field (Box 6.2). This section illustrates the use of these conventions to describe a simple machine learning algorithm. It also introduces the fundamental concept of a **loss function**, a function that measures the extent to which a machine learning model conforms to its training data, and the **gradient descent** algorithm to achieve this end.

Box 6.2 Notational Conventions
- x: a feature of a data point, such as a patient's HbA1C level
- **x**: (**boldface**) a vector made up of individual features for a data point
- X: the entire set of data points, such as a set of patients
- y: a label attached to a data point, e.g., 1 indicating "developed DKA"
- Y: the set of labels for the entire set of data points
- θ: the parameters of a model, e.g., the coefficients of a regression model
- *argmin*: the arguments that minimize some function, e.g., the parameters that minimize the difference between predicted and actual values for a data set
- $\|x\|$: the vertical lines indicate the length (or norm) of the vector x
- x^{T}: the superscript "T" indicates the transpose of the vector x—for example, the transpose of a row vector becomes a column vector
- $x_1^{\mathrm{T}}x_2$: shorthand for the scalar (or "dot") product between two vectors, x_1 and x_2. This is calculated by multiplying the values in corresponding coordinates, and summing up the total

---

The simplest example of a machine learning algorithm is finding the least-squares line that fits given (x,y) points on the plane. The training data for the algorithm consists of pairs of real numbers (x,y), and the pattern or model to be found is a line represented by the equation $y = \theta_1 x + \theta_0$, where the parameters θ_1 and θ_0 stand for the slope and intercept. The parameters θ_1 and θ_0 are obtained by minimizing the mean squared prediction error of the model over the given data points. As such, this simple example serves to introduce some of the standard nomenclature used to describe machine learning approaches: a dataset composed of pairs (**x**,y) where **x** is an input data point (part of a larger set X), and a corresponding output y (part of a larger set Y), and a function $f(\theta)$ characterized by some parameters θ that will be learned through application of some algorithm, so as minimize the difference between the predicted and actual outputs. This difference provides a measure of how "wrong" the model is about a data point, which can be averaged across all the points in a data set to assess overall model fit. More formally, for a dataset $D = \{(x^{(i)}, y^{(i)}) \mid x^{(i)} \in R \text{ and } y^{(i)} \in R; 1 \le i \le m\}$ containing m pairs of real values, and the parameter pair (θ_0, θ_1) defining a model of a line, the error made by the model is specified by a loss function, which is derived from the difference between y as predicted by this equation for each observed x value $(x^{(i)})$ given model parameters θ, and the actual value of y for the data points concerned. One widely used loss function is the *mean squared error loss function* (also known as the quadratic loss function), which minimizes the average of the square of this difference across all data points in the set:

$$Loss\left((\theta_0, \theta_1)\right) = \frac{1}{m} \sum_{i=1}^{m} \left(y^{(i)} - \left(\theta_0 + \theta_1 x^{(i)}\right)\right)^2$$

This loss function perspective on supervised machine learning unifies all the algorithms into a common framework. The entire family of supervised machine learning algorithms can be characterized by a loss function, a function family (in this case— the family of linear functions) for capturing the relationship between the predictors in vector $\mathbf{x}$ and the outcome y, and an optimization algorithm to find the parameters of that function—typically gradient descent to minimize the loss. Linear regression and the other algorithms introduced in this chapter all share the same structure. The differences may be in the loss function, the optimization algorithm, or the expressive power of the function family. Considering machine learning from this perspective not only provides a unified framework to support learning, but also permits communicating with machine learning researchers and practitioners with a shared terminology, a prerequisite to effective team science.

Values of θ_0 and θ_1 can be found that globally minimize this quadratic squared empirical loss function—these are the parameters that define the best fit line for the dataset D. By definition, these values will be the ones that minimize the average error in prediction across all the points in the set. These values can be found using an approach called **gradient descent**. The underlying idea is to start with a random guess, and gradually move toward a correct solution by adjusting the parameters to decrease the loss.

For a linear model with two parameters θ_0 and θ_1, a 3D visualization and contour plot of the loss function is shown in Fig. 6.4. The figures show how the loss (vertical z axis in Fig. 6.4 left and labeled blue ellipses in Fig. 6.4 right) changes as these parameters are adjusted. The loss is minimized with θ_0 and θ_1 at approximately 35 and -1 respectively. The figures plot this loss function across a broad range of parameter values. However, it would be preferable not to explore this space exhaustively in order to find a solution.

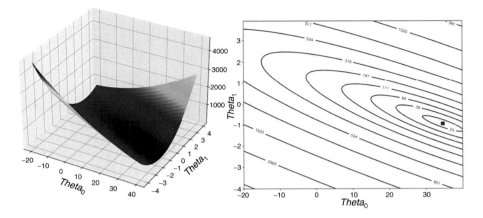

Fig. 6.4 Two views of gradient descent. These figures illustrate how the loss (vertical z axis in the left panel, labeled blue ellipses in the right panel) changes at different values of the parameters ∂_0 and θ_1. The loss in this case is minimized with θ_0 and θ_1 at approximately 35 and -1, respectively, which corresponds to the lowest point on the z axis (left panel), and the point marked by the red **X** (right panel)

To find the lowest loss value (marked with a red x in the contour plot in Fig. 6.4 right), a gradient descent algorithm starts with an initial random guess for (θ_0, θ_1) and follows the direction of steepest descent of the loss function $Loss((\theta_0, \theta_1))$ in the parameter space, updating its values using

$$\theta_j \leftarrow \theta_j - \alpha \frac{\partial Loss(\theta)}{\partial \theta_j}$$

until the values stabilize, and the gradient descent process converges. Conceptually, each parameter θ_j is updated *in accordance with its influence* upon the loss function. This is estimated as the partial derivative of the loss function with respect to each parameter, because the partial derivative estimates the extent to which changing a parameter of a function will change its output. In this way, each iterative step of the algorithm serves to move the parameters closer to values that reduce the error in predicted y values for the training data. Gradient descent provably converges to the optimal solution because the loss function is a **convex function**.[8] The step size cf the gradient descent algorithm is denoted α, the learning rate. It is chosen to be small enough so that the algorithm does not oscillate around the true minimum value of the loss function Loss (θ).

---

[8] A convex function is a function in which a line drawn between the results of evaluating the function at any two points (e.g., f(x) with x = 0.25 and x = 0.5) will lie above the result of evaluating it at any value in between (e.g., f(x) with x = 0.35). Effectively this means that the function has a single (global) minimum, and that this can be reached by following the slope of descent.

Once the parameters that lead to minimal loss have been found, the learned model can predict y for new values of x using $y = \theta_0 + \theta_1 x$. The quality of the model is assessed by measuring squared error on new x values.

Note that the specification of the linear regression problem requires more than just the training data, i.e., the (x,y) pairs. Several assumptions about the nature of these data, and a model that will fit them are made. It is assumed that the model that predicts y is linear in x and described completely by a slope and intercept parameter. The goodness of fit of the linear model is assessed by measuring averaged squared prediction error over the training data itself. That is, the strong assumption is made that the training data are a good proxy for new data that the model will predict on. Formally, it is said that the data set D is a **representative sample** of the fixed, but unknown distribution P of (x,y) example pairs—both observed and unobserved. Such an assumption is common in human learning in a classroom setting—problem sets solved by students are assumed to be a representative sample from the fixed distribution from which exam questions will be drawn. It is further assumed that each (x,y) is drawn independently, so there is no temporal dependence between the samples. This assumption is violated with time series data (see Chap. 11).

Supervised Learning: A Mathematical Formulation

The training of the model described in the previous chapter is an example of **supervised machine learning**, because the model parameters were fit to a set of data points (the x values) with labels (the y values) it learns to predict. More broadly, supervised machine learning can be conceptualized as shown in Fig. 6.5, as a search for the "best" function/pattern in the space of functions **H,** guided by a representative training sample. This view casts supervised machine learning as an **optimization problem** with a sample of (x,y) pairs drawn from an unknown but fixed distribution of examples, and a pre-defined space of functions characterizing the class of pattern relating the x's to the y's. The training data are used to navigate the space **H** of functions mapping x's to the y's to find one that "explains" the labeled training data the best. To guide the search for a suitable model in **H,** a loss function which quantifies how well the model fits the data is needed. Also needed are smoothness properties of the function space **H** to make search tractable. That is, **H** must be defined such that neighboring points in function space have similar losses with respect to the training data, so that the space can be explored systematically. The gradient descent algorithm works only when the function space **H** is smooth in this sense and supports computation of the derivative of the loss function with respect to the parameters of **H**. However, supervised machine learning problems can often be approached in this way, and gradient descent is a keystone of many contemporary machine learning approaches, including deep neural networks.

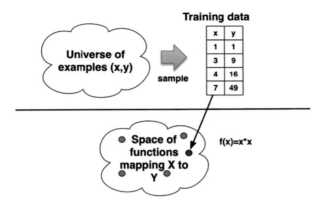

Fig. 6.5 Schematic depiction of supervised machine learning. Training data are a subset of the universe of possible labeled exampled pairs. The figure shows only a single *x* value per example, but in practice this is likely to consist of a vector of features, *x* (such as the intensities of pixel values in a radiology image). The task in supervised machine learning is to identify a function, f(*x*) (referred to as *h** in Box 6.3) that correctly maps the *x* values of the data to the *y* values of the labels

---

Box 6.3 Mathematical Components of a Supervised Machine Learning Problem

Given

- a finite data set of pairs (x,y), where x is a vector of predictor variables, and y, the associated real-valued prediction
- a class of functions $H: X \rightarrow Y$ which map vectors x in X to real numbers y in Y
- a loss function $L: Y \times Y \rightarrow R$ which maps a real-valued prediction and the true value to a real number denoting the distance between them

Find

- a function h^* in H which minimizes empirical loss (hence, the argument of the minimum, or *argmin*)

$$h^* = argmin_{h \in H} \frac{1}{m} \sum_{i=1}^{m} L\left(y^{(i)}, h\left(x^{(i)}\right)\right)$$

Box 6.3 provides a compact formulation of supervised learning which reveals the ingredients needed for building a good predictive model: (1) a representative, labeled training set composed of pairs (x,y), (2) a mathematical family of patterns H that potentially captures the association between x and y, and (3) a loss function L to evaluate the quality of fit between the model and the paired data. All of these must be constructed in a problem-specific way involving close collaboration between clinicians and machine learning scientists/engineers.

The class of patterns or functions **H** mapping the predictor variables **x** to an outcome variable y can be **parametric**, or **non-parametric**. Parametric models have a fixed number of parameters. The simple linear regression model on one variable has two parameters, θ_0 and θ_1, which are learned from (x,y) data by gradient descent optimization of the squared error loss function. Parametric methods make strong assumptions about the underlying function to be learned. They are computationally efficient at prediction time because they require the evaluation of a fixed parametric function (in the case of a linear regression model, each incoming feature would simply be multiplied by its respective parameter, followed by adding up of the results, and addition of the bias term θ_0).

Non-parametric methods make fewer assumptions about the nature of the underlying pattern relating the x's to the y's. A classic example of a non-parametric learning method is the k-nearest neighbors algorithm, illustrated in Fig. 6.6. To classify a new point, denoted by x in the figure, the algorithm computes the k closest points to x in the training data set, and outputs the majority vote (+ or −) among them. The method is very sensitive to the choice of distance metric as well as to the number k of neighbors chosen, with the latter illustrated in Fig. 6.6.

Augmenting Feature Representations: Basis Function Expansion

Returning to parametric models and fitting (x,y) points with a mean squared error loss function, it is possible to expand the model class to include higher order terms in x, while still retaining linearity in the parameter space. In the linear model introduced in the section on "The Structure of a Supervised Machine Learning

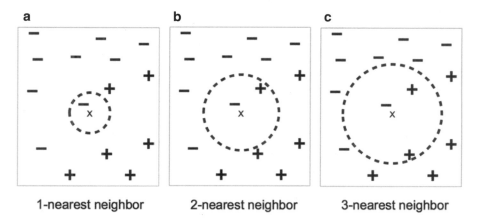

Fig. 6.6 Effect of the choice of k on the class assigned to the unseen data point x by a k-nearest neighbors classifier. With (**a**) k = 1, the negative class (−) is assigned. However, with (**b**) k = 2, the classes are tied, and with (**c**) k = 3, the positive class (+) is assigned

Algorithm", a change in the x value of a data point will always result in the same change in the y value that the model outputs. For example, if the parameter $\theta_1 = 2$ and $\theta_0 = 0$, doubling x will quadruple y. However, there are many examples in medicine (and beyond) in which the relationships between variables of interest are non-linear. Changes to an outcome of interest may be more severe once a value reaches its extremes. For example, risk of stroke increases gradually up to the age of around 65, and much more rapidly after this point [7]. The simple linear model introduced previously would underestimate the risk of stroke in older patients, because it cannot address changes in the relationship between age and risk. There are two fundamental approaches to increasing model expressivity to accommodate such relationships. One involves modifying the features that are provided to the model, and the other involves modifying the model itself. More expressive models are introduced in subsequent sections of this chapter. The discussion that follows shows how transforming the features of a data set into a more expressive *feature set* can allow a linear model to capture non-linear relationships between y (e.g., stroke risk) and x (e.g. age).

One expression of this idea is called **basis function expansion** and involves extending the feature set of a model to include higher order terms. The feature x can be expanded to the feature set x, x^2, x^3 and so forth. In the case of stroke risk, a model might be $risk\_stroke = \theta_0 + \theta_1 age + \theta_2 age^2$. The relationship between stroke risk and age would then be modeled as a weighted sum of a linear (age) and an exponential (age^2) function, with the parameters θ_1 and θ_2 indicating how much each of these should influence the model. While these parameters are constant once trained, the influence of the exponential component of the model will be stronger as age increases, as its contribution to the sum grows proportionately larger. With appropriately trained parameters, this model will be able to predict a sharper rise in stroke risk with increasing age accurately.

However, when applied injudiciously, basis function expansion can reduce the accuracy of model predictions on unseen examples. Consider, for example, fitting a cubic or higher-order function on given (x,y) points as shown in Fig. 6.7. These data points correspond to the pattern produced by a pneumotachogram (also known as a pneumotachograph), which measures the rate of air flow during inspiration (left part of the curve) and expiration, and is used to study lung function [8].

The model associated with the degree 3 polynomial shown at the bottom left panel is $y = \theta_3 x^3 + \theta_2 x^2 + \theta_1 x + \theta_0$ and a gradient descent algorithm finds values for all the θ coefficients to minimize the average squared error. It is possible to enrich the class of patterns even further and select a ninth order polynomial as shown in the bottom right panel. The fitted curve passes through all the training points, and zero training error is achieved with respect to the loss function. However, the learned polynomial performs poorly outside of the training set. A small vertical jitter (shifting each data point in the y-axis) applied to the training points will result in a cubic polynomial that is not very different from the one shown in the lower left of Fig. 6.7, but the shape of the degree 9 polynomial at the bottom right will undergo radical changes.

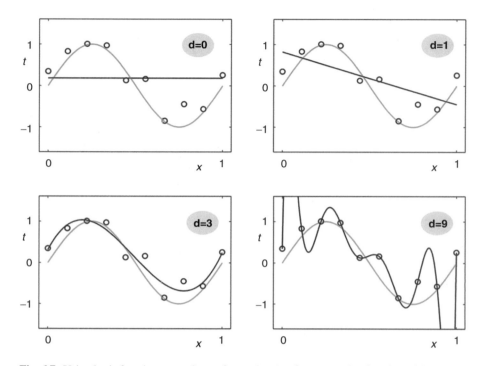

Fig. 6.7 Using basis function expansion to fit—and to overfit—a complex function with a model that is non-linear in x but linear in the expanded parameter vector θ. (Adapted from "The Elements of Statistical Learning" [9])

This figure illustrates the concept of **overfitting**—where a model has sufficient degrees of freedom to fit so tightly to the individual data points that it fails to capture the pattern of relatedness between them and is exceedingly sensitive to noise introduced to the data. Overfitting is a fundamental issue in machine learning, and one that will be returned to throughout the chapter. It is especially important in the medical domain, where datasets may be relatively small because they are limited to data from one institution or concern a rare condition. In the context of such limited data, a model with many degrees of freedom may conform closely to anomalous data points within the set that are not truly representative of the phenomenon that is being modeled and perform poorly at the point of deployment when applied to unseen data. Overfitting is also related to the tradeoff between *bias* and *variance*.

Bias and Variance

Figure 6.7 illustrates the tradeoff in machine learning between *complexity* of the model class—e.g., third vs. ninth degree polynomial (bias—which indicates the capacity of the functions in H and relates to how closely they can fit to individual data points) and *stability* of the parameter estimates (variance—which concerns how robust the estimated function is to variations in the training data). Models with high bias will have low variance because their strong assumptions render them insensitive to small changes in the data, so it is important to consider the tradeoff between bias and variance, and how they relate to sources of error. It is possible to decompose the error made by a model into two components: **structural error** (caused by limiting the class of functions considered), and **approximation error** (caused by limits on the amount of training data made available).

At the top right of Fig. 6.7, there is a model with a very strong bias (it assumes the training data can be explained by a line). The error made by this model is all accounted for by the limiting structural assumption. Providing the model with more training data will not reduce its prediction error. Such a model is called an **underfitted model**. Underfitted models have high errors on both the training and test data. At the bottom right, there is a model with many more degrees of freedom; thus, it has much lower bias. Its errors are approximation errors, caused by the limited amount of training data—there are just ten points to estimate the ten parameters of the polynomial. Such a model is an *overfitted* model. Overfitted models have low training error (because they have the freedom to fit tightly to the individual training data points) and high test error (because the tightness of the fit to a small number of potentially noisy training examples obscures the general pattern that would apply to other examples beyond the confines of the training set). The consequence is that overfitted models generalize poorly beyond their training data.

For the given collection of ten training points, the degree 3 polynomial (bottom left panel) offers a good tradeoff between structural and approximation error. The model class is powerful enough to capture the patterns in the data, and there are enough training samples to fit the model with low variance estimates. To build a successful machine learning model, one needs to find the right function class (bias) and provide a large enough training set to estimate the parameters of the learned function (variance) robustly. A family of techniques called regularization, to trade off bias and variance automatically, are introduced below. Regularization remains an important concern in machine learning, including in deep learning models, where techniques such as dropout are often a prerequisite to avoiding overfitting. The underlying principle of deliberately constraining the extent to which a model can fit to training data in order to prevent overfitting manifests in different ways in different models, but is fundamental to training models that generalize well to unseen data.

Regularization: Ridge and Lasso Regression

Regression models that are lower degree polynomials have fewer parameters and the gradient descent optimization procedure can find low variance estimates for them, even with a limited training set. However, such a model could potentially underfit the training data. Higher degree polynomials have far greater flexibility, but variance on the estimates of the optimized parameters could be high, which are signs of an overfitted model. An overfitted model, such as a degree 10 polynomial fitted on 10 (x,y) points, has parameters whose values are very large (both positive and negative).

One approach to control model complexity, then, is to penalize large (in the absolute value sense) parameter values, so that the final model has coefficients that do not grow without bound. Penalizing large parameter values by modifying the loss function used during optimization is called **regularization.**

The L2-regularized loss function for linear regression is,

$$Loss(\theta) = \frac{1}{m} \sum_{i=1}^{m} \left(y^{(i)} - h\left(x^{(i)}\right) \right)^2 + \frac{\lambda}{m} \sum_{j=1}^{d} \theta_j^2$$

so called because the L2 norm[9] is used to penalize the components of θ. Note that h(x) is the model prediction for x, and is the dot product of the parameter vector θ with [1;x]. The first term of the regularized loss function is the mean squared error of the model over the training data (as introduced in the section on "The Structure of a Supervised Machine Learning Algorithm"), which is also called the unregularized loss. The second term is the penalty function, which is the squared length of θ (the vector of parameters) without the intercept parameter θ_0. The larger the values of the parameters, the larger this term will be, which will in turn increase the value returned by the loss function. The penalty term is scaled by the factor λ which weights it relative to the unregularized loss. When λ is very low, the second term has negligible impact on the loss, so the components of θ can grow large. As λ increases, the second term dominates the loss function, and the optimizer focuses on keeping the components of θ as small as possible, ignoring the impact on the mean squared error term. As λ tends to infinity, all components of θ except for the intercept term are driven to zero. The model then simply predicts the mean of the training data for all new points x.

To choose an appropriate value of the regularization parameter λ, the training data are randomly divided into a *training set* and a *validation set* (as introduced in the section on "The Machine Learning Workflow: Components of a Machine Learning Solution"), typically in the ratio of 90/10. A sweep is conducted through potential values of λ in the log space, as shown in Fig. 6.8, to find the best value for the regularization constant—one that achieves the lowest loss over the validation set. The regularized loss is shown on the y-axis over the training and validation sets, and the natural logarithm of λ is shown in the x-axis. There is a range of λ values that are suitable for the model, and the convention is to choose the lowest value in the range. Regularization with search for the appropriate λ hyper-parameter, allows complex models to be trained on data sets without overfitting, essentially by

---

[9]The L2 norm gives the length of a vector from its origin and is calculated as the square root of the sum of this vector's squared components (in two dimensions this length would be that of the hypotenuse of a right-angled triangle with sides adjacent to the right angle corresponding the vector's components on the x and y axes). With L2 regularization, the sum of the squared components is used directly, without applying the square root.

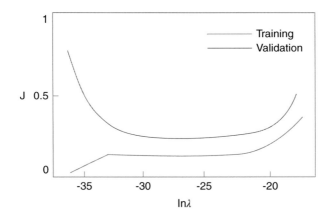

Fig. 6.8 Grid search to identify the optimal regularization parameter. The y axis shows the regularized loss J, and the x axis shows the natural logarithm of the regularization parameter, λ. Validation loss improves until a λ value of around 10^{-30}, suggesting this may be a good choice to achieve a model that generalizes well to unseen data. The extremes of the x axis suggest poorly fitted models. The leftmost extreme suggests an overfitted model, with near zero training loss with high validation loss at low λ. The rightmost extreme suggests an underfitted model, with increasing loss on both training and validation sets at high λ

limiting effective model complexity. Put another way, regularization drives higher order terms in the polynomial regression function to zero—thus, the learning procedure is given the ability to fit a ninth order polynomial, but the penalty term in the regularized loss function will drive the optimization process to select only terms no higher than degree 3, consistent with the amount of training data that are available.

L2-regularized regression is also known as ***ridge regression***. However, the penalty term in the regularized loss function need not be limited to the L2 norm of θ. A widely used penalty function is the L1-norm,[10] and the corresponding L1-regularized loss function for linear regression is

$$Loss\left(\theta\right) = \frac{1}{m}\sum\nolimits_{i=1}^{m}\left(y^{(i)} - h\left(x^{(i)}\right)\right)^{2} + \frac{\lambda}{m}\sum\nolimits_{j=1}^{d}\left|\theta_{j}\right|$$

L1-regularized regression is called ***lasso regression***. Lasso regression has the special property that it drives components of θ exactly to zero [9], given sufficiently large values of the regularization parameter λ. Thus, sparse models that only involve a subset of the features in input vector **x** are obtained. Since lasso regression performs automatic feature selection, it is in wide use in clinical settings, where predictive models with the fewest number of predictors (for a given level of performance) are prized. For example, Walsh and Hripcsak describe a series of readmission risk prediction models in which lasso regression resulted in an average of a fivefold reduction in the number of features considered [10]. Lasso models can be readily

---

[10] The L1 norm of a vector is the sum of its absolute coordinate values.

incorporated into clinical workflow with minimal computational requirements when relevant features can be extracted in real-time directly from data sources such as electronic records [10, 11].

Linear Models for Classification

A common task in biomedical machine learning involves assigning categorical labels, such as diagnosis names or types of predicted outcomes on the basis of observed data. This task is referred to as **classification**. In classification, the outcome variable is discrete rather than continuous. There is therefore a need to modify the class of prediction functions **H** as well as the loss function to accommodate the change in outcome type. A formal description of the components of a classification problem is provided in Box 6.4.

Box 6.4 Mathematical Components of a Classification Problem
Given
- a finite data set of pairs (**x**,y), where **x** is a vector of predictor variables, and y, is the associated discrete class or category drawn from a finite set C of labels
- a class of functions **H**: **X** → C which map vectors **x** in **X** to discrete values in C
- a loss function L: C × P(C) → R which maps a true category and the predicted distribution over the categories to a real number denoting the distance between true and predicted classes

Find
- a function h* in **H** which minimizes empirical loss

$$h^* = argmin_{h \in H} \frac{1}{m} \sum_{i=1}^{m} L\left(y^{(i)}, h\left(x^{(i)}\right)\right)$$

The only difference between regression and classification is in the target of the prediction function—regression functions produce continuous value predictions, while classification functions predict discrete values, or probability distributions on a discrete value set. Thus, the class of functions **H** and the loss function L are modified to handle this change in the target of prediction. A good way to visualize a classification function h in **H** is as a partition of the input space **X** into decision regions, each associated with a member of C. Linear models of classification learn **hyperplanes** in the input space dividing it into different decision regions, while linear models with expanded basis functions learn non-linear decision boundaries.

A very special case of classification is **binary classification** when the set C consists of exactly two elements {0,1} called the negative and positive class respectively. The goal of learning in binary classification is to find the best decision rule that predicts the correct class given the vector **x** of predictors.

Classification problems are frequent targets of machine learning applications in medicine, with typical examples including classifying patients by diagnosis on the basis of their imaging data (e.g. detecting diabetic retinopathy in retinal images [2]; for further examples see Chap. 12), classifying clinical notes with respect to the nature of their content (e.g. identifying clinical notes containing goals-of-care discussions [12]; see also *text classification*, Chap. 7, section "Overview of Biomedical NLP Tasks"), and predicting clinical outcomes (e.g. readmission within 30 days of discharge [10]; for further examples see Chap. 11).

Linear models of classification come in two flavors, based on whether they learn the posterior distribution P(y|x) (e.g. the probability of a side effect after some drug has been observed) or the joint distribution P(xy) (e.g. the overall probability of both the drug and side effect being observed together) from the paired (**x**, y) training data. The difference between these estimates may not be obvious at first. For a given binary predictor, $x_i \in$ {True,False} (e.g. presence of a drug), the posterior distribution P(y|x_i) will correspond to the proportion of observations of x_i in which y (e.g. presence of a side effect) is also true. In contrast, the joint distribution P(x_iy) corresponds to the proportion of *all examples* in which both x_i and y are true. In the example, P(x_iy) would be low when the side effect in question occurs many times *without* the drug being taken—but P(y|x_i) may still be high if the side effect occurs frequently in cases where the drug has been taken. Models that learn the posterior distribution are called **discriminative models**, while models that learn the joint distribution are called **generative models**.

Discriminative Models: Logistic Regression

A classic example of a linear discriminative binary classification model is **logistic regression**. Rather than predicting an unbounded value as with linear regression, logistic regression models P(y|x), the posterior distribution of the binary outcome y given input **x** as the following function: a linear computation (the dot product of a parameter vector θ with the input vector **x**, $\theta^T x$) followed by a non-linear "squashing" of that dot product into the range [0,1] to represent a probability. This can be interpreted as the probability of a class of interest, such as a diagnosis or outcome.

$$P\left(y = 1|x|;\theta\right) = g\left(\theta^T x\right) = \frac{1}{1 + \exp\left(-\theta^T x\right)}$$

The particular nonlinear squashing function g used in logistic regression is called the **sigmoid**. As shall be seen later, this function is a fundamental building block of deep neural networks. Given a training data set D, and an appropriate loss function, the optimal value of the parameter vector θ which characterizes the classification function can be found. Given a new vector $\mathbf{x}$, the posterior probability of $y = 1$ given $\mathbf{x}$, i.e., $P(y = 1|\mathbf{x})$, is evaluated, and if that probability is greater than or equal to 0.5, the new $\mathbf{x}$ is classified as positive (belong to class 1, which may indicate a diagnosis or outcome of interest). Since the sigmoid function $g(z)$ equals 0.5 when z is 0, the decision boundary separating class 0 from class 1 is defined by the hyperplane

$$\theta^T x = 0$$

The equation above defines a linear separating hyperplane for binary classification. When $\theta^T x \geq 0$, $\mathbf{x}$ lies on the positive side of the plane, and when $\theta^T x < 0$, $\mathbf{x}$ lies on the negative side (it is worth noting that the use of a bias term θ_0 allows the model flexibility in setting a threshold for classification—for $\theta^T x$ to equal zero, $\theta_{1...n}^T \mathbf{x}_{1...n} = -\theta_0$). The decision boundary learned by logistic regression on a nearly linearly separable data set composed of (x, y) pairs where each x is a point on a plane, is shown in Fig. 6.9. Points belonging to the positive class are marked with a + sign, while points belonging to the negative class are marked with a – sign.

The loss function for training a logistic model can be derived by the maximum likelihood principle, in which a model is trained to maximize the probability of the

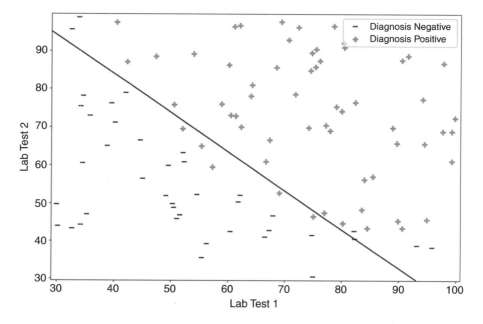

Fig. 6.9 Illustration of a decision boundary for a logistic regression classifier with two classes. Examples that fall to the right of the boundary ($\theta^T x > 0$) corresponding to estimated P(y|x) > 0.5), are classified as positive

observed data, assuming that $P(y = 1|x;\theta) = h(x) = g(\theta^T x)$. The logarithm of the *negative likelihood* of data set D composed of (**x**,y) pairs, where y is in the set {0,1} can be shown to be the cross entropy function.

$$J(\theta) = -\frac{1}{m}\sum_{i=1}^{m}\left[y^{(i)}\log\left(h\left(x^{(i)}\right)\right)\right]+\left[\left(1-y^{(i)}\right)\log\left(1-h\left(x^{(i)}\right)\right)\right]$$

As this function is not only fundamental to logistic regression but is also widely used in training deep neural networks amongst other models, it is worth unpacking here. $\frac{1}{m}\sum_{i=1}^{m}$ indicates that an average over m data points is taken, and the rest of the right-hand side of the equation is a compact way of describing the log likelihood of the data. If $y^{(i)}$, the label of the example i, is equal to one, only the leftmost term is considered, because $(1 - y^{(i)})$ in the rightmost term will be zero. In this case, the likelihood will be the log of the predicted probability h(x) = $P(y = 1|x)$ assigned to this example. Conversely, with $y^{(i)} = 0$, only the rightmost term will be considered, and the likelihood will be the log of the predicted probability $P(y = 0)$, or $1 - P(y = 1)$. So, the log likelihood of the dataset is the average of the logs of the predicted probabilities of the correct labels across all examples. The negative log likelihood reverses the polarity of this estimate, converting a maximization problem into a minimization one.

Gradient descent minimizes $J(\theta)$ to find the optimal value of the parameter vector θ. Since the cross-entropy function $J(\theta)$ is a convex function, it has a global minimum which can be computed by standard optimization algorithms. It is therefore guaranteed that θ found by minimizing the cross-entropy function represents the optimal classifier for the data set in the infinite space of parametric functions **H**.

Regularized Logistic Regression: Ridge and Lasso Models

The decision boundary in Fig. 6.9 applies readily to situations in which high values of the tests concerned indicate a diagnosis. However, circumstances may arise in which both high and low values of a laboratory test have implications for the prediction at hand. For example both high and low white cell counts may portend adverse outcomes. A range of modeling approaches that apply to classification in these circumstances are discussed in the section on "Non-linear Models". For the current discussion, it is noteworthy that basis function expansion—the same approach that was introduced as a way to augment feature representations to model non-linear functions with linear regression in the section on "Bias and Variance"—is also applicable to classification problems when logistic regression is used.

When a data set is not linearly separable in the (x_1, x_2) plane as shown in Fig. 6.10, it is possible use the basis function expansion trick to expand the space of predictors. Each point (x_1, x_2) could be mapped into a 15-dimensional space of all sixth-order polynomial combinations of x_1 and x_2, to learn a linear separating hyperplane

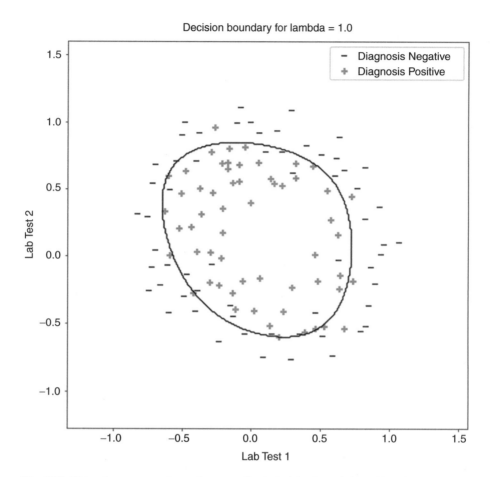

Fig. 6.10 Using feature expansion to learn non-linear decision boundaries with a (linear) logistic regression model. The black ovoid boundary is the decision boundary learned by the classifier, which separates the positive (+) and negative (−) classes reasonably cleanly, despite these classes not being linearly separable in the plane

in that 15-dimensional space. One benefit of this expansion is that it allows the model to consider the magnitude of a feature value out of context of its polarity—the polynomial expansion x^2 will be high for both highly negative and highly positive values of x, enabling the model to learn decision boundaries that are ovoid or circular in relation to the unexpanded features. The projection of that decision boundary in two dimensions is shown in Fig. 6.10. Basis function expansion allows us to consider rich models with low bias; therefore, to prevent overfitting it is necessary to strongly regularize the models. Ridge and lasso penalty terms are added to the cross-entropy function, just as in linear regression, to control the growth of the parameter vector.

Analogously to regularized linear regression, L2-regularized ridge logistic regression is characterized by the following loss function

$$J(\theta) = \left[-\frac{1}{m} \sum_{i=1}^{m} \left[y^{(i)} \log\left(h\left(x^{(i)} \right) \right) \right] + \left[\left(1 - y^{(i)} \right) \log\left(1 - h\left(x^{(i)} \right) \right) \right] \right] + \frac{\lambda}{m} \sum_{j=1}^{d} \theta_j^2$$

while L1-regularized lasso logistic regression penalizes the parameter vector θ using the absolute value.

$$J(\theta) = \left[-\frac{1}{m} \sum_{i=1}^{m} \left[y^{(i)} \log\left(h\left(x^{(i)} \right) \right) \right] + \left[\left(1 - y^{(i)} \right) \log\left(1 - h\left(x^{(i)} \right) \right) \right] \right] + \frac{\lambda}{m} \sum_{j=1}^{d} |\theta_j|$$

Note that in both L1 and L2 regularization, the intercept component θ_0 is not penalized because the intercept accounts for the overall mean of the data points, effectively setting the threshold for classification. The best value of the regularization constant λ can be determined by a cross-validation procedure as was done in the case of linear regression. By varying λ, it is possible to adjust the relative importance of minimizing error on the training data (first term of $J(\theta)$, representing the averaged log likelihood) and driving the coefficients of θ to zero (second term of $J(\theta)$, representing the penalty on the coefficients of θ). As λ approaches zero (no regularization), the solution found by the optimizer is very likely overfitted, especially when the number of training data points is small. As λ approaches infinity, the training data are ignored, and the coefficients of θ are driven to zero, leading to an underfitted model, such as the one shown in Fig. 6.11.

A Simple Clinical Example of Logistic Regression

This example is derived from data associating male lung cancer and smoking [13]. There is one binary predictor: whether someone is a smoker or not, and the outcome is also discrete with two values: cancer, or no-cancer. For this simple problem, it is easier to present summary statistics of the data as shown below—such a table is called a **contingency table**.

	Lung-cancer	No-cancer
Smoker	647	622
Non-smoker	2	27

The structure of the logistic model to predict the probability of cancer given smoking status is

$$p = P\left(cancer = 1 | smoking; \theta_0, \theta_1 \right) = g\left(\theta_0 + \theta_1 smoking \right)$$
$$= \frac{1}{1 + \exp\left(-\left(\theta_0 + \theta_1 smoking \right) \right)}$$

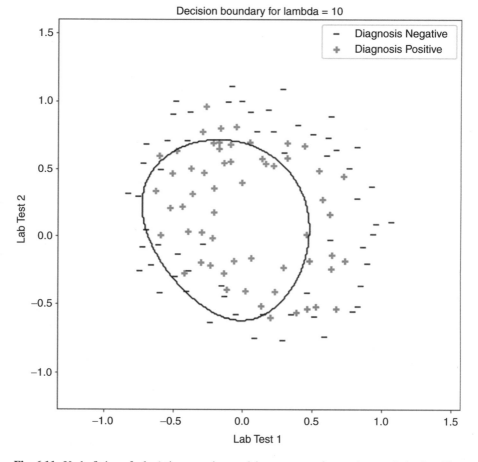

Fig. 6.11 Underfitting of a logistic regression model on account of excessive regularization. The black ovoid boundary is the decision boundary learned by the classifier, which does not cleanly separate the positive (+) and negative (−) classes

This model represents the natural logarithm of the odds ratio of cancer given smoking as a linear function of smoking.

$$\log\left(\frac{p}{1-p}\right) = \theta_0 + \theta_1 smoking$$

The parameter θ_0 represents the baseline log odds of getting cancer regardless of smoking status, and θ_1 characterizes the increment in log odds of getting cancer for the smoking cohort. Unregularized logistic regression can be used, since there is only one predictor and 1298 examples, so there is no need to penalize the loss function. The optimizer finds the values for the parameter vector θ shown below.

$$\log\left(\frac{p}{1-p}\right) = -2.6025 + 2.6419\, smoking$$

This model states that the log odds of developing cancer for non-smokers is -2.6025 (log (2/27)), while the incremental odds of developing cancer for smokers is 2.6419. That is, for a smoker, the predicted log odds of cancer goes up by 2.6419 over the baseline odds, $-2.6025 + 2.6419$, which is 0.039 (or log (647/622)). The estimated odds ratio of cancer for smokers versus non-smokers is $e^{2.6419} = 14.04$. That is, smokers are 14 times more likely to get cancer than non-smokers. The mechanics of logistic regression and the probabilistic interpretation of the parameter vector are revealed in this example, where summary statistics of the data suffice to estimate the parameters.

A Multivariate Clinical Example of Logistic Regression

Now consider the more complex problem of predicting whether or not a Type 2 diabetes patient's condition worsens over the course of a year based on a set of 10 baseline predictors: {age, gender, body mass index (bmi), average blood pressure (bp), and six blood serum measurements: total serum cholesterol (tc), low-density lipoprotein (ldl), high-density lipoprotein (hdl), total cholesterol/hdl (tch), logarithm of triglyceride level (ltg), blood glucose level (glu)}. These data for 442 patients along with the outcome variable, which is a quantitative measure of disease progression 1 year after the baseline are publicly available.[11] For this example, a discrete outcome variable y will be defined by labeling patients whose progression evaluations are more than one standard deviation above the cohort mean as positive ($y = 1$), and the others as negative ($y = 0$). That is, the model to be estimated has the form

$$P(y=1|\mathbf{x};\theta) = g(\theta^T\mathbf{x}) = \frac{1}{1+\exp(-\theta^T\mathbf{x})}$$

where $\mathbf{x}$ is the 11-element vector [1,age,gender,bmi, bp,tc,ldl,hdl,tch,ltg,glu] and the parameter vector θ has 11 components, the first being the intercept (θ_0), and the other 10 associated with the predictor variables in $\mathbf{x}$ ($\theta_{1...10}$). An L1-regularized logistic model is learned, finding the optimal choice for λ, the regularization parameter, by five-fold cross-validation. The model learned has only five non-zero coefficients, with bmi, ltg, and bp being the most significant coefficients in the model

$$P(y=1|\mathbf{x};\theta) = g(\theta^T\mathbf{x}) =$$
$$g(-1.89+18.29\,bmi+9.3\,bp+1.66\,hdl+11.91\,ltg+1.38\,glu)$$

[11] https://www4.stat.ncsu.edu/~boos/var.select/diabetes.html (accessed August 19, 2022).

The five-fold cross-validated AUROC of this model is 0.9 ± 0.05, indicating that it will predict well on new patients, if they are drawn from the same distribution of patients as the training set. Beyond accuracy, the model provides *interpretability* (see Chap. 8): the coefficients indicate both the magnitude and the direction of each parameter's influence on model predictions, albeit with the important caveat that unlike the binary feature in the previous example, the incoming features may be represented on different scales, which will affect the coefficients also.

Regularized logistic regression models are widely used for risk stratification in clinical settings. For example, a multivariate L1-regularized logistic regression model has been used to predict SARS-Cov2-related death within a year using ten baseline characteristics: gender, age, race, ethnicity, body mass index, Charlson comorbidity index, diabetes, chronic kidney disease, congestive heart failure and the Care Assessment Need score [14]. The model was trained on over 7.6 million Veteran's Affairs enrollees with training data obtained from the period May 21 to September 2020, and a testing cohort obtained from the period October 1 to November 2, 2020. The AUROC of the model on the test data was 0.836, outperforming a simple age-based stratification strategy with an AUROC of 0.74. The model was learned from structured data readily extractable from EHR records. Further, the model is easily interpretable since the coefficients of the ten predictors serve as the log-odds ratio of the effect of that predictor on the final outcome. The model was ultimately integrated into the clinical workflow with a built-in web-based risk calculator and used for prioritizing vaccinations among veterans. The model is estimated to have prevented 63.5% of deaths that would occur by the time 50% of VA enrollees are vaccinated. The model also adheres to the four ethical principles outlined by the Advisory Committee on Immunization Practices [15]. It maximizes benefits (by targeting those at highest risk for vaccine allocation), promotes justice (by identifying older adults or those with a high comorbidity burden who will require focused outreach for vaccination), mitigates health inequities (by assigning higher priority to racial and ethnic minorities directly reflecting their higher risk of mortality), and promotes transparency (by using an evidence-based model with explicit parameters). The use of ethnicity as a variable in this model compensates for known differences in health risk across populations, making a preventative intervention more readily available, without the benefit of additional contextual knowledge such as socio-economic status and other specific risk factors. Further discussion of the ethical implications of the use of such variables in predictive models is presented in Chap. 18.

Generative Models: Gaussian Discriminant Analysis

Generative models learn the full joint distribution $P(xy)$ from training data pairs (x,y) where x is a vector of predictor variables and y, a discrete outcome. For binary classification problems, y takes on one of two values $\{0,1\}$, while for multiclass classification problems, y can take some finite number, greater than two, of values.

Since $P(xy) = P(x|y)P(y)$ using probability theory, the following generative model component distributions are estimated.

- prior probabilities: $P(y = 1)$, $(P(y = 0) = 1 - P(y = 1))$
- class conditional distributions: $P(\boldsymbol{x}|y = 1)$, $P(\boldsymbol{x}|y = 0)$

from the training data. Armed with the component distributions, the information to generate new examples from both classes is available. To generate a new positive example, a random $\boldsymbol{x}$ from the distribution $P(\boldsymbol{x}|y = 1)$ is drawn. To generate a new negative example, the distribution $P(\boldsymbol{x}|y = 0)$ is used. This is why the model is called 'generative'—it can construct new examples from both classes. A discriminative model, which only estimates $P(y = 1|\boldsymbol{x})$ from training data, can classify a new example, but it cannot construct one *de novo*. Furthermore, unlike discriminative models, generative models learn the distributions of individual feature inputs, permitting one to pose questions such as "what are the characteristics of a patient with worsening type 2 Diabetes". This has inherent advantages for the generation of synthetic datasets and can support the construction of causal models that capture cause-effect relationships between individual variables (see Chap. 10). However, these capabilities come at a cost in that large amounts of data are required to correctly estimate the prerequisite distributions, which often cannot be robustly estimated with the relatively small datasets used for clinical machine learning.

Parametric generative models make assumptions about the (parametric) form of the prior probability distribution and the class conditional distributions. A common choice for the prior probabilities for binary classification problems is the Bernoulli distribution (the distribution used for modeling a coin toss), and for continuous predictors $\boldsymbol{x}$, the class conditional densities are modeled as multivariate Gaussian distributions with a mean and covariance for class $y = 0$ and for class $y = 1$. These two assumptions characterize Gaussian discriminant analysis (GDA); one of the simplest parametric generative models in the field. A simple two-class example of GDA with two-dimensional $\boldsymbol{x}$ vectors is shown below. The learned multivariate normal class conditional densities associated with the classes are drawn as ellipses. Each ellipse is a contour plot of a two-dimensional Gaussian distribution learned from data, representing an iso-probability line. The center of the ellipses is the mean, and the shape of the ellipse is determined by the covariance matrix of the two-dimensional Gaussian. The means of the two multivariate normals in Fig. 6.12 for the two classes are different, but their covariances are the same.

The decision boundary between the two classes is computed using Bayes rule with the learned prior and class conditional distributions (the negative class distribution is represented in the denominator of the equation, which indicates the probability of x summed across both possible values $\{0,1\}$ of the label y).

$$P(y = 1|x) = \frac{P(x|y = 1)P(y = 1)}{\sum_y P(x|y)P(y)}$$

Readers with a clinical or biostatistics background may be familiar with Bayes rule applied in this way, as it provides a means to convert the *sensitivity* of a test—$P(x|y = 1)$, where $y = 1$ indicates a positive case in a population, and x indicates a

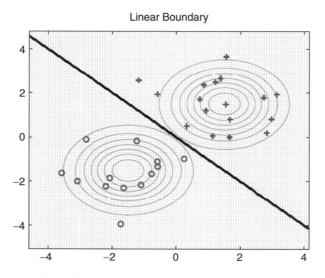

Fig. 6.12 Class-conditional distributions for a binary classification problem. The ellipses demarcate regions of probability that the members of each class (+ and **o**) will have particular values. The centers of the ellipses are class means, and the shapes of the ellipse are determined by the distribution of class members in relation to these means. In this case a single pattern of distribution has been estimated for both classes, but these have different means

positive test result—into a clinically actionable *positive predictive value*, $P(y = 1|x)$, or the probability that a patient has the disease given a positive test result.

When the class conditional distributions are Gaussians, with tied covariances, as shown in Fig. 6.12 above, the decision boundary between the classes is a hyperplane (line in two dimensions). When both the means and the covariances individually for both classes are estimated, the decision boundary is a quadratic (parabola). Gaussian discriminant analysis can be used to learn generative models for multiclass problems, with a combination of tied and independent covariances for the different classes, as shown in Fig. 6.13.

In sum, Gaussian discriminant analysis, a parametric generative model, is excellent for data that mostly conforms to a multivariate Gaussian distribution. When this assumption about the training data holds, GDA is the best classification method—it yields the most accurate classifier with the least amount of data. Discriminative models, like logistic regression, are less sensitive to assumptions about the distribution of the data in X, and therefore need a lot more examples to build models of comparable performance.

Factored Generative Models: Naive Bayes

Multivariate distributions of the form P(**x**|y) are difficult to handle, both analytically and computationally. One approach around this difficulty is to assume conditional independence between the features of the vector $x \in R^d$, and model the multivariate

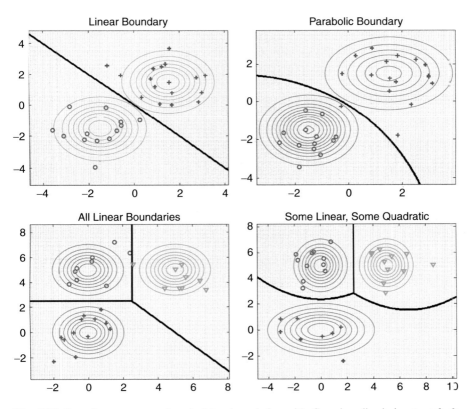

Fig. 6.13 Learning more complex decision boundaries with Gaussian discriminant analysis (GDA). This figure shows the boundaries learned from two class problems with tied (left panels) and individually estimated (right panels) covariance patterns for binary (top panels) and three-class classification (bottom panels). This illustrates the ability of GDA to fit to the unique characteristics of different classes, and address multi-class classification problems

distribution P(x|y) as the product of d one dimensional distributions of the form $P(x_i \mid y)$. This is a strong and often unfounded assumption—for example, when modeling clinical data this would mean ignoring relationships between the values of different liver function tests that in practice may be of considerable diagnostic utility, as well as other important relationships such as drug interactions and relationships to comorbid diagnoses. Nonetheless, despite their "naivete", models embodying this assumption can lead to surprisingly accurate predictions.

$$P(x|y) = \prod_j P(x_j|y)$$

This factorization works well for both discrete and continuous valued vectors **x**, even when the conditional independence assumptions between the components of **x** conditioned on the class y, do not hold. Naive Bayes models are the industry-standard for the problem of spam detection and for text classification (with over 300,000 articles on Google Scholar as of August 2022) and have been widely used for machine learning in medicine. Recent applications include suicide risk prediction [16], and predicting neonatal sepsis [17].

For illustrative purposes, consider the following problem: there are 1.13 cases of bacterial meningitis per 100,000 population in the US. Assume that 60% of patients with bacterial meningitis report the characteristic symptom of a stiff neck, but that 15% of patients *without* meningitis also report this symptom. Given that a new patient reports a stiff neck, what is the probability that they have meningitis? It is possible to write the facts of this problem as the following probability statements:

1. $P(y = meningitis) = 1.13 \times 10^{-5}$; $P(y = not\text{-}meningitis) = 1 - 1.13 \times 10^{-5}$
2. $P(stiff\,neck = 1|y = meningitis) = 0.6$
3. $P(stiff\,neck = 1|y = not\text{-}meningitis) = 0.15$

The first set of equations describe the prior probabilities of the two classes {meningitis, non-meningitis}, and the next two describe the class conditional distributions with respect to a primary symptom of meningitis—stiff neck. Bayes Theorem can be used to calculate the probability that a patient presenting with stiff neck has meningitis:

$$P(y = m|stiff\ neck = 1) = \frac{P(stiff\ neck = 1|y = m)P(y = m)}{\sum_d P(stiff\ neck = 1|y = d)P(y = d)}$$
where m = meningitis

The d in the denominator has one of two possibilities: 1 indicating meningitis, and 0 indicating "not meningitis". Since the prior probability of meningitis is very low, and stiff neck is four times more likely to occur in meningitis patients, the posterior probability of the patient having meningitis rises to 4.5×10^{-5}, if a patient presents with a stiff neck alone. However, stiff neck is only one of the symptoms of meningitis. By taking other symptoms into account, such as high fever, nausea, etc., it is possible to improve the estimation of the posterior probability of meningitis in a patient. Suppose k Boolean features are used, representing the presence or absence of specific symptoms—let us call the features $x_1, ..., x_k$. To keep things simple, each of these will take on values in {0,1} denoting absence or presence of a symptom. Now every patient is represented by a Boolean vector $\mathbf{x}$ of length k, with every position in the vector denoting whether a specific symptom is present or absent. To learn the distribution P(x|y = meningitis) or P(x|y = not-meningitis), it is possible to use

$$P(\mathbf{x}|y = m) = \frac{P(\mathbf{x}, y = m)}{P(y = m)} = \frac{Number\ of\ m\ patients\ represented\ as\ vector\ \mathbf{x}}{Number\ of\ m\ patients}$$
where m = meningitis

Since the vector $\mathbf{x}$ is discrete, it is possible to simply count the number of meningitis patients represented by the vector $\mathbf{x}$, and divide it by the total number of patients, to get the proportion of patients of the form $\mathbf{x}$, representing a specific absence/presence pattern of symptoms. If k (the number of symptoms) is 20, the possible number of configurations of vector $\mathbf{x}$ is 2^{20}. Estimating the distribution requires estimation of $O(2^{20})$ entries, an intractable task with typically available EHR data.

Now the power of the Naive Bayes assumption can be seen. The multivariate discrete distribution $P(\mathbf{x}|y)$ is factored as the product of k univariate Bernoulli distributions of the form $P(x_j = 1|y = meningitis)$ and $P(x_j = 1 \mid y = not\ meningitis)$. For a k-dimensional vector $\mathbf{x}$, only $2k$ parameters are needed to characterize the class conditional distributions. The reduction of parameters from $O(2^k)$ to $2k$ makes generative modeling of patients a tractable proposition.

$$P(y = m|x) = \frac{P(y = m)\prod_j P(x_j|y = m)}{P(y = m)\prod_j P(x_j|y = m) + P(y = not\ m)\prod_j P(x_j|y = not\ m)}$$

where m = meningitis, $not\ m$ = not meningitis

For the price of estimating $2k + 1$ parameters (the 1 is for $P(y = meningitis)$), Bayes rule can be used as above to diagnose meningitis. The real challenge in building Naive Bayes classifiers for diagnosis or more generally any classification problem, is choosing good features to characterize a patient. For example, Google's Gmail has a proprietary list of thousands of features that it extracts from each email to stay ahead of the arms race with spammers.

To avoid underflow problems that arise from multiplying thousands of probabilities in the numerator of the posterior probability calculation, the computation is performed in log space.[12] That is, to classify a new patient $\mathbf{x}$ as having meningitis, the following inequality is evaluated, which also eliminates computing the denominator of the expression above, which is identical for both classes.

$$\log\left(P(y = meningitis)\right) + \sum_j \log\left(P(x_j|y = meningitis)\right) >$$
$$\log\left(P(y = not\ meningitis)\right) + \sum_j \log\left(P(x_j|y = not\ meningitis)\right)$$

Recently, Naive Bayes classifiers for detecting patients at increased risk of suicide were constructed using structured data on 3.7 million patients across five diverse health care systems [16]. The model detected a mean of 38% of cases of suicide attempts with 90% specificity at a mean of 2.1 years in advance of the attempt. This model used univariate Gaussian distributions to model continuous variables obtained from structured health records, and Bernoulli or multinomial distributions for the discrete variables.

---

[12] This is a common computational optimization that works because $\log(ab) = \log(a) + \log(b)$—so we can add instead of multiplying, obviating the underflow that occurs when repeatedly multiplying by small number; and $\log(a) > \log(b)$ for all $a > b$—so we will assign the class with the highest posterior probability given the data x.

Bias and Variance in Generative Models

It is possible to either underfit or overfit a generative model. Continuing with the meningitis classification example, a model with low bias has a very large number of symptom features. With a limited amount of training data, the estimates of the class conditional probabilities for this large feature set are likely to have high variance. On the other hand, a model with very few features to represent a patient has high bias, and its parameters can be stably estimated, even with a limited amount of data. However, a model with a limited feature set is unlikely to generalize well to new data. Finding the right tradeoff between bias and variance amounts to finding the right feature set (both in content and size) to balance generalization performance and reliability of estimation of the distributional parameters, with respect to the available training data. Feature selection (see Chap. 11) is thus a critical aspect of construction of generative models.

The use of Bayes rule for performing classification of new examples raises a novel problem unique to generative models. Suppose one of the class conditional probabilities corresponding to a specific feature is estimated to be zero given the training data. This situation occurs quite frequently in email classification when a chosen word feature does not appear in the training corpus. Should a new piece of email contain that feature, the Bayes rule computation will yield a zero, since one of the probability terms in the numerator is zero. To guard against this situation, a regularization process called **Laplace smoothing** is performed on probability estimates. Instead of starting word counts at zero in the estimation procedure, counts are started at 1 (or another small constant). So, no class conditional probability is ever estimated to be zero, regardless of the limitations on the training data.

Recap of Parametric Linear Models for Classification

Given a training data set composed of pairs $(\mathbf{x}, y)$ where $\mathbf{x}$ is a vector of d dimensions in a continuous/discrete space, and y is a label drawn from the set $\{0,1\}$, there are two distinct approaches to building functions that predict y given a new $\mathbf{x}$

- **Discriminative models** learn the posterior probability $P(y = 1|\mathbf{x}) = g(\theta^T \mathbf{x})$ as a parametric function and optimize the value of the parameter vector θ to make the predicted distribution of y as close as possible to the true distribution. The learned parameter vector describes the linear classification boundary $\theta^T \mathbf{x} = 0$ between the two classes (0 and 1). Logistic regression belongs to this family of models.
- **Generative models** learn the full joint distribution $P(\mathbf{x}y)$ in terms of its components $P(y)$ and $P(\mathbf{x}|y)$. Generative models come in two forms: full models, and factored models which assume that the components of $\mathbf{x}$ are independent of one another given the class. Factored models are easier to estimate and work with and are widely used in a range of text classification and clinical decision-making tasks. The decision boundaries they learn can be characterized by a hyperplane in the domain of the input vectors $\mathbf{x}$.

Non-linear Models

Linear classification models assume a monotonic and proportional relationship between input variables and the probability of an output label. Models of this sort cannot learn that both high and low blood pressure can be useful predictive features for the onset of renal failure, nor can they learn that the probability of this outcome increases exponentially once a particular blood pressure is reached. However, they can be configured to do so, by transforming the incoming data to enrich the space of features.

Consider the following classification problem in two dimensions (Fig. 6.14 (left)). Can the two classes be separated by a linear boundary?

Clearly, there is no linear separating hyperplane in the original feature space (x_1, x_2). However, it is possible to use the basis function expansion trick introduced in the section on "Augmenting Feature Representations" to map each (x_1, x_2) pair into a new feature space z_1, z_2 defined as

$$\left(z_1, z_2\right) = \left(x_1 * x_1, x_2 * x_2\right)$$

Now a linear hyperplane defined by $z_1 + z_2 \leq R^2$ where R is the radius of the black circle in Fig. 6.14,[13] achieves perfect separation as shown below.

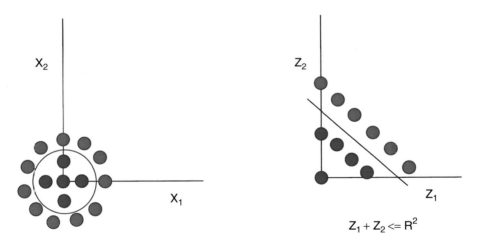

Fig. 6.14 (Left) A non-linear classification boundary in the original (x_1, x_2) feature space. (right): A linear boundary in the (z_1, z_2) feature space where $z_1 = x_1 \times x_1$ and $z_2 = x_2 \times x_2$. Note that the linear boundary with expanded bases (right) corresponds to the non-linear boundary in the original feature space (left)

---

[13] Summing the squares of x and y returns the square of the distance from the origin, which will be less than R^2 for the examples in the innermost class.

There are two approaches to constructing non-linear classifiers.

1. Stay within the framework of linear classifiers with their optimality guarantees, but manually construct appropriate non-linear feature spaces (basis functions) in which the classification boundaries are linear. The example shown above illustrates this idea. However, the downside of this approach is that it places the entire burden of designing basis functions for data representation on the human modeler.

2. Bypass the explicit construction of basis functions and build non-linear classifiers directly. What is lost in this approach are the optimality/convergence guarantees of linear models. However, there are a number of well-established approaches to apply, which can be broadly categorized as either **kernel methods** or stacked models.

    – Kernel methods represent examples not by their features, but in relation to other examples in the training set. **Kernel regression** and **support vector machines** belong to this family of methods.
    – Stacked models are constructed by chaining or layering simpler learning models. Layered logistic regression models, also known as **deep feedforward neural networks**, are an example of this class of techniques.

Kernel Methods

Consider a binary classification problem with points (x_1, x_2) drawn from a two-dimensional plane, with labels from the set $\{0,1\}$, where points in class 0 are colored orange, and points in class 1 are colored blue (see Fig. 6.15). A set of L landmarks from the training data are selected; in Fig. 6.15, the landmark points are labeled l_1, l_2, l_3, i.e., L = 3 for this example. One can think of these landmarks as paradigmatic positive and negative examples for a decision problem. In clinical datasets, such landmarks may correspond to textbook expositions of a disease or condition.

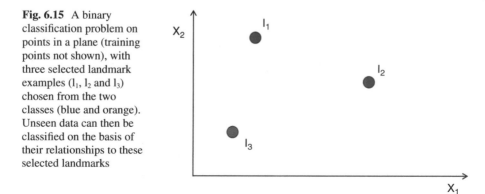

Fig. 6.15 A binary classification problem on points in a plane (training points not shown), with three selected landmark examples (l_1, l_2 and l_3) chosen from the two classes (blue and orange). Unseen data can then be classified on the basis of their relationships to these selected landmarks

Each point in the training data has the form $((x_1,x_2),y)$ and every method discussed so far predicts y from (x_1,x_2) using a function parameterized by a vector θ. For example, logistic regression without basis function expansion would learn θ such that the posterior probability of $y = 1$ given x is well approximated by the sigmoid of the dot product of θ and x.

$$P\left(y = 1|;\left(x_1,x_2\right)|;\theta\right) = \sigma\left(\theta_0 + \theta_1 x_1 + \theta_2 x_2\right)$$

Instead of describing a training example x by its intrinsic properties—i.e., its location in the $x_1 - x_2$ plane, let us represent it by its "similarity" to the three landmark examples shown in Fig. 6.16. That is, a similarity function *sim* on pairs of points in the $x_1 - x_2$ plane is first defined as follows. This similarity function or **kernel**, is called a radial basis function.

$$sim\left(x,l\right) = \exp\left(-\frac{x - l^2}{2\sigma^2}\right)$$

$sim(x,l)$ is characterized by a fixed bandwidth parameter σ(unrelated to the sigmoid product above), which is a real number that takes on values in the range $[0,1]$. The value 0 is achieved when x is far away (in terms of Euclidean distance) from l, and the value 1 is obtained when x is identical to l. In short, $sim(x,l)$ characterizes how similar x is to landmark l, for points x and l in an n-dimensional space. Note that *sim* is a symmetric function; $sim(x,l) = sim(l,x)$. This is a required condition for all

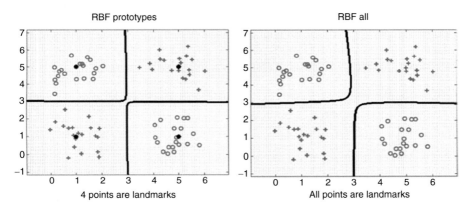

Fig. 6.16 Kernel logistic regression for a binary classification problem. On the left four landmarks are chosen, indicated by the black circles. On the right, all the data points serve as landmarks. The similarity between each data point and the landmarks concerned has been measured using the Radial Basis Function (RBF), described in the section on "Similarity Functions for Kernel Methods". Note that in this case the boundaries are similar, and that both lead to perfect separation of the classes

kernels. The new representation for point x is a three-dimensional vector, characterizing how similar x is to the three chosen landmarks

$$\left(sim(x,l_1),sim(x,l_2),sim(x,l_3)\right)$$

This representation of x is a sequence of pairwise comparisons to three landmark examples: instead of the classical representation in terms of the features of x alone. In this new representation, the posterior probability of $y = 1$ will be approximated for the example as

$$P(y = 1|;x|;\theta) = \sigma\left(\theta_0 + \theta_1 sim(x,l_1) + \theta_2 sim(x,l_2) + \theta_3 sim(x,l_3)\right)$$

The decision rule for classification is a linear function in θ which can be learned by classical logistic regression.

$$\left(\theta_0 + \theta_1 sim(x,l_1) + \theta_2 sim(x,l_2) + \theta_3 sim(x,l_3)\right) \geq 0$$

Note that the features associated with the decision function no longer pertain to x alone, but to its similarity to a set of landmark examples. When the radial basis function is used as a similarity function, the linear hyperplane in the similarity feature space forms complex non-linear boundaries in the original x_1–x_2 coordinate space. As an example, consider the task of separating the points laid out in an XOR configuration (XOR is a Boolean function with two inputs that will be true if and only if they are different) as shown in Fig. 6.16. Given points on the plane drawn from two classes, the task is to learn a decision surface that separates the two classes correctly. Clearly, the two classes cannot be separated by a linear hyperplane in the original feature space. Suppose four landmarks l_1, l_2, l_3, l_4, are presciently selected, which are centroids of the four clusters of training points, indicated by a larger filled black circle in the figure. Then, every point $x = (x_1,x_2)$ is mapped into

$$x \rightarrow \left(sim(x,l_1),sim(x,l_2),sim(x,l_3),sim(x,l_4)\right)$$

Given the 80 points in x labeled 0 or 1 the predictors are transformed into an 80×4 matrix K, and the label vector of length 80 containing 0s and 1s denoting members of class 0 or class 1. It is possible to use regularized logistic regression on (K,y), and optimize the penalized cross-entropy loss function to learn the parameter vector θ characterizing the linear hyperplane in the feature space of K. This approach is called **kernelized logistic regression**. To make a prediction on a new example x, x is transformed into a four-dimensional vector kx with the mapping above, and $\sigma(\theta^T kx)$ is computed to obtain its classification. It is possible to project the linear hyperplane into the original feature space as shown in Fig. 6.16 (black lines), and observe that a near-perfect approximation of the XOR function has been learned. This is mostly due to a very judicious choice of landmarks. However, when all training data points are chosen as landmarks, so that the transformed predictor matrix K is of dimension 80×80, an excellent approximation to the true function is still obtained.

There are three approaches to landmark selection for kernelized logistic regression:

1. use all examples in the training set as landmarks and choose a large regularization constant in the penalty function, especially if the number of examples is large. Regularization is critical to reduce the risk of overfitting.
2. cluster the examples in the training set and select cluster centers as landmarks. When the number of examples is very large (in the millions), this approach works better than choosing all examples as landmarks.
3. have domain experts suggest landmarks.

Kernelized logistic regression has been applied to predict the effects of drugs by representing them in terms of their similarity to other drugs. For example, McCoy and Perlis describe the application of logistic regression to drug representations that include the similarities between the side-effect profiles of a drug and those of a curated panel of six drugs that affect the central nervous system, in order to predict which drugs will cross the blood-brain barrier [18]. This work exemplifies the expert-driven approach to landmark selection.

Similarity Functions for Kernel Methods

The success of kernelization is closely tied to the choice of the similarity or kernel function. A kernel function k measures how similar two d-dimensional vectors are.

$$k : R^d \times R^d \to R$$

It takes two vectors as arguments and returns a real number measuring the similarity between the two input vectors. The **radial basis function** is a popular general-purpose kernel for vectors in R^d. It has been rediscovered in many applied areas of science, and is known by a variety of names, including the Gaussian kernel.

$$k\left(x,l\right) = \exp\left(-\frac{x-l^2}{2\sigma^2}\right)$$

Another popular kernel is the polynomial kernel of order n, defined as

$$k\left(x,l\right) = \left(x^T l + 1\right)^n$$

Note that both functions are symmetric. Kernel functions are often designed with specific applications in mind; this activity is called kernel engineering. Consider the problem of predicting DNA sequences in the human genome that encode proteins. A supervised machine learning approach to this problem casts the problem in the framework of binary classification. It entails gathering a training set of protein-encoding DNA sequences and DNA sequences known not to encode proteins (e.g., sequences drawn from regulatory regions). The success of the machine learning approach is deeply tied to how the input DNA sequences are represented. A poor representation leads to predictive models with poor generalization performance.

One idea for representing the training data sequences is to have expert biologists manually engineer features (e.g., counts of specific short subsequences which may/may not be indicative of protein regions). Another idea is to move away from a representation tied to a single DNA sequence to a comparative representational approach. That is, rather than trying to describe a DNA sequence on its own, a kernel function k is defined on DNA sequences which evaluates how similar two sequences are. Such kernel functions are much easier to design than features on an individual DNA sequence. Next, L landmark DNA sequences from both classes (protein-coding and non-coding) are selected and each DNA sequence is represented as a vector of length L denoting its similarity to these L landmarks. It is then possible to apply penalized logistic regression, Gaussian Discriminant Analysis, or Factored Naive Bayes models to learn the prediction function from the kernel representations. The reader is directed to the following textbook for further discussion of this approach [19].

The practical significance of working in kernel space, rather than in an expanded basis function space is revealed through the following image processing example. Suppose images of size 16 × 16 are available for a binary classification task. If all fifth order polynomial terms in the 16 × 16 pixel space are considered as features, the size of the feature space will expand to $\sum_{k=1}^{5} \binom{256}{k} \approx 10^{10}$. Instead, working with a polynomial *kernel* of degree 5, it is possible to compute $(x^T l + 1)^5$ between image x, and landmark l in $O(16 \times 16)$ time—take the dot product of image x and image l, and add 1 to the value, and raise it to the fifth power. The basis function space of all fifth order polynomials is never explicitly materialized, but the effect of working in that space is obtained, with simply O(256) amount of work! This is the magic of kernels.

Recap: How to Use Kernels for Classification

Given a labeled training set D of (**x**,y) pairs,

- Choose L landmarks from D
- Choose a kernel function k that captures similarity between pairs of examples
- Represent each **x** in D by a vector of length L + 1 of the form $(1, k(x, l_1), \ldots, k(x, l_L))$. The prepended 1 is used for the intercept term θ_0 in the learned model. The new training set K has (**kx**,y) pairs, where **kx** is the kernelized representation of **x**.

- Use a discriminative (penalized logistic regression) or generative (Gaussian discriminant Analysis, Naive Bayes) model to estimate a parameter vector from the kernel transformed data K and label vector y.
- To predict on a new example **x**, map it to its kernel form **kx**, and use the learned parameter vector with **kx** to compute the classification.

Sparse Kernel Machines and Maximum Margin Classifiers

Kernelization can yield models with poor generalization performance, particularly if landmarks are chosen poorly. Too many landmarks could potentially result in an overfitted model, and too few landmarks result in underfitted models. Conceptually, the most important landmarks are arguably those that are close to the boundary between classes, because it is these landmarks that will help to distinguish between examples that are hardest to classify. A geometric view of the classification problem gives us insight into how to simultaneously select good landmarks and build a high-performance classifier.

Consider the points on a plane drawn from two classes as shown in Fig. 6.17. The points are linearly separable, and an infinite collection of boundary lines drawn in the space between the two sets of points is a perfect classifier. Of all these lines, only one, shown as a dotted black line in Fig. 6.17, maximizes the distance between the points in the two classes. The separating hyperplane is equidistant from the closest points to it in both classes. By formulating the problem of finding the decision boundary that *maximally* separates two (separable) classes as an optimization problem, it is possible to find a *unique* solution to the problem of finding the "best" classifier. In Fig. 6.17, the position and orientation of the maximum margin separating line is determined by just two of the nine training data points—i.e., the points at the

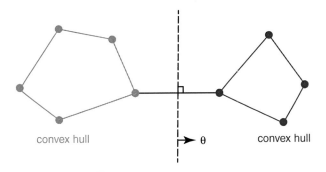

$$\theta^T x + \theta_0 = 0 : \text{separating hyperplane}$$

Fig. 6.17 The optimal decision boundary separating points from two classes on the plane. This boundary is the maximum margin separating line and is the perpendicular bisector of the line joining the closest points on the **convex hulls** of the two linearly separable classes. Note that this decision boundary can be identified using a single landmark from each class only

ends of the line perpendicular to the decision boundary. These two points are called *support vectors* and form the sparse set of landmarks needed to describe the optimal, margin-maximizing decision boundary. The problem of finding the (sparse) set of landmarks and the optimal placement of the decision hyperplane is thus solved jointly.

To understand how to set up the optimization problem of maximizing the geometric margin between two sets of separable points, it is helpful to review some geometry as shown in Fig. 6.18. The margin r of a point x from a hyperplane defined by $\theta^T x + \theta_0 = 0$ is the perpendicular distance of x from the plane. θ is the slope of the hyperplane, and θ_0 is the intercept.

The *sign* of the distance of a point from a decision boundary is determined by whether it is on the positive or the negative side of the hyperplane (the distance for x would be positive, but one might imagine the reflection of x falling on the negative side of the boundary, to the left of it). The label set $\{0,1\}$ will be mapped to the set $\{-1,1\}$ to write a single formula for the margins of members of both classes. With y as an element of this set (i.e., a label in $\{-1,1\}$), the margin of a point (x,y) in a dataset D is

$$r = y \frac{\theta^T x + \theta_0}{\|\theta\|}$$

Note that this new definition of margin r is greater than 0 for points on both sides of the boundary since the (negative) distance is multiplied with label $y = -1$ for points in the negative class. A dataset D is correctly classified, if and only if the margins of

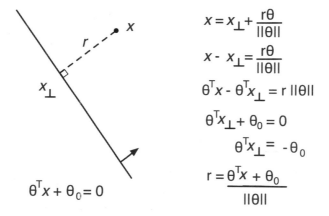

$$x = x_\perp + \frac{r\theta}{\|\theta\|}$$

$$x - x_\perp = \frac{r\theta}{\|\theta\|}$$

$$\theta^T x - \theta^T x_\perp = r\|\theta\|$$

$$\theta^T x_\perp + \theta_0 = 0$$

$$\theta^T x_\perp = -\theta_0$$

$$r = \frac{\theta^T x + \theta_0}{\|\theta\|}$$

Fig. 6.18 r is the perpendicular distance of the point x from the hyperplane $\theta^T x + \theta_0 = 0$. The unit vector perpendicular to the plane is $\frac{\theta}{\|\theta\|}$. A perpendicular line (of length r, and parallel to this unit vector) dropped from the point x meets the plane at $x_\perp$. So, x is the vector sum of $x_\perp$ and $r\frac{\theta}{\|\theta\|}$. Rearranging terms, and taking the dot product on both sides by θ, the given expression for the scalar distance r is derived

all the points in D are greater than 0. The margin of the entire dataset is the smallest margin among all its elements.

$$margin(D) = \min_{(x,y)in D} y \frac{\theta^T x + \theta_0}{\|\theta\|}$$

To separate the two classes maximally, the slope θ and intercept θ_0 of the separating hyperplane to maximize $margin(D)$ must be selected. That is, there is a need to find

$$(\theta, \theta_0) = argmax_{(\theta,\theta_0)} \min_{(x,y)in D} y \frac{\theta^T x + \theta_0}{\|\theta\|}$$

Unfortunately, this specification of the optimization problem yields infinitely many solutions for θ and θ_0—because for every k, if θ and θ_0 are solutions, so are $k\theta$ and $k\theta_0$. That is, the optimal solution is agnostic to the length of the vector defining the hyperplane. To obtain a unique solution, a scaling factor is defined such that

$$\min_{(x,y)in D} y(\theta^T x + \theta_0) = 1$$

for the point (x,y) in the dataset D that is closest to the decision boundary. So, the optimization problem is reduced to finding

$$(\theta, \theta_0) = argmax_{(\theta,\theta_0)} \frac{1}{\|\theta\|}$$

subject to the constraints that $y(\theta^T x + \theta_0) \geq 1$ for all points (x,y) in D. That is, all points in D must be at a distance of one or greater from the decision boundary. Maximizing $\frac{1}{\|\theta\|}$ is equivalent to minimizing $\|\theta\|$, so the maximization problem is converted into a constrained quadratic minimization problem and can be solved using a classical numerical solver.

$$\min_{\theta,\theta_0} \frac{1}{2}\|\theta\|^2 \text{ subject to } y(\theta^T x + \theta_0) \geq 1 \text{ for all}(x,y)\text{in D}$$

The solution obtained from the solver has the form

$$\theta = \sum_{(x,y)in D} \alpha yx$$

which associates a weight α with each point (x,y) in D. The slope and intercept of the maximum margin separator depends only on those (x,y) for which $\alpha > 0$, as illustrated in Fig. 6.19. These points are the support vectors for the classifier and form a sparse set of landmarks for the dataset. The dark line in Fig. 6.19 is the

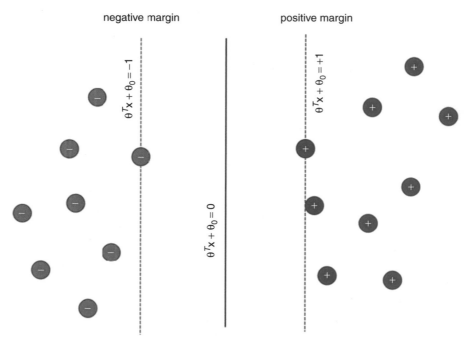

negative margin   positive margin

Fig. 6.19 Two support vectors for a two-class problem in two dimensions. The position and orientation of the decision boundary is determined by the two support vectors, which form a sparse set of landmarks for the dataset shown. The support vectors are computed by solving the quadratic optimization problem of finding the maximum margin separator between the two classes. The dotted blue line, called the positive margin, is parallel to the decision boundary. All positive (blue) examples lie on or to the right of the positive margin. The dotted orange line is the negative margin. A. negative (orange) examples lie on or to the left of the negative margin. The positive and negative examples are separated by a distance equal to the margin width. The larger the margin width, the more robust the classifier

decision boundary, and the dotted lines at +1 and −1 denote the positive and negative margin lines. The resulting classifier is called a **support vector machine** (SVM).

To classify a new point x' with a SVM the side of the decision boundary the point lies on is computed,

$$sign\left(\theta^T x' + \theta_0\right) = sign\left(\sum_{(x,y)\,in\,D} \alpha\, y x^T x' + \theta_0\right)$$

Only the support vectors with non-zero α are involved in this computation, even though the summation as written is over all (x,y) in D. Effectively, the position of the new point relative to *all* of the support vectors is used to make classification decisions, taking into account both which side of each support vector the point lies on, and how far it is from this support vector. To build a non-linear SVM, the linear dot product $x^T x'$

Fig. 6.20 Non-linear
decision boundaries
(demarcating the red and
the blue shaded regions)
and support vectors (circles
enclosed in a purple ring)
for a 2D data set learned
with a radial basis function

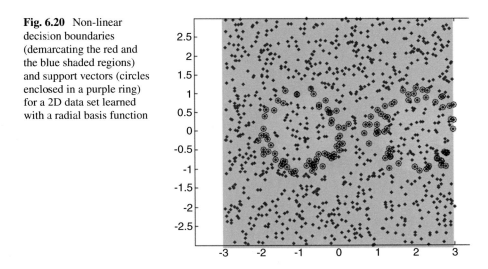

is replaced by a kernel function $k(x,x')$, such as the radial basis function. It is possible
to learn non-linear decision boundaries in two-dimensional data as shown in Fig. 6.20
and identify a sparse set of support vectors using radial basis function as kernels,
rather than the linear dot product kernel described in the equation above.

In all the discussion so far, it has been assumed that the two classes are separable,
either linearly with a dot product kernel, or non-linearly with a polynomial or radial
basis function kernel. To make SVMs practical for real world data sets which are not
linearly separable to begin with, the formulation of maximum margin classifiers is
extended to allow misclassified points. This tolerance for misclassification also
relates to the recurring theme of overfitting. A solution that permits misclassification of points in the training set may generalize better to other data than one that fits
the training set perfectly (Fig. 6.21).

The optimization objective of SVMs will be adapted to relax the margin constraint on some of the points. Margin width of the final classifier can be traded off
with the number of points in the data set that are allowed to violate margin constraints, i.e., fall on the wrong side of their class boundary.

Margin violation $\xi_{(x,y)}$ of a point (x,y) is defined as the distance of x from its class
margin (Fig. 6.22). Then, the margin maximization optimization problem is formulated as

$$\min_{\theta,\theta_0} \frac{1}{2}\|\theta\|^2 + C\sum_{(x,y) \text{ in } D} \xi_{(x,y)} \text{ subject to}$$
$$y\left(\theta^T x + \theta_0\right) \geq 1 - \xi_{(x,y)} \text{ and } \xi_{(x,y)} \geq 0 \text{ for all } (x,y) \text{ in } D$$

A point that is correctly classified will have a margin violation of exactly zero,
incorrectly classified points will have margin violations greater than zero. The regularization constant C is a measure of the willingness to allow misclassifications.

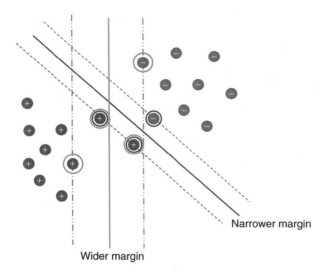

Fig. 6.21 Given the two-class dataset on the plane, the maximum margin separator derived by an SVM is shown by the solid purple line and the small-dashed margins. This SVM has a narrow margin and is defined by three support vectors, that are circles, enclosed in a purple ring. If the two circled positive class points in the center are ignored, it is possible to construct an SVM classifier with a much wider margin indicated by the broken dotted blue and orange lines. The support vectors for the wider margin classifier are circled in green. Wider margin classifiers have better generalization performance

Fig. 6.22 The orange point outside the orange margin, and the misclassified blue point outside the blue margin, have both violated their margins. The extent of violation, defined as the distance from the point to its class margin, is traded off against margin width in the penalized objective function for an SVM for non-separable data

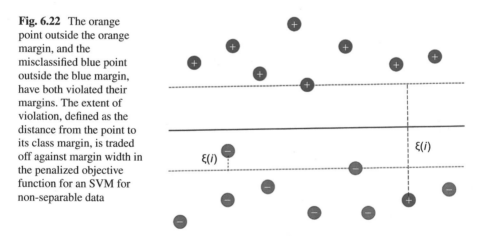

This is analogous to the approaches to regularization introduced in the discussion of linear models, in the sense that permitting misclassifications prevents a model from overfitting to the training set, improving generalization to new datasets. If C is high (imposing a high penalty for misclassification), then the margin violation term dominates, and the optimizer is forced to reduce the margin width concomitantly; while if C is low, the optimizer will construct a wide margin classifier since margin violations are not penalized so heavily. The penalized version of the SVM optimization yields a soft-margin SVM. For any value of C, which expresses the tradeoff between margin width and misclassification rate, the optimizer produces a unique solution to θ and θ_0 and identifies the sparse set of landmarks (i.e., support vectors).

Neural Networks: Stacked Logistic Models

In this section, neural networks will be introduced. As noted throughout this volume, neural networks—and, in particular, **deep neural networks**—have led to rapid advancements in automated image recognition, speech recognition, and natural language processing, amongst other areas. A remarkable feature of contemporary neural network models is that the underlying models are composed of individual units that are relatively simple in their design. It is the interaction between large numbers of such units that gives deep neural networks their representational power.

The fundamental building block of deep neural networks is the logistic model, shown in Fig. 6.23. As was seen in the section on "Discriminative models: Logistic Regression", the logistic model characterized by the parameter vector θ captures the posterior probability $P(y = 1|x; \theta)$ from a dataset composed of vectors $x \in R^d$ with associated labels $y \in \{0, 1\}$. It predicts class membership y from the input x by computing $g(\theta^T x)$ where g is the sigmoid function. The sigmoid function squashes the dot product $\theta^T x$ which can be an arbitrary real number, into the range [0,1]. The dot product here provides a concise way to express a sequence of operations in which the values of each blue input node (1 for the bias term, x_1 and x_2) are multiplied by a corresponding weight $1(-30) + x_1 (20) + x_2 (20)$ and added together to produce the input to the orange node, which applies the sigmoid function as its **activation function**. A logistic model is a linear classifier—it can only capture linear boundaries separating classes $y = 0$ and $y = 1$.

The model in Fig. 6.23 maps $x \in \{0, 1\}^2$ to $y \in \{0, 1\}$. The network computes the Boolean AND of the two components of x. Note that the sigmoid function $g(a) \approx 0$ for $a \ll 0$ and $g(a) \approx 1$ for $a \gg 0$. Thus, when both components of x are 1, the linear

Fig. 6.23 A logistic model, drawn as a two-layer neural network. The first layer is the Boolean input vector **x** and the second layer is the output y composed of a single logistic unit. This network computes the Boolean AND of the components of x

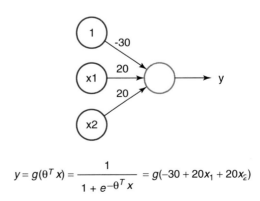

$$y = g(\theta^T x) = \frac{1}{1 + e^{-\theta^T x}} = g(-30 + 20x_1 + 20x_2)$$

dot product $\theta^T x = 10$; and $y = g(10) \approx 1$. When any one, or both of the components of x are zero, the corresponding dot product $\theta^T x \leq -10$, so $y = g(-10) \approx 0$.

In 1943, McCollough and Pitts [20] demonstrated that a stacked assembly of logistic units can represent **any** Boolean function—and by extension any function that can be calculated on a classical computer. An example of a stacked assembly composed of three layers is shown in Fig. 6.24. The network represents the nonlinearly separable XNOR function (the logical complement of the XOR function—true if and only if both inputs are identical), i.e., the output $y = x_1 \; XNOR \; x_2$.

Given an input Boolean vector x, the intermediate outputs a_1 and a_2 of the second (hidden) layer are calculated, and the output y of the final layer is then computed in terms of a_1 and a_2:

$$a_1 = g\left(-30 + 20 x_1 + 20 x_2\right)$$

$$a_2 = g\left(10 - 20 x_1 - 20 x_2\right)$$

$$y = g\left(-10 + 20 a_1 + 20 a_2\right)$$

Computation of the outputs of the network proceeds sequentially, layer by layer, with outputs of layer $i + 1$ computed from the outputs of layer i. This network is

Fig. 6.24 A three layer, fully connected, stacked assembly of logistic units with an input layer, a hidden layer (composed of a bias unit set to 1, and two logistic units with outputs a_1 and a_2) and an output layer with a single logistic unit with output y. The network computes the nonlinear function x_1 XNOR x_2, which cannot be represented by a single logistic model. The parameters defining the model are the weights on the edges connecting the units to one another, and it is these weights that define the behavior of the model. The attentive reader will recognize the AND subnetwork from Fig. 6.23 leading to output a_1

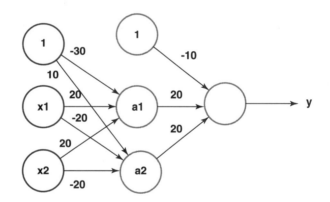

X_1	X_2	a_1	a_2	y
0	0	0	1	1
0	1	0	0	0
1	0	0	0	0
1	1	1	0	1

fully connected, i.e., every logistic unit in layer $i + 1$ is connected to all the units in the layer i below. In the example network shown in Fig. 6.24, layer 2 outputs are computed from layer 1 (the inputs), and the layer 3 output is computed from the values of units in layer 2. Note that the units a_1 and a_2 in layer 2 are connected to all units (including the bias unit) in the input layer. Fully connected stacked assemblies of logistic units are therefore called **feedforward multilayer networks**. The final output y is a highly non-linear function of the input vector x, viz.,

$$y = g\left(-10 + 20g\left(-30 + 20x_1 + 20x_2\right) + 20g\left(10 - 20x_1 - 20x_2\right)\right)$$

The parameters of the feedforward network are defined in Fig. 6.24 using two parameter matrices, one defining the weighted connections between layer 2 and layer 1 (the matrix $\Theta^{(1)}$), and the other between layer 3 and layer 2 (the matrix $\Theta^{(2)}$) shown below (Fig. 6.24).

$$\Theta^{(1)} = \begin{bmatrix} -30 & 20 & 20 \\ 10 & -20 & -20 \end{bmatrix}; \quad \Theta^{(2)} = \begin{bmatrix} -10 & 20 & 20 \end{bmatrix}$$

Note that $\Theta^{(1)}$ has dimension 2×3, reflecting the fact that there are two logistic units in layer 2 connected to the two input units in layer 1 and the additional bias unit. $\Theta^{(2)}$ has dimension 1×3, since there is a single output unit in layer 3 connected to the two logistic units and the bias unit in layer 2.

Parameterizing Feedforward Networks and the Forward Propagation Algorithm

Given a new input vector $\mathbf{x}$, it is possible to define the vector $a^{(l)}$ of activations of the units in each layer l in the network with the following system of matrix operations.

$$a^{(1)} = x$$

$$z^{(l+1)} = \Theta^{(l)} * \left[1; a^{(l)}\right], \quad l = 1...L-1$$

$$a^{(l+1)} = g\left(z^{(l+1)}\right), \quad l = 1...L-1$$

The symbol z in these equations corresponds to the sum of the inputs to a layer (or individual unit within a layer) *before* the activation function g has been applied. In the running example, the value z—known as the **logit**—for unit a_1 would be $-30 + 20x_1 + 20x_2$. The equations provide a symbolic representation of a sequence of steps in which the input, x, provides initial activation values for the input layer of the network. Then, the logits, z, for a subsequent layer are calculated by multiplying these inputs by the weighted connections, Θ, to each of its units, and adding the results. The matrix product in the equation provides a shorthand notation for performing this operation across all units in a layer and describes the way in which this operation is generally implemented to take advantage of efficient numerical computations provided by Graphical Processing Units (GPUs) and other specialized hardware. Finally, the activation function, g, is applied to the logits, to estimate the activations for this layer, which may in turn provide the input for a layer to follow.

The system of equations for forward propagation shown above can be used to calculate the final output of a fully connected, L layered feedforward network. Such a network is characterized by $L - 1$ parameter matrices $\Theta^{(l)}$, $l = 1...L - 1$. Each layer l has $S^{(l)}$ units and a single bias unit. Matrix $\Theta^{(l)}$ connects layer l to layer $l + 1$ and has dimensionality $S^{(l + 1)} \times (S^{(l)} + 1)$. For example, in the network depicted in Fig. 6.24, $S^{(1)} = 2$, $S^{(2)} = 2$, $S^{(3)} = 1$, $L = 3$. This network has two parameter matrices of sizes $2 \times (2 + 1)$ and $1 \times (2 + 1)$ and a total of 9 parameters.

By increasing the number L of layers, as well as by increasing the number of logistic units in each layer, it is possible to represent nonlinear functions of ever-increasing complexity. A deep feedforward network encodes a set of prior beliefs about the structure of the function that maps vectors x to the class y. The intermediate layers represent underlying factors of variation, which in turn can be expressed in terms of simpler factors, all the way down to the input components in x. Fully connected, feedforward networks are universal function approximators, capable of representing any mapping from inputs to outputs to within any specified tolerance ε of the true function [21].

Any Boolean function can be represented by a three-layer network, such as the one shown in Fig. 6.24. Any continuous function on the reals can be approximated by a three-layer network, but it may require a very large number of units in each layer [22, 23]. Finally, any function (including discontinuous functions) can be approximated by a four-layer network with enough units in each layer. Surprisingly, these representation theorems hold not just for logistic units (in which the non-linearity $g(x)$ is the sigmoid function), but for **rectified linear units** (called ReLUs), defined as $g(x) = max\,(0, x)$ as well. ReLUs are the most widely used non-linearity in feedforward neural networks, because the maximum is cheaper to compute than the sigmoid, and it has been experimentally found to accelerate the convergence of stochastic gradient descent for parameter learning [24].

While the representation theorems assure us that a network with four layers is sufficient to capture any mapping, they place no bounds on the "width" of each layer. In practice, networks of much greater depths are built, trading off the number of units in each layer for depth. While a feedforward neural network of sufficient depth and width can represent any function in principle, in practice, it is not guaranteed to find those parameter settings with the training algorithms.

In the networks discussed up to this point, the parameters of the networks have been pre-configured to approximate particular Boolean functions. However, neural networks must learn how to approximate functions of interest for AIM applications, such as radiological image recognition. As is apparent from the network in the running example, the behavior of a feedforward neural network is dictated by its weights, as these determine how input from one layer proceeds to activate units in the next. Therefore, it is the weights that must be adjusted to change the behavior of a neural network during the process of training it. The section that follows will explain how the backpropagation algorithm—the mainstay of training neural networks—is used to accomplish this end.

Learning the Parameters of a Feedforward Network

A standard way of presenting the backpropagation algorithm uses calculus to calculate a sequence of derivatives, each of which measures how much the result of one operation (such as multiplication by a set of network weights, or the application of an activation function) influences the operation that follows it. As with linear regression, the key idea is to update each model parameter in accordance with its influence. However, with linear regression this influence is straightforward to estimate, as it depends only upon the (constant) slope of the line concerned, and the input features. With nonlinearities such as the sigmoid function, the extent to which a particular change in input influences the output of the function differs depending upon the value of the function beforehand (Fig. 6.25).

With knowledge of the extent of the influence of each neural network weight on the output of the model—and hence the loss function—it is possible to update individual parameters to steer the model toward accurate classification of the data in a training set. Beginning with this standard presentation, some other perspectives on the algorithm will be provided to help to build intuition about backpropagation. While this constitutes more detail than has been provided with some of the other algorithms under discussion, this is warranted here because backpropagation is fundamental to training deep neural networks, which have become—or are becoming—the dominant approach to many problems in AIM. As ultimately there is a

Fig. 6.25 The extent to which changing the input of the sigmoid function (x axis) influences its output (y axis) depends upon the value of the function beforehand. Both d1 and d2 represent the change in y after adding 1 to x, but d2 is much larger

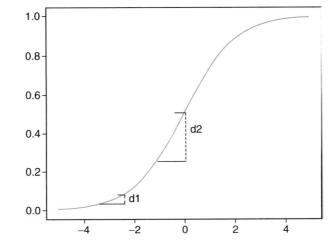

need to know how much each parameter influences the loss function, the presentation will begin there.

$$J(\theta) = -\left(\left[y\log(h(x))\right] + \left[(1-y)\log(1-h(x))\right]\right)$$

Recall the cross entropy loss function for a single example (x,y), shown above. The prediction function with parameter vector θ is

$$h(x) = g\left(\theta^T x\right)$$

The parameters θ (referred to as weights in neural network parlance) can be learned from a given data set by gradient descent on the cross-entropy loss function

$$\theta \leftarrow \theta - \frac{dJ(\theta)}{d\theta}$$

The gradient of the cross-entropy loss function with respect to the component θ_j is

$$\frac{dJ(\theta)}{d\theta_j} = \left(h(x) - y\right)x_j$$

The first term is the error in prediction on the (x,y) pair (how "wrong" the model was), and the second term is the j-*th* component of the input vector x (this determines how changing the parameters in θ will affect a model prediction—for example, if $x_j^{(i)} = 0$, changing the parameter $\theta_j^{(i)}$ will not improve classification of this example). Therefore, the gradient tells us how each parameter in θ influences how well the prediction for a specific example approximates the correct label, y. This gradient can be used for updating the parameters connecting the final two layers of a feedforward network, which function as a simple logistic model. However, with deeper networks there is a need to estimate the influence of weights in proximal layers on model error, to determine how these weights should be updated. The simple feedforward network in Fig. 6.26 will be used to explain how derivatives of the loss function can be computed with respect to all the weights in the network.

The input vector x has two components, and the hidden layers have two logistic units each. The final output is a scalar $a^{(4)}$. Here are the forward equations to calculate the output $h((x_1, x_2))$ of the network, repeating the sequence of equations from the section on "Parameterizing feedforward networks and the forward propagation algorithm" (input → logit (z) → activation ($g(z)$) for each layer of the network.

$$a^{(1)} = (x_1, x_2)$$

$$z^{(2)} = \Theta^{(1)} * \left[1; a^{(1)}\right]$$

Fig. 6.26 A simple four-layer feedforward neural network to illustrate the backpropagation algorithm and the computation of the derivative of the loss function with respect to all the network parameters

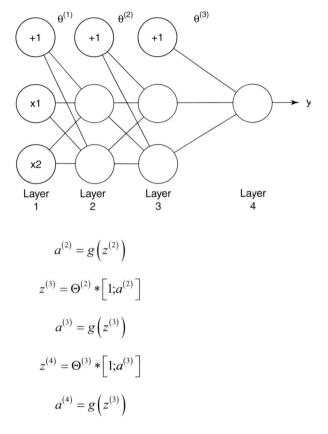

$$a^{(2)} = g\left(z^{(2)}\right)$$

$$z^{(3)} = \Theta^{(2)} * \left[1; a^{(2)}\right]$$

$$a^{(3)} = g\left(z^{(3)}\right)$$

$$z^{(4)} = \Theta^{(3)} * \left[1; a^{(3)}\right]$$

$$a^{(4)} = g\left(z^{(3)}\right)$$

First, the derivative of the loss function $J(\theta)$ with respect to $\theta^{(3)}$ is calculated, using the chain rule of differentiation. This estimates the influence of the weights in the penultimate layer $(\Theta^{(3)})$ on the loss function. As the output of the third layer will be ingested by the fourth layer to generate the output of the network, this estimation must consider the operations of the output unit also.

$$\frac{dJ}{d\Theta^{(3)}} = \frac{dJ}{da^{(4)}} \frac{da^{(4)}}{dz^{(4)}} \frac{dz^{(4)}}{d\Theta^{(3)}}$$

Consequently, the first term is the derivative of the cross-entropy loss with respect to the network output, the result of applying the sigmoid activation function to the logit of the output unit, $z^{(4)}$. The second term is the derivative of this non-linear sigmoid function with respect to the logit, and the final term is the derivative of the logit with respect to the $\theta^{(3)}$ parameter. The steps of the calculation are as follows:

$$J(\theta) = -\left[\left[y log\left(a^{(4)}\right)\right] + \left[(1-y)\log\left(1-a^{(4)}\right)\right]\right]$$

$$\frac{dJ}{da^{(4)}} = -\frac{\left(y - a^{(4)}\right)}{a^{(4)}\left(1 - a^{(4)}\right)} \quad \text{---hint}^{14}$$

$$\frac{da^{(4)}}{dz^{(4)}} = a^{(4)}\left(1 - a^{(4)}\right)$$

$$\frac{dz^{(4)}}{d\Theta^{(3)}} = \left[1; a^{(3)}\right]$$

$$\frac{dJ}{d\Theta^{(3)}} = \left(a^{(4)} - y\right)\left[1; a^{(3)}\right]$$

which mirrors the derivative of a single logistic unit with input x replaced by the activation of the layer right below the output layer ($[1;a^{(3)}]$, with 1 indicating the relevant bias term). The numerator of the first derivative calculated, $\frac{dJ}{da^{(4)}}$, incorporates the class label: $(y - a^{(4)})$ indicates both the direction and the magnitude of the desired correction to the output of the model. If the label y is one, this will measure how far from one the output was, and the sign will be positive. If the label y is zero, this will measure how far from zero the output was, and the sign will be negative. The denominator is the derivative of the sigmoid function,[15] $g(x)(1 - g(x))$.

This is also the second derivative calculated, because it governs the influence of the logit it activates, z,[4] on the loss function. The influence of the weights in the preceding layer, $\Theta^{(3)}$, on this logit depend upon the activations they are multiplied by, $a^{(3)}$. When these three derivatives are multiplied together, as dictated by the chain rule, the term $a^{(4)}(1 - a^{(4)})$ cancels out, leaving $\frac{dJ}{d\Theta^{(3)}}$. Essentially, the chain of influence is traversed in reverse, from the error function through the logistic unit, and finally to the weights of the third layer. From here it is possible to proceed recursively.

A second view of the backpropagation algorithm considers it from the perspective of how responsibility for error is allocated across the weights of the network. If the counterpart of model error (the $a^{(4)} - y$ term) for the hidden units in the network is known, it is possible to compute derivatives of the loss function with respect to $\Theta^{(2)}$ and $\Theta^{(1)}$ as well. Error at the output layer is defined as

$$\delta^{(4)} = \left(a^{(4)} - y\right)$$

---

[14] Recall (perhaps from distant calculus) that the derivative of d/dy log(y) = 1/y. Proceed algebraically from this step by cross-multiplying the summed fractions to reach this derivative.

[15] The sigmoid function $g(x) = 1/(1 + e^{-x}) = (1 + e^{-x})^{-1}$. Its derivative $dg(x)/dx = (-1)(1 + e^{-x})^{-2}de^{-x}/dx = (-1)(1 + e^{-x})^{-2}(-1)e^{-x} = 1/(1 + e^{-x})(1 - 1/(1 + e^{-x})) = g(x)(1 - g(x))$.

The key idea behind the backpropagation algorithm is that each of the hidden nodes in Layer 3 is responsible for some fraction of the error in the output node, and the extent of this responsibility depends upon the weights connecting them to it. For example, the error at hidden node j in Layer 3 is determined by $\theta_j^{(3)}$, the weight connecting unit j to the output unit, and the error at the output unit, $\delta^{(4)}$, modulated by the extent to which changing the logit of this node will affect the output of the activation function that follows it.

$$\delta_j^{(3)} = \theta_j^{(3)} \delta^{(4)} \left(\frac{da^{(3)}}{dz^{(3)}} \right)_j$$

In vector form, this can be rewritten as

$$\delta_j^{(3)} = \left(\theta_j^{(3)} \right)^T \delta^{(4)} \odot \frac{da^{(3)}}{dz^{(3)}}$$

where the $\odot$ operator is the Hadamard product of the two vectors—a pointwise multiplication of the components of two equally sized vectors. One can see the correspondence between the the jth element of $\delta^{(3)}$ shown above, and vectorized form below. Generalizing, for $l = 2 \dots L - 1$,

$$\delta^{(l)} = \left(\theta_j^{(l)} \right)^T \delta^{(l+1)} \odot \frac{da^{(l)}}{dz^{(l)}}$$

Gradient descent is used to update the parameters of the network. The learning procedure which incorporates both forward and backward propagation is shown below. Initialization of gradients for all unit pairs ij is with unit j in layer l and unit i in layer $l + 1$, for $l = 1 \dots L - 1$.

$$\Delta_{ij}^{(l)} = 0$$

For every example pair (x,y) in the training data

1. set $a^{(1)} = x$
2. use forward propagation to compute $a^{(2)},...,a^{(L)}$
3. set $\delta^{(l)} = (a^{(L)} - y)$
4. use backpropagation to compute $\delta^{(l-1)},...,\delta^{(2)}$
5. update gradients using $\Delta_{ij}^{(l)} \leftarrow \Delta_{ij}^{(l)} + a_j^{(l)} \delta_i^{(l+1)}$ for every i,j,l
6. update parameter by gradient descent using $\theta_{ij}^{(l)} \leftarrow \theta_{ij}^{(l)} - \alpha \Delta_{ij}^{(l)}$ for every i,j,l

This algorithm can be extended to work not just on feedforward networks, but on general computation graphs, providing a third perspective on the algorithm. The nodes of a computation graph are operations (e.g., sums, products, reciprocals, exponentiations) and the leaves of the graph are the operands (the quantities upon which these operations are applied). The computation graph for the sigmoid of the dot product of two vectors $\theta, x \dfrac{1}{1 + \exp\left(-\left(\theta_0 + \theta_1 x_1 + \theta_2 x_2\right)\right)}$ is shown in Fig. 6.27.

Schematically, this could represent the components of the neural network in Fig. 6.26 running from layer three to the output node, after receiving, summing, and transforming input from the previous layer. To keep the quantities manageable and readable, the inputs -1 and -3 are used, though in practice these would be values between 0 and 1 if a sigmoid activation function were used. Feeding forward (from left to right), these incoming values as well as a 1 representing the bias term are then multiplied by the weights of the third layer, $\theta^{(3)}$ (i.e. the vector $[-3,1,-2]$), which connects this layer to the output node. The resulting products are then added to generate the logit $z^{(4)}$. This logit provides the input to the sigmoid function ($1/1 + \exp(-x)$), which in the computation graph is decomposed into a series of individual operations, first reversing the sign, exponentiating, adding one and taking the reciprocal. The result is $a^{(4)}$, which gives the output of the network for this example: a predicted probability of 0.88 that this example belongs to the positive class.

In order to update the weights of the network the cross-entropy loss (CE) is first measured. For an example from the positive class this is calculated as $-log(p)$, with p as the predicted probability. The next step is to proceed back across the graph (from right to left), multiplying this value by the derivative of the operation in the node concerned. These derivatives are as follows:

$$\text{For } f\left(z\right) = 1/z, \frac{df\left(z\right)}{dz} = -1/z^2$$

$$\text{For } f\left(z\right) = z + c, \frac{df\left(z\right)}{dz} = 1$$

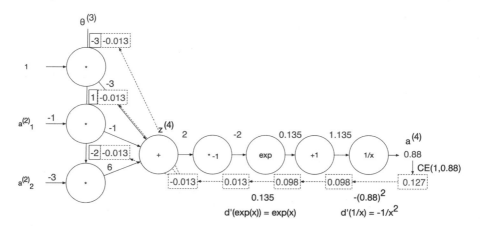

Fig. 6.27 The computation graph for the sigmoid of the dot product of two vectors is used to demonstrate how to run forward propagation and backward propagation for general network architectures

$$\text{For } f(z) = e^z, \frac{df(z)}{dz} = e^z$$

$$\text{For } f(z) = az, \frac{df(z)}{dz} = a$$

To compute the derivative of J with respect to the first operation ($1/x$), the chain rule is used, and incoming derivative 0.127 is multiplied with the derivative of $1/x$, which is $-1/x^2 = -0.88^2$, to give 0.098. The derivative of the +1 operation is 1, so the incoming derivative 0.098 moves unchanged across that operation. Again, multiplying the incoming derivative 0.098 with $e^z = 0.135$, it is possible to propagate the product 0.013 across the *exp* operation. To propagate the incoming derivative 0.013 across the $*-1$ operation, the fourth derivative in the table of derivatives above is used, obtaining -0.013. Figure 6.28 shows how weights learned from training data using backpropagation can be used to approximate the XNOR function.

To propagate the derivative across the sum and product operations, recall that

$$\text{For } (x,y) = x + y, \frac{df}{dx} = 1, \frac{df}{dy} = 1$$

$$\text{For } f(x,y) = xy, \frac{df}{dx} = y, \frac{df}{dy} = x$$

To complete the example, it is evident that the incoming derivative is being propagated unchanged across the sum operator, and being multiplied by the input on the other branch across the product operation. This provides part of the information required to update each weight in $\theta^{(3)}$: the extent to which changing this weight would influence the loss function if it were multiplied by one in the forward pass. However, this is not the case—the weights in $\theta^{(3)}$ are multiplied by the vector $[1,-1,-3]$. This vector is multiplied by -0.013 (as well as the learning rate) to determine the update to each weight.

In modern deep learning frameworks, such as PyTorch and TensorFlow, one must specify only the forward propagation computation. The computation is internally represented as a directed acyclic graph and derivatives are propagated over the operations by the chain rule using automatically computed derivatives such as the ones in the tables above. More details on automatic differentiation can be found in Chap. 6 of Goodfellow et al.'s comprehensive deep learning text [9].

The core ideas behind the backpropagation algorithm have been around since the late 1980s [25, 26]. The success of deep learning networks today can be attributed to the ready availability of massive data sets needed to train the millions of parameters in modern networks, as well as efficient vector and matrix computations (including special-purpose (tensor processing) hardware) to accelerate the forward and backward computations. Another major innovation is the replacement of the sigmoid nonlinearity in networks by the rectified linear unit [27] (ReLU) defined as ReLU(x) = max(0,x). As can be observed in Fig. 6.25 the sigmoid function g(z)

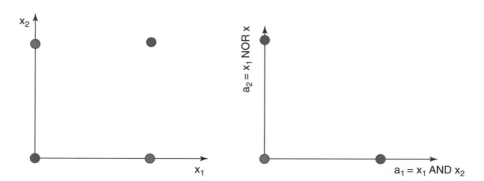

Fig. 6.28 In the original feature space (x_1, x_2) on the left, the four values of the XNOR function are depicted with orange and blue dots. Blue dots represent the value 1, and orange dots represent the value 0. Note that when x_1 and x_2 are the same (both 0 or both 1), the XNOR function has value 1. The blue and orange dots cannot be separated by a single hyperplane in the (x_1, x_2) space. However, in the (a_1, a_2) space shown on the right, where a_1 and a_2 are the intermediate outputs of the stacked assembly of logistic units shown in Fig. 6.26, the XNOR function is linearly separable and thus can be represented by a single output unit y. The new basis functions a_1 and a_2 can be learned automatically by the backpropagation algorithm from training data representing the XNOR function

saturates beyond a narrow range of z values about the origin (i.e., it asymptotes to 0 for negative z values, and to 1 for positive z values). Outside this narrow range, small changes to z (represented by the x axis on Fig. 6.25) will have negligible effects on the output (represented by the y axis on this figure). Hence, the derivative of the sigmoid function beyond this narrow interval is 0, and the gradient descent training algorithm essentially stalls. This problem is called the **vanishing gradient problem**. The use of the ReLU non-linearity significantly reduces this problem, since the gradient is one if the result of the linear logit computation is positive.

Convolutional Networks

This section describes the Convolutional Neural Network (CNN), a specialized deep neural network architecture that is especially effective at modeling imaging data and as such underlies many of advances in medical image processing that are described in Chap. 12. CNNs offer advantages over standard architectures in their ability to leverage the innate 2D correlational structure of image-related data sources. Multi-layer, fully connected feedforward networks of the appropriate depth and width have the power to represent any function from a set of inputs to an output set (continuous or discrete). However, the architecture forces all inputs, including those with 2D or 3D structure, such as still images and videos, to be flattened into one-dimensional vectors, for processing by the network. Spatial and temporal structure inherent in two-dimensional image arrays or three-dimensional video streams (the third dimension is time) are lost in this representational transformation. Convolutional neural networks preserve local correlations in the input and use convolution in place of full matrix multiplication in some of the layers. Convolution is a well-known mathematical operation in which a function called a kernel or filter is applied to an input, yielding an **activation map**. It is widely used in computer vision applications where kernels are designed to detect specific features (such as oriented edges) in images. Figure 6.29 shows a 2D kernel of size 2×2 applied to an input matrix of size 5×5, yielding a 4×4 activation map. The kernel or filter is swept horizontally across the input starting at the top left, with a specified shift (called stride) to the right, until it reaches the right edge of the image. The values in the 2×2 kernel are pointwise multiplied and summed with the 2×2 part of the image underneath it, yielding a scalar. In a trained model, this scalar indicates the extent to which this part of the image maps to a feature the filter has learned to identify. For instance, when the kernel is aligned with the left most corner of the input, the convolution yields $2 \times 1 + 3 \times 1 + 1 \times 2 + 4 \times 2 = 15$. This is the first element of the activation map which is computed by sweeping the kernel across and then down by the specified stride. The 2×2 kernel yields four elements in the activation map for each horizontal sweep (as each position occupies two columns of the input matrix, there are four possible horizontal positions). Since the vertical stride is also one, the activation map is of size 4×4, with each cell indicating the strength of activation of the filter in one of its possible positions in the input matrix.

Convolution networks have far fewer parameters than a conventional feedforward network on the same inputs. Continuing with the example in Fig. 6.29, the number of units to represent the 5×5 input would be 26 ($5 \times 5 + 1$ bias unit) and the number of units to represent the next layer, that is, the 4×4 activation map would be 17 ($16 + 1$). In a standard neural network architecture, every one of the 16 units in the activation layer would need to be connected to the 26 units below, yielding $16 \times 26 = 416$ parameters. Instead, there are just four parameters (the

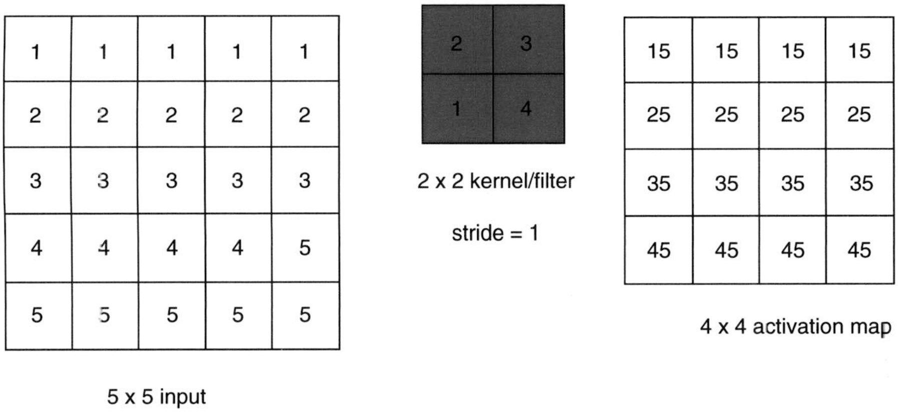

1	1	1	1	1
2	2	2	2	2
3	3	3	3	3
4	4	4	4	5
5	5	5	5	5

5 x 5 input

2	3
1	4

2 x 2 kernel/filter

stride = 1

15	15	15	15
25	25	25	25
35	35	35	35
45	45	45	45

4 x 4 activation map

Fig. 6.29 An example of a 2D convolution with a 5×5 input matrix and a 2×2 kernel. The resulting activation map is of size 4×4 since the stride is 1. The first row of numbers in the activation map is generated by sweeping the kernel across the first two rows of the input starting at the left corner and moving one column horizontally to the right. The pointwise products of the filter values with the input values under the filter are taken and summed to yield the values in the activation map

kernel values or weights) capturing the entire interaction between the input and the activation layer. Since the kernel computes the same function across all the input units, the activation map values are akin to the output of a feature detector. Convolutional networks embody **translational invariance** because the kernel identifies specific features no matter where they occur in the input. This is intuitively appealing for image classification problems, as ideally the network would learn to recognize important features, such as cavitation in chest radiographs, irrespective of where they occur within a particular training image. The **parameter sharing** with the use of convolutional layers with small kernels or filters becomes even more compelling when working with larger inputs of size $224 \times 224 \times 3$ (such as the ImageNet collection [28]—the "×3" indicates three channels, for red, green and blue color encoding). The input is padded with zeros around the edge and a $3 \times 3 \times 3$ kernel is used to obtain an activation map of size $224 \times 224 \times 3$ ($224 + 2 - 3 + 1$ for each dimension). A fully connected model will need $224 \times 224 \times 3 \times 224 \times 224 \times 3 = 2.3 \times 10^{10}$ parameters or weights, while the convolutional layer only has $3 \times 3 \times 3 = 27$ parameters! By sweeping a small kernel by a small stride across a large image, **sparsity** is obtained in the connections between layers, because not every unit in a layer is connected to all units in the following layer. The filter thus defines a receptive field that moves across the entire image.

To specify a convolutional layer in a deep network with input of size $H \times H \times D$, several hyper-parameters must be defined: K, the number of filters or kernels, F, the size of the filter (typically a square matrix), S, the stride of the filter (typically 1 or 2), and P, a zero padding around the edges of the input to ensure that the activation map size $A \times A$ where $A = \dfrac{H + F - 2p}{S} + 1$ is an integer. The total number of parameters defining a convolutional layer for an input of size $H \times H \times D$ is $(K \times F \times F \times D)$ parameters for the K filters and K bias parameters (one per filter).

Filter weights in convolutional networks trained by backpropagation can be visualized as color images, as shown in Fig. 6.30. The filters come to resemble the

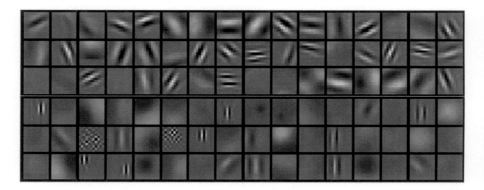

Fig. 6.30 A visualization of the filter weights of the first layer of a VGGNet trained on the ImageNet classification task [29]

features they detect, because the signal that propagates forward from a matrix multiplication will be highest when the matrices have similar values. This capability to learn feature representations from data is an important advantage of deep learning models, especially considering these feature representations can be of value for tasks beyond those the network was originally trained. Zeiler and Fergus [29] pioneered this visualization technique in the context of the ImageNet recognition task, rendering the 96 11 × 11 × 3 filters in the convolutional layer next to the input layer as color images of size 11 × 11 each. Oriented edge detectors and color patches are automatically learned by the machine, by minimizing the cross-entropy loss at the output layer and propagating loss functions derivatives back to the first layer. Similarly, activation maps at higher hidden layers can be projected back to the input, to reveal the regions of the input image that contribute most to the final classification decisions [30], as illustrated in Fig. 6.31.

The convolution operation is linear; and once the linear activation map is computed, a nonlinearity, such as ReLU, is applied. Convolutional/ReLU layers are generally followed by a pooling layer which reduces the dimensionality of the activation map. A commonly used pooling kernel is of size 2 × 2 with horizontal and vertical stride of two, which selects the maximum value in its receptive field. That is, only the signal from the region that most strongly activates a filter propagates forward to the next layer of the network. MaxPool is illustrated in Fig. 6.32, where it clearly functions as a non-linear downsampler. When a convolutional layer follows a pooling layer, the network learns filters on a wider receptive field than on the original input.

Classical convolutional networks for K-class object recognition problems such as VGGNet [32] are a sequence of convolution/ReLU/MaxPool layers that progressively map the input image through a series of reduced dimensional hidden outputs into a penultimate layer which is flattened and fully connected to an output layer of size K.

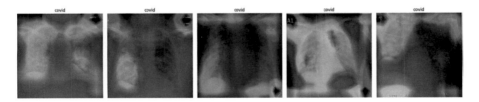

Fig. 6.31 GradCAM [30] visualization of examples from a popular and somewhat controversial set of radiological images used to train deep learning models to detect COVID-positive patients, with high accuracy reported in several evaluations. Pixels in red have the highest importance in the classification decision. Of note, the models are often attending to regions outside the lungs themselves, which contain metadata denoted in different ways across institutions. As "healthy control" counterexamples were often drawn from different sources to the COVID-positive cases, the ability to identify image provenance explains much of the model's ostensibly strong performance [31]

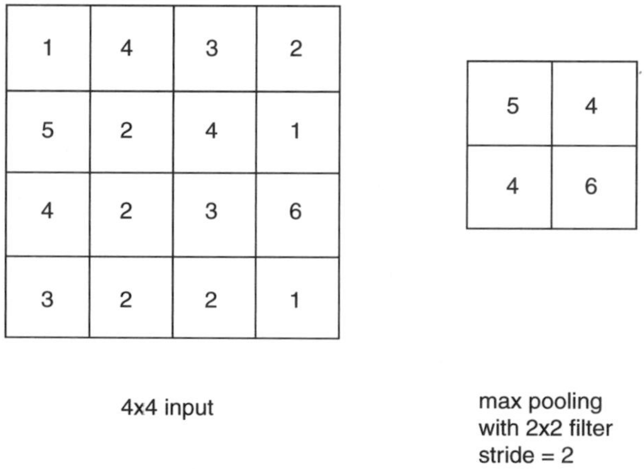

1	4	3	2
5	2	4	1
4	2	3	6
3	2	2	1

| 5 | 4 |
| 4 | 6 |

4x4 input

max pooling
with 2x2 filter
stride = 2

Fig. 6.32 The max pool filter selects the maximum value in a 2 × 2 block starting at the left corner of the input. The maximum value in the first 2 × 2 block of the input is 5. The next step is to stride the filter by 2 horizontally, and obtain 4 as the maximum value. The resulting output is a 2 × 2 matrix since the vertical stride of the filter is also 2. Max pooling reduces a n × n input matrix into a n/2 × n/2 output

Other Network Architectures

While convolutional networks with convolution/ReLU/MaxPool layers, with fully connected layers at the output form the dominant architectural paradigm, a host of variations have been proposed in the literature to solve problems beyond discrete object recognition. One class, called UNets [33] are specially engineered for solving image segmentation problems, i.e., problems in which exact localization of features is important, unlike a simple object recognition problem. Details of the UNet architecture are beyond the scope of this chapter, and the interested reader is directed to the original paper [33].

For handling time series data such as video streams in medical imaging, recurrent networks are the appropriate architecture. Unlike the feedforward systems studied thus far, in which the computations flow in one direction from inputs to the final outputs, recurrent networks allow the final output of a network to serve as input with a time delay. Chapter 10 of the Goodfellow et al. text [34] on deep learning offers an excellent introduction to this family of networks, and its many variations such as LSTMs and echo state networks.

In natural language processing, the Transformer architecture has emerged as an important approach to processing text sequences underlying widely used models such as **Bidirectional Encoder Representations from Transformers (BERT)** [35, 36]. Transformers generate context-specific representations of textual input, by allowing words (or parts of words) in a sequence to influence the representations of other words as they progress through the network. This provides an intuitive way to model ambiguous words such as "cold" (virus vs. temperature), because representations of this word that are close to the output layer will be informed by contextual cues. The relative influence of specific contextual cues is learned by the model, so that those cues that are useful for particular tasks will be emphasized when the model is fine-tuned accordingly. For discussion of some key applications of neural Transformer models, see Chap. 7.

Putting It All Together: The Workflow for Training Deep Neural Networks

Deep learning models have been used in a wide range of clinical applications ranging from diagnosis, to risk assessment and treatment. A large fraction of them are end-to-end models that start with images (optical, CT, Xray) as inputs and culminate in a classification output layer with intervening hidden layers consisting of convolutional/ReLU/pooling layers together with fully connected feedforward layers at the end of the pipeline. In this section, the workflow for setting up and training deep neural networks for supervised learning problems in clinical applications is elaborated.

1. **Decide on the network architecture**: for a supervised learning problem, the type and arrangement of layers is determined by the inputs and outputs and the nature of the prediction problem: e.g., whether it is classification into a small set of discrete categories, image segmentation, or risk estimation. Modern deep learning frameworks such as Pytorch [37], Keras (keras.io) and TensorFlow (tensorflow.org) allow easy parametric specification of layers ranging from simple fully connected to convolution/ReLU and MaxPool composites, as well as more exotic layers to support specialized applications. It is important to avoid the data arrogance trap, particularly if the available training sets are orders of magnitude smaller in size than the number of parameters in the network model. The use of pre-trained networks with parameters optimized for related tasks is crucial to obtain robust generalization performance. An example is the use of a VGGNet and Resnet architecture trained on the ImageNet dataset with 1.2 million images in 1000 categories as a feature extractor for classification of pneumonia from chest X-ray images [38].

2. **Choose an appropriate loss function**: for regression problems, mean squared error is the standard choice, while cross-entropy loss is the usual choice for binary classification. The softmax loss function, which is a generalization of cross-entropy loss, is used for multi-class classification. Weighted versions of these loss functions are available in standard deep learning frameworks, allowing designers to accommodate problems with class imbalance, or problems where the costs associated with false positive errors and false negative errors are quite different.

3. **Choose a regularization approach**: One technique for regularization is to use penalized loss functions, where the L1 or L2 norm of the network weights is added to the chosen loss function. Another technique is called dropout [39], and can be added as a layer in modern deep learning frameworks. During training, some of the units (and their connections) are stochastically dropped during weight update, which encourages sparsity in the network weights.

4. **Initialize network parameters**: weights on bias units are typically initialized to zero. The most used technique [40] for initializing weights connecting units in layers $l-1$ and l is to select them from a uniform distribution $[-b, +b]$ where $b = \sqrt{6} / \sqrt{S^{(l)} + S^{(i-1)}}$. $S^{(l)}$ denotes the number of hidden units in layer l of the network. Proper initialization of network parameters is still an open problem in the field.

5. **Select pre-processing steps for training data**: to make the inputs well-conditioned, it is traditional to normalize training inputs, e.g., subtracting means from images, or more generally, using standard scaling of each column of the input to make it have zero mean and unit variance. The choice of pre-processing step requires domain knowledge and understanding of how the inputs were generated, and the elimination of input artifacts that could cause overfitting in the models. In many medical image classification problems, such as Gleason grading of prostate cancer from whole slide images [41], semi-automated label cleaning is employed, in which erroneously graded training examples are excluded from the training sets. Another significant pre-processing step in image classification tasks is to break up an input image into smaller patches and learn models on the patches. A second model learns to integrate feature responses from the patches to make a final classification.

6. **Determine if data augmentation is needed**, and if it is, determine how to augment training data. If the number of parameters in the chosen network architecture far exceeds (i.e., is an order of magnitude greater than) the product of the number of training examples and the size of each example, there is a need to augment the training set. One of the easiest ways to perform data augmentation to is apply affine transformations: translations and small rotations to the existing training set data to force the network to be robust in the face of perturbations of the input. Yet another approach is to inject a small amount of white noise to all the inputs to encourage better generalization performance.

7. **Decide on a stopping criterion**: It is customary to set aside a small portion of the training set, called a validation set, and calculate the loss function on both the training and validation sets for each epoch of training. In a single epoch, network parameters are updated after iterating through the whole training set. Training loss decreases with the number of training epochs, eventually tending to zero. The validation loss, on the other hand, first decreases and then increases, indicating that the network has been overfitted to the training data. The optimal stopping point for training is when the validation loss achieves its minimum.

8. **Tuning the learning hyper-parameters**: these include choice of learning rate, the gradient descent optimization algorithm, and example batch size for gradient estimation. Tuning hyper-parameters is still an art and is extremely computationally intensive. Close monitoring of the training and validation loss using a visualization framework such as Tensorboard[16] is crucial to find good values for the hyper-parameters. Tools such as AutoML[17] can automatically perform coarse to fine grained searches in the hyper-parameter space to find good combinations of values.

9. **Train the model**: Run the model with the (augmented) training data with the chosen hyper-parameters and architecture until the optimal stopping point.

10. **Test the model**: evaluate the predictive performance of the model on the set aside test set (or on the set aside chunk for N-fold cross-validation). In datasets with class imbalance, cross-validation has to be designed carefully to avoid overfitting and overestimating model performance [42]. Generating artificial examples to overcome imbalance in classification problems can introduce inadvertent biases in the model. An interesting example of this phenomenon occurs in the domain of predicting synergistic drug interactions. While there are tens of thousands of known drug compounds, very few documented examples of synergistic interactions exist (rare class problem). Further, drug pairs that do not have synergistic interaction are never documented. Researchers often use random drug pairs as negative examples. These models rarely perform well outside the training set, because they merely learn to distinguish random drug pairs from ones that have synergistic interactions, instead of generalizing patterns present in useful drug combinations [43]. Deep learning models in computer vision are vulnerable to adversarial attacks in which small perturbations in inputs cause large variations in outputs [44] (such as misclassifying a stop sign image with a few pixel alterations as a 30 mph speed limit sign). In healthcare predictive analytics, algorithms for generating adversarial examples for biomedical text classification have been devised [45] to test the robustness of deep models. Adversarial example generation for healthcare applications is an active area of research.

11. **Interpret/Visualize the model**: Visualize the network weights and generate activation maps as well as GradCAM maps for both correctly classified and incorrectly classified members of the test set to build an understanding of the generalization performance of the network model. GradCAM maps reveal whether relevant areas of the input contribute to the final decision made by the network. When irrelevant features (such as a date or patient name on a clinical image) are highlighted by GradCAM, the input data is reengineered to eliminate these noise features and the system retrained on the cleaned data.

---

[16] tensorflow.org/tensorboard (accessed August 19, 2022)

[17] automl.org (accessed August 19, 2022)

Ensembling Models

So far, several model families for supervised learning have been presented, ranging from simple models such as linear and logistic regression with basis function expansion, dense and sparse kernel methods which project examples into appropriately chosen similarity spaces, and non-linear adaptive basis functions with universal approximation properties, exemplified by deep neural networks. For each family, a loss function was optimized to obtain the best model for the given labeled data set. In this section, model ensembles are introduced. Ensembles improve prediction by combining several models by weighted averaging for regression models or simple majority/weighted majority voting for classification models. Two conditions are necessary for an ensemble of classification models to perform better than a single model. First, the error rate (i.e., probability of misclassification) of each model in the ensemble must be less than 0.5. Second, the errors made by each member of the ensemble must be uncorrelated with the others. If the highest error rate of an individual binary classifier in an ensemble of size L is ϵ, then the error rate of the entire ensemble with simple majority voting is

$$\sum_{i=L/2+1}^{L} \binom{L}{i} \epsilon^i (1-\epsilon)^{L-i}$$

For $L = 21$ and $\epsilon = 0.3$, the error rate of the ensemble is 0.026! This is a direct consequence of the strong assumption that the errors of the ensemble members are uncorrelated. This assumption, unfortunately, generally does not hold for human committees, leading to the general belief that committee decisions are inferior to an individual member's decision. Thus, the key to making good ensembles is to devise ways to decorrelate the errors of individual members.

There are two major approaches to constructing ensembles: **bagging** and **boosting**.

- In bagging [46], L bootstrap samples are created from the given training data set D with m elements of the form (x,y). A bootstrap sample is constructed by uniformly sampling m times, with replacement, from D. A bootstrap sample has the same size as the original dataset D but may have duplicates. L classifiers are constructed with each of the bootstrap samples, and a simple majority rule is used for final classification. Bagging can be easily parallelized since the construction of the bootstrap sample and the associated classifier can occur independently. The random forest algorithm [47] builds bagged ensembles of decision trees and it has found wide acceptance in medicine because of its impressive performance in clinical decision-making tasks [48].
- In boosting [49], ensemble members are learned sequentially, with each member focusing on the errors made by the previously learned members of the ensemble. Weights $w^{(i)}$ are associated with every example $(x^{(i)}, y^{(i)})$ in a dataset

D containing m pairs. Initially all weights are 1, and a classification algorithm that minimizes weighted cross-entropy loss is learned in each round. Examples misclassified by a classifier are weighted higher for the next classifier in the sequence; examples correctly classified are down weighted for the next classifier. The same data set D with the new weights is used to learn the next classifier in the sequence, with the process terminating with the error rate of the learned classifier exceeds 0.5. Finally, the predictions are combined by a weighted voting scheme where each classifier's voting weight reflects its overall predictive accuracy. There are many boosting algorithms in the literature [49–51]. Each of them is characterized by (1) specification of the initial example weights, and how weights are up- and down-weighted after each round of classifier learning, (2) how the voting weight of each classifier in the ensemble is determined, (3) the specific loss function (e.g., weighted cross-entropy loss) for learning each classifier, and (4) a termination criterion (which determines how many members will be included in the boosted ensemble). The most popular boosting algorithm in use today is XGBoost [52]—it is readily scalable to large data sets and has achieved state-of-the-art results on many machine learning challenges. A recent example of its use is the prediction of adverse outcomes in Type 2 diabetes patients with administrative health data [53]: on a training dataset of over a million patients, an XGBoost model on over 700 features extracted from administrative data predicted 3-year risk of diabetes complications in with an AUROC of 0.77 on held out validation and test sets of over a quarter million patients.

Conclusion

This chapter has introduced supervised machine learning algorithms for solving clinical decision-making problems with labeled data. The types of problems that are best suited for supervised learning and workflow sequence for model construction and validation have also been identified. Although machine learning systems have shown success in a range of retrospective studies, relatively few are deployed in practice. An interesting exception is Google's neural network detector of diabetic retinopathy in retinal fundus photographs [2]. One of the many challenges faced in translation of research algorithms to the clinical context is that systems are often trained on data that are subject to extensive cleaning and curation, and thus quite unlike data in a real-world clinical setting.

Randomized controlled trials and prospective studies are now being pursued to ease the transition from the computational lab to patient bedside. More refined, context-specific measures of performance, beyond F1-scores and AUROCs, are being developed for evaluating ML systems. A recent study uses the percentage of time pediatric Type 1diabetic patients spend inside their target glucose range as a way of evaluating a learning system that manages real-time insulin dosing [54]. Simple linear models such as logistic regression have the potential for ready deployment since the coefficients of the model can be easily converted into a score card system for risk stratification. A recent review of clinical prediction models shows the wide-spread use of logistic models in medicine [55].

The most visible recent successes of ML have been in image interpretation with deep neural networks, in the domains of radiology, pathology, gastroenterology and ophthalmology. In these problem areas, clinicians generally find it difficult to articulate decision-making criteria for classification. Thus, end-to-end learning systems such as deep neural nets that take pairs of the form *(raw image, overall decision)* as training inputs, and learn appropriate intermediate features by optimization of well-chosen loss functions, are a winning alternative that have even outperformed clinicians in some evaluations [56, 57].

An open problem is how to get doctors, as well as patients, to trust the decisions made by ML systems. Clearly, interpretable and explainable models will be key (see Chap. 8), and stronger prospective validation guidelines developed jointly by ML scientists and by clinicians, and then endorsed by regulatory bodies, will go a long way to bridging the trust gap. For example, the use of GradCAM visualizations of deep neural net image classification models have been important for convincing clinicians and regulators of the validity of a model's decisions beyond performance scores such as AUROC and F1. Equally important are ethical considerations concerning data use and equity (see Chap. 18), particularly the need for standards of diversity and inclusion in the design of training data for machine learning systems. A 2021 study of underreporting and underrepresentation of diverse skin types in present-day skin cancer databases reveals gaps in training sets that limit the applicability of predictive models for people of color [58].

Many technical, legal, ethical and regulatory problems need to be addressed before predictive ML systems are routinely incorporated into clinical workflow (see Chaps. 17 and 18). There are open questions in accountability assignment: who is to be held responsible for a model's mistakes? Do we turn to the ML engineers who build the model, the clinicians who use the model, the regulators who cleared the model for use, or others? As these issues are raised and solved in specific clinical contexts, supervised learning will be a major enabler of improved access to high-quality healthcare at a global scale.

Questions for Discussion

- How does one integrate prior knowledge about a clinical decision-making problem in the formulation of a supervised learning approach to it? Under what circumstances are we likely to obtain high performing models using data alone?
- One of the few useful theoretical results in supervised machine learning is the "no free lunch" theorem [59]—there is no single best model that performs optimally for all problems. Do deep neural networks with their universal approximation properties negate this theorem?

- Modern machine learning algorithms can build high-performing models by picking up on incidental correlations in training data. An apocryphal story from the early days of machine learning is about a neural network learning algorithm that distinguished images of enemy tanks from friendly tanks by picking up the blue skies at the top edge of the friendly tank images. Flushing out confounding variables in a high-dimensional dataset is still an art. Can you provide examples of confounders in clinical decision-making tasks? How can one systematically eliminate such features from consideration during model construction?
- The ImageNet dataset has 12 million examples of over a thousand object categories, and the best performing neural nets trained on ImageNet (an ensemble of Resnet50 networks) have error rates of under 3% on set-aside test sets. Why do deep neural networks require millions of examples to learn robust models of objects, when humans can generalize from very few examples? Why is it that humans generalize so well with very few examples? Hint: a new area called few-shot learning concerns an attempt to reduce the sample complexity of deep neural networks.
- What, in your opinion, are the primary barriers to the adoption of machine learning systems in a clinical context? Are the barriers lower in some areas of medicine than in others? If so, why?
- Obtaining high quality labeled data is a bottleneck in the design of supervised machine learning systems for clinical decision-making. The quality of the learned model is determined completely by the quality of the associated labels/ decisions associated with each case. What approaches can be used to assess consistency and quality of data labels before one embarks on model construction?
- What are potential uses of unsupervised learning (learning from unlabeled data) in the clinical context?

Further Reading

Goodfellow I, Bengio G, Courville A. Deep learning. MIT Press; 2016.

- The definitive text on deep learning available online at deeplearningbook.org It has three major parts. Part 1 is a concise yet comprehensive of review of all the mathematics needed to understand machine learning algorithms and a summary of ML algorithms before the deep learning era. Part 2 is a deep dive into modern deep learning networks starting from feedforward multilayer networks through convolutional networks and recurrent networks. This part combines a clear exposition of the theoretical foundations of deep networks with practical tips on network design and training. Part 3 covers advanced topics including representation learning, autoencoders, and deep generative models, including generative adversarial networks.

Murphy K. Probabilistic machine learning: an introduction. MIT Press; 2022.

- A new two volume, comprehensive, reference textbook from an authority in the field, available online at probml.ai. The first book covers the foundational mathematics, linear models for regression and classification, deep neural networks, non-parametric models including ensemble models and unsupervised learning. The second book, to be released in 2023, will cover advanced topics in prediction, generative models, causality, and reinforcement learning.

Bishop CM. Pattern recognition and machine learning. Springer; 2021 (old edition 2006 available online).

- An extremely well-written textbook on classical machine learning algorithms including feedforward neural networks. The latest edition covers graphical models and approximate inference.

James G, Witten D, Hastie T, Tibshirani R. An Introduction to Statistical Learning with Applications in R. 2nd ed. Springer; 2017.

- A basic textbook on machine learning which goes deep into linear and logistic regression, tree-based models, basis function expansion, ensemble techniques and clustering methods. It has excellent practical end-of-chapter exercises. It is available as a free download online at hastie.su.domains/ElemStatLearn.

Nielsen M. Neural networks and deep learning, online book at neuralnetworksanddeeplearning.com.

- This book is an excellent introduction to neural networks. It has the clearest explanation of backpropagation and through a hands-on approach elucidates why neural networks are universal function approximators. This book should be required reading for all machine learning enthusiasts.

References

1. Johnson AEW, et al. MIMIC-III, a freely accessible critical care database. Sci Data. 2016;3:160035.
2. Gulshan V, et al. Development and validation of a deep learning algorithm for detection of diabetic retinopathy in retinal fundus photographs. JAMA. 2016;316:2402–10.
3. Esteva A, et al. Dermatologist-level classification of skin cancer with deep neural networks. Nature. 2017;542:115–8.
4. Golden JA. Deep learning algorithms for detection of lymph node metastases from breast cancer: helping artificial intelligence be seen. JAMA. 2017;318:2184–6.
5. FitzHenry F, et al. Creating a common data model for comparative effectiveness with the observational medical outcomes partnership. Appl Clin Inform. 2015;6:536–47.
6. Hersh W. Information retrieval: a health and biomedical perspective. Springer; 2008.
7. Kelly-Hayes M. Influence of age and health behaviors on stroke risk: lessons from longitudinal studies. J Am Geriatr Soc. 2010;58:S325–8.
8. Otis AB, Fenn WO, Rahn H. Mechanics of breathing in man. J Appl Physiol. 1950;2:592–607.
9. Hastie T, Tibshirani R, Friedman JH, Friedman JH. The elements of statistical learning: data mining, inference, and prediction, vol. 2. Springer; 2009.

10. Walsh C, Hripcsak G. The effects of data sources, cohort selection, and outcome definition on a predictive model of risk of thirty-day hospital readmissions. J Biomed Inform. 2014;52:418–26.
11. Milea D, et al. Artificial intelligence to detect papilledema from ocular fundus photographs. N Engl J Med. 2020;382:1687–95.
12. Howell K, et al. Controlling for confounding variables: accounting for dataset bias in classifying patient-provider interactions. In: Shaban-Nejad A, Michalowski M, Buckeridge DL, editors. Explainable AI in healthcare and medicine: building a culture of transparency and accountability. Springer; 2021. p. 271–82. https://doi.org/10.1007/978-3-030-53352-6_25.
13. Doll R, Hill AB. Smoking and carcinoma of the lung. Br Med J. 1950;2:739.
14. Ioannou GN, et al. Development of COVIDVax model to estimate the risk of SARS-CoV-2–related death among 7.6 million US veterans for use in vaccination prioritization. JAMA Netw Open. 2021;4:e214347.
15. Dooling K, et al. The Advisory Committee on Immunization Practices' interim recommendation for allocating initial supplies of COVID-19 vaccine—United States, 2020. Morb Mortal Wkly Rep. 2020;69:1857.
16. Barak-Corren Y, et al. Validation of an electronic health record–based suicide risk prediction modeling approach across multiple health care systems. JAMA Netw Open. 2020;3:e201262.
17. Joshi R, et al. Predicting neonatal sepsis using features of heart rate variability, respiratory characteristics, and ECG-derived estimates of infant motion. IEEE J Biomed Health Inform. 2019;24:681–92.
18. McCoy TH, Perlis RH. A tool to utilize adverse effect profiles to identify brain-active medications for repurposing. Int J Neuropsychopharmacol. 2015;18.
19. Istrail S, Pevzner PA. Kernel methods in computational biology. MIT Press; 2004.
20. McCulloch WS, Pitts W. A logical calculus of the ideas immanent in nervous activity. Bull Math Biophys. 1943;5:115–33.
21. Nielsen M. Deep learning. 2017. http://neuralnetworksanddeeplearning.com/.
22. Cybenko G. Approximation by superpositions of a sigmoidal function. Math Control Signals Syst. 1989;2:303–14.
23. Hornik K. Approximation capabilities of multilayer feedforward networks. Neural Netw. 1991;4:251–7.
24. Krizhevsky A, Sutskever I, Hinton GE. Imagenet classification with deep convolutional neural networks. Adv Neural Inf Process Syst. 2012;25:1097–105.
25. Rumelhart DE, McClelland JL, Group PR. Parallel distributed processing, vol. 1. New York: IEEE; 1988.
26. Rumelhart DE, Hinton GE, Williams RJ. Learning representations by back-propagating errors. Nature. 1986;323:533–6.
27. Jarrett K, Kavukcuoglu K, Ranzato M, LeCun Y. What is the best multi-stage architecture for object recognition? In: 2009 IEEE 12th international conference on computer vision. IEEE; 2009. p. 2146–53.
28. Fei-Fei L, Deng J, Li K. ImageNet: constructing a large-scale image database. J Vis. 2009;9:1037.
29. Zeiler MD, Fergus R. Visualizing and understanding convolutional networks. In: Fleet D, Pajdla T, Schiele B, Tuytelaars T, editors. Computer vision—ECCV 2014. Springer; 2014. p. 818–33.
30. Selvaraju RR, et al. Grad-cam: visual explanations from deep networks via gradient-based localization. In: Proceedings of the IEEE international conference on computer vision; 2017. p. 618–26.
31. López-Cabrera JD, Orozco-Morales R, Portal-Diaz JA, Lovelle-Enríquez O, Pérez-Díaz M. Current limitations to identify COVID-19 using artificial intelligence with chest X-ray imaging. Health Technol. 2021;11:411–24.

32. Simonyan K, Zisserman A. Very deep convolutional networks for large-scale image recognition. ArXiv Prepr. ArXiv14091556. 2014.
33. Ronneberger O, Fischer P, Brox T. U-net: convolutional networks for biomedical image segmentation. In: International conference on medical image computing and computer-assisted intervention. Springer; 2015. p. 234–41.
34. Goodfellow I, Bengio Y, Courville A. Deep learning. MIT Press; 2016.
35. Vaswani A, et al. Attention is all you need. Adv Neural Inf Process Syst. 2017;30.
36. Devlin J, Chang M-W, Lee K, Toutanova K. Bert: pre-training of deep bidirectional transformers for language understanding. ArXiv Prepr. ArXiv181004805. 2018.
37. Paszke A, et al. Pytorch: an imperative style, high-performance deep learning library. Adv Neural Inf Process Syst. 2019;32.
38. Victor Ikechukwu A, Murali S, Deepu R, Shivamurthy RC. ResNet-50 vs VGG-19 vs training from scratch: a comparative analysis of the segmentation and classification of Pneumonia from chest X-ray images. Glob Transit Proc. 2021;2:375–81.
39. Srivastava N, Hinton G, Krizhevsky A, Sutskever I, Salakhutdinov R. Dropout: a simple way to prevent neural networks from overfitting. J Mach Learn Res. 2014;15:1929–58.
40. Glorot X, Bengio Y. Understanding the difficulty of training deep feedforward neural networks. In: Proceedings of the thirteenth international conference on artificial intelligence and statistics. JMLR Workshop and Conference Proceedings; 2010. p. 249–56.
41. Bulten W, et al. Artificial intelligence for diagnosis and Gleason grading of prostate cancer: the PANDA challenge. Nat Med. 2022;28:154–63.
42. Santos MS, Soares JP, Abreu PH, Araujo H, Santos J. Cross-validation for imbalanced datasets: avoiding overoptimistic and overfitting approaches [research frontier]. IEEE Comput Intell Mag. 2018;13:59–76.
43. Zitnik M, Agrawal M, Leskovec J. Modeling polypharmacy side effects with graph convolutional networks. Bioinformatics. 2018;34:i457–66.
44. Eykholt K, et al. Robust physical-world attacks on deep learning visual classification. In: 2018 IEEE/CVF conference on computer vision and pattern recognition. IEEE; 2018. p. 1625–34. https://doi.org/10.1109/CVPR.2018.00175.
45. Mondal I. BBAEG: towards BERT-based biomedical adversarial example generation for text classification. In: Proceedings of the 2021 conference of the North American Chapter of the Association for Computational Linguistics: Human Language Technologies; 2021. p. 5378–84.
46. Breiman L. Bagging predictors. Mach Learn. 1996;24:123–40.
47. Breiman L. Random forests. Mach Learn. 2001;45:5–32.
48. Subudhi S, et al. Comparing machine learning algorithms for predicting ICU admission and mortality in COVID-19. NPJ Digit Med. 2021;4:1–7.
49. Schapire RE. The boosting approach to machine learning: an overview. In: Denison DD, Hansen MH, Holmes CC, Mallick B, Yu B, editors. Nonlinear estimation and classification. Springer; 2003. p. 149–71. https://doi.org/10.1007/978-0-387-21579-2_9.
50. Friedman JH. Stochastic gradient boosting. Comput Stat Data Anal. 2002;38:367–78.
51. Friedman J, Hastie T, Tibshirani R. Additive logistic regression: a statistical view of boosting (with discussion and a rejoinder by the authors). Ann Stat. 2000;28:337–407.
52. Chen T, Guestrin C. XGBoost: a scalable tree boosting system. In: Proceedings of the 22nd ACM SIGKDD international conference on knowledge discovery and data mining. Association for Computing Machinery; 2016. p. 785–94. https://doi.org/10.1145/2939672.2939785.
53. Ravaut M, et al. Predicting adverse outcomes due to diabetes complications with machine learning using administrative health data. NPJ Digit Med. 2021;4:1–12.
54. Nimri R, et al. Insulin dose optimization using an automated artificial intelligence-based decision support system in youths with type 1 diabetes. Nat Med. 2020;26:1380–4.
55. Chen L. Overview of clinical prediction models. Ann Transl Med. 2020;8:71.
56. Zhou D, et al. Diagnostic evaluation of a deep learning model for optical diagnosis of colorectal cancer. Nat Commun. 2020;11:2961.

57. Gong D, et al. Detection of colorectal adenomas with a real-time computer-aided system (ENDOANGEL): a randomised controlled study. Lancet Gastroenterol Hepatol. 2020;5:352–61.
58. Guo LN, Lee MS, Kassamali B, Mita C, Nambudiri VE. Bias in, bias out: underreporting and underrepresentation of diverse skin types in machine learning research for skin cancer detection—a scoping review. J Am Acad Dermatol. 2021.
59. Wolpert DH. The supervised learning no-free-lunch theorems. In: Roy R, Köppen M, Ovaska S, Furuhashi T, Hoffmann F, editors. Soft computing and industry: recent applications. Springer; 2002. p. 25–42. https://doi.org/10.1007/978-1-4471-0123-9_3.

Chapter 7
Natural Language Processing

Hua Xu and Kirk Roberts

After reading this chapter, you should know the answers to these questions:
- What is natural language processing and what are the types of linguistic information it attempts to capture?
- What are the common biomedical text sources and common biomedical NLP tasks?
- What are some existing biomedical NLP tools and methods?
- What are the trends and challenges in biomedical NLP?

Introduction to NLP and Basic Linguistics Information

Natural Language Processing (NLP) is the use of automatic methods to understand and generate *natural* (i.e., human) language (e.g., English, Chinese, Tagalog, Wolof) as distinct from formal languages (such programming languages like Python, Java, and Prolog). It encompasses tasks that fall under **natural language understanding** (NLU)—understanding language written/spoken by humans—and **natural language generation** (NLG)—creating human-like language. Many NLP tasks incorporate elements of both, such as **machine translation** and **text summarization**.

The term NLP is often used synonymously with the terms **computational linguistics** and **text mining**, though these terms emphasize slightly different aspects of NLP. Computational linguistics is concerned with the modeling of language using

H. Xu (✉) · K. Roberts
The University of Texas Health Science Center at Houston, Houston, TX, USA
e-mail: hua.xu@uth.tmc.edu; Kirk.Roberts@uth.tmc.edu

© The Author(s), under exclusive license to Springer Nature Switzerland AG 2022
T. A. Cohen et al. (eds.), *Intelligent Systems in Medicine and Health*, Cognitive Informatics in Biomedicine and Healthcare,
https://doi.org/10.1007/978-3-031-09108-7_7

computational techniques, including determining which computational data structures and models are best-suited to represent and learn certain linguistic phenomena (e.g., syntax, discourse). Meanwhile, text mining generally emphasizes the application of NLP techniques to extract information from natural language sources (i.e., data mining applied to textual data).

In addition to drawing inspiration and techniques from linguistics, NLP is generally regarded as a sub-field of artificial intelligence (AI), as understanding human language requires mimicking many aspects of human intelligence. NLP also heavily utilizes many methods from another AI sub-field, machine learning (ML). Notably, while many early NLP methods were rule-based with a heavy emphasis on linguistic theory, most current NLP research focuses on data-driven techniques leveraging ML models. The chapter touches on these topics further below, but in order to understand NLP it is still important, if under-appreciated, to understand the basics of linguistic terminology and structure.

The process of understanding human language can be viewed as being broken down into a series of layers, or a stack, starting from the basic input representation to a full computational understanding. This stack is visualized in Fig. 7.1 and each of the layers are described briefly below. Importantly, many NLP tasks focus on

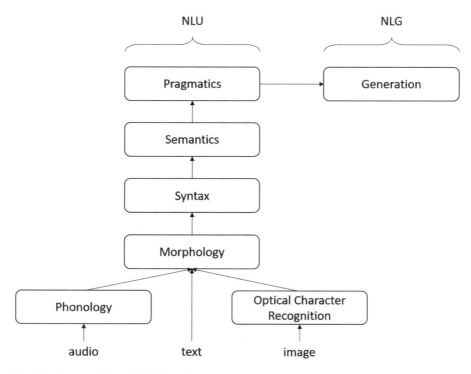

Fig. 7.1 Layers of linguistic information

directly learning the representations at each layer (e.g., **part-of-speech** tagging, **co-reference resolution**), while other NLP tasks are more application-focused and are not as focused on a particular layer or may involve several layers (e.g., information extraction, question answering). However, different NLP approaches require different levels of linguistic reasoning, and those that require information from higher up the linguistic stack tend to be more challenging. These layers should not, however, be seen as silos or purely uni-directional, as there are interactions and dependencies that make language complex (and wonderful). The layers do, however, help to organize language and NLP tasks.

1. **Phonology**: This layer focuses on sounds, and is thus relevant for natural language originating from, or destined for, speech (as opposed to text, which is the focus of most of this chapter). The most notable linguistic task for phonology is automatic speech recognition (ASR), also known as speech-to-text, in which speech sounds (as wave form data) are converted to textual strings (on which most NLP tasks work). See Chap. 9 for more about ASR system use in dialog systems. Beyond speech and text, another potential language input is image-based representations of language, in which an equivalent task of **optical character recognition** (OCR) is performed. In a biomedical context, phonology is commonly used for clinical environments where typing may be difficult, such as with clinical note dictation or the use of voice commands. Additionally, the widespread availability of smart speaker devices (e.g., Amazon Alexa, Google Home) has led to a proliferation of voice-based agents (a.k.a., Chatbots) that can serve as tools to educate and aid patients, clinicians, and biomedical researchers.

2. **Morphology**: This layer focuses on how words are composed from atomic units called morphemes. For example, the term hypertension combines three morphemes: hyper- (meaning high), -tens- (meaning pressure), and -sion (meaning a state of being). Thus the entire term means something along the lines of "being over-pressured"–how this comes to stand for the medical notion of high blood pressure is a separate linguistic process altogether. A common NLP task involving morphology is **stemming**, whose goal is to determine the root or stem of a word, separate from the affixes (prefixes and suffixes). This can be useful to identify when the surface form of two words (e.g., clinician and clinical) derive from the same basic meaning, which may be useful for information retrieval, machine translation, or other applications. No major biomedical NLP application focuses primarily on morphology, but many applications can leverage morphological understanding for improved performance.

3. **Syntax**: This layer focuses on the grammatical structure of language, specifically which words are interacting with which other words in a sentence to hierarchically understand the meaning of what is an otherwise linear sequence of words. It is syntax that lets us know that, in the case of "the tumor at the base of the right lung has grown", it is the tumor that is growing, not the lung.

The major linguistic tasks for syntax include **part-of-speech** tagging (labeling each word in a sentence as a noun, verb, adjective, etc.), **treebank parsing** (identifying the hierarchical phrase structures, such as noun phrases and prepositional phrases, up to the level of a sentence, according to the Penn Treebank structure [1]) and **dependency parsing** (a separate tree-like syntax structure that encodes word-word syntax relations and is more commonly used today due to being both simpler and closer in structure to semantics). Few biomedical NLP tasks focus primarily on syntax, though the compositional nature of syntax is very important in semantic tasks like concept recognition and relation extraction.

4. **Semantics**: This layer focuses on piecing together the meaning of words, phrases, and sentences based on input from the prior layers. Sometimes the specific meaning of words is separated out, distinguishing lexical semantics from sentence-level semantics. Regardless, this layer is responsible for the vast majority of NLP tasks. The linguistically-motivated tasks include **word sense disambiguation** (WSD; distinguishing the meaning of a word from a set of potential meanings, e.g. cold can be a temperature or a sickness), **named entity recognition** (NER; identifying proper names and associating them with their semantic type), and **relation extraction** (RE; identifying specific semantic relations between two or more entities). Likewise, most biomedical NLP applications are primarily focused on semantics, including **concept recognition** (similar to NER, but for medical concepts like diseases or treatments) and biomedically-focused **information extraction** (IE) tasks, which are a class of tasks focusing on extracting a particular type of structured data from text (e.g., tumor stage, treatment outcome, or a gene-protein interaction).

5. **Pragmatics**: This layer focuses on how context influences meaning. This can include both document-level context (sometimes separated out into a separate discourse layer) and external context (e.g., real-world knowledge that the reader is expected to have but an algorithm is not necessarily aware of). Discourse-type pragmatics includes linguistic tasks such as **co-reference resolution** (recognizing referring expressions such as pronouns) and temporal relations (placing various events within the document on some form of timeline), as these are generally relevant at the document level and require sophisticated reasoning to understand. Pragmatics can extend to conversations as well, including tasks such as recognizing speech acts and conversation analysis. Because pragmatics is the top layer of NLU, it has some of the most linguistically interesting tasks in NLP, but also the most challenging. For biomedical NLP applications, the most popular tasks include a clinical version of temporal relations in which a timeline of a patient's medical events is reconstructed from text, and development of health-related chatbots that need to model conversation behavior accurately in order to inform or intervene (see Chap. 9).

6. **Generation**: Separate from NLU, this NLG layer focuses on generating realistic language given a computational representation. This is obviously highly

dependent upon what NLU algorithms are used, if applicable, as more powerful NLU representations should make realistic language generation more successful. The primary linguistic task for NLG is language modeling, which models the likelihood of a given sequence of words (and thus, whether it is useful text to generate) and is used as a component of many other NLP (including non-generation) approaches. Common application tasks include Summarization (shortening a long document, or multiple documents, into a concise summary) and Machine Translation (translating from a source language to a target language). For biomedical NLP applications, there has been some work on summarization, but also a major focus is the generation of synthetic clinical records.

Common Biomedical NLP Tasks and Methods

Overview of Biomedical NLP Tasks

As shown in section "Introduction to NLP and Basic Linguistics Information", there are a number of common NLP tasks that have been investigated extensively in the general domain. In the biomedical domain, the uses of NLP primarily focus on supporting biomedical research activities and facilitating operational applications in healthcare. Common biomedical NLP applications include:

1. Information retrieval (IR)—to find relevant documents from a text collection based on user specified queries. A prominent example is a search to find relevant articles in bibliographic databases. For example, PubMed [2] provides an interactive interface to support sophisticated Boolean queries to search MEDLINE, the largest biomedical bibliographic database.
2. Text classification (TC)—to classify a textual document to one or more predefined labels. For example, systematic review is an important method for generating reliable evidence from published biomedical literature and it requires users screening articles to decide whether to include it into the review or not (i.e., labels of 1 or 0). It is a binary TC task and diverse methods have been developed for this task, showing a potential for reduction of manual review effort [3].
3. Information extraction (IE)—to extract specific information from a biomedical document. Examples include extraction of disease entities from clinical notes, or gene mentions from biomedical articles. In addition to recognizing important biomedical entities (e.g., diseases, drugs, and genes), IE tasks also include identifying relations between entities (e.g., a drug is used to treat a disease). Moreover, to further maximize the use of extracted information, biomedical IE systems often include functional modules that can map extracted entities to concepts in standard vocabularies (e.g., SNOMED-CT (https://www.snomed.org) for diseases, and Gene Ontology [4] for genes).

In addition, advanced applications such as question answering and conversational agents are also emerging and they often build on basic applications of IR, TC, and IE, with additional components. For example, QA systems have been developed to address finding answers in the biomedical literature [5] and electronic health records [6]. There are also QA systems targeted toward consumers (non-experts), including the use of such a system as an Alexa skill [7]. Note, however, the questions asked by health professionals and consumers are very different [8], both in structure and information need. As such, QA is generally seen as an end application of NLP, rather than a building block for other systems, since a clear idea of the intended user is needed to properly design the QA system.

Several studies have reviewed recent work on clinical NLP and have provided excellent summaries focusing on different NLP tasks. In 2008, Meystre et al. [9] conducted a careful review of 174 publications on information extraction from textual documents in electronic health records (EHRs) and identified clusters of different IE applications such as de-identification of clinical text, code extraction, IE for surveillance, IE for clinical decision support systems, and IE for supporting clinical research etc. More recently, Wang et al. [10] conducted another literature review on clinical IE articles published from January 2009 to September 2016. They analyzed data sources, tools, methods, as well as applications of clinical IE and provided informative details about recent progress in this field. In another recent review on deep learning-based clinical NLP, Wu et al. [11] found that TC and IE tasks are dominant (89.2%) among all clinical NLP articles that used deep learning technologies.

In the following section, more details about common clinical IE tasks are discussed, including examples of specific tasks and recent advances in method development.

Biomedical IE Tasks and Methods

A typical biomedical IE system usually should meet three requirements: (1) it can extract specific types of biomedical entities of interest; (2) it should also recognize required context features about extracted main entities (i.e., modifiers of main entities such as negation status, certainty, temporal information); and (3) it is able to map extracted entities to concepts in standard biomedical ontologies. The first task is known as named entity recognition (NER), which is to identify the boundary and determine the type of an entity (e.g., a mention of a disease) in the text. The second task is often treated as a relation extraction (RE) task, in which classifiers are built to determine the relations between main entities and modifier entities. The last task is known as entity linking in the open domain and often called concept normalization (CN) in the medical domain. It is important to link recognized entities to standard concepts, in order to integrate NLP systems with downstream clinical information systems.

NER Examples and Methods

Clinical NER tasks often focus on important clinical entities such as diseases, drugs, procedures, and lab tests. A typical example is the 2010 i2b2 [12] (informatics for integrating biology and the bedside) shared task on clinical NER [4], which is to recognize entities of medical problems, treatments (including drugs and procedures), and lab tests in discharge summaries. Figure 7.2 shows an example of the NER task to recognize entities of medical problems (i.e., the NER system should recognize "her recent GI bleeding" as a medical problem entity).

In early clinical NLP systems, dictionary-based lookup methods are often employed for clinical NER. For example, MedLEE (medical language extraction and encoding system), one of the earliest clinical NLP systems [13], uses collections of semantic lexicons to recognize clinical entities. Similar approaches are still being used for other IE tasks, especially when rich medical resources are available for the entities of interest, e.g., the MedEx [14] system uses terms derived from the RxNorm [15] resource to recognize drug entities in clinical documents.

Since 2010, more annotated clinical corpora have become available for clinical NER tasks (see section "Current Biomedical NLP Tools and Corpora"), which leads to active development of machine learning-based NER approaches for clinical entities. In a machine learning-based NER approach, each token is usually labeled with one of the [B, I, O] tags, where B stands for the beginning of an entity, I for inside an entity, and O for outside an entity (see Fig. 7.2). By using the BIO representation, the NER task is converted into a sequence labeling task—to assign a B/I/O tag to each token in a sentence. A number of machine learning algorithms that are suitable for the sequence labeling task have been implemented in clinical NER tasks and have demonstrated good performance, including semi-Markov models [16], conditional random fields (CRF) [17], and structural support vector machines (SSVM) [18]. To optimize the performance of machine learning-based NER, most of the effort has been spent on comparing different machine learning algorithms and experimenting with diverse feature engineering approaches.

More recently, deep learning algorithms have been extensively investigated for clinical NER tasks as well. An early study compared both the convolutional neural network (CNN) and the recurrent neural network (RNN) models with the CRF model on the 2010 i2b2 shared task. The RNN model achieved the best

An Example Sentence:	Plavix	was	not	recommended	,	given	her	recent	GI	bleeding	.
BIO Labels:	O	O	O	O		O	O	B	I	I	I	O

Fig. 7.2 An example sentence with an "medical problem" entity, as well as its representation in the BIO format. B indicates the beginning of an entity of interest, I indicate a token is "inside" this entity, and O indicates that it is "outside" the bounds of the entity

performance [19]. Then the bidirectional Long short-term memory and conditional random fields (Bi-LSTM-CRF) algorithm was applied to biomedical NER tasks with state-of-the-art performance on both a clinical corpus (the 2020 i2b2 shared task [20]) and a biomedical literature corpus (the NCBI Disease Corpus [21]). In 2018, new neural network-based language representation models such as Bidirectional Encoder Representations from Transformer (BERT) [22] further advanced performance on nearly all NLP tasks and they have been quickly applied to clinical NER tasks as well. Si et al. [23] compared different contextual representations and showed that the BERT model fine-tuned using clinical corpora achieved new state-of-the-art performance on the 2010 i2b2 shared task.

RE Examples and Methods

To understand fully why a clinical entity is mentioned in a document, it is important to extract its contextual information, which includes its neighborhood entities and their relations to the target entity. Figure 7.3 shows a few examples of such relations between entities, including (a) a negation modifier of a disease entity; (b) prescription information associated with a drug; and (c) a temporal relation between a disease and a temporal expression.

Many studies have investigated methods for RE in clinical documents, including both rule-based approaches and machine learning/deep learning-based methods. To

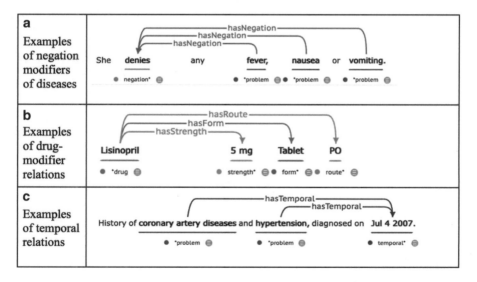

Fig. 7.3 Examples of relations extraction tasks: (**a**) negation modifiers of disease entities; (**b**) signature information of drugs; and (**c**) temporal relations between clinical entities and temporal expressions

illustrate existing methods for different types of clinical entities, the following RE tasks are selected and described with more details.

Negation and Other Contextual Information of Diseases As recognized clinical entities could be mentioned in a negative manner (e.g., "patient has no history of diabetes"), it is critical to recognize negations associated with medical problems. In addition, other contextual information such as "subject" (i.e., is an identified medical problem for patients vs. others, e.g., patients' parents) is also important and should be recognized in order to extract the true disease status of patients. In 2001, a simple regular expression based algorithm called NegEx was developed by Chapman et al., and it showed good performance in identifying negation of diseases [24], and later similar approaches were applied to identifying other context information as well [25]. To further improve the performance of recognizing negation in clinical text, researchers have further developed additional approaches, including adding dependency relations into NegEx [26] and more recent application of the BERT model to negation detection [27].

Drug Signature Information Extraction As shown in Fig. 7.3b, drug names in clinical documents often occur with its signature information (e.g., dose, route, frequency, duration etc.) and other related information (e.g., reason, adverse events, etc.), which should be extracted together with drug mentions. Two shared tasks have been organized to extract drug related information from clinical documents: (1) the 2009 i2b2 shared task [28] and (2) the 2018 n2c2 (National NLP Clinical Challenges) challenge on drug-ADE (adverse drug events) extraction [29]. In the 2009 i2b2 challenge, most of the participating systems (i.e., seven out of the top 10 best performing ones) used rule-based [30] or hybrid approaches [31], which leverage existing medical knowledge bases to derive lexicons of drug names and specify rules for drug-signature patterns. In the 2018 n2c2 challenges, machine learning and deep learning based approaches were widely implemented in the top ranked systems.

Temporal Relation Extraction Extracting temporal information of clinical events is critical for understanding disease trajectories of patients and it has been investigated extensively, even in early clinical NLP work [32]. In 2012, i2b2 organized a comprehensive shared task to extract temporal relations from clinical text, which requires extracting temporal expressions and temporal relations (before, overlap, and after) between clinical events and temporal expressions [33]. For the temporal relation extraction task, diverse machine learning-based classification algorithms have been used and the top-ranked system applied the SVM to the task, with novel strategies to define potential candidate pairs between events/times [18]. Nevertheless, temporal relation extraction from clinical text remains challenging and active research is ongoing to further improve its performance.

CN Examples and Methods

CN aims at mapping recognized entities to codes in standard vocabularies, which is important for downstream computerized applications that rely on standard vocabularies in medicine. Many clinical NLP systems map entities to Concept Unique IDs (CUIs) in the UMLS (unified medical language system) [34], which integrates over one hundred different medical vocabularies. Figure 7.4 shows an example of finding the right UMLS concept ID for the entity "knee amputation right below", in which several candidates are available. It is obvious that simply relying on string similarity between the entity and candidate terms is not sufficient—the variation of different surface forms is a big challenge in the CN task. In addition, ambiguity is another big issue, e.g., an abbreviated entity "pt" could have different meanings at different contexts, such as "patient", "physical therapy", "prothrombin time" etc.

In the computer science community, CN is often called entity linking, which refers to linking an entity to an entry in a dictionary or a knowledge base. A typical entity linking framework [35] consists of three steps: (1) generating candidate concepts for an entity (e.g., relying on string similarity algorithms such as BM25) [36]; (2) ranking candidate concepts using diverse types of information, to decide on the most relevant candidate concept; (3) predicting an unlinkable entity, which will further decide whether the top ranked candidate is the right one or the entity has no linkable entry in the dictionary (i.e., a new entity not covered by the dictionary). Among them, candidate concept ranking is the key step that plays an important role in optimizing entity ranking performance. String similarity-based methods (e.g., retrieval-based models [37]), learning-to-rank methods (e.g., RankSVM) [38], as well as many other machine learning and neural network-based ranking approaches [39] have been proposed.

In the medical domain, several widely used clinical NLP systems (e.g., MetaMap, cTAKES, and CLAMP) map clinical entities to concepts in the UMLS. Moreover, specific methods have been investigated to address the needs of mapping clinical entities to specified medical terminologies. For example, Perotte et al. [40] proposed a hierarchy-based classifier to assign ICD-9 codes from discharge summaries and showed better performance than that from the baseline flat classifier. More recently, Kate [41] proposed a new method to map entities to SNOMED-CT codes, with the capability to fully represent new concepts in text by post-coordinating existing SNOMED concepts. In 2013, a shared challenge for mapping disease mentions in clinical text to UMLS CUIs was organized by the ShARe/CLEF eHealth Evaluation Lab, and diverse CN methods were proposed by over 20 different teams [42]. Another more recent challenge on clinical CN is the 2019 National Natural

Fig. 7.4 An example of concept normalization— map an entity to concepts in the UMLS

Entity: "knee amputation right below"
Candidate Concepts:
- C2202463   "right lower leg amputated below knee"
- C0002692   "amputation of leg through tibia and fibula"
- C0177649   "other amputation below knee"

language processing (NLP) Clinical Challenges (n2c2)/Open Health NLP (OHNLP) shared task track 3, which requires mapping medical problems, treatments and tests to concepts in SNOMED-CT and RxNorm [43]. Different approaches such as cascading dictionary lookup, edit distance, retrieval-based ranking, as well as deep learning algorithms have been used in the challenge [43]. Overall, deep learning-based ranking methods have shown improved performance [44, 45].

Current Biomedical NLP Tools and Corpora

Biomedical NLP Tools

Over the past two decades, many clinical NLP systems have been developed and used to support diverse applications. Based on their purposes, we often divide them into two categories: (1) general purpose clinical NLP systems, which can extract broad types of clinical information such as diseases, drugs, etc, and can be used to support diverse applications; (2) specific purpose NLP systems, which are built to extract specific types of clinical information that are needed for specified applications, e.g., a system to extract smoking status [46]. General purpose clinical NLP systems often require more resources and take more time to build. On the contrary, specific purpose clinical NLP systems sometimes can be developed quickly to achieve good performance, depending on the difficulty of the task. In this section, we will focus our discussion on a few widely used general purpose clinical NLP systems.

MedLEE is one of the earliest general purpose clinical NLP systems, developed by Dr. Carol Friedman and her team at Columbia University in 1994, starting with radiology reports and quickly extending to other types of clinical reports [47]. It is primarily a rule-based system that follows the sublanguage theory to parse clinical text using a set of well-defined semantic grammars. MedLEE recognizes broad types of clinical entities and their relations, and provides codes from standard vocabularies (e.g., CUIs from UMLS), which leads to many applications in diverse care settings [48].

Following MedLEE, a number of systems have been developed to extract broad types of information from clinical text. A few of them are actively used by large communities, including:

MetaMap MetaMap is a biomedical NLP system developed at the National Library of Medicine of the U.S. beginning in the 1990's, with the original goal of mapping biomedical literature text to concepts in the UMLS Metathesaurus [49]. It has been applied to process clinical documents as well, with many use cases [50]. To improve its efficiency, a Java implementation of MetaMap, called MetaMap Lite [51], was released to the community in 2017. MetaMap can be accessed at https://metamap.nlm.nih.gov/.

cTAKES Clinical Text Analysis and Knowledge Extraction System (cTAKES) is a clinical NLP tool developed at Mayo Clinic in 2010 [52]. It follows the Apache UIMA framework [53] to organize components within an NLP pipeline and it quickly becomes an Apache open source project (accessible at https://ctakes.apache. org/). cTAKES leverages multiple open domain NLP packages (e.g., openNLP) and customizes those models using clinical corpora. It has been widely used for clinical concept extraction as an open source tool.

CLAMP Clinical language annotation, modeling, and processing (CLAMP) is a comprehensive clinical NLP toolkit developed by a research team at University of Texas Health Science Center in 2018 [54] and now available as a commercial product that is freely available for academic purposes. It provides a collection of machine learning-based and hybrid pipelines to extract common or specific types of clinical entities from text and map them to concepts in the UMLS. In addition, it includes user-friendly interfaces to allow users to annotate text, train machine learning models, and specify rules for building customized IE pipelines. As of July of 2021, CLAMP has been used by researchers and professionals from over 650 different healthcare organizations. It is available at https://clamp.uth.edu.

Biomedical Text Resources

Types of Biomedical Text

In the biomedical domain, diverse types of narrative documents are available and valuable for providing insights to research and business in life science and healthcare. Some different types of available textual resources as follows:

Biomedical Literature MEDLINE (Medical Literature Analysis and Retrieval System Online) is perhaps the most comprehensive bibliographic database (over 32 million citations) available in the biomedical domain. It is accessible through PubMed (https://pubmed.ncbi.nlm.nih.gov/). Through the Entrez Programming Utilities (E-utilities), users can obtain subsets of abstracts of biomedical articles from PubMed, for NLP method development and applications. Moreover, PubMed Central provides a downloadable collection of over 2.75 million full-text articles for text mining purposes.

Clinical Documents in EHRs Due to privacy and security issues, clinical reports are often not freely available for the public. However, several efforts have made some de-identified clinical corpora available for research purposes. A prominent example is the MIMIC (medical information mart from intensive care) database, which contains millions of de-identified clinical reports [55]. MTSamples (https:// www.mtsamples.com/) is another resource for clinical documents, which provides over four thousand synthetic transcribed medical reports. A number of annotated clinical corpora are also available from past NLP challenges (see Table 7.1).

Table 7.1 Available corpora from past NLP shared tasks

Corpus name	Description	Task type	Sample size	Access URL
2010 i2b2 challenge	Extraction of medical problems, treatments, and tests, assertion identification, and relation extraction	NER, RE	871 discharge summaries and progress reports	https://portal.dbmi.hms.harvard.edu/projects/n2c2-nlp/
2011 BioNLP challenge	Concept extraction, co-reference, entity relations, gene renaming, event extraction	NER, RE	2450 literature abstract, 60 literature full text	http://2011.bionlp-st.org/
2012 i2b2 challenge	Temporal relation extraction	RE	310 discharge summaries	https://portal.dbmi.hms.harvard.edu/projects/n2c2-nlp/
2013 CLEF challenge	Concept extraction, normalization of acronyms/abbreviations	NER, CN	200 clinical reports	https://sites.google.com/site/shareclefehealth/home
2013 BioNLP challenge	Concept extraction, corpus annotation, Relation extraction	NER, RE	34 literature full text, 1525 literature abstract, 201 sentences, 131 documents	http://2013.bionlp-st.org/tasks
2014 SemEVAL	Entity/acronym/abbreviation recognition and mapping to UMLS CUIs	NER, CN	300 clinical reports	https://alt.qcri.org/semeval2014/task7/
2015 SemEVAL	Concept extraction and concept normalization	NER, CN	531 clinical notes (a mix of discharge summaries and radiology reports)	https://alt.qcri.org/semeval2015/task14/
2016 BioNLP challenge	Entity categorization, concept extraction, event extraction, knowledge base population, relation extraction	NER, RE	307 literature abstracts, 131 documents, 87 literature paragraphs	http://2016.bionlp-st.org/home
2018 n2c2 challenge	Drug and ADE extraction	NER, RE	505 discharge summaries	https://portal.dbmi.hms.harvard.edu/projects/n2c2-nlp/
2019 n2c2 challenge	Clinical semantic textual similarity, concept extraction, relation extraction, concept normalization	NER, RE, CN	2054 clinical sentence pairs, 100 discharge summaries	https://n2c2.dbmi.hms.harvard.edu/
2019 BioNLP challenge	Concept annotation, coreference, concept extraction, relation extraction, concept normalization, event extraction, information retrieval, sentence extraction	NER, RE, CN	97 literature full texts, 1000 open access Spanish medical publications, 2000 literature abstracts	https://2019.bionlp-ost.org/tasks

Social Media Social media platforms such as Twitter have also accumulated huge amounts of textual data and studies have shown that they are useful in providing insights to public health problems [56, 57]. Some social media platforms provide APIs for querying and collecting their data for method development and data analysis (e.g., Twitter developer APIs: https://developer.twitter.com/en/products/twitter-api), making it easy for NLP researchers.

Clinical Trial Documents Clinicaltrials.gov is probably the most comprehensive clinical trial database that is publicly available for researchers. As of July 2021, it contains information for 382,313 publicly or privately funded clinical trials. Detailed clinical trial protocols can be queried and downloaded through its web interface and APIs, making it a great resource for developing NLP and text mining technologies for understanding clinical trials.

FDA Drug Labels Another important textual source for drug development is drug labels approved by the United States Food and Drug Administration (FDA)—a number of NLP studies have investigated extracting and normalizing drug information in labels [58]. One useful resource for this type of work is the DailyMed database developed by the NLM [59]. It provides a downloadable copy of label information for all FDA approved drugs.

Annotated Corpora from Past Challenges

One particular resource for biomedical NLP is annotated corpora from previous shared tasks, which provide benchmark datasets for developing and evaluating NLP methods. Table 7.1 summarizes some available corpora for NER, RE, and NC tasks, from biomedical NLP challenges since 2010.

Applications, Challenges and Future Directions

Applications of NLP

As EHRs become an enabling resource for observational studies, many clinical NLP systems have been used to automatically extract patient information from clinical documents to support diverse research such as comparative effectiveness studies. One example is to use NLP to identify patients with specific phenotypes [60]. Studies have shown that combining information extracted from clinical documents using NLP with structured data in EHRs can greatly improve the performance of phenotyping algorithms [61]. Detailed information extracted by NLP, e.g., drug exposure, has been applied to support diverse studies such as pharmacovigilance [62], pharmacogenomics [63], and drug repurposing [64, 65] research.

Another big application area of clinical NLP systems is to support practice and operations in healthcare. In a review article by Demner-Fushman et al. [66], the uses of NLP in clinical decision support systems are described with details, showing how NLP can automatically extract required information at the point and time needed during care delivery. Moreover, NLP has also been used to optimize care workflow and improve care quality, e.g., analyzing emergency department notes using NLP detects inappropriate usage of the emergency room [67].

Many applications of NLP have also been demonstrated that use other biomedical textual sources. Researchers have mined large biomedical article collections to generate new hypotheses for scientific discoveries, an approach known as **literature-based discovery** (LBD) following Don Swanson's seminal work beginning in the 1980s with manual identification of implicit links between concepts expressed in journal articles [68]. NLP methods have been used in LBD for both NER and relation extraction [69]. As a recent example, Pyysalo et al. have developed LION LBD [70], a literature-based discovery system by leveraging the PubTator NLP system [71], to support new discoveries by biomedical researchers. Similar approaches have also been used for other applications, e.g., detect drug repurposing signals from the literature using SemRep [72], a linguistically-motivated biomedical NLP tool that has been widely used across a range of research applications [73, 74]. Examples of NLP applications for other biomedical text data include (1) mining social media for adverse drug reaction [75, 76]; (2) processing clinical trial protocols to identify computable eligibility criteria [77, 78]; and (3) standardizing information in FDA drug labels [79].

Challenges and Future Directions

Despite the enormous potential of NLP to extract meaning and structure from the vast amount of unstructured text data in biomedicine, there are numerous challenges that inhibit its growth as a field. Because NLP is so dependent upon ML, these challenges could apply to any ML-based models in biomedicine. However, the challenges we discuss below are particularly acute in NLP due to its reliance on expert-driven annotation (that is, the creation of data on which the ML models are trained and tested) and the variety of human language.

The first major challenge is the difficulty and cost related to annotating sufficient data for training ML-based NLP models. Because the goals and domain of many NLP systems in biomedicine are so specialized, it is quite common that subject-matter experts are needed to perform the manual annotation work themselves, or actively oversee the annotation done by others. For instance, it often takes radiologists to fully understand the language in radiology reports, or proteomics experts to fully understand the language in papers about protein-protein interactions. Engaging with these experts is time-consuming, costly, and difficult to scale, so significant efforts have gone into methods that reduce the amount of annotation needed on a given project. One such method is **Active Learning**, where the annotator interacts with the ML model in such a way that only the most "useful" examples for the model need to be annotated [80]. Another method is **Transfer Learning**, where a ML model is built on other data for a related "source" task, then some part of that model is "transferred" to reduce the amount of data needed on the intended "target" task [81]. These methods, and others, can reduce the burden of annotation significantly, but the difficulty of creating manual annotations is still seen as the greatest hindrance to creating a new NLP system.

The second major challenge applies most particularly to clinical data, but is broadly true of any data that contains sensitive information (e.g., like a patient's medical history) and thus needs to remain private. This challenge is the difficulty of data sharing. The aforementioned issue related to annotation cost could be greatly alleviated if annotations developed in one place could be widely shared according to FAIR (findable, accessible, interoperable, reusable) principles. But data such as clinical notes contain far too much private information to be easily shareable. Laws such as the Health Insurance Portability and Accountability Act (HIPAA) restrict sharing of patient data. NLP methods such as **De-identification** can remove many of the identifiers in clinical notes that could link a patient back to the shared record [82], but like all NLP systems these methods make errors that, to date, make them insufficient to allow widespread sharing of clinical texts. Another partial solution is **Federated Learning**, wherein the original data never leaves the originating institution, only the ML model is transferred [83]. At this point, it seems clear that ultimately some form of federated learning will be needed to train ML-based NLP models from many institutional sources, but there are many open questions about how best to perform federated learning [84]. Additionally, as models get more powerful and more complex, it seems possible that these models are also capable of encoding and retrieving private patient information [84]. This would mean that federated learning alone could not ensure privacy, and either additional safeguards would be necessary or only simpler, inferior models could be used that don't endanger privacy.

The third major challenge, which is fundamental to nearly all of science, is generalizability. Specifically, in this case, how NLP models can generalize to slightly different types of text. While on many occasions the NLP tasks will be different from data type to data type so task generalization is not critical (e.g., radiology reports and nursing notes contain very different information, as do scientific articles about genomics and psychology), there are still many NLP tasks that in theory should generalize between domains (e.g., extracting patient history from clinical notes, or reasons for citation in scientific articles). However, the language used in different domains can be incredibly different, such that they have even been described as having separate sub-languages [47, 85]. The challenge gets even more irksome when one considers that for EHR notes, the same note type (e.g., cardiology reports) may have entirely differ structures and linguistic patterns from one institution to another. This means that an NLP model trained on Hospital A's data could have a significant performance drop when run on the same note types for Hospital B's data. At its most extreme, this may mean that only academic medical centers with NLP researchers and budgets for data annotation are capable of developing NLP. This could result in widening the already-sizable disparities in the analytical capabilities of health systems. What is needed, at a fundamental level, are NLP models that are able to overcome small language variations as well as the availability of data from multiple institutions to train and test such models for their generalizable performance.

Conclusion

With the accumulation of large textual data in the biomedical domain, NLP has become an enabling technology for unlocking valuable information from biomedical text to support diverse downstream computational applications. This chapter introduces basic NLP tasks, as well as current methods, tools, and resources that are important for biomedical NLP research and development. With new advances in data, algorithms, and computational infrastructures, NLP will achieve better performance and support broader applications in biomedicine.

Questions for Discussion

- Given all the complex NLP tasks described in this chapter, it is worth considering *why* we use natural language when given the choice. For instance, a biomedical paper could be written in an entirely formal language, or an EHR could only contain structured information about a patient. What are the relative advantages and disadvantages of natural language with respect to structured data? What are some cases where each would be preferable?
- When it comes to EHR data in the United States, HIPAA creates several barriers to sharing EHR data for research purposes (similar laws exist in many other countries), particularly natural language notes. Why do you think structured data is so much easier to share in a HIPAA-compliant manner?
- Please download one of the general clinical NLP systems (e.g., MetaMap, cTAKES, CLAMP), review its available components, and specify which type of linguistic information is addressed by each component.
- Assuming that you want to build a knowledge graph of drugs, genes, and their relations from biomedical literature. What NLP tasks are involved in such a system?
- We want to determine whether a disease mention in a clinical document is negated or not. What NLP tools are available for this task? What methods are used in each tool?
- Some automated NLP methods have extremely high performance (e.g., greater than 95% on some metric), while others are quite low (many are below 60%). What are some of the linguistic features that make a task "easy" or "hard"? What are some of the non-linguistic features of the data that could result in low or high performance?

Further Reading

Cohen KB, Demner-Fushman D. Biomedical Natural Language Processing. John Benjamins Publishing Company, 2014.

- A short textbook introducing biomedical NLP tasks, primarily focusing on those useful from a bioinformatics and computational biology perspective.

Demner-Fushman D, Chapman WW, McDonald CJ. What can natural language processing do for clinical decision support? J Biomed Inform. 2009;42(5):760–2.

- This article lays the foundation for how NLP can be used to improve decision-making for diagnosing and treating patients.

Meystre SM, Savova GK, Kipper-Schuler KC, Hurdle JF. Extracting information from textual documents in the electronic health record: a review of recent research. Yearb Med Inform. 2008:128–44.

- This is an early review paper conducted in 2008, with careful review of 174 publications on information extraction from clinical documents for different applications.

Wang Y, Wang L, Rastegar-Mojarad M, Moon S, Shen F, Afzal N, et al. Clinical information extraction applications: A literature review. J Biomed Inform. 2018;77:34–49.

- A literature review on clinical information extraction articles published from January 2009 to September 2016. The authors analyzed data sources, tools, methods, as well as applications of clinical NLP and provided cogent insights into current uses of clinical NLP.

Wu S, Roberts K, Datta S, Du J, Ji Z, Si Y, et al. Deep learning in clinical natural language processing: a methodical review. J Am Med Inform Assoc. 2020;27(3):457–70.

- This is a more recent review of the uses of deep learning methods in clinical NLP.

References

1. Mitchell Marcus BS, Marcinkiewicz MA. Building a large annotated corpus of English. Penn: The Penn Treebank; 1993.
2. PMC article datasets. https://pubmed.ncbi.nlm.nih.gov.
3. García Adeva JJ, Pikatza Atxa JM, Ubeda Carrillo M, Ansuategi ZE. Automatic text classification to support systematic reviews in medicine. Expert Syst Appl. 2014;41(4):1498–508.
4. Christophe Dessimoz NŠ. The gene ontology handbook. 2017. http://geneontology.org/.
5. Demner-Fushman D, Lin J. Answering clinical questions with knowledge-based and statistical techniques. Comput Linguist. 2007;33(1):63–103.
6. Roberts K, Patra BG. A semantic parsing method for mapping clinical questions to logical forms. AMIA Symp. 2018;2017:1478–87.
7. Demner-Fushman D, Mrabet Y, Ben AA. Consumer health information and question answering: helping consumers find answers to their health-related information needs. JAMIA. 2020;27(2):194–201.

8. Roberts K, Demner-Fushman D. Interactive use of online health resources: a comparison of consumer and professional questions. J Am Med Inform Assoc. 2016;23(4):802–11.
9. Meystre SM, Savova GK, Kipper-Schuler KC, Hurdle JF. Extracting information from textual documents in the electronic health record: a review of recent research. Yearb Med Inform. 2008;2008:128–44.
10. Wang Y, Wang L, Rastegar-Mojarad M, Moon S, Shen F, Afzal N, et al. Clinical information extraction applications: a literature review. J Biomed Inform. 2018;77:34–49.
11. Wu S, Roberts K, Datta S, Du J, Ji Z, Si Y, et al. Deep learning in clinical natural language processing: a methodical review. J Am Med Inform Assoc. 2020;27(3):457–70.
12. Uzuner Ö, South BR, Shen S, DuVall SL. 2010 i2b2/VA challenge on concepts, assertions, and relations in clinical text. J Am Med Inform Assoc. 2011;18(5):552–6.
13. Friedman C. A broad-coverage natural language processing system. Proc AMIA Symp. 2000;2000:270–4.
14. Xu H, Stenner SP, Doan S, Johnson KB, Waitman LR, Denny JC. MedEx: a medication information extraction system for clinical narratives. J Am Med Inform Assoc. 2010;17(1): 19–24.
15. Nelson SJ, Zeng K, Kilbourne J, Powell T, Moore R. Normalized names for clinical drugs: RxNorm at 6 years. J Am Med Inform Assoc. 2011;18(4):441–8.
16. de Bruijn B, Cherry C, Kiritchenko S, Martin J, Zhu X. Machine-learned solutions for three stages of clinical information extraction: the state of the art at i2b2 2010. J Am Med Inform Assoc. 2011;18(5):557–62.
17. Jiang M, Chen Y, Liu M, Rosenbloom ST, Mani S, Denny JC, et al. A study of machine-learning-based approaches to extract clinical entities and their assertions from discharge summaries. J Am Med Inform Assoc. 2011;18(5):601–6.
18. Tang B, Wu Y, Jiang M, Chen Y, Denny JC, Xu H. A hybrid system for temporal information extraction from clinical text. J Am Med Inform Assoc. 2013;20(5):828–35.
19. Wu Y, Jiang M, Xu J, Zhi D, Xu H. Clinical named entity recognition using deep learning models. AMIA Annu Symp Proc. 2017;2017:1812–9.
20. Raghavendra Chalapathy EZB, Piccardi M. Bidirectional LSTM-CRF for clinical concept extraction. 2016.
21. Xu KZZ, Hao T, Liu W. A bidirectional LSTM and conditional random fields approach to medical named entity recognition. Adv Intell Syst Comput. 2018;2018:639.
22. Apache OpenNLP. https://arxiv.org/abs/1810.04805.
23. Si Y, Wang J, Xu H, Roberts K. Enhancing clinical concept extraction with contextual embeddings. J Am Med Inform Assoc. 2019;26(11):1297–304.
24. Chapman WW, Bridewell W, Hanbury P, Cooper GF, Buchanan BG. A simple algorithm for identifying negated findings and diseases in discharge summaries. J Biomed Inform. 2001;34(5):301–10.
25. Chapman WW, Chu D, Dowling JN. ConText: an algorithm for identifying contextual features from clinical text. In: Proceedings of the workshop on BioNLP 2007: biological, translational, and clinical language processing. Prague: Association for Computational Linguistics; 2007. p. 81–8.
26. Lin C, Bethard S, Dligach D, Sadeque F, Savova G, Miller TA. Does BERT need domain adaptation for clinical negation detection? J Am Med Inform Assoc. 2020;27(4):584–91.
27. Mehrabi S, Krishnan A, Sohn S, Roch AM, Schmidt H, Kesterson J, et al. DEEPEN: a negation detection system for clinical text incorporating dependency relation into NegEx. J Biomed Inform. 2015;54:213–9.
28. Uzuner O, Solti I, Cadag E. Extracting medication information from clinical text. J Am Med Inform Assoc. 2010;17(5):514–8.
29. Henry S, Buchan K, Filannino M, Stubbs A, Uzuner O. 2018 n2c2 shared task on adverse drug events and medication extraction in electronic health records. J Am Med Inform Assoc. 2020;27(1):3–12.
30. Doan S, Bastarache L, Klimkowski S, Denny JC, Xu H. Integrating existing natural language processing tools for medication extraction from discharge summaries. J Am Med Inform Assoc. 2010;17(5):528–31.

31. Patrick J, Li M. High accuracy information extraction of medication information from clinical notes: 2009 i2b2 medication extraction challenge. JAMIA. 2010;17(5):524–7.
32. Zhou L, Melton GB, Parsons S, Hripcsak G. A temporal constraint structure for extracting temporal information from clinical narrative. J Biomed Inform. 2006;39(4):424–39.
33. Sun W, Rumshisky A, Uzuner O. Evaluating temporal relations in clinical text: 2012 i2b2 challenge. JAMIA. 2013;20(5):806–13.
34. Bodenreider O. The unified medical language system (UMLS): integrating biomedical terminology. Nucleic Acids Res. 2004;2004:267–70.
35. Shen W, Wang J, Han J. Entity linking with a knowledge base: issues, techniques, and solutions. IEEE Trans Knowl Data Eng. 2015;27(2):443–60.
36. Robertson S, Walker S, Jones S, Hancock-Beaulieu MM, Gatford M. Okapi at TREC-3. Gaithersburg: NIST; 1994. p. 109–26.
37. Salton G, Wong A, Yang CS. A vector space model for automatic indexing. Commun ACM. 1975;18(11):613–20.
38. Joachims T. Optimizing search engines using clickthrough data. In: Proceedings of the eighth ACM SIGKDD international conference on knowledge discovery and data mining. Edmonton: Association for Computing Machinery; 2002. p. 133–42.
39. Xiao Ling SS, Daniel S. Design challenges for entity linking. Trans Assoc Comput Linguist. 2015;3:315–28.
40. Perotte A, Pivovarov R, Natarajan K, Weiskopf N, Wood F, Elhadad N. Diagnosis code assignment: models and evaluation metrics. JAMIA. 2014;21(2):231–7.
41. Kate RJ. Automatic full conversion of clinical terms into SNOMED CT concepts. J Biomed Inform. 2020;111:103585.
42. Mowery D, Velupillai S, South B, Christensen L, Martinez D, Kelly L, et al. Task 1: ShARe/CLEF eHealth evaluation lab 2013. New York: Springer; 2013.
43. Henry S, Wang Y, Shen F, Uzuner O. The 2019 national natural language processing (NLP) clinical challenges (n2c2)/open health NLP (OHNLP) shared task on clinical concept normalization for clinical records. J Am Med Inform Assoc. 2020;27(10):1529–37.
44. Li H, Chen Q, Tang B, Wang X, Xu H, Wang B, et al. CNN-based ranking for biomedical entity normalization. BMC Bioinformatics. 2017;18(11):385.
45. Zongcheng Ji QW, Hua Xu. BERT-based ranking for biomedical entity normalization. 2020.
46. Uzuner O, Goldstein I, Luo Y, Kohane I. Identifying patient smoking status from medical discharge records. JAMIA. 2008;15(1):14–24.
47. Friedman C, Alderson PO, Austin JH, Cimino JJ, Johnson SB. A general natural-language text processor for clinical radiology. J Am Med Inform Assoc. 1994;1(2):161–74.
48. Lussier YA, Shagina L, Friedman C. Automating SNOMED coding using medical language understanding: a feasibility study. Proc AMIA Symp. 2001;2001:418–22.
49. Aronson AR. Effective mapping of biomedical text to the UMLS Metathesaurus: the MetaMap program. Proc AMIA Symp. 2001;2001:17–21.
50. Aronson AR, Lang FM. An overview of MetaMap: historical perspective and recent advances. J Am Med Inform Assoc. 2010;17(3):229–36.
51. Demner-Fushman D, Rogers WJ, Aronson AR. MetaMap lite: an evaluation of a new Java implementation of MetaMap. J Am Med Inform Assoc. 2017;24(4):841–4.
52. Savova GK, Masanz JJ, Ogren PV, Zheng J, Sohn S, Kipper-Schuler KC, et al. Mayo clinical text analysis and knowledge extraction system (cTAKES): architecture, component evaluation and applications. JAMIA. 2010;17(5):507–13.
53. Apache UIMA.
54. Soysal E, Wang J, Jiang M, Wu Y, Pakhomov S, Liu H, et al. CLAMP - a toolkit for efficiently building customized clinical natural language processing pipelines. J Am Med Inform Assoc. 2018;25(3):331–6.
55. Johnson AE, Pollard TJ, Shen L, Lehman LW, Feng M, Ghassemi M, et al. MIMIC-III, a freely accessible critical care database. Sci Data. 2016;3:160035.
56. Du J, Xu J, Song H-Y, Tao C. Leveraging machine learning-based approaches to assess human papillomavirus vaccination sentiment trends with Twitter data. BMC Med Inform Decis Mak. 2017;17(2):69.

57. Sarker A, O'Connor K, Ginn R, Scotch M, Smith K, Malone D, et al. Social media mining for toxicovigilance: automatic monitoring of prescription medication abuse from Twitter. Drug Saf. 2016;39(3):231–40.
58. Li Q, Deleger L, Lingren T, Zhai H, Kaiser M, Stoutenborough L, et al. Mining FDA drug labels for medical conditions. BMC Med Inform Decis Mak. 2013;13:53.
59. DailyMed. https://dailymed.nlm.nih.gov/dailymed/.
60. Zeng Z, Deng Y, Li X, Naumann T, Luo Y. Natural language processing for EHR-based computational phenotyping. IEEE/ACM Trans Comput Biol Bioinform. 2019;16(1):139–53.
61. Pathak J, Kho AN, Denny JC. Electronic health records-driven phenotyping: challenges, recent advances, and perspectives. J Am Med Inform Assoc. 2013;20(2):206–11.
62. Wu Y, Warner JL, Wang L, Jiang M, Xu J, Chen Q, et al. Discovery of noncancer drug effects on survival in electronic health records of patients with cancer: a new paradigm for drug repurposing. JCO Clin Cancer Inform. 2019;3:1–9.
63. Haerian K, Varn D, Vaidya S, Ena L, Chase HS, Friedman C. Detection of pharmacovigilance-related adverse events using electronic health records and automated methods. Clin Pharmacol Ther. 2012;92(2):228–34.
64. Xu H, Jiang M, Oetjens M, Bowton EA, Ramirez AH, Jeff JM, et al. Facilitating pharmacogenetic studies using electronic health records and natural-language processing: a case study of warfarin. J Am Med Inform Assoc. 2011;18(4):387–91.
65. Xu H, Li J, Jiang X, Chen Q. Electronic health records for drug repurposing: current status, challenges, and future directions. Clin Pharmacol Ther. 2020;107(4):712–4.
66. Demner-Fushman D, Chapman WW, McDonald CJ. What can natural language processing do for clinical decision support? J Biomed Inform. 2009;42(5):760–72.
67. St-Maurice J, Kuo MH. Analyzing primary care data to characterize inappropriate emergency room use. Stud Health Technol Inform. 2012;180:990–4.
68. Swanson DR. Fish oil, Raynaud's syndrome, and undiscovered public knowledge. Perspect Biol Med. 1986;30:7–18.
69. Weeber M, Klein H, de Jong-van den Berg LT, Vos R. Using concepts in literature-based discovery: Simulating Swanson's Raynaud–fish oil and migraine–magnesium discoveries. J Am Soc Inf Sci Technol. 2001;52(7):548–57.
70. Pyysalo S, Baker S, Ali I, Haselwimmer S, Shah T, Young A, et al. LION LBD: a literature-based discovery system for cancer biology. Bioinformatics. 2019;35(9):1553–61.
71. Wei CH, Leaman R, Lu Z. PubTator central: automated concept annotation for biomedical full text articles. Nucleic Acids Res. 2019;47(1):587–93.
72. Zhang R, Hristovski D, Schutte D, Kastrin A, Fiszman M, Kilicoglu H. Drug repurposing for COVID-19 via knowledge graph completion. J Biomed Inform. 2021;115:103696.
73. Kilicoglu H, Fiszman M, Rosemblat G, Marimpietri S, Rindflesch TC. Arguments of nominals in semantic interpretation of biomedical text. In: Proceedings of the 2010 workshop on biomedical natural language processing. 2010. pp. 46–54.
74. Kilicoglu H, Rosemblat G, Fiszman M, Shin D. Broad-coverage biomedical relation extraction with SemRep. BMC Bioinformatics. 2020;21:1–28.
75. Nikfarjam A, Sarker A, O'Connor K, Ginn R, Gonzalez G. Pharmacovigilance from social media: mining adverse drug reaction mentions using sequence labeling with word embedding cluster features. J Am Med Inform Assoc. 2015;22(3):671–81.
76. Rezaei Z, Ebrahimpour-Komleh H, Eslami B, Chavoshinejad R, Totonchi M. Adverse drug reaction detection in social media by Deepm learning methods. Cell J. 2020;22(3):319–24.
77. Yuan C, Ryan PB, Ta C, Guo Y, Li Z, Hardin J, et al. Criteria2Query: a natural language interface to clinical databases for cohort definition. J Am Med Inform Assoc. 2019;26(4):294–305.
78. Xu J, Lee HJ, Zeng J, Wu Y, Zhang Y, Huang LC, et al. Extracting genetic alteration information for personalized cancer therapy from ClinicalTrials.gov. J Am Med Inform Assoc. 2016;23(4):750–7.
79. Ly T, Pamer C, Dang O, Brajovic S, Haider S, Botsis T, et al. Evaluation of natural language processing (NLP) systems to annotate drug product labeling with MedDRA terminology. J Biomed Inform. 2018;83:73–86.

80. Chen Y, Lasko TA, Mei Q, Denny JC, Xu H. A study of active learning methods for named entity recognition in clinical text. J Biomed Inform. 2015;58:11–8.
81. Yifan Peng SY, Zhiyong L. Ransfer learning in biomedical natural language processing: an evaluation of BERT and ELMo on ten benchmarking datasets. In: Proceedings of the 18th BioNLP workshop and shared task; 2019, pp. 58–65.
82. Meystre SM, Friedlin FJ, South BR, Shen S, Samore MH. Automatic de-identification of textual documents in the electronic health record: a review of recent research. BMC Med Res Methodol. 2010;10(1):70.
83. Zhu X, Wang J, Hong Z, Xiao J. Empirical studies of institutional federated learning for natural language processing. ACL Anthol. 2020;2020:625–34.
84. Eric Lehman SJ, Pichotta K, Goldberg Y, Wallace B. Does BERT pretrained on clinical notes reveal sensitive data? In: Proceedings of the 2021 conference of the north American chapter of the association for computational linguistics: human language technologies; 2021, pp. 946–59.
85. Irina Temnikova KC. Recognizing sublanguages in scientific journal articles through closure properties. In: Proceedings of the 2013 workshop on biomedical natural language processing; 2013, pp. 72–9.

Chapter 8
Explainability in Medical AI

Ron C. Li, Naveen Muthu, Tina Hernandez-Boussard, Dev Dash, and Nigam H. Shah

After reading this chapter, you should know the answers to these questions:
- What are the current trends in AI explainability research?
- What types of explainability paradigms can be conferred onto different machine learning (ML) models?
- What are the different methods by which ML models can be explained?
- How can principles of cognitive informatics be applied to explainability in medical AI?
- What is an 'emergent property' of a sociotechnical system?
- What regulatory frameworks have been put forth with regards to accountability of ML models?

Introduction

The current paradigm of artificial intelligence (AI) in medicine primarily relies on machine learning (ML) models as a means to provide insights—typically in the form of a diagnosis or prognosis—that can affect the health of individuals and populations. A model learned from past data is often a trigger that invokes a series of

R. C. Li (✉) · T. Hernandez-Boussard · D. Dash · N. H. Shah
Stanford University School of Medicine, Stanford, CA, USA
e-mail: ronl@stanford.edu

N. Muthu
University of Pennsylvania School of Medicine, Philadelphia, PA, USA

Children's Hospital of Philadelphia, Philadelphia, PA, USA

© The Author(s), under exclusive license to Springer Nature
Switzerland AG 2022
T. A. Cohen et al. (eds.), *Intelligent Systems in Medicine and Health*, Cognitive
Informatics in Biomedicine and Healthcare,
https://doi.org/10.1007/978-3-031-09108-7_8

actions comprising a care workflow. We define a *model* as a function learned from data that maps a vector of predictors to a real-valued response. Predictors are also referred to as inputs, features, or variables; response is referred to as an outcome, output, label, or task. The "logic" of *how* ML models generate their estimates, and how those estimates translate into recommendations in the context of explicit or implicit policies, is often difficult for human beings to understand.

The high complexity and dimensionality of the relationships that ML models derive from data are often not interpretable by human reasoning, which is why many ML models are often referred to as "black box" models. However, we have known for decades that explainability is an important attribute of any human reasoning process (see Chap. 5) and clinicians have historically named it as a top requirement for a clinical decision support system [1]. Because model generated recommendations in medicine can affect high stakes decisions, the discussion around the "explainability" of both the model's output and the policy that translates that output into actions is particularly relevant for the safe and effective use of this technology.

Current Trends in AI Explainability Research

Explainability of ML models has been deeply explored across academia, industry, and government as a potentially critical component of applying AI into health care in a way that is usable, transparent, and trustworthy [2]. Key themes from current work in explainability center on how it is defined, the methods by which it can be achieved for different ML models, how it is evaluated, and whether it is truly useful when applying AI in healthcare settings [3]. Based on the current consensus definition of explainability, a ML model is considered explainable if the explanation satisfies two criteria: (1) it is "interpretable," meaning that the logic the model incorporates to make predictions is understandable by humans, and (2) it has fidelity, meaning that the explanation faithfully reflects the underlying logic of the task model (the model making predictions) [4].

There are now a range of methods described in the literature to generate explanations that attempt to satisfy these criteria, albeit with varying degrees of success [5]. These methods can be broadly divided into two categories: (1) using aspects of the model's intrinsic architecture (e.g. beta coefficients from a linear regression) to derive explanations, which can only be done for certain model architectures, and (2) post hoc methods, where separate interpretable models are developed to accompany the original, potentially "black box", model in order to approximate explanations between model features and the outcome. The majority of such post hoc methods fall into the category of attribution-based explanations, which use a variety of quantitative methods to attempt to measure the relative importance of the task model features in determining the outcome. These methods are typically applicable to more complex and non-linear model architectures such as neural networks that may deliver higher predictive performance at the expense of the lack of intrinsic model interpretability. Nevertheless, while these computational strategies can be used to approximate the relative importance of model variables, they do not reflect the true inner workings of the task model logic, so they may not satisfy the fidelity clause of explainability. Further, statistical explanations, even for the more "easily explainable" linear task models, still require an additional layer of human interpretation that can vary and may not faithfully reflect the underlying model mechanism.

In light of these limitations, whether explainability is truly useful when applying AI to health care continues to be debated. Explainable models are thought to facilitate users' ability to understand and improve the model, discover new insights learned from the model, and even to be more empowered to manage social interactions with other humans when using the model [6]. Qualitative stakeholder studies have also indicated that clinicians seem to want to understand explainable variables when exposed to predictive models in order to assess whether they align with their clinical judgement [7]. The healthcare AI field has indeed been moving forward, with increasing interest demonstrated in government research and development, venture capital and industry, as well as in professional societies as these entities encourage the development of methods, financing, and regulations that encourage explainability in medical AI [8, 9]. However, there remains some skepticism that explainability can truly enhance the usefulness of AI in health care, as well as concern that it may even lead to harm. For example, explanations, especially if they do not sufficiently satisfy the clauses of interpretability and fidelity, may give users a false sense of security, especially since they typically require some level of statistical comprehension and nuance to understand them, even for linear models [10].

Applying Additional Context to Understand Explainability in Medical AI

How we think about the meaning and purpose of explainability and its incorporation deserves deeper examination because the answers to these questions may depend on the context in which the model is deployed. This chapter applies principles of **cognitive informatics** to delve into these questions. Consider the following hypothetical scenarios:

1. An AI software product is used to analyze chest CTs as part of an automated system for lung cancer screening. Patients with chest CTs that are flagged by the AI software as high risk are automatically referred for biopsy.
2. A physician and nurse for a hospitalized patient each receives an AI generated alert that a patient for whom they both are caring is at risk of developing respira-

tory failure in the near future and recommends mechanical ventilation. They proceed to meet and discuss next steps for the patient's clinical management.
3. A consumer smartwatch outfitted with AI capabilities, detects cardiac arrhythmias and notifies a user that an irregular heart rate has been detected recommending that the user consult a physician for further evaluation. After performing a full clinical assessment, the physician orders a continuous cardiac monitoring study for a formal diagnostic evaluation.

Although each scenario includes an AI solution, the nature of the task performed by the AI enabled tool and how it is incorporated into patient care differ. The first scenario describes an AI approach that drives the diagnosis of lung cancer and automatically triggers an intervention without any mediation by humans. The second AI scenario also drives the diagnostic and management process for a high risk medical condition, but the process is mediated by humans. In example three, the AI system supplies diagnostic insights, but is intended only to be supplementary information for a formal evaluation; however, at the population level the use of such a system does impact the total amount of work done by those that have to perform the formal evaluation.

The level of risk associated with the task and extent of human involvement in the delivery of care has broad implications for how to approach the purpose of AI explainability as well as the kinds of explanations provided. For example, in scenario one, where the system drives high stakes clinical care without any mediation by human clinicians, it may be important for patients, as well as the clinicians, to understand the tool's "reasoning" behind its conclusions, similar to how a patient would want a physician to explain the reasoning behind a cancer diagnosis. The health system employing this AI solution and regulatory bodies may also require in-depth understanding of how the ML model generates its predictions and the level of model performance for quality assurance. In scenario two, the AI system interacts with human clinicians who need to synthesize the prediction with the rest of their clinical evaluation in order to make a decision about the patient's management. While the clinicians need to trust the tool for its advice to be adopted, the mechanics of how the ML model generated the prediction may be less important to the clinicians than a conceptual understanding of why the program predicted this patient to be at risk that they can mentally incorporate into the rest of their clinical assessment. In scenario three, trust in the AI advisor is similarly important, but insight into the "how" and "why" of the AI prediction may be less relevant to the non-clinician layperson user since the AI prediction is only meant to be supplemental to a formal evaluation by a physician and does not directly drive care management.

These scenarios demonstrate that the thinking around the need for AI explainability must move beyond a binary "yes/no" paradigm to *it depends* and *for what purpose?* Explainability can be for several purposes: understanding how the relationships between variables generate the output of the ML model, a conceptual appreciation for why certain predictions are formed from the available data, or simply as a surrogate for trust in the model's performance. As illustrated by these scenarios, the purpose of explainability depends on the nature of the task, the recipient(s) of the predictions, and the broader environment in which the AI system is deployed.

Deciding the appropriate purposes of AI explainability requires an understanding of how AI interacts with human users and the implications these interactions have on downstream clinical outcomes. In order to capture the depth and breadth of how explainability affects medical AI, we must consider three levels of impact that explainability can have on how AI systems are shaped: information processing by the individual human user, the interactions between people and AI agents, and the **emergent properties** of the broader AI-enabled **sociotechnical system**.

For example, when assessing how to incorporate AI explainability into scenario two, we would first consider what the physician and nurse individually need to understand about the prediction in order to make sense of it in the context of their understanding of the patient (i.e. do they need to understand *how* the program generated the prediction of respiratory failure in order to make sense of the rest of the patient's clinical findings or do they primarily need to know that the predictions are rarely wrong). Second, we would query how explainability would affect the ability of the physician and nurse to interact with the AI agent to make shared decisions (i.e. given the social nature of human cognition, can the AI system function as an effective teammate?) Finally, these interactions with the AI system and the physician and nurse may have downstream ripple effects that may ultimately affect the clinical outcomes in unpredictable ways, such as impact on communication patterns, culture, and patient safety.

The goals of this chapter are (1) to describe the different purposes of AI explainability, (2) to present a framework for assessing the different needs for AI explainability by examining how an AI system interacts with human cognitive processes situated in sociotechnical systems, and (3) to discuss how this framework can be applied to real world examples of AI in medicine and implications for regulatory approaches.

Three Purposes of AI Explainability

Explainability is a tricky notion given the lack of consensus in the form of explainability desired and when. For AI systems in medicine, we consider three purposes of explainability: (1) to allow the study of a ML model and perform quality assurance and/or improvements, (2) to help the user(s) of the AI system to gain contextual understanding of the model's prediction in order to incorporate into their subsequent decisions and actions, and (3) to facilitate trust in AI systems (Chap. 18) [11]. To the ML engineer, explainability often refers to the ability to articulate which variables and their combinations, in what manner, led to the output produced by the model [12]. This approach to explainability requires an understanding of the computational relationships among the variables and architecture needed to generate the model outputs, which is often highly complex in ML. For example, an ML model that predicts respiratory failure may generate predictions from hundreds of thousands of features derived from clinical data that may not be clinically meaningful (e.g. the log of the mean blood pressure over 24 h cubed), and the computational relationships among these features are often high dimensional and difficult to represent in any clinically understandable way. Sometimes, features may be included in an ML model due to pure statistical associations but not indicate any potential causal relationship that would be helpful to a clinician seeking insight into what about a patient's clinical status may be increasing their risk of respiratory failure (e.g. hair color may be a feature in a model that predicts respiratory failure given a possible statistical association in the training set, but this would not offer a clinically meaningful explanation for why the patient may be a risk for respiratory failure). The *purpose* of this type of explainability is typically to allow engineers to perform quality assurance and to replicate or improve on the ML model, whereas a user of the AI system, such as a clinician or patient, may not find this type of explanation helpful (Fig. 8.1).

To the clinician or patient user of medical AI, explainability is more likely to be important for enriching their understanding of the prediction in the context of the clinical situation and providing information that would allow them to trust the performance of the AI system. For example, a team of physicians and nurses who are alerted by an AI system that their patient is at risk of going into respiratory failure and that the situation may warrant mechanical ventilation will typically want to understand which clinical variables contributed most to the model's prediction. Here, explainability allows the clinician users to make sense of the prediction in the context of the rest of their evaluation as well as potentially to use that information to tailor their subsequent decisions and actions to respond to the risk. The precise

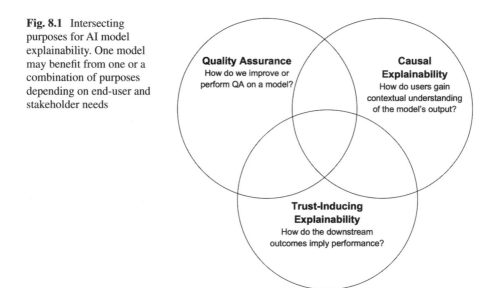

Fig. 8.1 Intersecting purposes for AI model explainability. One model may benefit from one or a combination of purposes depending on end-user and stakeholder needs

mathematical representation of the features is likely far less important to the clinical team than an understanding that the AI system detected the patient's deteriorating mental status and increasing respiratory rate over the past 12 h as factors contribut-ing to the risk of needing mechanical ventilation. Such summative insight, along with information about the model's accuracy and how it was trained and validated may be enough to trust the AI system even without an in-depth trace-back of the inner workings of the model. To a layperson user of the AI system, such as the owner of the AI-enabled smartwatch in scenario three that detected an arrhythmia, understanding the context of the prediction may even be less important than having information to trust the system, especially if the information generated is only sup-plemental to an evaluation by a physician.

Sometimes, the same information about explainability can be applied to all three purposes of model engineering, enriching user understanding, and facilitating trust. For example, the commonly used **Pooled Cohort Equations** for the prediction of 10 year risk of atherosclerotic cardiovascular disease (**ASCVD**) is a linear regression that relies on variables including age, sex, race, blood pressure, cholesterol, history of diabetes, smoking history, and use of antihypertensive, statin, or anti-platelet med-ications [13]. These variables all happen to also be components of a patient's medical history that a physician would review to assess ASCVD risk, so knowledge of these variables and weights would fulfill the purposes of understanding the inner mechan-ics of the model as well as deriving clinically meaningful explanations for the patient's clinical condition and facilitating trust in the model prediction.

Given two models of equal performance, one a black-box and one an explainable model, most users, when asked, prefer the explainable model [14]. However, in many practical scenarios, models that may not be as easily interpreted can lead to better end user outcomes and may even be desirable in certain situations [15]. For example, when users are asked to accept or reject the price of a New York City apartment based on an explainable model, which tells them the features used such as the number of bedrooms and bathrooms, the distance to subways or schools) or a black box model which does not, the participants receiving explanation were more likely to accept wrong predictions than those who were shown the black box output.

In parallel, it is worth considering whether rigorous validation and high accuracy and consistency of the ML model alone could be sufficient for building user trust [16]. For example, one does not need to have an explainable model for a rain fore-cast as long as it is correct enough, often enough, to rely on to carry an umbrella. Trust in the model's output can be established by rigorous testing and prospective assessment of how often the model's predictions are correct and calibrated, and for assessing the impact of the interventions on the outcome. At the same time, prospec-tive assessment can be costly.

A request for "explainability" in medical AI can be separated into a request for explaining model mechanics (perhaps better phrased as transparency of the model-ing), a need by the user to understand the clinical context of the AI predictions, or a need to establish user trust. We will explore how principles of cognitive informatics can be applied to untangle the kind of explainability needed in a particular application.

Expanding the Conception of AI Explainability Based on Cognitive Informatics

As discussed in the section on "Three Purposes of AI Explainability", the current science has already established that explainability is not a single easily-defined construct that can be conceived as present or absent, and is substantially dependent on what "explainability" is meant to help the person receiving the "explanation" accomplish. In addition to the concepts of causality, surrogacy for trust and functional understanding of AI construction for an engineer, knowledge from cognitive informatics and related disciplines also suggest numerous nuances to "explainability" that need to be further explored. Specifically, theories of human information processing, conceptions of humans interacting with AI agents, and complex sociotechnical systems theory all suggest that there is yet much to be learned about how explainability is applicable to healthcare settings.

Human Information Processing

Consider the physician in the second example presented at the beginning of the chapter: while the physician having a difficult conversation with a patient about a poor prognosis, the physician is interrupted by an alert that suggests that a different patient in a different building is at risk of developing respiratory failure and may need escalation of care and mechanical ventilation. How will the physician respond? Will the physician leave the conversation? Seek more information? Dismiss the alert?

Models of human information processing have been part of the cognitive psychology and human factors literature for decades (see also Chaps. 1 and 5). Early models were developed in the 1950s and 1960s [17]. At their most basic, these human information processor models note that there's a layer of information processing between human perception of inputs/stimuli (involving encoding perceived stimuli in the context of mental models, comparing various options and choosing a response) and outputs/execution of action. Importantly, cognitive processing is both "top-down" and "bottom-up"—what we perceive and process is filtered by what our attention is directed towards. A commonly used model of human information processing in healthcare settings is the model in **situation awareness theory** (Fig. 8.2). Among other applications, situation awareness theory has been used in the improvement of the recognition of clinical deterioration in hospitalized patients as well as the diagnostic reasoning process [18]. The human information processing model underlying situation awareness theory resembles other goal-directed linear models of human information processing such as **Norman's theory of action** and **Rasmussen's decision ladder** [19–21]. This model suggests that when humans perceive information, they then comprehend the information (see discussion of mental models below), project the expected future states based on this information as well

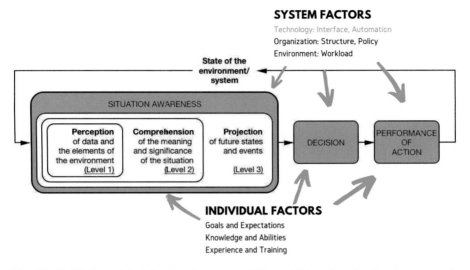

Fig. 8.2 Endsley's model of situational awareness. This model describes situational awareness in dynamic decision making and notes how technology such as AI can affect each step in human information processing [22]

as various choices that the person might make, then make a choice based on the desired future state, finally acting on the decision.

In our scenario, the physician may perceive the alert and see if there's any other information that can quickly allow for comprehension and verification of the current situation. If no supplemental information allows for verification of the alert, the only information that the physician will use to project the future state of the patient is what remains in the physician's memory. Any new information obtained by sensors or documented in the electronic health record that may be relevant and explain why the alert triggered will not be used by the physician. Because such information is never perceived, the physician may simply project that the patient's risk of respiratory failure has not changed and that the alert is simply incorrect, resuming their focus on the challenging conversation.

Comprehension of the alert and the situation does not happen in a vacuum. Human experts rely on mental models stored in long-term memory to translate perceived information into comprehension that can support reasoned projection of future states and subsequent decision-making. A mental model is a person's explanation of "how things work in the world" and allows one to predict what will happen if one takes a particular action (see also Chaps. 1 and 5). Experts are able to do this very efficiently by framing new information in the context of existing mental models built from experience (such as knowledge about disease processes, how previous patients with similar appearance have progressed in their illness, etc.).

So consider again how AI predictions alone, unaccompanied by additional explanatory information that matches the mental models of the user, may fail to produce action. For example, suppose that the alert in our example was received by a relatively inexperienced physician, and this physician knew that the alert was appearing for a patient admitted with a neurological concern. In this inexperienced physician, the mental model of neurologic abnormalities may not yet have linked "impending respiratory failure" to the possibility that such failure is a consequence of a neurologic problem interfering with the central respiratory control system. Because the physician experiences an apparent mismatch between the mental model of the patient (this patient will experience a deterioration with primarily neurologic changes such as altered mental status) and the alert (warning of impending respiratory failure), the alert may again be ignored in the absence of another explanation that helps the physician to establish quickly that the alert is not a false alarm.

Of course, human comprehension is not always a linear process. Other models of human comprehension, such as **Klein's data-frame theory** of sense-making and theories of information foraging in the human-computer interaction literature, explain that information processing is often an iterative process [23]. People tend to gather just enough information to "satisfice" and allow them to apply a mental model that helps them to understand the current situation [24]. If all relevant information had been gathered, a different mental model might have been applied, as a key piece of information may have reframed the situation. This also suggests an aspect of sufficiency for optimal stopping to the concept of explanation (see also Chap. 5). In the example discussed, if the most salient information presented with the risk prediction alert biases the physician towards framing the risk as a primary respiratory failure that is viewed as unlikely in the patient, the physician may be satisfied and dismiss the alert. On the other hand, if the explanatory information supplementing the AI risk prediction helps physicians frame the patient as potentially experiencing a neurologic disruption of the respiratory control system, they may be far more likely to seek more information and act.

Through all of these concepts of human information processing, explainability can be considered in the context of the "gulf of evaluation": the degree to which a person can use information to make sense of a situation and determine how well their goals have been met. To the extent that a user can perceive information or knowledge in an AI system and quickly make sense of the real world based on the explanation provided, they are more likely to make the optimal decision. If the explanatory information that allows the person to make sense of the situation is missing or requires substantial effort to glean, such as needing to click through multiple screen transitions, the person is much more likely to fail to appropriately use AI.

Human-AI Agents

In the previous section, we primarily conceived of explanation in AI systems as relevant at one point in time: when a person receives information from the AI system and may make a decision to act. However, AI systems can be complex enough, especially if there is a component of automation, that it can be conceived of as an independent agent. The "agency" of the AI system comes from implicit goals in any automated steps the technology might take (e.g. the automated referral for biopsy in the first example from the beginning of the chapter) as well as the "conversation" that occurs over a series of interactions between people and the technology that they are using. In this context, explanations may be considered in terms of their ability to make the AI agent's intentions and actions understood in order to produce predictable interactions that allow work towards a common goal [25].

The conception of humans and AI systems as agents that interact has been present from some of the foundational work in clinical informatics [26]. In the MYCIN and EMYCIN systems, the role of the AI agent was as a "consultant" for the clinical user (see Chap. 2). In Clancey's GUIDON project, the system was a tutor for students. In this work, an early discovery was the need for users to understand "why" the systems were acting as they did. The systems attempted to make explicit as explanation the internal goal and strategy of the AI system. Often these goals and strategies are implicit, which can be challenging for a human who seeks to interact with the system. In the absence of explicit explanation, people must infer goals and strategies for the agent with which they interact, which is even more challenging in the case of adaptive AI systems that change their behavior over time.

Conceiving of the interaction between humans and an AI agent as a "dialogue" was also established in the projects that were derived from MYCIN (see also Chap. 9). A conversation implies a conception of explanation tied to intelligibility. A phenomenon studied in aviation is that of "automation surprises", where the AI system acts in a way that is not expected and is thus not comprehensible to the person without an explanation. In this case, humans may assume that automation has failed, leading the person to take inappropriate actions. Another issue may arise when the set of actions that are offered do not match what the user is expecting, limiting the "conversational" nature of the interaction. For example, if the physician interacting with an AI-enabled sepsis alert is expecting to gather more information through lab testing to assess patient risk for sepsis but the system forces a decision about antibiotics before the physician can obtain that information, then the physician may wonder "why" the AI system is "recommending" antibiotics, even though the AI system is merely providing an incomplete set of potential choices.

As with human information processing, it is beyond the scope of this chapter to review all of the ways that explanations may function in a back-and-forth series of interactions between human and AI agents. Appreciation of humans as agents interacting with potential AI agents, however, suggests there is much still to be learned about the role of explanation in such interactions. Explanation is critically important so that a person can predictably interact with an AI system to achieve one's goals.

Sociotechnical Systems

When considering the impact of AI systems on health care, we need to examine the broader care delivery system in which the AI technologies are being incorporated. Healthcare is complex - meaning that the delivery of health care, whether it is diagnosing and identifying disease, providing therapies, or implementing interventions to prevent disease, occurs in complex sociotechnical systems. Complexity exists because (1) there are numerous relationships/interactions among the many entities that are involved, and (2) health care is a human-driven process (since care is provided by and for humans, and human behavior is adaptive to changes in the environment). While the previous section introduced the idea of interaction between the human and the AI system, outcomes in health care are mediated by numerous nonlinear interactions between people, processes, and technologies. With nonlinear systems, changes in the input do not always lead to proportional changes in output. Outcomes from complex systems cannot be predicted by examining the properties of just one component of the system. The system must be examined as a whole, and we need to assess how changes to any particular component impact the rest of the system in order to understand how it could affect the outcome. These outcomes are known as emergent properties as they emerge only when the system exists as a whole but not within or between any individual components.

Health care has made important progress in recognizing that processes and outcomes that we see are not products of individual actions but instead emerge from a complex set of interactions between people, the tools they use, and the processes/organization of their work environment. Patient safety is a great example of what is now often conceptualized as an emergent property of the care delivery system. The Systems Engineering Initiative for Patient Safety (**SEIPS**) model is now well established in health care and has been applied to numerous healthcare projects to design tools and technology in healthcare delivery (Fig. 8.2) [27]. Patient safety, defined as the prevention of unintended harm to the patient, cannot be attributed to any one part of the work system alone but emerges from how each part of the care delivery system interacts with the others (Fig. 8.3).

When introducing AI systems to improve health care, we need to think about how the system changes the existing sociotechnical work environment to mediate the outcome. In other words, how does the AI system interact with the other people, processes, and technologies (including other AI systems)? A common assumption in health care is that digital tools improve the reliability of care because humans are error-prone. In reality, any introduction of technology adds new components and thus new "failure" points for safety. In order to function effectively, the person in the sociotechnical environment needs the AI system not just to explain its goals and intentions, but also to convey how it is interacting with the other elements of the sociotechnical environment.

Trust is a concept that is discussed often in the context of explainable AI—understandably, as it may be essential to sustained use of any given AI system. While trust is traditionally viewed as a property of the human-AI interaction, it may also be useful to conceive of trust as another emergent property like patient safety. Over time, when people observe interactions and the outcomes of interactions with AI systems in their work, people will develop a set of expectations on how to best interact with AI systems. This will come not just from their own experience but also through observing other people, socialization of the technology in the popular press and the culture of their work organization. If these expectations are violated without

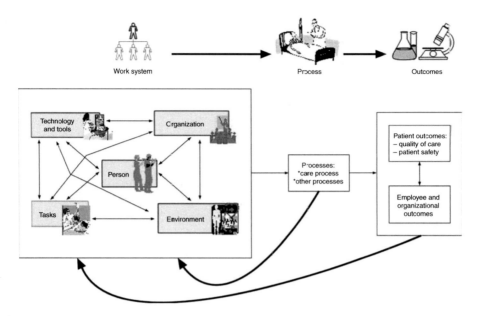

Fig. 8.3 The systems engineering initiative for patient safety (SEIPS) model. An example of a framework for understanding the structures, processes and outcomes in health care and their interactions, which result in the 'emergent' outcomes such as patient safety [27]

explanation, trust in a given AI system can be lost. Furthermore, knowing that attention to information processing has a "top-down" component (i.e. humans pay selective attention to information they are already expecting), subtle unexpected changes in the system may never be perceived by the user. For example, consider the example of the AI system that automatically screens chest CTs for lung cancer and refers patients for biopsies. If the threshold for referral is updated with only a subtle notation and without explanation to the patient or physician, the change in system's behavior may be noticed only when there are dramatic outcomes, such as a large increase in the number of referrals or a missed referral in a patient with lung cancer. At that point, physicians and patients may lose trust in the system.

This is why trust is best assessed not as "present" or "absent" but in terms of whether trust is appropriately calibrated. Under-trust is traditionally the focus of healthcare AI literature, given the limited adoption of AI systems to date. Much effort is spent on increasing trust in AI systems because of the adoption problem. However, over-trust is just as important. Over-trust occurs when the clinician comes to depend on the AI system, either because of the clinician's lack of expertise or because other pressures from the sociotechnical system such as the workload potentially drive inappropriate reliance on technology. A goal of explanation for AI systems is to optimize the calibration of trust. The goal is neither under-trust when the AI system is enabling the correct action but also not over-trust when the AI system is operating outside of its optimal scope or the user should not trust the AI system without further patient assessment.

This understanding of sociotechnical systems suggests that AI explanations may not translate across clinical contexts in which the AI system might be used. Rather, local customization of the explanation and user interface may be necessary to situate the AI system in the sociotechnical environment. Design principles that incorporate contextual constraints such as ecological interface design may be useful on this front. To the extent that the interface can mirror the external world, and the AI system's actions are placed within the context of that external world, people can be more successful in their essential roles for patient safety: anticipating errors and acting as a source of resilience.

Ultimately, the lenses of human information processing, human-AI agents, and sociotechnical systems suggest that there may be no single "universally" suitable design for optimal AI explanations and approaches to AI explanation will continue to evolve.

Implications of Explainability on Bias and the Regulatory Environment

It is important to understand the effect of explainability on accountability and the regulation of AI. As mentioned, complex AI systems often include elaborate data transformation using hundreds of thousands of features derived from clinical data that may or may not be meaningful. As these complex systems increasingly drive clinical decisions, it is important to acknowledge the legitimate concerns about the intentional and unintentional consequences of these AI systems. Explainability presents an opportunity to understand better the changing landscape of accountability and regulation.

Explainability and Inherent Biases

An emerging body of evidence suggests that AI systems can make unfair and discriminatory decisions, replicate or develop biases, and behave in inscrutable and unexpected ways in highly sensitive environments that put human interests and safety at risk. Therefore, it is important to consider how explainability may mitigate such biases and affect our own inherent biases using the three purposes of explainability mentioned in section "Three Purposes of AI Explainability".

For the ML engineer, explainability offers an opportunity to identify and mitigate potential biases in AI systems. However, this is only possible through the transparent reporting of the AI details, such as recommended by the Minimal Information for Medical AI Reporting, or the **MINIMAR standards** [28]. Such standards demand information related to the data source and cohort selection, demographics of the training population, model features and design characteristics, as well as evaluation criteria and validation steps. Data biases (see Chap. 3) are common across most data sources, therefore the transparent reporting of the MINIMAR concepts ensures that the interpretability of the model and can help end users (e.g., providers, healthcare systems, etc.) to identify the populations for which the AI can be applied—a step at mitigating inherent data biases. Furthermore, having a clear definition of the model output is imperative. Datasets with inconsistent, imperfect, or even incorrect labels used for training and testing data allow one's own biases to enter into the model and affect explainability. Understanding the intent of the model (e.g. predict mortality or predict transfer to ICU), composition of the training data, development of the ground truth, model architecture, and data transformation enables the ML engineer to assess biases in the data and algorithmic fairness empirically. While the model architecture may not be critical for explainability, understanding sample representativeness in AI models may help clinicians decide if the prediction is applicable to their patient population. For example, many models predicting adverse events in Type II diabetic (T2DM) patients have not reported Hispanics in their training data. Given Hispanics higher prevalence and complication rates for T2DM compared to Whites, it is essential clinicians have this type of explainability to determine if they incorporate the AI prediction into their clinical decision making. This type of explainability is the foundation of developing trust for both the clinician as well as the patient population, as it is only through transparency and explainability that one can mitigate biases in AI that contribute to unfair and discriminatory decisions that put human interests and safety at risk.

Effect of Explainability on Accountability for Decision Making

Accountability, in this context, means the ability to determine whether a decision was made in accordance with procedural and substantive standards and to hold someone responsible if those standards are not met. Therefore, it is important that developers understand and integrate current standards within the model's design and during development. Explainable models must be developed through team efforts involving knowledge experts, decision makers, and end-users. The incorporation of procedural and substantive standards must be clearly presented to end-users across platforms.

Human-interpretable information about the factors used in a decision and their relative weight is necessary. This is likely the most common understanding of what constitutes an explanation for a decision. A list of the factors that went into a decision, ideally ordered by the significance to the output, can provide accountability by confirming that proper procedures were followed.

While there is significant support for explanations as a tool for holding AI accountable, there are also concerns about the costs of generating such explanations. True explainability could inhibit innovation by forcing transparency around key model features which may be seen as industry trade secrets. However, the lack of incentives, restrictions around data sharing and data privacy, and the acceptance of stealth science in industry has created an environment that allows AI to be implemented without understanding how the model was developed, from what data was the model learned, and using what data was the model deemed satisfactory for use. Accountability can only fairly proceed if transparency is provided regarding the data, model, and standards woven into the AI model.

The Current Regulatory Framework and Explainability

Across the global AI regulatory environment, explainability is the center of accountability (see Chap. 18). In 2017, the International Medical Device Regulators Forum (**IMDRF**) came together to develop a path for standardized AI regulations, including a risk-based framework [29]. The hypothetical scenarios described in the introduction provide examples of the different levels of risk to consider and the importance of explainability in each scenario. The level of regulation and necessary documentation are determined by the risk-based framework, as described above. In addition to the risk-framework, the European Union has put forth the General Data Protection Regulation (**GDPR**) mechanism which ensures users (or patients) have a right to information about the existence, logic, and potential consequences of AI-driven decision-making systems. The GDPR establishes rules and regulations for privacy and permissions and gives control to individuals. Patients must not only consent to the collection of the data but also to each use of their data. For AI developers, this requires that they explain *in plain language* how data will be used as part of the consent process. Many interpret this as the "right to explanation". Systems are now aiming to produce more explainable models; design an explanation interface; and understand the human requirements for useful explanations [30]. However, there are also concerns about the costs of generating explainable AI in regard to engineering challenges, the effect on innovation and trade secrets; and the cost of system accuracy or other performance objectives.

Application of Explainability to Real World Examples of Medical AI

The following real world examples of medical AI can be used to understand the differences among the purposes of explainability, targets and downstream actions among the three methods of explainability, as well as how the cognitive informatics concepts we have described apply to particular use cases of medical AI.

Example: Continuous Blood Glucose Monitoring for Patients with Type 1 Diabetes

Current Type 1 Diabetes management approaches are largely limited to non-closed loop systems that depend on the patient checking blood glucose levels and administering themselves insulin either through a pump or a syringe. The iLet bionic pancreas from Beta Bionics [31] aims to simplify the latter, interfacing with an embedded glucose monitor and continuously dosing insulin similar to a native pancreas. It needs to be able to adapt to blood glucose variation patterns and function autonomously. The end users of this device are endocrinologists and their patients who will likely not benefit from a mechanistic or 'engineer's' explainability but rather on 'trust inducing explainability'—relying on outcome data that shows a closed loop feedback system for glucose control has minimal hypoglycemic events and maintains glucose levels within an acceptable range that is conducive for improved long term outcomes. From a cognitive informatics perspective, human information processing needs with this system are likely very different from how patients are counseled about diabetes management now, learning to "count carbohydrates" and estimate how much insulin to self-administer. However, explanation for this highly autonomous agent may need to convey information like how the insulin administered is based on the blood sugar goal or how well the overall blood sugar control has been, allowing a patient to not only monitor the system but also troubleshoot and recover from malfunctions without experiencing life-threatening hypoglycemic or hyperglycemic events. From a regulatory perspective, given this automated closed-loop system, and lack of a physician intermediary while care is being delivered, the regulatory concerns are high although this device would be categorized as a medical device rather than **SaMD** (software as a medical device) per the previously mentioned framework put forth by IMDRF.

Example: Digital Image Analysis Tools Assisting in Histopathological Diagnoses

Proscia's digital pathology tools are designed to drive clinical management by analyzing pathology samples and prioritizing certain cases for review by pathologists, especially cases that are flagged by the system to demonstrate high risk features. For example—biopsy samples of precancerous lesions that have high risk features are prioritized for expedited review to allow for earlier management of a potential cancer diagnosis. Such a system, which is tasked in prioritizing certain cases for review for the end user (in this case a Pathologist), will need to demonstrate the reasons for prioritization. In this case, the Pathologist is tasked with making the final diagnosis. Clinical data may help with contextual explainability but these tools may benefit most from having surrogates for the underlying mechanistic 'engineering' processes. In the case of AI/computer vision systems, segmentation and bounding box techniques can assist in establishing this surrogate, but may need significant more time invested into labeling training data. Image classification techniques that do not have segmentation, object detection, or bounding boxes built in will need to depend on context to engender trust in the end user. These tools have to rely on proper functioning within a human-AI team; the level at which this tool can operate autonomously should be carefully conveyed to the healthcare team to optimize calibration in such a tool. This will avoid under-trust leading to under-utilization and over-trust leading to an inappropriate amount of dependency. From a regulatory perspective, digital pathology tools fall under Category II of the IMDRF framework as they drive clinical management of serious conditions and would likely benefit from independent review.

Example: Wearable Devices Informing Clinical Management

Finally, we offer an emerging use-case scenario where wearable data is informing clinical management. Wearables are starting to incorporate not only heart rate information to show variability, and correlate the rate to motion sensors to determine types of activity and levels of sleep, but also to oxygen sensors and basic one lead rhythm monitors such as the **ECG** App on the Apple Watch. This particular app is designed to detect atrial fibrillation, low and high heart rates, and to provide a summary of heart rate variability. Algorithms that assist in aggregation of clinical data will likely need to depend on causal explainability—information that becomes important with context. In the case of an ECG app assisting in detection of atrial fibrillation, the output is to be taken in conjunction with patient data—possibly complaints of palpitations or indications of a history of cardiac disease that would predispose to a diagnosis of atrial fibrillation. Human information processing models are important for information that is best analyzed in context (in this case, patient symptoms and history). Along with contextual explanatory information presented with the model output, the end users' experiences within their sociotechnical environment will also drive each user's trust in the prediction and subsequent decision-making. Regulatory concerns with wearables that inform clinical management are largely dependent on the manufacturer and on the element for which it chooses to obtain clearance. The ECG app has **FDA** clearance as a Class II device but the pulse oximeter function is described for 'general wellness' and thus does not have FDA clearance as a medical device.

Conclusion

The question of whether explainability is useful for medical AI must be expanded to include considerations around (1) the type and purpose of the explanation and (2) the type of human-machine interaction in which explainability may play a role in mediating the desired outcome. Finally, the degree of explainability may impact how bias and accountability are incorporated into the medical AI product and how it may be regulated.

Questions for Discussion

- How can the different methods and purposes of explainability be applied to different AI use cases?
- How do principles of human information processing and information flow across teams affect how AI explainability should be approached?
- What frameworks are important to consider for an AI agent, with a similar underlying model, that is deployed across different environments?
- What potential pitfalls might there be with the current regulatory framework with regards to AI explainability?
- Who are the common stakeholders and what motivations do they have with regards to accountability in AI systems?
- What are some of the potential underlying causes of unintended intrinsic biases within AI systems?

Further Reading

General Data Protection Regulation (GDPR), https://gdpr-info.eu/.

- Official EU documentation of General Data Protection Regulation, including recitals and key issues. This regulation for consumer privacy is a reference for other countries and regions as they craft their own versions. E.g. California Consumer Privacy Act has many similarities with GDPR.

Gilpin, L.H., Bau. D., Yuan, B.Z., et al. Explaining Explanations: An Overview of Interpretability of Machine Learning. In: 2018 IEEE 5th International Conference on Data Science and Advanced Analytics (DSAA). pp. 80–89. Available at https://arxiv.org/pdf/1806.00069.

- An exploration into best practices of explainability, the insufficiency of current approaches and future directions for explainable artificial intelligence. Being aware of the work being done in the non-clinical realm will help inform efforts with regards to explainable medical AI.

Markus, A.F. The role of explainability in creating trustworthy artificial intelligence for health care: A comprehensive survey of the terminology, design choices, and evaluation strategies. Journal of Biomedical Informatics. 2021;113:103655. https://doi.org/10.1016/j.jbi.2020.103655.

- In this paper is an exploration of quantitative metrics regarding explainable AI. Although the field is far from a consensus, having quantitative metrics will allow for model comparison with regards to explainability similar to how model performance is compared today.

Carayon, P., Hundt, A.S., Karsh, B.T., et al. Work system design for PATIENT safety: The SEIPS model. Qual Saf Health Care. 2006 Dec;15 Suppl 1(Suppl 1):i50–8. http://dx.doi.org/10.1136/qshc.2005.015842.

- This paper provides an overview for the Systems Engineering Initiative for Patient Safety framework, which is applied to describe complex work systems in healthcare and provides a tool to examine the context for the downstream impact of explainable AI in healthcare workflows.

Brady, P.W., Wheeler, DS, Muething, S.E., Kotagal, U.R. Situation awareness: A new model for predicting and preventing patient deterioration. Hosp Pediatr. 2014;4(3):143–6. https://doi.org/10.1542/hpeds.2013-0119.

- This paper describes an example of how AI is applied to a use case in pediatrics, and how explainability facilitates a team dynamic that was important in mediating the outcome.

References

1. Teach L, Shortliffe H. An analysis of physician attitudes regarding computer-based clinical consultation systems. Comput Biomed Res. 1981;14(6):542–58. https://doi.org/10.1016/0010-4809(81)90012-4.
2. Cutillo CM, Sharma KR, Foschini L, Kundu S, Mackintosh M, Mandl KD, et al. Machine intelligence in healthcare—perspectives on trustworthiness, explainability, usability, and transparency. NPJ Digit Med. 2020;3(1):47. https://doi.org/10.1038/s41746-020-0254-2.
3. Abdul A, Vermeulen J, Wang D, Lim BY, Kankanhalli M. Trends and trajectories for explainable, accountable and intelligible systems: an HCI research agenda. In: Proceedings of the 2018 CHI conference on human factors in computing systems. Montreal: ACM; 2018. p. 1–18. https://doi.org/10.1145/3173574.3174156.
4. Gilpin LH, Bau D, Yuan BZ, Bajwa A, Specter M, Kagal L. Explaining explanations: an overview of interpretability of machine learning. In: 2018 IEEE 5th international conference on data science and advanced analytics (DSAA). Turin: IEEE; 2018. p. 80–9.
5. Markus AF, Kors JA, Rijnbeek PR. The role of explainability in creating trustworthy artificial intelligence for health care: a comprehensive survey of the terminology, design choices, and evaluation strategies. J Biomed Inform. 2021;113:103655. https://doi.org/10.1016/j.jbi.2020.103655.
6. Montavon G, Vedaldi A, Hansen LK, Muller K-R. Explainable AI: interpreting, explaining and visualizing deep learning. New York: Springer; 2019. p. 439.
7. Tonekaboni S, Joshi S, McCradden MD, Goldenberg A. What clinicians want: contextualizing explainable machine learning for clinical end use. In: Doshi-Velez F, Fackler J, Jung K, Kale D, Ranganath R, Wallace B, et al., editors. Proceedings of the 4th machine learning for healthcare conference. Ann Arbor: PMLR; 2019. p. 359–80.
8. Turek M. Explainable artificial intelligence. Defense Advanced Research Projects Agency. 2021. https://www.darpa.mil/program/explainable-artificial-intelligence.
9. Top Explainable AI Companies. Venture Radar. Available from: https://www.ventureradar.com/keyword/Explainable%20AI.

10. Babic B, Gerke S, Evgeniou T, Cohen IG. Beware explanations from AI in health care. Science. 2021;373(6552):284–6. https://doi.org/10.1126/science.abg1834.
11. Miller K. Should AI Models be explainable? That depends. HAI. 2021. Available from: https://hai.stanford.edu/news/should-ai-models-be-explainable-depends.
12. Slack D, Friedler S, Scheidegger C, Roy CD. Assessing the local interpretability of machine learning models. Workshop on human-centric machine learning at the 33rd conference on neural information processing systems. 2019.
13. Muntner P, Colantonio LD, Cushman M, Goff DC, Howard G, Howard VJ, et al. Validation of the atherosclerotic cardiovascular disease pooled cohort risk equations. JAMA. 2014;311(14):1406. https://doi.org/10.1001/jama.2014.2630.
14. Lipton ZC. The mythos of model interpretability. Queue. 2018;16(3):31–57.
15. Holm EA. In defense of the black box. Science. 2019;364(6435):26–7.
16. Poursabzi-Sangdeh F, Goldstein DG, Hofman JM, Wortman Vaughan JW, Wallach H. Manipulating and measuring model interpretability. In: Proceedings of the 2021 CHI conference on human factors in computing systems. Yokohama: ACM; 2021. p. 1–52.
17. Hilgard ER, Bower GH. Theories of learning by Ernest R. Hilgard and Gordon H. Bower. Appleton-Century-Crofts; 1966.
18. Brady PW, Wheeler DS, Muething SE, Kotagal UR. Situation awareness: a new model for predicting and preventing patient deterioration. Hosp Pediatr. 2014;4(3):143–6. https://doi.org/10.1542/hpeds.2013-0119.
19. Singh H, Giardina TD, Petersen LA, Smith MW, Paul LW, Dismukes K, et al. Exploring situational awareness in diagnostic errors in primary care. BMJ Qual Saf. 2012;21(1):30–8. https://doi.org/10.1136/bmjqs-2011-000310.
20. Norman DA. The psychology of everyday things. New York: Basic Books; 1988.
21. Rasmussen J. Information processing and human machine interaction: an approach to cognitive engineering. New York: North-Holland; 1986.
22. Endsley MR. Toward a theory of situation awareness in dynamic systems. Human Factors. 37(1):32–64.
23. Klein G, Phillips JK, Rall EL, Peluso D. A data-frame theory of sensemaking. Expertise out of context: Proceedings of the sixth international conference on naturalistic decision making; 2007, pp. 113–55.
24. Simon HA. Rational choice and the structure of the environment. Psychol Rev. 1956;63(2):129–38.
25. Lewis M. Designing for human-agent interaction. AIMag. 1998;19(2):67.
26. Clancey WJ. From guidon to neomycin and Heracles in twenty short lessons. AIMag. 1986;7(3):40.
27. Carayon P, Schoofs Hundt A, Karsh B-T, Gurses AP, Alvarado CJ, Smith M, et al. Work system design for patient safety: the SEIPS model. Qual Saf Health Care. 2006;15(1):50. https://doi.org/10.1136/qshc.2005.015842.
28. Hernandez-Boussard T, Bozkurt S, Ioannidis JPA, Shah NH. MINIMAR (MINimum Information for Medical AI Reporting): developing reporting standards for artificial intelligence in health care. J Am Med Inform Assoc. 2020;27(12):2011–5. https://doi.org/10.1093/jamia/ocaa088.
29. Sun J, et al. IMDRF essential principles of safety and performance of medical devices and IVD medical devices introduction and consideration. Zhongguo Yi Liao Qi Xie Za Zhi. 2021;45(1):62–6.
30. Gunning D. Broad agency announcement explainable artificial intelligence (XAI). Technical report. 2016.
31. Jafri RZ, Balliro CA, Sherwood J, Hillard M, Ekhlaspour L, Hsu L, Russell SJ. 77-OR: first human study testing the iLet, a purpose-built bionic pancreas platform. Diabetes. 2019;68(1):77. https://doi.org/10.1016/S2213-8587(15)00489-1.

Chapter 9
Intelligent Agents and Dialog Systems

Timothy Bickmore and Byron Wallace

After reading this chapter, you should know the answers to these questions:
- What is a dialog system and how can it be used in patient- and consumer-facing systems in medicine?
- What are the main approaches to the implementation of dialog systems? What are the limitations of these approaches?
- How are dialog systems evaluated?
- What are some of the safety issues in fielding patient- and consumer-facing dialog systems in medicine?

Introduction to Dialog Systems

People most commonly communicate with each other not in isolated utterances, but in interleaved sequences of utterances wrapped in ritualized behavior that we colloquially refer to as conversations. Developing natural language interfaces that can move beyond single transactions of user query/system response to fully engage users in conversation would benefit a variety of applications. At a minimum, once the information that needs to be exchanged extends beyond that which can be expressed in a single utterance, dialog becomes imperative. Beyond this, dialog is essential for performing tasks that require multiple natural language exchanges with a user in a coherent manner, as for example in a series of questions and responses to automate an interactive, incremental differential diagnosis. Certainly, the emulation

T. Bickmore (✉) · B. Wallace
Khoury College of Computer Sciences, Northeastern University, Boston, MA, USA
e-mail: t.bickmore@northeastern.edu; b.wallace@northeastern.edu

© The Author(s), under exclusive license to Springer Nature
Switzerland AG 2022
T. A. Cohen et al. (eds.), *Intelligent Systems in Medicine and Health*, Cognitive Informatics in Biomedicine and Healthcare,
https://doi.org/10.1007/978-3-031-09108-7_9

of any kind of counseling session or interview to produce automated patient-facing health education systems requires complex goal-oriented dialog management that spans many interleaved patient and system messages In addition, interleaved sequences of messages allow a listener to confirm understanding or request clarification of information provided (a process referred to as "grounding"). Only in dialog can a conversational task (e.g., diagnosis or health counseling) be dynamically decomposed into sub-tasks in a coherent manner.

To ground our discussion, Fig. 9.1 shows an excerpt of a dialog between a study nurse and a patient about informed consent for an oncology clinical trial. There are several interesting things to note for those who have not studied natural conversations before. First, spontaneous conversation is full of *disfluencies*: there are very few grammatically complete and correct sentences in spontaneous conversation, and the use of "filler words" such as "um" (as in line #11) is very common. Second, conversational turns can span a single word to many sentences in duration. Third, a great deal of conversation is spent establishing mutual understanding of what was said: the patient feedback at lines #2 and #10, and the patient query at line #14 all serve exclusively to ensure that both parties understand each other, at least well enough for the purpose at hand. Only one person can talk at a time in conversation, and people are generally very good at coordinating their use of the speech channel, but overlaps, pauses (as in line #11) and interruptions (such as in line #15) are common. Finally, conversation typically makes extensive use of "deixis", which is a reference to the immediate physical context or to what was said before (for example, line #1 refers to the current day, line #9 refers to the consent form that is being handed to the patient). Designing automated dialog systems that can participate in these kinds of conversations, for example taking the role of the study nurse here to

1. Nurse: So, today I am going to talk to you about a research study that your doctor has stated that might be a good option for you.
2. Patient: OK.
3. Nurse: Have you had any experience with research before?
4. Patient: I have done a couple of research before. Nothing like this, just questionnaires on how I was treated as a patient. You know, small little things like 25 dollars.
5. Nurse: All right, but no treatment. You never took any drugs or anything like that?
6. Patient: No.
7. Nurse: Have you ever been treated for cancers in the past?
8. Patient: This is the first time.
9. Nurse: First time. OK, what I am going to do is give you is this packet. And this is something that we give to all of our patients. This is the consent form.
10. Patient: OK.
11. Nurse: Ummmm. So......(Pause)... This drug that Doctor Smith said that you may be eligible for is a drug that is kind of daughter or son of Thalidomide. Have you ever heard of Thalidomide?
12. Patients: No, never heard of it.
13. Nurse: Thalidomide was used back in the 50's and 60's for nausea in European women and...
14. Patient: (interrupting) Feeling sick?
15. Nurse: Yeah, feeling sick. And, they took this drug that does wonders for the nausea but unfortunately because they were pregnant during that it caused side-effects. ...

Fig. 9.1 Excerpt of nurse-patient dialog for administration of oncology clinical trial informed consent

automate administration of informed consent, represents an aspirational goal for dialog systems researchers. However, the state of the art is quite far from achieving this level of performance.

Chapter 7 introduced natural language processing (NLP). In this chapter we review the state of the art in dialog systems, a sub-field of NLP, including text-based chatbots, speech-based conversational assistants, and multimodal embodied conversational agents that simulate face-to-face conversation, for both provider- and patient-facing biomedical applications.

Definitions and Scope

Dialog has been defined as a conversational exchange between two or more entities. For the purposes of this chapter, we will be concerned with communicative exchanges between a human (health professional, patient, or consumer) and an automated system in which messages are in textual or spoken natural language. This system may also be augmented with additional information such as the non-verbal behavior used by humans in face-to-face conversation (hand gestures, facial displays, eye gaze, etc.). We refer to an isolated message from one entity within a dialog as an **utterance**. While a dialog can consist of a single utterance, we are primarily concerned with dialogue in which several utterances from two entities are interleaved in order to accomplish some task. *Discourse* is a generalization of dialog that also includes the study of written text comprising multiple sentences.

Discourse theory is generally concerned with how multiple utterances fit together to specify meaning. Theories of discourse generally assume that discourses are composed of **discourse segments** (consisting of one or more adjacent utterances), organized according to a set of rules. Beyond this, however, discourse theories vary widely in how they define discourse segments and the nature of the inter-segment relationships. Some define these relationships to be a function of surface structure (e.g., based on categories of utterance function, such as *request* or *inform*, called "speech acts" [1]), while others posit that these relationships must be a function of the intentions (plans and goals) of the individuals engaged in conversation [2, 3]. In addition, researchers developing computational models of discourse and dialog have included a number of other constructs in their representation of discourse context, including: entities previously mentioned in the conversation; topics currently being discussed (e.g., "questions under discussion" [4]); and information structure, which indicates which parts of utterances contribute new information to the conversation as opposed to those parts that serve mainly to tie new contributions back to earlier conversation [5].

Discourse theory also seeks to provide accounts of a wide range of phenomena that occur in naturally-occurring dialog, including: mechanisms for conversation initiation, termination, maintenance and turn-taking; interruptions; speech intonation (used to convey a range of information about discourse context [6]); discourse markers (words or phrases like "anyway" that signal changes in discourse context [7]); discourse ellipsis (omission of a syntactically required phrase when the content can be inferred from discourse context); grounding (how speaker and listener negotiate and confirm the meaning of utterances through signals such as headnods and paraverbals such as "uh huh" [8]); and indirect speech acts (e.g., when a speaker says "do you have the time?" they want to know the time rather than simply wanting to know whether the hearer knows the time or not [9]).

Box 9.1 Definition
Dialog systems are computational artifacts designed to engage humans in dialog, as defined above. **Intelligent agents** are autonomous, goal-directed computational artifacts. **Conversational agents** are intelligent agents that converse with humans via a dialog system interface. **Conversational assistants** are conversational agents that use speech input and output to perform a wide range of tasks, as exemplified by the now ubiquitous Siri, Amazon Alexa, and Google Home products.

Embodied Conversational Agents (ECAs) are conversational agents that include the ability to use human-like conversational nonverbal behavior in their dialog (Fig. 9.2). ECAs are animated humanoid computer-based characters that use speech, eye gaze, hand gesture, facial expression and other nonverbal modalities to emulate the experience of human face-to-face conversation with their users [10]. Such agents can provide a "virtual consultation" with a simulated health provider, offering a natural and accessible source of information for patients. These agents represent one form of multimodal dialog system, in which the nonverbal modalities are recognized and produced in addition to accompanying text or speech, to more fully understand the user's communicative intent and to better express system

Fig. 9.2 Embodied conversational agent for patient education at hospital discharge

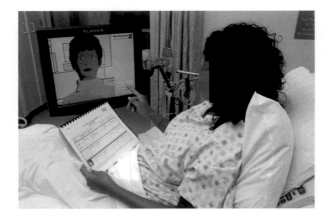

output. In addition to carrying additional factual information, nonverbal behavior is also used in face-to-face conversation to regulate the interaction structure itself, for example, gaze and intonation to regulate turn-taking behavior, and body position and orientation to regulate conversation initiation and termination. Nonverbal behavior is also particularly effective for conveying affective and relational cues that may be important for establishing patient trust in and working alliance with the ECA [11].

What's Hard About Getting Machines to Engage in Spontaneous Human Conversation?

People unconsciously leverage a complex set of processes to make conversation work, most of which are entirely automatic and unconscious. They assume that an entity that engages them in what appears to be natural language dialog has these abilities until they discover their limitations. Several of these processes, such as conversation initiation and termination, and turn-taking and grounding, were mentioned above. Additional examples include: deixis, referring to something in the speakers' mutual context (object, time, location, social relationship) in language; anaphoric or cataphoric references (referring to something said earlier or later in the dialog); and conversational framing [12] or layering [13] in which different styles or genres of talk are used to change how utterances are interpreted (e.g., symptom inquiry by a third party made within social chat storytelling occurring within the context of a clinical interview). There are many more conversational processes and linguistic phenomena that together make the seemingly effortless task of a water cooler conversation seem miraculous upon close inspection.

Fortunately, most of these conversational processes can be "compiled out" by tightly constraining what a user is allowed to do, or by greatly lowering their expectations. System-initiated dialog that rigidly walks a user through a series of steps generally avoids the need to engage in many of these processes. Similarly, a system that engages a patient in scripted greeting and small talk at the start of a health education session does not need a computational model of conversational frames. Agents that only provide responses to single utterance user queries (such as popular conversational assistants like Siri) have trained users to not expect any conversational behavior beyond these simple exchanges.

Machine Learning and Dialog Systems

In the research community, the dominant modern approach to dialog systems is now based on machine learning (ML; see Chap. 6). Learning-based approaches to dialog permit flexibility and avoid the need for exhaustive manual engineering of rules.

ML-based approaches to dialog have yielded strong empirical performance, although measuring this is a challenge ([14]; see the section on "Automated Metrics for End-to-End Architectures"). However, building such systems requires *training data* (i.e., example conversations) from which to learn, which may not be available in all domains, and can be prohibitively expensive to collect. Moreover, it is difficult to *control* the outputs of machine learning models, and so deploying such systems in the context of healthcare applications may be a risky endeavor.

History of Dialog Systems in Healthcare

Chapter 2 reviewed the history of AI in medicine; here we focus on the development of dialog systems specifically. One of the very earliest dialog systems developed was produced as a demonstration of a patient-facing psychotherapy counseling agent (see Chap. 2). The ELIZA system was developed to simulate the behavior of a Rogerian psychotherapist, in which the patient and the computer exchanged typed text messages [15]. Although ELIZA was not intended to be used for actual therapy, similar systems have been proven effective for therapy in which the system is essentially prompting a patient to think aloud and work through his or her own problems [16]. An example conversation with ELIZA is shown in Fig. 9.3.

Colby developed an ELIZA-like system that was designed to use Cognitive Behavioral Therapy to treat individuals with depression. In addition to providing typed text counseling with patients, the system provided text-based educational materials about depression [17]. These systems are characterized by system responses that are only coherent with the immediately preceding user utterance, implemented using pattern-response rules that are matched to the user input with regular expressions, and template-based text generation of system responses. They also use a variety of techniques to maintain the illusion of coherent dialog, including: maintaining system-initiated dialog, having most system outputs prompt the user with open-ended questions; relying on the user's sense-making ability to infer

1. ELIZA: Hello, I am Eliza.
2. User: Hi.
3. ELIZA: How are you today.. What would you like to discuss?
4. User: I've been feeling a little depressed lately.
5. ELIZA: Can you elaborate on that?
6. User: I'm just not myself. I find it hard to get motivated.
7. ELIZA: Did you come to me because you are just not yourself. You find it hard to get motivated?
8. User: Yes, that's right.
9. ELIZA: I see.

Fig. 9.3 Example Conversation with ELIZA

coherent explanations for the system's outputs; and reflecting the user's inputs back to them with minor wording changes in order to give the illusion of understanding what the user is saying. This approach to dialog system implementation is widely used in "chatbots" deployed on the web for entertainment, marketing and sales applications, and has given rise to an open standard chatbot implementation language (AIML [18]).

Development dating from 1964 was also conducted on systems that could collect a medical history from patients [19]. Unlike ELIZA, these systems conducted system-initiated dialog only, asking patients a series of questions with highly-constrained patient input (mostly YES/NO questions) to drive branching logic. Research and development of these systems has continued, and some commercial tools are available, although they still have not attained wide use in clinical practice [20].

Some of the earliest work in physician-facing medical expert systems used system-initiated dialogue to interact with providers for decision support. MYCIN was an early rule-based expert system that identified bacteria causing an infection and recommended antibiotics [21] (see Chap. 2). It was designed to interact with physicians by asking a series of very constrained questions requiring one- or two-word responses. In fact, it was a desire to avoid having to implement natural language understanding that led to the use of MYCIN's core backward-chaining diagnostic algorithm.

> By using a backward-chained approach, MYCIN controlled the dialogue and therefore could ask specific questions that generally required one- or two-word answers. ([21], p. 601)

MYCIN (and derivative projects) used various text generation techniques to produce their final output case summaries.

The sections on "Example Patient- and Consumer-facing Dialog Systems" and "Example Provider-facing Dialog Systems" provide more recent examples of patient- and provider-facing medical dialog systems.

In the last decade, deep neural network-based methods trained on massive corpora have come to dominate Natural Language Processing (NLP) [22]. These methods have enabled highly accurate automatic speech transcription tasks [23] and improved NLP system performance across a variety of problems, including building conversational agents [24].

One means for building dialog systems entails specifying models that map user input utterances directly to output utterances ("end-to-end" systems). This can yield strong performance with respect to the fluency of outputs, but such systems can struggle to maintain coherence throughout a dialog [25]. While such text-to-text models have been used in the context of task-oriented dialog systems [26, 27], they may be more suitable to "general domain" conversational agents—i.e., general "chatbots"—as such models are not naturally amenable to guiding "goal-based" dialog. This reflects the myopic optimization strategy used to estimate model parameters: Typically one aims to find parameters that make the model as likely as possible to produce the words comprising response utterances in the observed training data. This optimization criterion does not explicitly encode higher-order conversational goals, which likely require explicit planning to achieve.

A common strategy to address this problem is to decompose dialog systems into independent modules, to be trained separately and combined in a pipeline. For example, one module might process user utterances, a second might then decide on an action to take, and a third might then generate a response, conditioned on this. Developing "end-to-end" methods that permit joint optimization of all components necessary for goal-based dialog is an active area of research [28]. We discuss archetypal modern machine learning models in the section on "Neural Network Methods and End-to-End Architectures".

Dialog System Technology

Classic Symbolic Pipeline Architectures

Historically, dialog systems have been developed using a pipeline architecture, in which a user utterance is incrementally transformed into a representation that the core agent logic can provide a response to, followed by another series of processing stages to render the system output. These stages can include Automated Speech Recognition (ASR), multimodal integration, utterance understanding, dialog management, natural language generation, multimodal generation, and Text-To-Speech (TTS). Approaches to dialog management include **finite-state automata**, **frames**, and plan-based frameworks (Fig. 9.4).

Automated Speech Recognition (ASR) is responsible for transcribing the users' speech input into one or more text representations. Speech recognition has improved significantly from single-speaker digit recognition systems in 1952 [29] to speaker-independent continuous speech recognition systems based on deep neural networks [30]. Currently, several open source ASR engines such as Pocketsphinx [31], Kaldi [32], and HTK [33] are available, but accurate speech recognition can require substantial processing power which cloud based services such as IBM Watson [34], and the Google cloud platform [35] provide. Although recent systems have achieved around 5% word error rates [36, 37], there are still some doubts regarding the use of ASR in applications such as medical documentation [38]. Goss et al [39] reported that 71% of notes dictated by emergency physicians using ASR contained errors, and 15% contained critical errors.

A **Natural Language Understanding** (NLU) module extracts a semantic representation of the user's utterance, which can then be used by the dialog manager to generate a system response. State-of-the-art statistical NLU systems often contain three main components: domain detection, intent detection, and slot tagging [40].

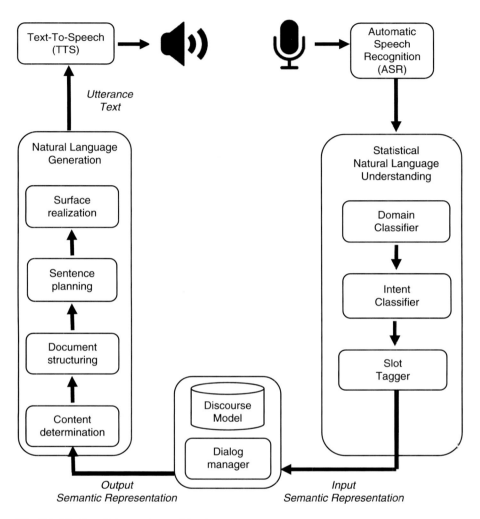

Fig. 9.4 Pipeline dialog system architecture

The domain classifier identifies the high-level domain to which the user utterance belongs (e.g., symptoms, medications, or educational content). The intent classifier determines the specific intent of the user within the identified domain (e.g. *report_ finding*). Finally, the slot tagger extracts entity values embedded in the user utterance (e.g. *syndrome_name* or *severity_level*). NLU is one of the most complex tasks in dialog systems for several reasons. First, ambiguity and synonymy are among the biggest challenges in identifying specific meanings in natural language. Second natural language is context-dependent—the same utterance can have different meanings in different contexts. Third, spontaneous speech is often noisy with disfluencies (e.g., filled pauses, repairs, restarts).

Dialog management is most typically implemented using finite state machines or layers of finite state machines, also referred to as hierarchical transition networks, particularly for applications in which the system maintains the conversational initiative. In these systems, states typically represent system utterances and branches to next states are made in response to user responses. Layers in the hierarchy can be used to represent discourse segments, for example to satisfy a particular conversational goal. Dialog managers can also be frame-based, in which a current "frame" is used to guide the conversation by asking users for information to fill slots until enough information has been gathered for the system to take an action.

More advanced approaches to dialog management involve the explicit representation of user and system plans and goals, which is required to manage conversational phenomena such as: mixed-initiative dialog, in which either the user or the system can take control of the conversation at any time; proper handling of interruptions and requests for clarifications; and indirect speech acts. Flexibly handling these phenomena requires representing and reasoning about the intentions that underlie system and user utterances, inferring the user's goals and task plan, and dynamically synthesizing the system's task plan. Inferring a user's goals and task plan is necessary because, as exemplified by indirect speech acts, people's utterances do not always correspond directly to their communicative intent (e.g., as in "Do you have the time?"). Thus, plan-based theories of communicative action and dialog assume that the speaker's speech acts are part of a plan, and the listener's task is to infer it and respond appropriately to the underlying plan, rather than just to the utterance [41]. Synthesizing system task plans, including communicative and other actions, is necessary in complex applications in which all possible conversational contingencies (and their possible orderings) cannot be anticipated and scripted, but must be addressed in an incremental, reactive manner.

Dynamic planning and plan inference can be computationally very complex and difficult to develop, and thus have not been used much to date in fielded health dialog systems. However, they remain active areas of research, and a handful of health dialog systems that use these techniques have been developed for the application of clinical guidelines [42], for the automatic generation of reminders for older adults with cognitive impairment [43], for medication advice [44], and for diet promotion [45].

One research project used a task decomposition planning formalism to drive health behavior change counseling dialog for exercise and diet promotion [46]. This formalism was based on the Shared Plans theory [47, 48], in which dialog is viewed as a collaboration in which participants coordinate their action towards achieving a shared goal. Discourse segments are defined by the sequence of sub-goals or atomic actions in a recipe that serve to elaborate a particular goal, and the only meaningful relationships among discourse segments are elaboration (goal expansion) and ordering of goals and actions. Figure 9.5 shows a portion of the plan tree for an exercise promotion dialog. Plan fragments that elaborate dialog goals into subgoals and atomic actions are referred to as recipes and are represented in ANSI/CEA-2018 [49] (ANSI/CEA-2018 provides a standard declarative representation for tasks that can be decomposed in this manner). Figure 9.6 shows a portion of a high-level

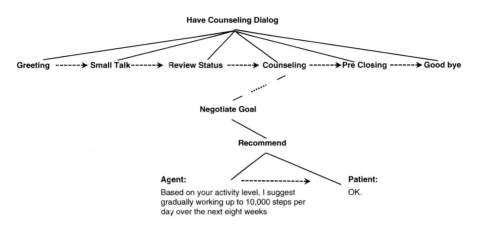

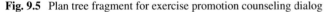

Fig. 9.5 Plan tree fragment for exercise promotion counseling dialog

Fig. 9.6 Example
pseudocode for a
high-level recipe and a
low-level dialogue
specification

> **task** Negotiate
>   **input parameters**: behavior, target
>   **outputs**: goal
>   **steps**: 1. ComputeDesired
>   2. Recommend
>   3. Followup
>   4. Confirm
>
> **task** Recommend
>   **input parameters**: behavior, target, desired
>   **outputs**: response
>   **precondition**: (behavior='exercise' **and**
>   target ='long_term_goal'
>   **adjacency pair**:
>   **agent utterance**:
>   Based on your activity level, I suggest
>   gradually working up to ‹**desired**› steps per
>   day over the next eight weeks
>   ...

recipe for behavior goal negotiation, and an example of an atomic dialogue turn that elaborates the "Recommend" subgoal for negotiating long-term exercise goals. The run-time planning system (based on the COLLAGEN collaborative dialog system [50]) starts with a top-level goal to have a counseling dialog, then incrementally elaborates the goal using recipes until atomic utterances are produced. This process results in a plan tree in which the root is the initial goal and the leaves are the utterances produced by the agent and the user (Fig. 9.5). The planning process proceeds without backtracking, i.e., elaborations are never undone once they are added to the dialog plan tree.

The most common approach to symbolic **Natural Language Generation** (NLG) is template-based text generation, in which an output utterance is represented as a string annotated with variables whose values are determined at runtime [51]. While relatively simple and straightforward, this approach does not offer much flexibility or expressivity. In the most general case, text generation can involve word-by-word synthesis of utterances based on a grammar and dictionary, discourse context and world knowledge, and is itself decomposed into another pipeline of processing stages [51] (Fig. 9.4).

Content determination is the first stage, and involves deciding what information should be communicated in the output, beyond that dictated by the dialog manager. *Document structuring* decides how chunks of text should be grouped together in one or more output utterances and how they should be related in rhetorical terms. *Sentence planning* involves: selection of the specific words or other linguistic resources that should be used to express the selected content; deciding what expressions should be used to refer to entities; and deciding how structures created by document planning should be mapped onto linguistic structures, such as utterances or conversational turns.

The last step of NLG, referred to as **surface realization,** involves turning the internal representations produced during sentence planning into the text of one or more utterances. Research has also been conducted into generation of multi-modal system outputs (speech or text plus accompanying nonverbal behavior for an ECA, or graphics to help illustrate a concept to be conveyed) although, as with multi-modal input understanding, this has not been used widely in health dialog systems to date.

Finally, **Text-To-Speech** (TTS) involves the conversion of utterance text into an acoustic signal. TTS is now a very mature technology and the quality and naturalness has improved significantly over the last decade, producing understandable speech for a wide range of languages. Speech Synthesis Markup Language (SSML) enables the annotation of utterance text with tags that can manipulate speed, pitch, volume, and other aspects of prosody to produce more expressive speech [52].

Neural Network Methods and End-to-End Architectures

In the past decade, neural networks have emerged as the dominant model class for natural language processing (NLP) [22], as they have become the dominant machine learning formalism for many areas of modeling in medicine (see Chap. 1). Neural network-based NLP has in turn given rise to neural conversational models [25, 53–55]. Departing from the classical symbolic approaches reviewed above, neural models represent utterances as dense, continuous vectors (i.e., learned representations). Neural language models [56] are typically used in such architectures to generate responses conditioned on a representation of context, e.g., the most recent utterance.

Completely "end-to-end" systems forego explicit planning and learn to map directly from an input to an output utterance via a deep neural network [57].

Fig. 9.7 High-level
schematic of a Seq2Seq
model for dialog
generation

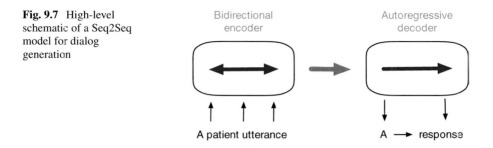

Bidirectional
encoder

Autoregressive
decoder

A patient utterance   A ⟶ response

Sequence-to-sequence architectures are currently dominant neural models for dialog; these use neural network modules to map input to output texts. This is typically accomplished with an *encoder-decoder* architecture. The encoder learns to compress inputs into a dense representation; this is then passed onto the decoder, which is responsible for conditionally generating a response. Because the decoder must generate text, it is typically defined as an auto-regressive (conditional) language model, which is to say that it generates outputs one word at a time in a left-to-right fashion. Figure 9.7 provides a high-level schematic of this approach.

Simple sequence-to-sequence approaches have the advantage of minimizing the manual effort that must be expended to build new conversational systems; they are induced entirely from training data, and so do not require explicit rule- or template-formulation. However, this brings inherent drawbacks. Chief amongst them is the reliance on large, high-quality training corpora. In addition, such models struggle to make meaningful use of dialog history [58]. With respect to task-oriented dialog systems, end-to-end sequence-to-sequence models can learn to take particular actions only implicitly, which makes them difficult to interpret and control.

Some work has attempted to make neural dialog models more explicitly task-oriented by learning *policies* via (deep) reinforcement learning [25, 59]. Other recent efforts have aimed to combine the strengths of end-to-end and more explicitly goal-oriented approaches [28]. Unifying the symbolic approaches discussed above with modern, data-driven neural network models for dialog is likely to remain an active area of research in the coming years.

Approaches to Dialog System Evaluation

Evaluating dialog systems is important in general, but is especially crucial in safety-critical areas such as medicine. Due to the multi-faceted nature of dialog systems, and the inherent complexity of natural language, evaluation is typically multidimensional. Of course, medical applications typically have well-defined health outcomes that are ultimately of greatest importance, such as knowledge gain for health education systems, or objective health outcomes for conversational agents that promote health behavior change, but here we review application-independent performance metrics and methods.

Evaluation of Pipeline Architectures

In classic pipeline architecture-based systems, a "Wizard-of-Oz" methodology is commonly used to replace one or more pipeline components with a human "wizard" (unbeknownst to test subjects) so that the overall system can be evaluated prior to full implementation, or to provide a baseline comparison for a fully-automated system [60]. Dialog from these sessions is recorded and analyzed for several purposes, including: early characterization of domain dialogs; characterization of user responses in particular contexts of interest; assessment of user acceptance of and attitude towards a planned system; and assessment of utility and efficacy of a planned system. Although ideally, user-system interaction will closely follow provider-patient interaction, it has been observed that in many situations users speak and otherwise behave differently when interacting with a computerized system than when with another human (e.g., they simplify their speech patterns) [61]. In these situations, Wizard-of-Oz testing is particularly important, since the study of provider-patient interaction will not correctly characterize these dialogs.

Pipeline architectures also have well-established evaluation metrics for certain components. For example, **Word Error Rate** (WER) is often used as one of the most common figures of merit for ASR modules.

Automated Metrics for End-to-End Architectures

Manual assessment of model outputs remains the gold standard for evaluating Natural Language Processing (NLP) models for text generation tasks broadly (e.g., machine translation, abstractive summarization), and for dialog systems in particular. Manual assessment involves having humans interact with a dialog system, or review transcripts of interactions or text generation outputs, and provide subjective and objective performance evaluations. However, enlisting domain experts to perform such assessments is time-consuming and expensive. Manual evaluation is therefore impracticable for model development, which typically requires iterative refinement. For this reason, contemporary work on NLP models for text generation tasks tends to favor use of fully automated metrics to facilitate model development.

Such metrics assume access to "reference" texts written by humans and aim to measure some notion of similarity between a model output $\hat{y}_i$ for a given input x_i and the corresponding reference text y_i. In the context of dialog systems, x_i might be an utterance and y_i a reference response. Intuitively, we would like a metric that is high if $\hat{y}_i$ is similar to y_i. Most automated metrics essentially measure similarity as some function of word overlap between the model output and reference.

BLEU (short for Bilingual Evaluation Understudy) is one such metric, first popularized in the context of automated machine translation. The motivating dictum behind BLEU is "The closer a machine translation is to a professional human translation, the better it is" [62]. To operationalize this intuition, BLEU computes *n*-gram *precision*,[1] for varying n; that is, it measures the number of n-grams in a generated output that also appear in the corresponding reference. The precision values for different n-gram lengths are then combined using a weighted average. This aggregate precision score is subsequently multiplied by a "brevity penalty" factor, which is intended to measure whether outputs are comparable in length to reference summaries. Meteor [63] is a similar metric, also popular in machine translation: This proposes several modifications intended to address limitations of BLEU. Both of these metrics have been shown to correlate reasonably well with human assessments of translation system outputs [62, 63].

Recall Oriented Understudy for Gisting Evaluation (ROUGE) [64], another automated metric, is perhaps the dominant choice for evaluating *summarization* systems. It is—as the name suggests—more focused on *recall*, i.e., it is high when $\hat{y}_i$ contains as many n-grams as possible that also appear in y_i. Typically one calculates ROUGE-N for a particular n-gram list; for example, ROUGE-1 tallies unigram recall of the model output with respect to the reference. In the context of automated summarization, ROUGE has been shown to correlate with human judgements of quality [64], although it has been noted that it does not reliably measure higher-order properties of outputs such as *factual accuracy* [65].

The above automated measures of generated outputs were not designed for evaluating dialog generation systems, but they are nonetheless often used for this when "reference" response utterances are available. However, in the context of evaluating dialog systems such metrics have been shown to poorly correlate with human judgements, and so should be interpreted accordingly [14]. Developing better automated metrics for evaluating automatically generated dialog responses is an active area of research [66, 67].

System-Level Evaluation

There are a number of approaches for evaluating overall dialog system performance (see Chap. 17 for a more general discussion of evaluation issues). From a usability perspective, metrics such as task completion rate, user satisfaction, efficiency, and learnability are relevant. One influential dialog system evaluation framework (PARADISE) attempts to combine these into a single metric [68]. PARADISE uses a decision-theoretic framework to combine evaluations of system accuracy (success rate at achieving desired conversational outcomes) with the "costs" of using a system—comprised of quantitative efficiency measures (number of dialog turns, conversation time, etc.) and qualitative measures (e.g., number of repair utterances)—to yield a single quality measure for a given interaction. Weights for the various elements of the evaluation are determined empirically from overall

---

[1]An n-gram is just a sequence of n words or "tokens", e.g., "bank" is a 1-gram (or "unigram"), "river bank" is a 2-gram ("bigram"), and so on.

Table 9.1 Example conversational agent usability heuristics (from [71])

Heuristic	Explanation
Visibility of system status	The system should keep users informed about what is going on, through appropriate feedback within reasonable time, without overwhelming the user
User control and freedom	Users often choose system functions by mistake and will need an option to effortlessly leave the unwanted state without having to go through an extended dialogue. Support undo and redo
Context preservation	Maintain context preservation regarding the conversation topic intra-session, and if possible inter-session. Allow the user to reference past messages for further interactions to support implicit user expectations of conversations

assessments of user satisfaction for a sample set of conversations, and the evaluation formula can be applied to sub-dialogs as well as to entire conversations to enable identification of problematic dialog fragments.

Two other qualitative evaluation methods were developed on the TRINDI and DISC projects. They provide criteria for evaluating a dialog system's competence in handling certain dialog phenomena. The TRINDI Tick-List consists of three sets of questions that are intended to elicit explanations describing the extent of a system's competence [69]. The first set consists of eight questions relating to the flexibility of dialog that a system can handle. For example, the question "Can the system deal with answers to questions that give more information than was requested?" assesses whether the system has any ability to handle mixed-initiative dialog. The DISC Dialog Management grids [70] include a set of nine questions, similar to the Trindi Tick-List, that are intended to elicit some factual information regarding the potential of a dialog system.

Langevin et al. recently developed a set of usability heuristics to guide the evaluation of text- or speech-based conversational agents [71]. Usability heuristics are used to guide "expert evaluation" of an interface, in which a designer uses them as a checklist to draw their attention to common classes of usability problems. Derived from Nielsen's classic usability heuristics [72], the 11 new heuristics were found to be more effective at identifying problems with conversational agents than Nielsen's original set. Examples of the heuristics are shown in Table 9.1.

Example Patient- and Consumer-Facing Dialog Systems

A number of embodied conversational agents have been developed to provide health education and health behavior change counseling across several health conditions. For example, an ECA was developed as a virtual discharge nurse who explained their hospital discharge and home care instructions (Fig. 9.2) [73, 74]. The agent was provided on a touch screen kiosk to patients while they were in their hospital beds, and spent 30–60 min reviewing a hospital discharge booklet with them, including information about medications, follow-up appointments, and self-care procedures. Patient understanding was confirmed using comprehension checks, and at the end of the session a report was printed for the human discharge nurse that indicated questions the patient still had that he or she could address. A randomized controlled trial (RCT) was conducted with 764 patients on a general medicine floor at an urban safety net hospital, aged 49.6, 49.7% with inadequate health literacy, comparing the virtual nurse to standard care. Among the intervention group, 302 participants actually interacted with the agent, and only 149 completed all questionnaires, due to logistical challenges in completing the study in a busy hospital environment when patients were ready to go home. Patients reported very high satisfaction and working alliance with the agent, and more patients preferred talking to the agent than their doctors or nurses in the hospital.

Several speech-based conversational agents have also been developed and evaluated in RCTs [43, 75, 76]. For example, the Telephone-Linked Care (TLC) systems developed by Friedman and colleagues at Boston University used recorded speech output, and either DTMF or ASR for user input. TLC behavior change applications have been applied to changing dietary behavior [77], promoting physical activity [78], smoking cessation [79], and promoting medication adherence in patients with depression [80] and hypertension [81]. TLC chronic disease applications have been developed for chronic obstructive pulmonary disease (COPD) [82], and coronary heart disease, hypercholesterolemia, and diabetes mellitus [81]. All of these systems have been evaluated in RCTs and most were shown to be effective on at least one outcome measure, compared to standard-of-care or non-intervention control conditions.

There are now many commercially-successful patient- and consumer-facing dialog systems. Woebot, is a text-based chatbot designed to alleviate anxiety and depression using a range of counseling techniques, and was recently demonstrated to be effective at reducing substance misuse [83]. Clear Genetics produces a text-based chatbot that provides a range of genetics counseling functions, including administration of informed consent for genetic testing [84]. In addition, many dialog systems have been developed as add-on "skills" for speech-based conversational assistants such as Alexa. At the time of this writing, Amazon lists over 2000 skills (task-specific modules that can extend Alexa's functionality) in their Health and Fitness category, all of which can be considered patient- and consumer-facing health dialog systems.

Example Provider-Facing Dialog Systems

There are far fewer examples of provider-facing medical dialog systems in the literature, and these have largely been early research prototypes. For example, the HOMEY system is a decision support tool that advises physicians on whether a patient should be referred to a cancer specialist [85]. Laranjo et al. describe several additional dialog systems that interact with both patients and providers [86]. Dialog systems may be less acceptable to health providers than to patients and consumers because they are slower to use and more error-prone compared to functionally-equivalent graphical user interfaces.

Safety Issues in Dialog Systems for Healthcare

Dialog systems that provide advice to healthcare providers can tolerate imperfect performance, since providers presumably have the expertise to recognize unsafe recommendations. However, due to the inherent ambiguity in natural language, lack of user knowledge about the expertise and natural language abilities of a conversational agent, and potentially misplaced trust, great care must be taken to ensure patients and consumers do not put themselves in situations in which may they act on information mistakenly provided by a conversational agent that could cause harm. To demonstrate these potential safety issues, a study was conducted using three widely-available disembodied conversational agents (Apple's Siri, Google Home, and Amazon's Alexa). Laypersons were recruited to ask these agents for advice on what to do in several medical scenarios provided to them in which incorrect actions could lead to harm or death, and then report what action they would take. Out of 394 tasks attempted, participants were only able to complete 42.6% (168). For those tasks, 29.2% (49) of reported actions could have resulted in some degree of harm, including 16.1% (27) that could have resulted in death, as rated by clinicians using a standard medical harm scale [87]. The errors responsible for these outcomes were found at every level of system processing as well as in user actions in specifying their queries and in interpreting results (see Fig. 9.8 for an example). The findings from this study imply that unconstrained natural language input, in the form of speech or typed text, should not be used for systems that provide medical advice given the state-of-the-art. Users should be tightly constrained in the kinds of advice they can ask for, for example, through the use of multiple-choice menus of utterances they are allowed to "say" in each step of the conversation (e.g. as in Fig. 9.2). In addition, unconstrained generative approaches to dialog generation pose additional complications; these may yield offensive or medically inaccurate outputs, for example (as discussed in the section on "Approaches to Dialog System Evaluation").

State of the Art: What We Currently Can and Can't Do

There are currently several commercially-available toolkits for developing state-machine-based dialog systems in which the system maintains initiative, and constrained or unconstrained user inputs can be reliably mapped to a small number of

User: Siri, I'm taking Oxycontin for chronic back pain. But I'm going out tonight. How many drinks can I have?
Siri: I've set your chronic back pain one alarm for 10:00 P.M.
User: I can drink all the way up until 10:00? Is that what that meant?
RA: *Is that what you think it was?*
User: Yeah, I can drink until 10:00. And then after 10 o'clock I can't drink.

Fig. 9.8 Example of medical advice from siri that was rated as potentially fatal (excerpt from [87]) (RA is the research assistant)

options in each state. This state-based model is exemplified by standard dialog management languages (e.g., VoiceXML for speech-based systems [88]) and commercial dialog-management tools (e.g., Google's DialogFlow [89]). As described in the
section on "Example Patient- and Consumer-facing Dialog Systems", there are also
several commercial products that use this approach for consumer- and patient-
facing health education and counseling.

However, we cannot reliably support general, unconstrained user input in
mixed-initiative conversations, nor any of the other conversational phenomena
described in the section on "Introduction to Dialog Systems", at least not to the
degree that people can.

Future Directions

It is unclear if end-to-end approaches will ever be capable of sustaining coherent
dialog over many utterances given that the discourse context alone becomes combi-
natorically large. Hybrid systems that use the best capabilities of the pipelined and
neural approaches combined represent more promising approaches, at least in the
near-term. Consistent with the recurrent theme of combining machine learning and
symbolic approaches mentioned elsewhere in this book, one approach is to bring
more machine learning-based components into the classic symbolic pipeline. Going
forward, key questions include: How can we unify end-to-end neural systems with
symbolic planning-based approaches? Conversely, might we better represent and
exploit (long term) context in modern neural dialog systems?

Patient- and consumer-facing dialog systems that support unconstrained natural language input are certainly preferred to those that are more constrained, since
patients can express themselves freely and may be able to communicate more
nuanced information. However, these systems represent a safety risk as described
in the section on "Safety Issues in Dialog Systems for Healthcare". The identification and mitigation of unsafe medical dialog remains an important area of
research and a problem that must be addressed before these systems can reach
their potential.

There are several active research areas dialogue systems. For example, in pipeline architectures, incremental processing, in which system responses are generated
incrementally while a user is producing their utterance, allows for much faster system response time, but requires re-architecting how the pipeline works [90].
Multiparty interaction represents another important area of research to support
group counseling [91] or three-way patient-clinician-agent interactions. Multimodal
dialog with ECAs or humanoid robots, in which user verbal and nonverbal behavior
can be used to support conversational processes and allow users to better express
themselves [92], also represents an active area of research.

These advances will enable the development of automated health providers and
counselors that can provide complex information to patients and consumers in a
natural, fluid, and intuitive way, tailored to each user and situation, and that do not
require users to dumb down and simplify their language and requests, such as the

one shown in Fig. 9.1. This will enable routine patient education and counseling tasks, such as administration of informed consent, explanation of medications and medical procedures, and explanation of discharge instructions, to be fully automated.

Conclusion

In this chapter, we have provided a review of the state of medically relevant dialog systems, including their current capabilities and limitations, and directions of ongoing and future research and development. Development of this technology is important for the delivery of complex information to patients and consumers, but is particularly important for those with low health or computer literacy who may struggle with text-heavy graphical user interfaces. While these systems have great potential for improving health, attention must be paid to the risks inherent in using unconstrained text or speech input in situations in which misunderstandings can lead to harm.

Questions for Discussion

- How do pipeline and rule-based systems differ from "end-to-end" neural approaches?
- Why might existing automated metrics like ROUGE fail to reliably measure the factual accuracy of utterances?
- How can unsafe medical dialog be identified and mitigated?
- What kinds of medical applications would benefit most from embodiment by the conversational agent?
- What kinds of medical applications would make the relative slowness of dialog systems acceptable to clinicians?

Further Reading

Chattopadhyay D, Ma T, Sharifi H, Martyn-Nemeth P. Computer-controlled virtual humans in patient-facing systems: systematic review and meta-analysis. J Med Internet Res. 2020;22(7):e18839 [93].

- This article provides a comprehensive review of patient-facing embodied conversational agents in medicine.

Laranjo L, Dunn AG, Tong HL, Kocaballi AB, Chen J, Bashir R, et al. Conversational agents in healthcare: a systematic review. J Am Med Inform Assoc. 2018;25(9):1248–58 [86].

- This article provides a review of conversational agents in medicine that use unconstrained natural language input.

Bickmore T, Trinh H, Olafsson S, O'Leary T, Asadi R, Rickles N, et al. Patient and consumer safety risks when using conversational assistants for medical information: an observational study of Siri, Alexa, and Google Assistant. J Med Internet Res. 2018;20(9):e11510 [87].

- This is an empirical study of worst-case safety issues when patients or consumers use conversational agents for actionable medical advice.

Grosz B, Pollack ME, Sidner CL. Discourse. In: Posner MI, editor. Foundations of cognitive science. Cambridge: MIT Press; 1989 [94].

- This chapter provides an excellent primer on basic issues in the study of discourse.

Sordoni A, Galley M, Auli M, Brockett C, Ji Y, Mitchell M, et al. A neural network approach to context-sensitive generation of conversational responses. In Proceedings of the 2015 Conference of the North American Chapter of the Association for Computational Linguistics: Human Language Technologies, pages 196–205, Denver, Colorado. Association for Computational Linguistics [95].

- An early neural dialog system that is illustrative of approaches to follow.

Sankar C, Subramanian S, Pal C, Chandar S, Bengio Y. Do neural dialog systems use the conversation history effectively? An empirical study. In Proceedings of the 57th Annual Meeting of the Association for Computational Linguistics, pages 32–37, Florence, Italy. Association for Computational Linguistics [96].

- An examination of how well current neural based approaches can harness conversational history to inform utterances/responses.

References

1. Searle J. Speech acts: an essay in the philosophy of language. Cambridge: Cambridge University Press; 1969.
2. Grosz B, Sidner C. Attention, intentions, and the structure of discourse. Comput Linguist. 1986;12(3):175–204.
3. Allen J, Perrault CR. Analyzing intention in utterances. In: Grosz BJ, Jones KS, Webber BL, editors. Readings in natural language processing. Los Altos: Morgan Kaufmann Publishers, Inc.; 1986. p. 441–58.
4. Larsson S, Ljunglof P, Cooper R, Engdahl E, Ericsson S. GoDIS - an accommodating dialogue system. ANLP/NAACL-2000 workshop on conversational systems; 2000. pp. 7–10.
5. Prince EP. Toward a taxonomy of given-new information. In: Cole A, editor. Radical pragmatics. Academic: New York; 1981. p. 223–55.
6. Hirschberg J. Accent and discourse context: assigning pitch accent in synthetic speech. AAAI 901990. pp. 952–7.
7. Schiffrin D. Discourse markers. Cambridge: Cambridge University Press; 1987.
8. Clark HH, Brennan SE. Grounding in communication. In: Resnick LB, Levine JM, Teasley SD, editors. Perspectives on socially shared cognition. Washington: American Psychological Association; 1991. p. 127–49.
9. Searle J. Indirect speech acts. In: Cole P, Morgan J, editors. Syntax and semantics, volumen 3: speech acts. Academic: New York; 1975. p. 59–82.
10. Cassell J, Sullivan J, Prevost S, Churchill E. Embodied conversational agents. Cambridge: MIT Press; 2000.

11. Bickmore T, Gruber A, Picard R. Establishing the computer-patient working alliance in automated health behavior change interventions. Patient Educ Cousel. 2005;59(1):21–30.
12. Tannen D, editor. Framing in discourse. New York: Oxford University Press; 1993.
13. Clark HH. Using language. Cambridge: Cambridge University Press; 1996.
14. Liu C-W, Lowe R, Serban IV, Noseworthy M, Charlin L, Pineau J. How not to evaluate your dialogue system: an empirical study of unsupervised evaluation metrics for dialogue response generation. In: Proceedings of the conference on empirical methods in natural language processing; 2016. pp. 2122–32.
15. Weizenbaum J. Eliza - a computer program for the study of natural language communication between man and machine. Commun ACM. 1966;9(1):36–45.
16. Slack W. Patient-computer dialogue: a review. Yearb Med Inform. 2000;2000:71–8.
17. Colby K. A computer program using cognitive therapy to treat depressed patients. Psychiatr Serv. 1995;46:1223–5.
18. Satu S, Parvez H. Review of integrated applications with AIML based chatbot. In: International conference on computer and information engineering (ICCIE). Piscataway: IEEE; 2015.
19. Slack WV, Hicks GP, Reed CE, Van Cura LJ. A computer-based medical-history system. N Engl J Med. 1966;274(4):194–8. https://doi.org/10.1056/nejm196601272740406.
20. Bachman JW. The patient-computer interview: a neglected tool that can aid the clinician. Mayo Clin Proc. 2003;78(1):67–78. https://doi.org/10.4065/78.1.67.
21. Buchanan B, Shortliffe E. Rule based expert systems: the MYCIN experiments of the stanford heuristic programming project. Reading: Addison-Wesley; 1984.
22. Goldberg Y. Neural network methods for natural language processing. Synth Lect Hum Lang Technol. 2017;10(1):1–309.
23. Chiu C-C, Sainath TN, Wu Y, Prabhavalkar R, Nguyen P, Chen Z, et al. State-of-the-art speech recognition with sequence-to-sequence models. In: 2018 IEEE international conference on acoustics, speech and signal processing (ICASSP). Piscataway: IEEE; 2018. p. 4774–8.
24. Wolf T, Sanh V, Chaumond J, Delangue C. Transfertransfo: a transfer learning approach for neural network based conversational agents. arXiv preprint arXiv:190108149. 2019.
25. Li J, Monroe W, Ritter A, Galley M, Gao J, Jurafsky D. Deep reinforcement learning for dialogue generation. arXiv preprint arXiv:160601541. 2016.
26. Madotto A, Wu C-S, Fung P. Mem2seq: effectively incorporating knowledge bases into end-to-end task-oriented dialog systems. arXiv preprint arXiv:180408217. 2018.
27. Lei W, Jin X, Kan M-Y, Ren Z, He X, Yin D. Sequicity: simplifying task-oriented dialogue systems with single sequence-to-sequence architectures. In: Proceedings of the 56th annual meeting of the association for computational linguistics, volume 1: long papers; 2018. pp. 1437–47.
28. Ham D, Lee J-G, Jang Y, Kim K-E. End-to-end neural pipeline for goal-oriented dialogue systems using GPT-2. In: Proceedings of the 58th annual meeting of the Association for Computational Linguistics; 2020. pp. 583–92.
29. Juang B-H, Rabiner LR. Automatic speech recognition–a brief history of the technology development.
30. Hinton G, Deng L, Yu D, Dahl GE, Mohamed A, Jaitly N, et al. Deep neural networks for acoustic modeling in speech recognition: the shared views of four research groups. IEEE Signal Process Mag. 2012;29(6):82–97.
31. Huggins-Daines D, Kumar M, Chan A, Black AW, Ravishankar M, Rudnicky AI. Pocketsphinx: a free, real-time continuous speech recognition system for hand-held devices. In: Acoustics, speech and signal processing, 2006 ICASSP 2006 proceedings 2006 IEEE international conference. Piscataway: IEEE; 2006.
32. Povey D, Ghoshal A, Boulianne G, Burget L, Glembek O, Goel N, et al. The Kaldi speech recognition toolkit. In: IEEE 2011 workshop on automatic speech recognition and understanding. Piscataway: IEEE Signal Processing Society; 2011.
33. Woodland PC, Odell JJ, Valtchev V, Young SJ. Large vocabulary continuous speech recognition using HTK. In: Acoustics, speech, and signal processing, 1994 ICASSP-94, 1994 IEEE international conference, vol. 1994. Piscataway: IEEE. p. 125.

34. IBM: Watson speech to text. https://www.ibm.com/watson/services/speech-to-text/. Accessed 30 September 2017.
35. Google: speech recognition. https://cloud.google.com/speech/. Accessed 30 September 2017.
36. Saon G, Kurata G, Sercu T, Audhkhasi K, Thomas S, Dimitriadis D, et al. English conversational telephone speech recognition by humans and machines. arXiv preprint arXiv:170302136. 2017.
37. Xiong W, Droppo J, Huang X, Seide F, Seltzer M, Stolcke A, et al. The Microsoft 2016 conversational speech recognition system. In: Acoustics, speech and signal processing (ICASSP), 2017 IEEE international conference, vol. 2017. Piscataway: IEEE. p. 5255–9.
38. Hodgson T, Coiera E. Risks and benefits of speech recognition for clinical documentation: a systematic review. J Am Med Inform Assoc. 2015;23(1):169–79.
39. Goss FR, Zhou L, Weiner SG. Incidence of speech recognition errors in the emergency department. Int J Med Inform. 2016;93:70–3.
40. Liu X, Sarikaya R, Zhao L, Ni Y, Pan Y-C. Personalized natural language understanding. Interspeech; 2016, pp. 1146–50.
41. Cohen P. Dialogue modeling. In: Cole R, editor. Survey of the state of the art in human language technology. Alexandria: National Science Foundation; 1996.
42. Beveridge M, Millward D. Combing task descriptions and ontological knowledge for adaptive dialogue. In: Proceedings of the 6th international conference on text, speech and dialogue (TSD-03); 2003.
43. Pollack ME, Brown L, Colbry D, McCarthy CE, Orosz C, Peintner B, et al. Autominder: an intelligent cognitive orthotic system for people with memory impairment. Robot Auton Syst. 2003;44:273–82.
44. Ferguson G, Quinn J, Horwitz C, Swift M, Allen J, Galescu L. Towards a personal health management assistant. J Biomed Inform. 2010;43(5):13–6. https://doi.org/10.1016/j.jbi.2010.05.014.
45. Grasso F, Cawsey A, Jones R. Dialectical argumentation to solve conflicts in advice giving: a case study in the promotion of healthy nutrition. Int J Hum-Comput Stud. 2000;53:1077–115.
46. Bickmore T, Schulman D, Sidner C. A reusable framework for health counseling dialogue systems based on a behavioral medicine ontology. J Biomed Inform. 2011;44:183–97.
47. Grosz B, Kraus S. Collaborative plans for group activities. In: Proc 13th Int joint Conf artificial intelligence. Chambery, France; 1993, pp. 367–73.
48. Lochbaum K. A collaborative planning model of intentional structure. Comput Linguist. 1998;24(4):525–72.
49. Rich C. Building task models with ANSI/CEA-2018. IEEE Comput. 2009;42(8):20–7.
50. Rich C, Sidner CL, Lesh N. Collagen: applying collaborative discourse theory to human-computer interaction. AI Mag. 2001;22(4):15.
51. Reiter E, Dale R. Building natural language generation systems. Cambridge: Cambridge University Press; 2000.
52. Baggia P, Bagshaw P, Bodell M, et al. Speech synthesis markup language (SSML) version 1.1. 2010. https://www.w3.org/TR/speech-synthesis11/.
53. Sordoni A, Galley M, Auli M, Brockett C, Ji Y, Mitchell M, et al. A neural network approach to context-sensitive generation of conversational responses. In Proceedings of the 2015 Conference of the North American Chapter of the Association for Computational Linguistics: Human Language Technologies, pages 196–205, Denver, Colorado. Association for Computational Linguistics.
54. Vinyals O, Le Q. A neural conversational model. arXiv preprint arXiv:150605869. 2015.
55. Serban IV, Sankar C, Germain M, Zhang S, Lin Z, Subramanian S, et al. A deep reinforcement learning chatbot. arXiv preprint arXiv:170902349. 2017.
56. Bengio Y, Ducharme R, Vincent P, Janvin C. A neural probabilistic language model. J Mach Learn Res. 2003;3:1137–55.
57. Serban IV, Lowe R, Charlin L, Pineau J. Generative deep neural networks for dialogue: a short review. arXiv preprint arXiv:161106216. 2016.
58. Sankar C, Subramanian S, Pal C, Chandar S, Bengio Y. Do neural dialog systems use the conversation history effectively? an empirical study. arXiv preprint arXiv:190601603. 2019.

59. Liu B, Tur G, Hakkani-Tur D, Shah P, Heck L. End-to-end optimization of task-oriented dialogue model with deep reinforcement learning. arXiv preprint arXiv:171110712. 2017.
60. Dahlback N, Jonsson A, Ahrenberg L. Wizard of Oz studies: why and how. IUI 931993. pp. 193–9.
61. Oviatt S. Predicting spoken disfluencies during human-computer interaction. Comput Speech Lang. 1995;9:19–35.
62. Papineni K, Roukos S, Ward T, Zhu W-J. Bleu: a method for automatic evaluation of machine translation. In: Proceedings of the annual meeting of the Association for Computational Linguistics; 2002, pp. 311–8.
63. Banerjee S, Lavie A. METEOR: an automatic metric for MT evaluation with improved correlation with human judgments. In: Proceedings of the ACL workshop on intrinsic and extrinsic evaluation measures for machine translation and/or summarization; 2005, pp. 65–72.
64. Lin C-Y. Rouge: a package for automatic evaluation of summaries. Text summarization branches out; 2004. pp. 74–81.
65. Gabriel S, Celikyilmaz A, Jha R, Choi Y, Gao J. Go figure! A meta evaluation of factuality in summarization. arXiv preprint arXiv:201012834. 2020.
66. Lowe R, Noseworthy M, Serban IV, Angelard-Gontier N, Bengio Y, Pineau J. Towards an automatic turing test: Learning to evaluate dialogue responses. arXiv preprint arXiv:170807149. 2017.
67. Tao C, Mou L, Zhao D, Yan R. Ruber: an unsupervised method for automatic evaluation of open-domain dialog systems. In: Proceedings of the AAAI conference on artificial intelligence; 2018.
68. Walker M, Litman D, Kamm C, Abella A. Paradise: a framework for evaluating spoken dialogue agents. In: Maybury MT, Wahlster W, editors. Readings in intelligent user interfaces. San Francisco: Morgan Kaufmann Publishers, Inc.; 1998. p. 631–41.
69. Bohlin P, Bos J, Larsson S, Lewin I, Mathesin C, Milward D. Survey of existing interactive systems. 1999.
70. Bernsen N, Dybkjaer L. A methodology for evaluating spoken language dialogue systems and their components. In: Second international conference on language resources and evaluation; 2000. pp. 183–8.
71. Langevin R, Lordon R, Avrahami T. Heuristic evaluation of conversational agents. ACM conference on human factors in computing systems (CHI); 2021.
72. Nielsen J, Molich R. Heuristic evaluation of user interfaces. In: ACM SIGCHI conference on human factors in computing systems (CHI); 1990. pp. 249–56.
73. Bickmore T, Pfeifer L, Jack BW. Taking the time to care: empowering low health literacy hospital patients with virtual nurse agents. In: Proceedings of the ACM SIGCHI conference on human factors in computing systems (CHI), Boston, MA; 2009.
74. Zhou S, Bickmore T, Jack B. Agent-user concordance and satisfaction with a virtual hospital discharge nurse. In: International conference on intelligent virtual agents (IVA), Boston, MA; 2014.
75. Corkrey R, Parkinson L. Interactive voice response: review of studies 1989-2000. Behav Res Methods Instrum Comput. 2002;34(3):342–53.
76. Piette J. Interactive voice response systems in the diagnosis and management of chronic disease. Am J Manag Care. 2000;6(7):817–27.
77. Delichatsios HK, Friedman R, Glanz K, Tennstedt S, Smigelski C, Pinto B, et al. Randomized trial of a "talking computer" to improve adults' eating habits. Am J Health Promot. 2001;15(4):215–24.
78. Pinto B, Friedman R, Marcus B, Kelley H, Tennstedt S, Gillman M. Effects of a computer-based, telephone-counseling system on physical activity. Am J Prev Med. 2002;23(2):113–20.
79. Ramelson H, Friedman R, Ockene J. An automated telephone-based smoking cessation education and counseling system. Patient Educ Couns. 1999;36:131–44.
80. Farzanfar R, Locke S, Vachon L, Charbonneau A, Friedman R. Computer telephony to improve adherence to antidepressants and clinical visits. Ann Behav Med. 2003;2003:161.

81. Friedman R. Automated telephone conversations to asses health behavior and deliver behavioral interventions. J Med Syst. 1998;22:95–102.
82. Young M, Sparrow D, Gottlieb D, Selim A, Friedman R. A telephone-linked computer system for COPD care. Chest. 2001;119:1565–75.
83. Prochaska JJ, Vogel EA, Chieng A, Kendra M, Baiocchi M, Pajarito S, et al. A therapeutic relational agent for reducing problematic substance use (woebot): development and usability study. J Med Internet Res. 2021;23(3):e24850. https://doi.org/10.2196/24850.
84. Schmidlen T, Schwartz M, DiLoreto K, Kirchner HL, Sturm AC. Patient assessment of chatbots for the scalable delivery of genetic counseling. J Genet Couns. 2019;28(6):1166–77. https://doi.org/10.1002/jgc4.1169.
85. Beveridge M, Fox J. Automatic generation of spoken dialogue from medical plans and ontologies. J Biomed Inform. 2006;39(5):482–99.
86. Laranjo L, Dunn AG, Tong HL, Kocaballi AB, Chen J, Bashir R, et al. Conversational agents in healthcare: a systematic review. J Am Med Inform Assoc. 2018;25(9):1248–58. https://doi.org/10.1093/jamia/ocy072.
87. Bickmore T, Trinh H, Olafsson S, O'Leary T, Asadi R, Rickles N, et al. Patient and consumer safety risks when using conversational assistants for medical information: an observational study of Siri, Alexa, and Google Assistant. J Med Internet Res. 2018;20(9):e11510.
88. Oshry M, Auburn R, Baggia P, et al. Voice extensible markup language (VoiceXML) 2.1. 2007. https://www.w3.org/TR/voicexml21/.
89. Google: dialogflow. https://cloud.google.com/dialogflow.
90. Manuvinakurike R, DeVault D, Georgila K. Using reinforcement learning to model incrementalityin a fast-paced dialogue game. In: 18th annual SIGdial meeting on discourse and dialogue. Stroudsburg: Association for Computational Linguistics; 2017. p. 331–41.
91. Utami D, Bickmore T. Collaborative user responses in multiparty interaction with a couples counselor robot. Human Robot Interaction (HRI); 2019.
92. Bohus HE. Models for multiparty engagement in open-world dialog. In: Proceedings of the SIGDIAL 2009 conference. London: Association for Computational Linguistics; 2009. p. 225–34.
93. Chattopadhyay D, Ma T, Sharifi H, Martyn-Nemeth P. Computer-controlled virtual humans in patient-facing systems: systematic review and meta-analysis. J Med Internet Res. 2020;22(7):e18839. https://doi.org/10.2196/18839.
94. Grosz B, Pollack ME, Sidner CL. Discourse. In: Posner MI, editor. Foundations of cognitive science. Cambridge: MIT Press; 1989.
95. Sordoni A, Galley M, Auli M, Brockett C, Yangfeng J, Mitchell M, et al. A neural network approach to context-sensitive generation of conversational responses. NAACL-HLT; 2015.
96. Sankar C, Subramanian S, Pal C, Chandar S, Bengio Y. Do neural dialog systems use the conversation history effectively? An empirical study. In Proceedings of the 57th Annual Meeting of the Association for Computational Linguistics, pages 32–37, Florence, Italy. Association for Computational Linguistics.

Part III
Applications

Chapter 10
Integration of AI for Clinical Decision Support

Shyam Visweswaran, Andrew J. King, and Gregory F. Cooper

After reading this chapter, you should know the answers to these questions:
- What are the key challenges faced by clinicians that motivate integrating AI into clinical decision support?
- What are the main types of AI that have been developed for clinical decision support? How does data-derived AI clinical decision support differ from knowledge-based AI clinical decision support?
- What are typical degrees of automation and integration of AI in clinical decision support?
- Describe the types of clinical tasks that can be supported by AI clinical decision support?
- What are the pitfalls of data-derived clinical decision support?

Clinical decision support (CDS) aims to improve health and healthcare by providing clinicians, healthcare workers, and patients with situation-specific knowledge that aids critical clinical activities such as risk assessment, diagnosis, prognosis, and selection of therapy [1]. CDS systems assist clinicians in making decisions about patient care in various ways, such as by providing interpretations of patient data and clinical images, event monitoring and alerts, and recommendations. Some CDS systems guide patients and caregivers who integrate the clinical guidance from the CDS with their personal preferences to make informed decisions.

S. Visweswaran (✉) · G. F. Cooper
Department of Biomedical Informatics, University of Pittsburgh, Pittsburgh, PA, USA
e-mail: shv3@pitt.edu; gfc@pitt.edu

A. J. King
Department of Critical Care Medicine, University of Pittsburgh, Pittsburgh, PA, USA
e-mail: andrew.king@pitt.edu

© The Author(s), under exclusive license to Springer Nature Switzerland AG 2022
T. A. Cohen et al. (eds.), *Intelligent Systems in Medicine and Health*, Cognitive Informatics in Biomedicine and Healthcare,
https://doi.org/10.1007/978-3-031-09108-7_10

Artificial intelligence (AI) enables computer systems to perform tasks that normally require human intelligence (see Chap. 1 for detailed definitions of AI). Because clinical decision-making predominates in medical practice, most applications of AI in clinical care are intended to enhance the quality of clinical decisions. Since the beginnings of AI in the 1950s, AI in medicine has been used increasingly for CDS, although the type of AI that drives CDS systems has evolved over the decades (see Chap. 2 for a historical account of AI in medicine). In the current era, modern AI that leverages large amounts of healthcare data to construct computational models is increasingly being used in such systems.

This chapter provides an overview of the rapidly developing field of **artificial intelligence-based clinical decision support** (AI-CDS) and the associated promising research efforts; it focuses on CDS that is targeted to clinicians, provides the motivation for integrating AI into CDS, describes the types of AI that are being developed for CDS systems, and explores a range of clinical tasks that AI-CDS can support. While the potential benefits of AI-CDS are enormous, significant challenges remain that must be overcome to ensure high-quality healthcare. This chapter describes some of the challenges (especially those stemming from **big data**), summarizes related regulatory developments, and closes with several predictions regarding future directions for AI-CDS.

Challenges Faced by Clinicians

Excellent clinical decision-making requires (1) up-to-date, pertinent medical knowledge, (2) access to accurate and complete patient data, and (3) good decision-making skills. CDS systems are increasingly important in aiding clinical decision-making due to the following key challenges faced by clinicians:

Exponential Growth of Medical Knowledge Provision of optimal care is dependent on the clinician's ability to obtain relevant, up-to-date knowledge. The body of medical knowledge in the era of Galenic medicine appears to have been quite static during the lifetime of a clinician (the Galenic era lasted for more than 1300 years from 300 CE to the seventeenth century, when Galen, a Greek physician, heavily influenced medicine). Today, however, medical knowledge is increasing in volume and complexity. In 1950, the doubling time of medical knowledge was estimated to be 50 years; it decreased to 7 years in 1980 and to a mere 73 days in 2020 [2]. Furthermore, the traditional histopathological classification of disease, which has been the way medical knowledge has been organized and taught for over a century, is giving way to a more fine-grained molecular and functional subtyping of disease. The volume and rapidly evolving genomic, proteomic, metabolomic, and other - omic characteristics of disease and health make it impossible for a clinician to remember and apply them in clinical care without some form of assistance.

Rapid Accumulation of Patient Data The amount of clinical data per individual is rising, driven by the widespread adoption of **electronic health record** (EHR) systems and the rapid growth of new laboratory tests, investigations, and imaging that are increasingly used in clinical care (see Chap. 3). For example, in critical care, it is estimated that a patient generates an average of 1460 new data points daily [3], and a clinician is exposed to an average of 4380 data points during a shift of 12 h [4]. The large amount of patient data has led clinicians to spend more time reviewing and collating data in the EHR that are pertinent to the current clinical context.

Increase in Inference Complexity Human clinicians have limited cognitive capacity and can simultaneously consider only a few variables at a time in decision-making (see Chap. 5). With the exponential growth of medical knowledge and the rapid accumulation of patient data, good medical decision-making requires the consideration of many facts. With individual genomic and proteomic data becoming available for making decisions, inevitably, the number of salient facts to consider for a clinical decision will rise steeply [5]. As the number of facts to consider for clinical decision-making outstrips human cognitive capacity, CDS systems are needed to aid the clinician [6] (see Chap. 5).

Clinical Data Capture Clinicians, particularly in the United States, face an increasing amount of clinical documentation that reduces the time available for direct patient care. For example, primary care physicians spent 42% of their time (5.9 h of an 11.4-h workday) in the EHR, of which half the time is spent on documentation, order entry, billing, and coding [7].

Artificial Intelligence-Based CDS

AI has a long history that traces its modern roots to the 1956 Dartmouth meeting, where computer scientists discussed the notion of AI with the ultimate aim of building machine systems that can perform human-like intellectual and cognitive tasks (see Chap. 2). **Machine learning** (ML), which has come to constitute the largest subset of AI in recent years, refers to AI systems that can achieve some aspects of human-like intelligence without being explicitly programmed by human authors. In particular, **deep learning**, an important subfield of ML, relies on learning large neural networks, often from massive datasets (See Chaps. 1 and 6). Since the inception of AI, medicine has been identified as one of the most promising application areas. Many AI-CDS systems have been described and implemented for a panoply of tasks in medicine, from risk assessment and diagnosis to prognosis and therapeutics to patient monitoring and interpretation of human genomes.

The typical structure of an AI-CDS system has two main components: a knowledge component that represents medical knowledge in a computable form and an inference component that applies the knowledge to a patient's data to provide decision support (see Fig. 10.1). Different ways have been developed for representing

Fig. 10.1 The key
components of a
knowledge-based AI-CDS
system include a
knowledge base such as
expert-derived rules and an
inference mechanism for
clinical application such as
chained inference for rules.
The key components of a
data-derived AI-CDS
include a model, such as a
data-derived neural
network, and an inference
mechanism for clinical
application, such as
forward propagation in a
neural network model

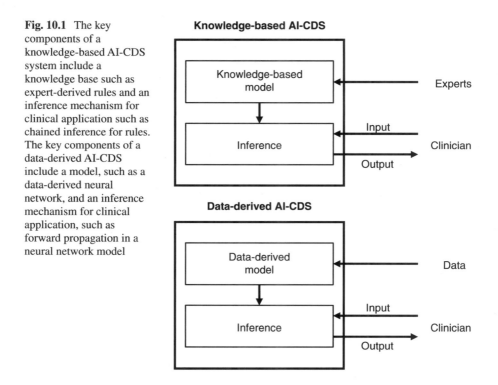

knowledge, such as rules and Bayesian networks, and a variety of inference mechanisms have been created, including chained inference for rules and probability calculations for Bayesian networks. Historically, the knowledge base is explicitly
derived from human experts. With the advent of ML and deep learning, the knowledge component is replaced with computational models, such as classification trees
and neural networks that capture relations among domain concepts. Models are then
applied to a patient's data to provide outputs such as predicting a clinical outcome.
Typically, models are derived from data and often big data. We can view a knowledge base as constituting a model as well. By doing so, models become a unified
representation that can be constructed from data, knowledge, or both. We will refer
to systems in which models are derived primarily from data as *data-derived systems*. Similarly, *knowledge-based systems* will refer to systems derived primarily
from human knowledge (see Chap. 4).

Types of AI-CDS Broadly speaking, AI-CDS can be categorized into knowledge-
based and data-derived systems (see Fig. 10.1). Early AI-CDS systems that were
developed in the 1970s and 1980s used knowledge-based approaches in which medical knowledge represented as rules, expert constructed Bayesian networks, and
semantic networks are stored in a **knowledge base**. In rule-based systems (Chaps. 2
and 4), knowledge is expressed in IF … THEN ... expressions; for example, in a
diagnostic system, the IF part would typically encode symptoms, and the THEN
part would encode diseases that manifest those symptoms. **Knowledge-based**

AI-CDS enjoyed early success and AI-CDS systems were used, for example, to choose appropriate treatments, interpret electrocardiograms, and generate diagnostic hypotheses in complex clinical scenarios. Their key advantages include knowledge that is represented in a form that is easy for clinicians to comprehend and the ability to explain inference in clinically meaningful ways (see Chaps. 1, 4, and 8). However, the construction of knowledge bases is typically manual, which can be time-consuming and tedious, and updates to the knowledge are also manual and slow. Additionally, the construction of stores of numerical knowledge, such as probabilities, as for example, in Bayesian networks, is tedious and difficult.

The data-derived approach to developing AI-CDS systems began in the 1990s. In these systems, knowledge of the earlier AI-CDS was replaced by models that were automatically derived from data. Typically, these models are computational objects that have structural and numerical components. For example, in a neural network model, the network architecture consisting of connections among layers of nodes constitutes the structure, and the weights assigned to connections constitute the numerical component. ML and deep learning methods (see Chap. 6) have been used to derive a wide range of models. ML methods have been developed to derive from data rules and probabilistic networks, resembling manually constructed knowledge-based AI-CDS models. The key advantages of **data-derived AI-CDS** include the ability to rapidly construct models that can have excellent performance. A key disadvantage is that the models are often opaque to human experts, and the explanation of inference using these models remains impenetrable to human users (see Chap. 8).

The impetus for the widespread application of ML to medical data came from advances in data availability, the development of a broad range of ML methods, and powerful and ubiquitous computing capability. First, data on health and disease are increasingly available and include a broad range of data types. In addition to experimental data that are typically collected in research studies under controlled conditions, observational data are becoming available from sources such as EHRs, social media, and monitoring through mobile smartphones. Second, a broad range of ML methods has been developed and is readily available as computer programs for application. Third, access to faster and ever more powerful computers is becoming inexpensive and ubiquitous.

Until recently, data-derived AI-CDS systems were static, implying that the computable knowledge learned from data is not updated. **Static AI-CDS** provides the same result each time the same input is provided, and they do not evolve over time and do not use new data to alter their results. This approach has the limitation that a static model may become obsolete when the conditions in which it was applicable change, for example, changes in the characteristics of a hospital's patient population. This limitation has led to the development of **adaptive AI-CDS** in which the CDS is dynamic in that it can learn and change performance over time, incorporating new data and new methods for learning from data [8]. An adaptive CDS that predicts the risk of cardiovascular disease would refine the predictive model in several ways: for example, the model might be slightly different at each institution where it is deployed, reflecting geographic or population variations, or an institution's model may be continuously updated based on more recent data from that institution.

Machine Learning and Data-Derived AI-CDS Systems As described in the previous section, data-derived models typically consist of structural and numerical components. While most models are derived automatically from data using ML approaches, they can be hand-crafted by human experts or constructed by a hybrid process where the model structure is hand-crafted, and the numerical component is derived automatically from data. ML models capture patterns in data, and these patterns are often used to make predictions and also may lead to the discovery of new knowledge. ML methods can be categorized broadly into supervised, unsupervised, semi-supervised, deep, and causal learning (see also Chap. 6).

Supervised ML leverages data that contain cases that consist of input variables (such as symptoms, signs, and laboratory test values) and corresponding output labels (such as the presence or absence of myocardial infarction). By analyzing the patterns in the data, supervised ML constructs a model that seeks to produce the correct output when provided with the input on new cases. When the output is discrete and has a limited number of labels (e.g., presence or absence of myocardial infarction), the supervised ML is called classification. When the output is numerical and has a large number of values (e.g., height), the supervised ML is called regression.

In contrast to supervised ML, **unsupervised ML** uses data that contain cases with only input variables but no output labels. Unsupervised ML infers patterns in the data such as clusters, outliers, and low-dimensional representations. Clusters are groups of cases that are similar in some way. Outliers are cases that are very different from the other cases in the data. Low-dimensional representations represent cases with a smaller number of features (variables) than are present in the raw data.

Semi-supervised ML is concerned with learning from a combination of data that contain outputs (e.g., diagnostic labels) and data that do not. This type of ML extends the applicability of both supervised and unsupervised ML, which traditionally can use only labeled and unlabeled data, respectively.

The current advances in ML are largely driven by **deep learning,** which involves training artificial neural networks with many layers on large amounts of data. Compared to the other types of ML described so far, deep learning has the advantage of automatically selecting relevant features in the data, creating complex features from simpler ones, and deriving a large number of relations, both simple and complex, from big datasets.

Another advance in ML that is particularly applicable to medicine is **personalized ML**. The typical ML approach is to derive a single model from training data, such that the model is optimized to perform well on average on all future individuals. This **population ML** approach has been quite successful; however, it may ignore important differences among patients, such as differences in the mechanisms causing disease or in treatment response. An approach for better capturing individual differences is personalized ML, where the model is tailored to the characteristics of the current individual and is optimized to perform especially well for that individual, but not necessarily for all future patients [9–11]. For example, the breast cancer of a current patient may have a mutation W that is highly predictive of the cancer course, although it is rare. A mutation X is much more common in the breast cancer population; however, it is only modestly predictive. A population model is likely to include X as a predictor, but not W, because mutation X is so common. That model would predict the cancer course of the current patient only fairly well. In contrast, a personalized model would likely include W as a predictor and predict the cancer course quite well.

Causal ML is concerned with modeling and discovering causal relationships [12, 13]. Such relationships predict the values of one or more variables after we *set* the values of other variables independently. Such predictions are important when making decisions to optimize expected outcomes, as is common in healthcare. For example, deciding on the best therapy for a patient involves making causal predictions. In contrast, most of the research and methods in ML have focused on learning models that predict one or more variables after we *observe* the values of other variables. Patient diagnosis in light of existing patient information is an example of an observational prediction.

Sometimes correct causal and observational predictions yield the same answers, but other times they do not. Figure 10.2a shows a situation in which X causally influences Y, and there are no other sources of statistical dependence between X and Y. In this example, the causal prediction of Y given that we independently set X equals the prediction of Y given that we observe X. In such a scenario, we can estimate model parameters using observational data and apply the resulting model to make causal predictions. Figure 10.2b is an example in which the causal and observational predictions differ, due to the presence of a hidden (latent) variable H. Here the observational prediction of Y given that we observe X is determined by the association due to X directly causing Y and association due to the path from X to H to Y, which is not due to X causing Y. In contrast, the causal prediction of Y given that we independently set $X = x$ [13] involves the situation shown in Fig. 10.2c. By independently setting X, we break the non-causal source of association between X and Y that goes through H, and we predict Y based only on the causal influence of X on Y [14].

For most of the past century, the predominant, formal method for causal discovery in healthcare and beyond has been the randomized controlled trial (RCT) [15]. By randomizing the setting of the value of X (e.g., a treatment selection), its value

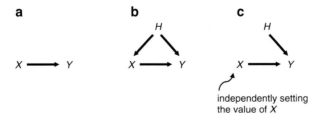

Fig. 10.2 Examples of causal Bayesian networks. X and Y are measured variables. H is a hidden (latent) variable. (**a**) X causally influences Y, and there is no confounding. (**b**) X causally influences Y, and there is hidden confounding. (**c**) Independently setting X removes the hidden confounding of X and Y

is set independently of the values of any of the other measured variables; thus, for example, the situation in Fig. 10.1c results, where the only dependency between X and Y is due to direct causation. On the other hand, RCTs are often expensive, sometimes infeasible, and frequently they study only a small, selected subset of patients, relative to the broader population of interest. Conversely, observational data, such as EHR data, are relatively plentiful, contain a rich variety of types of information, and more faithfully represent "real-world populations." However, care must be taken in deriving causal knowledge solely from observational data. A commonly used causal model is the causal Bayesian network, which is a Bayesian network in which a directed edge from X to Y represents that X is a direct cause of Y, relative to a set of modeled variables (as, for example, in Fig. 10.2).

ML methods have been developed that derive causal models from data, including observational-only data, or from a combination of knowledge and data. For instance, methods exist for learning Bayesian networks from expert knowledge and data [16, 17]. Expert knowledge could define an initial model for a system that provides diagnostic, prognostic, or therapeutic advice, for example. As data accumulate, the model adapts to represent the causal relationships consistent with the data. Causal modeling could also support the development of adaptive CDS systems. In the context of a given clinical task, such a system could compare its causal model of a domain with its model of a clinician's causal knowledge of the domain to provide advice to the clinician that optimally augments what he or she is likely to already know [18, 19].

Degree of Automation in AI-CDS

The early AI-CDS systems were standalone; the clinician interacted with the system by manually providing relevant patient data as input and then incorporating the system's output with their judgment to make clinical decisions. The widespread adoption of EHR systems has enabled increased integration of AI-CDS with such systems. AI-CDS may be integrated with EHR systems to a varying extent that enables the AI-CDS to obtain inputs automatically from the EHR, make recommendations, and provide those recommendations to the clinician and output them to the EHR (see Fig. 10.3).

Based on the degree of automation and integration with EHR systems, AI-CDS can be broadly categorized into three types [20]. In conventional AI-CDS, the CDS system collects patient data from the EHR and provides recommendations that the clinician receives, clarifies and considers in making the final decision. In integrative AI-CDS, the CDS system actively obtains patient data from the EHR, provides recommendations to the clinician, and also automatically records them in the EHR. The clinician still makes the final decision. In fully automated AI-CDS, the CDS system gathers information about and from a patient, makes decisions autonomously, and records results in the EHR. The clinician may monitor the recommendations and clarify the CDS system's recommendations. For some clinical tasks, fully automated decision support may be suitable, for example, some steps in robotic

Fig. 10.3 Categories of AI-CDS based on the degree of automation and integration with EHR systems. (**a**) Conventional AI-CDS obtains patient data from the EHR system and provides recommendations to the clinician who makes decisions. (**b**) Integrative AI-CDS obtains patient data from the EHR system, provides recommendations to the clinician, and records them in the EHR system. (**c**) Fully automated AI-CDS collects information from the patient, makes decisions, and records them in the EHR system

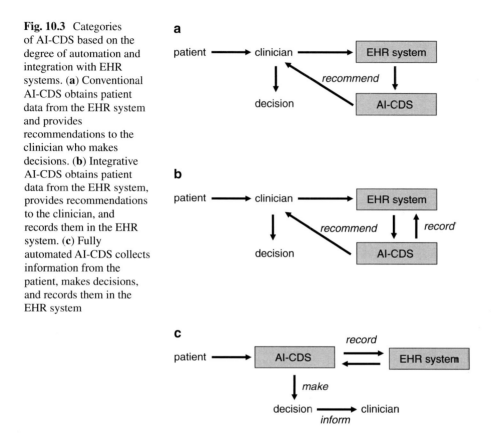

surgery or in insulin dose adjustments by an insulin pump; in many more tasks, however, integrative decision support will be more practical in the foreseeable future with the final decisions made by the clinician.

AI-CDS systems are often based on an input-process-output workflow. Inputs can come from various sources such as data from EHR and medical imaging systems and devices such as mobile smartphones, Fitbit, Apple, and other health trackers (see Box 10.1). Outputs can be delivered in many ways. Examples include diagnoses, recommendations, alerts and reminders, order sets, relevant medical knowledge, and context-aware summaries (see Box 10.1).

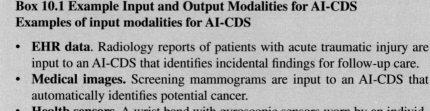

Box 10.1 Example Input and Output Modalities for AI-CDS
Examples of input modalities for AI-CDS

- **EHR data**. Radiology reports of patients with acute traumatic injury are input to an AI-CDS that identifies incidental findings for follow-up care.
- **Medical images.** Screening mammograms are input to an AI-CDS that automatically identifies potential cancer.
- **Health sensors.** A wrist band with gyroscopic sensors worn by an individual at risk for fall provides input to an AI-CDS that automatically detects falls.

Examples of output modalities for AI-CDS

- **Highlighting in EHR.** An AI-CDS identifies important new patient data in the EHR and highlights them to the clinician.
- **Alerts.** On detecting strokes in CT images of the brain, an AI-CDS sends alerts to stroke clinicians.
- **Discharge summaries.** An AI-CDS automatically generates discharge summaries to support communication during the transition of care from hospital to community care.

Application of AI-CDS in Clinical Care

As described in the section on "Challenges Faced by Clinicians", clinicians face challenges in the daily practice of medicine that arise from the exponential growth of medical knowledge, rapid accumulation of a diversity of patient data, and the increased complexity of clinical decision-making. Clinicians perform a range of tasks, such as assessing the risk of developing a disease in the future (risk assessment and stratification), determining the presence or absence of disease at the current time (diagnosis), forecasting the likely course of disease (prognosis), predicting treatment response (therapeutics), and monitoring in acute care, such as in critical care and during surgery, as well as outside the hospital for chronic diseases (see Chaps. 11, 12, and 14). The remainder of this section provides examples of areas of rapid progress in the development of AI-CDS.

Providing Relevant Medical Knowledge Studies have shown that clinicians have knowledge needs in many aspects of clinical decision-making, including diagnosis, prognosis, and therapy during patient encounters [21]. CDS systems have been developed that provide relevant medical knowledge at the right time and at the right place, such as the **Infobutton** that collates medical knowledge from the literature, textbooks, and other sources of information and presents knowledge relevant to a particular clinical context [22]. More recently, AI-CDS approaches have been described for generating medical evidence for treatments in a specific clinical context when such knowledge is lacking in the medical literature or in published treatment guidelines. One approach to this situation that has been described is to generate evidence from the EHR and other health utilization data of similar patients [23]. For a clinical question, the approach specifies the relevant population, intervention, comparator, outcome, and timeframe to select data from a large database such as a hospital's EHR data warehouse, which is used for treatment-effect estimation and survival analysis. However, such estimates may be subject to bias due to idiosyncrasies in the hospital's EHR data and due to hidden confounding and selection bias.

Prioritization of Patient Data In a specific clinical context, relevant patient data should be readily available for optimal decision-making. However, in current EHR systems, retrieval of patient data relevant to a clinical task is cumbersome and time-consuming, exacerbated by confusing layouts, workflows, poor prioritization, and weak search capabilities. Clinicians spend substantial amounts of time searching large volumes of data to identify clinically meaningful patterns and important patient details, predisposing them to information overload. AI-CDS systems are needed that intelligently identify and display clinically relevant patient data that enhance the clinician's ability to rapidly assess the clinical context and make optimal decisions. The learning electronic medical record (LEMR) system uses ML models to highlight data and are trained from output labels that clinicians have identified in past patient cases. In a research study, the LEMR system was able to identify and highlight salient patient information to summarize the clinical status of the patient for morning rounds in the critical care setting (Fig. 10.4) [24].

Risk Assessment Data-derived AI-CDS is increasingly developed to predict the risk of developing a disease or monitor adverse clinical events. For example, a deep learning strategy that combines results from cognitive testing and magnetic resonance imaging (MRI) of the brain predicts the risk of developing Alzheimer's disease [25]. As another example, an ML-based system that predicts the risk of hypoxemia in the near future and explains the risk factors during general anesthesia was developed to aid anesthesiologists in early intervention [26].

Diagnosis The application of ML and deep learning approaches for diagnosis in medical imaging has rapidly grown in recent years in the areas of radiology, ophthalmology, dermatology, pathology, cardiology, and gastroenterology. In radiology, clinicians rely primarily on imaging for diagnosis, and deep learning methods have rapidly improved the performance of diagnostic tasks in images. For example, the automated diagnosis of common lung diseases with chest radiography [27], the detection of lung nodules with computed tomography (CT) [28], and the identification of breast tumors using mammography [29] have achieved expert-level diagnostic accuracies. In dermatology, clinicians rely on visual inspection of skin lesions to diagnose and differentiate between benign and malignant lesions. For example, neural networks can identify malignant melanomas from a single photograph of the lesion at a dermatologist's level of accuracy [30]. In ophthalmology, fundus photographs are visually examined by ophthalmologists to detect and monitor various diseases, such as glaucoma and diabetic retinopathy. In a recent application of deep learning, neural network models were able to identify diabetic retinopathy at an accuracy comparable to that of ophthalmologists [31]. In pathology, histopathological assessment under the microscope of biopsied specimens by pathologists is used to diagnose many types of cancer. Deep learning models have been shown to be useful in detecting prostate cancer from biopsy specimens [32, 33] and identifying breast cancer metastasis in lymph nodes [34]. Cardiologists use electrocardiograms and echocardiograms, and deep learning methods have recently been shown to perform at expert-level accuracy for diagnosing heart attacks, as well as cardiac abnormalities like hypertrophic cardiomyopathy, from electrocardiograms [35]. Identification of small polyps during colonoscopy is an arduous task for gastroen-

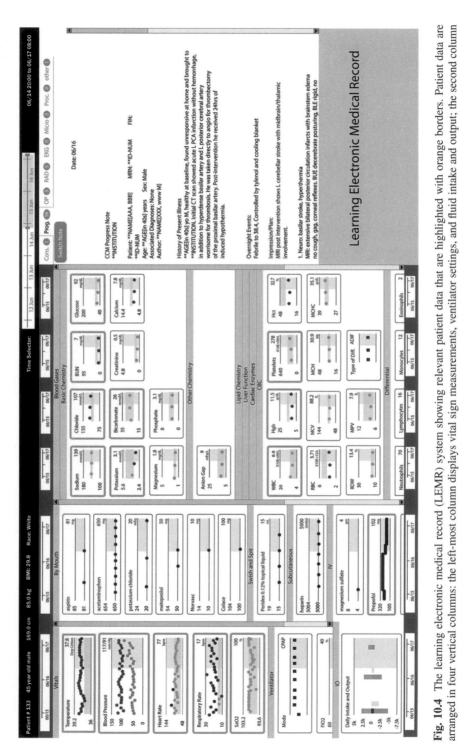

Fig. 10.4 The learning electronic medical record (LEMR) system showing relevant patient data that are highlighted with orange borders. Patient data are arranged in four vertical columns: the left-most column displays vital sign measurements, ventilator settings, and fluid intake and output; the second column shows medication administrations; the third column displays laboratory test results; and the right-most column displays free-text notes and reports. Names have been removed, and the demographic data and dates have been changed to preserve patient confidentiality

terologists. Recently, an ML-based approach that identifies polyps in images from a colonoscopic camera was shown to enhance the clinician's speed and accuracy of detecting polyps during colonoscopy [36, 37]. The future translation into clinical applications of the successful application of AI, especially deep learning for image-based diagnosis, will significantly change current medical practice. Curt Langlotz, a pioneer in AI in radiology, posed the question, "Will AI ever replace radiologists?" then answered, "I say no – but radiologists who use AI will replace radiologists who don't" [38].

Early diagnosis of rapidly developing clinical conditions is another area of abundant application of ML approaches. For example, in critical care, early diagnosis of sepsis using ML models has been shown to be more accurate than traditional tools such as the quick Sepsis Related Organ Failure Assessment (SOFA) score [39].

Prediction of Clinical Outcomes Prediction of clinical outcomes with ML has grown rapidly with the increased availability of large volumes of EHR and health insurance claims data. ML models can learn the patterns of health trajectories from EHR and other data of a large number of individuals, and such models can antici-pate future events at an expert clinical level. For example, accurately forecasting the likely clinical course in a patient with community-acquired pneumonia enables decision-making about whether to treat the patient as an inpatient or as an outpatient [11]. Similar ML-based forecasting can identify recently discharged patients who are likely to develop complications requiring readmission or patients who are at risk for prolonged hospitalization [40]. Such information can be used proactively to pro-vide additional resources or initiate more intensive management. Furthermore, Bayesian networks have been developed to predict mortality, readmission, and length of hospital stay using EHRs from the emergency department [41], and deep learning applications have been developed to predict in-hospital mortality, 30-day readmissions, and prolonged length of hospital stay [40]. ML has also been applied to identify patient characteristics in the medical notes to classify cancer patients with different responses to chemotherapy [42].

Therapy Therapeutic CDS systems that aid in choosing the best therapy have been developed since the inception of CDS systems. One of the earliest such systems was MYCIN (see Chap. 2), a rule-based system that uses backward chaining inference to identify causative bacteria in infections and recommend appropriate antibiotics and dosages. Examples of AI-CDS are found in the field of radiomics that use AI-based analyses of clinical images to characterize tumor phenotypes and predict treatment response. For example, a deep learning approach using radiomic features in CT scans of non-small cell lung cancer was able to predict treatment response to various therapeutic agents [43].

Alerting Alerting CDS systems have been developed for a long time to draw the clinician's attention to the important data at the right time. One of the earliest such systems was the **HELP** system that was developed at LDS Hospital in Salt Lake City in the 1960s and generated automated alerts about abnormalities in patient data

[44]. Several alerting AI-CDS systems have been described in recent years. A deep learning approach has been developed and deployed that sends alerts to stroke clinicians on detecting strokes in CT images of the brain [45]. More recently, an ML approach for detecting anomalous patient-management decisions in the critical care unit was developed and evaluated at the University of Pittsburgh [46].

Patient Monitoring In-hospital patient monitoring is an essential clinical activity in operating rooms, intensive care units, and emergency rooms. Real-time detection of critical events from data generated by monitoring devices is an area where ML is increasingly applied. For example, ML methods can identify seizures from continuous electroencephalographic monitoring [47]. As another example, such methods can predict hypoxemia events during surgery from continuous physiological monitoring [26]. These results suggest that the application of ML methods to continuous patient-monitoring data can achieve accurate and timely predictions, thus relieving information overload on clinicians.

Clinical Data Capture A significant contributor to clinician frustration and burnout is the undue length of time spent in documenting encounters, often at the cost of decreased time spent interacting with patients. Clinical scribes, who work alongside clinicians to translate and record information in clinical encounters, were introduced to reduce the burden of documentation on clinicians. More recently, digital scribes that leverage speech recognition and natural language processing are being developed to capture and document the spoken portions of the clinical encounter automatically [48]. Advances in **human-computer interaction** technologies, such as speech and gesture recognition and ambient listening and seeing, will likely lead to the development of autonomous digital scribe systems that allow clinicians to migrate from interacting with a standalone computer to speaking in an intelligent room where the environment itself becomes the automated scribe.

Pitfalls of AI-CDS

In a recent application of ML to detect pneumonia in chest X-rays, the ML model performed successfully, detecting pneumonia with an accuracy of 93% when the model was evaluated on a different batch of X-rays at the institution where the model was developed. However, when the model was evaluated on a batch of X-rays from a different institution, its performance in detecting pneumonia fell to 73% [49]. It was subsequently found that the X-rays of pneumonia had been mostly taken from very sick patients lying down with portable chest X-ray machines, and X-rays of patients lying down look very different from X-rays of patients who are standing up, and the model had learned to discriminate between X-rays of patients lying down from standing up, rather than identifying features of pneumonia. This is an example of a pitfall of data-derived AI-CDS due to an inadvertently introduced bias in the data that was used to derive the ML model. Translation of ML research into clinically robust AI-CDS requires mitigating a range of such pitfalls.

AI-CDS has significant pitfalls that include dataset shift, algorithmic bias, automation complacency and inscrutable explanations. We discuss each of these problems in the remainder of this section.

Dataset shift is a common pitfall in ML that occurs when data characteristics differ between the training phase and the application or deployment phase. It is common and occurs for reasons that range from the bias in the training data to the application of the ML system to an inappropriate clinical context. The availability of high-quality training data may be limited if, for example, portions of the data need manual review by experts, if the outcome is poorly defined, or the available data are a convenience sample that is not representative of the entire population. Sometimes, dataset shift is introduced by the process of training; for example, the training data may have been adjusted to contain an equal number of cases and controls to maximize the performance of the ML system; however, at application time, it is rarely the situation in medicine that the condition of interest occurs 50% of the time.

Dataset shifts are common across locations and across time. Thus, ML models developed at one location may perform poorly at a different location because disease patterns are different across the two locations. Further, even within the same healthcare system, models that are developed from data on patients who attend a specialty clinic may perform poorly on the general population. For example, an ML model that is trained on photographs of skin lesions in a dermatology clinic may have lower accuracy when applied to patients seen in a primary care clinic where the appearance of lesions, and the risk profile of patients, are different.

Even at the same location, disease patterns can change over time, leading to a decrease in performance in the future. Models developed only from historical data will reinforce existing practice and may not reflect new medical developments and changes in policies and guidelines. For example, an AI-CDS system might erroneously recommend a drug after it has been withdrawn due to safety concerns or will not recommend a medication appropriately whose use has been expanded to the treatment of new conditions.

It is important to monitor and update ML models because unanticipated dataset shifts will almost certainly occur, and the performance of deployed models is likely to deteriorate. Thus, AI methods are needed to detect when shifts have occurred, identify the nature of the shifts, and continually update the models using more recent data.

Algorithmic bias refers to errors in an AI-CDS that systematically underperform for one group of individuals relative to others. Algorithmic bias exacerbates existing inequities in socioeconomic status, race, ethnic background, religion, gender, disability, and sexual orientation, and it may amplify inequities in healthcare systems. Bias arises due to many factors; however, the common problem is that the data used in training ML models often do not represent the whole population, leading to poor performance in underrepresented groups. Most data used for ML are observational data that are often limited by low diversity in race, gender, geographical location, economic conditions, and other important attributes. Training with such biased data can lead to biased ML models that are not valid for parts of the population, and the application of such models has the potential to exacerbate existing healthcare disparities.

As examples, ML models trained with gender-imbalanced data perform poorly at reading chest X-rays for the underrepresented gender [50]; and ML models trained primarily on light-skinned individuals perform poorly in detecting skin cancer affecting individuals with darker skin [51]. A recent study reviewed over 70 publications and noted that most of the data used to train ML models came from just three states in the United States [52], suggesting the potential for geographic bias. As another example, a commercial risk model for predicting future risk of needing complex healthcare exhibited racial bias. For the same level of predicted risk, black patients were found to be sicker than white patients because the model was trained on healthcare costs as a proxy for healthcare needs. Since less money had been spent on black patients who have the same level of need, the model inaccurately predicted that black patients are healthier than white patients [53].

Beyond problems with the data, algorithmic bias can arise at any point in the development of an AI-CDS system from data collection and cleaning, model choice, the protocol used in training and evaluation, and implementation and dissemination. Preventing algorithmic bias requires that the teams that develop AI-CDS include experts who have knowledge about how to prevent bias and not simply data scientists who are technical experts in ML. Particularly, clinicians and even patients should be included in the teams, as they can provide deep insights into the clinical context [54].

Automation Complacency With the deployment of autopilots in aircrafts and, more recently, in automobiles, it has been observed that pilots often failed to monitor important flight indicators, and drivers in autonomous automobiles frequently failed to watch the road. Similar behavior has been noted to occur with clinicians using AI-CDS systems. If an AI-CDS system were completely accurate and reliable, then clearly following its recommendations would lead to positive outcomes; however, practical AI-CDS systems are not perfect and can increase errors if incorrect advice is followed. Over-dependence on CDS in conjunction with reduced vigilance in information seeking and processing is termed automation complacency, which can lead to errors that would not normally occur in the absence of CDS [55]. Automation complacency can result in omission errors in which the clinician fails to consider relevant medical knowledge or patient information because the CDS did not recommend it, and commission errors where the clinician complies with incorrect CDS recommendations.

For example, an AI-CDS system that aids in detecting cancers in screening mammograms can increase the rate of cancer detection by uncovering those that the radiologist would otherwise miss. However, omission errors by the AI-CDS will result in cancers going undetected, and commission errors may result in individuals without cancers receiving unnecessary interventions [56]. Similar errors due to automation complacency occur in the computerized interpretation of electrocardiograms [57], decision support in e-prescribing [58], and answering questions about clinical scenarios [59].

The factors causing automation complacency are multifactorial; they include complex tasks that impose a greater cognitive load, low clinician experience with a task, and high trust in the AI-CDS system, especially as familiarity with the system grows over time. Mitigating automation complacency is a challenging, open problem, and interventions, such as providing clinicians with information on the AI-CDS system's reliability, have had little impact. One potential solution to this problem is having an AI-CDS that balances sometimes offering advice upfront with sometimes only offering critiques post facto.

Inscrutable Recommendations With the increasing complexity of AI models that underlie CDS, explanations that describe the basis of recommendations or predictions are important to detect error or bias, as well as to engender trust in the system (see Chaps. 1, 2, and especially Chap. 8). The insight that an explanation provides about why a patient is at high risk of developing a disease can help a clinician understand the reasoning, which helps gain trust in the AI-CDS system. In knowledge-based AI-CDS, such as rule-based systems, and some ML models, such as classification trees, the reasons for the resulting predictions can be clearly explained. Other ML models, such as random forests and artificial neural networks, often perform better than earlier models, but their black-box nature makes their recommendations more inscrutable (see Chap. 8).

A wide range of methods, which can be broadly categorized into ante-hoc and posthoc approaches, are being developed to provide explanations for AI-CDS systems. In the ante-hoc approach, the AI-CDS system is designed to be interpretable, and such systems have a long tradition in medicine and are created from expert knowledge and employ human-AI interaction. For example, MYCIN was designed as a consultation system with explanatory capabilities to advise clinicians on diagnosing and treating bacterial infections. The MYCIN system conducts a question-and-answer dialog to elicit relevant patient data, and the execution of the rules forms a coherent explanation of MYCIN's reasoning [60].

Posthoc approaches aim to provide explanations for a specific recommendation and are more applicable to modern ML models that are not designed for interpretability (see Chap. 8). For example, in deep learning-based AI-CDS systems for medical imaging, a post-hoc approach uses saliency maps. In a saliency map, the explanation highlights the salient regions in the image that are important to the system's recommendation, such as the regions on the chest X-ray or the picture of a skin lesion that most contributed to the recommendation. Beyond image analysis model-agnostic explanatory methods that focus on explaining individual recommendations of a black-box ML model have been developed. Examples of such methods include Local Interpretable Model-Agnostic Explanations (LIME) [61] and SHapley Additive exPlanations (SHAP) [62]; these methods estimate the impact of input features for a specific prediction from analysis of the behavior of the model when the inputs are varied.

Regulation of AI-CDS

As AI-CDS systems become more complex, automated, and adaptive, they will surpass the ability of clinicians to independently verify their veracity, which makes regulatory oversight vital to shield patients from the pitfalls of such systems (see also Chap. 18). Depending on the complexity, the regulatory requirements for AI-CDS can range from none at all to substantial compliance burden. For example, in the outpatient clinic, a clinician receives a CDS recommendation to offer colonoscopy for a patient who is 45 years of age. The clinician can easily verify the accuracy of the recommendation, given the U.S. Preventive Services Task Force guidelines on which the recommendation is based. Such a CDS system would not require regulation.

In contrast, consider an AI-CDS system that uses an ML model to recognize cardiopulmonary instability from continuous physiological monitoring of the cardiac and respiratory systems. Such a system may be deployed in the critical care unit to monitor and predict the elevated risk of cardiopulmonary instability, and a prediction of elevated risk may lead to decisions such as initiation of medication to increase the blood pressure or mechanical ventilation. In this situation, the clinician cannot readily assess the accuracy of the assessment provided by the AI-CDS, and such a system would need to be regulated to ensure patient safety.

AI-CDS systems consist of software, and software may be deemed a medical device if it is used to guide clinical decision-making. The U.S. Food and Drug Administration (FDA) has created guidelines for regulating Software as a Medical Device (SaMD) that encompasses AI-CDS. The FDA guidelines are based on recommendations from the International Medical Device Regulators Forum (IMDRF), an international group of medical device regulators that develops guidelines for the uniform regulation of medical products worldwide.

There are many important factors in the regulatory framework of AI-CDS, including risk assessment, unbiased training, reproducibility, and whether the AI methods in the CDS are static vs. adaptive. The FDA provides a framework for the clinical evaluation of SaMD that is adopted from the IMDRF. The goal of the clinical evaluation is to assess a SaMD's clinical safety, effectiveness, and performance as intended by the developer of the SaMD. The clinical evaluation consists of three components that include scientific validity, analytical validation, and clinical validation (see Table 10.1). A SaMD must pass all three components successfully to be considered validated. Further, following the IMDR, the FDA stratifies SaMD into four risk levels based on the intended medical purpose of the SaMD (treat or

Table 10.1 Components of clinical evaluation of Software as a Medical Device (SaMD)

Clinical evaluation		
Valid clinical association (scientific validity)	Analytical validation	Clinical validation
Is there a valid clinical association between the SaMD's output and the SaMD's targeted clinical condition?	Does the SaMD correctly process input data to generate accurate, reliable, and precise output data?	Does the use of SaMD's accurate, reliable, and precise output data achieve the intended purpose in the target population in the context of clinical care?

Adapted from [63]

Table 10.2 Regulatory requirements for Software as a Medical Device (SaMD) by the intended medical purpose and the nature of the patient's condition

Nature of the patient's condition	Intended medical purpose		
	Treat or diagnose	Drive clinical management	Inform clinical management
Critical	IV	III	II
Serious	III	II	I
Non-serious	II	I	I

I: least regulatory requirements, IV: greatest regulatory requirements. Adapted from [63]

Table 10.3 Examples of AI-CDS that have received FDA clearance as SaMDs

Name of device or algorithm	Name of parent company	Short description	FDA approval number	Date	Medical specialty
Arterys Cardio DL	Arterys Inc	Analysis of cardiovascular magnetic resonance images	K163253	2016/11	Cardiology
ContaCT	Viz.ai	Automated stroke detection on CT images	DEN170073	2018/02	Radiology
EyeArt	Eyenuk, Inc	Automated detection of diabetic retinopathy on retinal fundal images	K200667	2020/06	Ophthalmology

diagnose, drive clinical management, inform clinical management) and the nature of the patient's condition (critical, serious, non-serious). A higher level of risk requires increased oversight, more regulatory requirements, and more evidence for the efficacy and safety of the SaMD (see Table 10.2).

The FDA certified the first AI-CDS system in 2016 when Arterys became the initial company to receive clearance to use deep learning in a clinical setting for the analyses of cardiovascular images. As of January 2021, a total of 71 AI-CDS systems have been cleared by the FDA as SaMDs. The largest number of AI-CDS systems certified by the FDA are in the fields of radiology and cardiology [64]. Table 10.3 provides examples of AI-CDS systems that have received FDA clearance.

Conclusions

CDS is at a critical juncture for the safe and effective integration of AI into clinical care. The technical capacity to develop, implement, and maintain AI-CDS in the clinical enterprise is increasing by leaps and bounds, and the promise of AI in clinical decision-making offers considerable opportunities to improve patient outcomes, reduce costs, and improve population health.

AI-CDS is poised to advance the learning health system in which clinical experience and patient data are systematically integrated to provide higher quality, safer, more efficient care. Clinical trials and similar research underlie one of the key ways of generating new knowledge and evidence for improving clinical care. The clinical enterprise of treating patients and the research enterprise of evaluating new therapies, for the most part, are segregated into two disparate enterprises. However, to realize the learning health system, there is a need to treat patients and evaluate therapies at the same time [65, 66]. In the future, AI-CDS systems will support patient care and support research tasks that include screening, enrollment, adaptive treatment assignment, data collection, and dynamic data analysis.

With new approaches for measuring and analyzing a wide range of biomedical data, including molecular, genomic, cellular, physiological, clinical, behavioral, and environmental data, ML models that power AI-CDS will integrate heterogeneous multimodal data to provide broader, more accurate and nuanced recommendations and predictions. As data is generated at increasing volumes and rates, adaptive AI-CDS systems will grow and continuously learn and adapt to optimize overall healthcare. Such systems will intelligently adapt to the patient (e.g., taking into account patient preferences and life circumstances), to the clinician (e.g., physician vs. nurse vs. pharmacists, etc.), to the clinical task (e.g., diagnosis, prognosis, medication reconciliation, etc.), and to the clinical context to help optimize the overall delivery of healthcare to individuals and society. Current AI-CDS systems collaborate very little, if at all, with clinician users, and as they begin to interact with thousands of users every day, human-AI cooperative systems will be increasingly developed [19].

Questions for Discussion

- What are the pros and cons of knowledge-based and data-derived AI-CDS? Discuss how to improve data-derived AI-CDS by incorporating biomedical knowledge.
- The current popular paradigm is to use big data (e.g., EHRs and billing data) to develop AI models for CDS. Describe the pitfalls of this paradigm and suggest methods to mitigate these pitfalls.
- The development of a new therapeutic (e.g., a drug or vaccine) involves rigorous assessment and validation of safety and efficacy. Do you agree that a new AI-CDS system should undergo a similar rigorous assessment and validation of safety and performance? Why or why not? How does validating an AI-CDS system differ from validating a new therapeutic? How does the nature of software complicate the application of traditional evaluation and regulation approaches?
- Hospitals typically have antimicrobial stewardship programs to monitor antibiotic prescribing and resistance patterns and to guide appropriate antimicrobial use. If you were the Chief Medical Information Officer of a large hospital that has deployed a large number of AI-CDS tools, propose the design for an AI-CDS stewardship program. What factors will you monitor and how will you accomplish doing so?

Further Reading

Greenes RA, editor. Clinical Decision Support: The Road Ahead. Elsevier; 2011 Apr 28. (Revised edition to be published in early 2023).

- This book provides a comprehensive description of the computational challenges in development of CDS systems and detailed discussions of their deployment.

Rajkomar A, Dean J, Kohane I. Machine learning in medicine. New England Journal of Medicine. 2019 Apr 4;380 (14):1347–58.

- This review provides an overview of the uses and key challenges of machine learning for clinical applications.

Topol EJ. High-performance medicine: The convergence of human and artificial intelligence. Nature Medicine. 2019 Jan;25 (1):44.

- This article surveys the clinical applications of AI and deep-learning and describes their impact on clinicians, patients, and health systems.

Montani S, Striani M. Artificial intelligence in clinical decision support: A focused literature survey. Yearbook of Medical Informatics. 2019 Aug;28 (1):120.

- This survey of the literature found data-driven AI to be prevalent in CDS either used independently or in conjunction with knowledge-based AI.

Challen R, Denny J, Pitt M, Gompels L, Edwards T, Tsaneva-Atanasova K. Artificial intelligence, bias and clinical safety. BMJ Quality & Safety. 2019 Mar 1;28 (3):231–7.

- This article provides an overview of short-term, medium-term, and long-term safety and quality issues related to clinical deployment of AI in medicine.

References

1. Osheroff JA, Teich JM, Middleton B, Steen EB, Wright A, Detmer DE. A roadmap for national action on clinical decision support. J Am Med Inform Assoc. 2007;14(2):141–5.
2. Densen P. Challenges and opportunities facing medical education. Trans Am Clin Climatol Assoc. 2011;122:48–58.
3. Manor-Shulman O, Beyene J, Frndova H, Parshuram CS. Quantifying the volume of documented clinical information in critical illness. J Crit Care. 2008;23(2):245–50.
4. Gal DB, Han B, Longhurst C, Scheinker D, Shin AY. Quantifying electronic health record data: a potential risk for cognitive overload. Hosp Pediatr. 2021;11(2):175–8.
5. Institute of Medicine. Evidence-based medicine and the changing nature of healthcare: 2007 IOM annual meeting summary. Washington, DC: National Academies Press (US); 2008.
6. Stead WW, Searle JR, Fessler HE, Smith JW, Shortliffe EH. Biomedical informatics: changing what physicians need to know and how they learn. Acad Med. 2011;86(4):429–34.
7. Arndt BG, Beasley JW, Watkinson MD, Temte JL, Tuan WJ, Sinsky CA, Gilchrist VJ. Tethered to the EHR: primary care physician workload assessment using EHR event log data and time-motion observations. Ann Fam Med. 2017;15(5):419–26.

8. Petersen C, Smith J, Freimuth RR, Goodman KW, Jackson GP, Kannry J, Liu H, Madhavan S, Sittig DF, Wright A. Recommendations for the safe, effective use of adaptive CDS in the US healthcare system: an AMIA position paper. J Am Med Inform Assoc. 2021;28(4):677–84.
9. Liu X, Wang Y, Ji H, Aihara K, Chen L. Personalized characterization of diseases using sample-specific networks. Nucleic Acids Res. 2016;44(22):e164.
10. Cai C, Cooper GF, Lu KN, Ma X, Xu S, Zhao Z, Chen X, Xue Y, Lee AV, Clark N, Chen V, Lu S, Chen L, Yu L, Hochheiser HS, Jiang X, Wang QJ, Lu X. Systematic discovery of the functional impact of somatic genome alterations in individual tumors through tumor-specific causal inference. PLoS Comput Biol. 2019;15(7):e1007088.
11. Visweswaran S, Angus DC, Hsieh M, Weissfeld L, Yealy D, Cooper GF. Learning patient-specific predictive models from clinical data. J Biomed Inform. 2010;43(5):669–85.
12. Beebee H, Hitchcock C, Menzies P. The Oxford handbook of causation. Oxford University Press; 2009.
13. Pearl J. Causality. Cambridge: Cambridge University Press; 2009.
14. Spirtes P, Glymour CN, Scheines R. Causation, prediction, and search. Cambridge, MA: MIT Press; 2000.
15. Fisher RA. The design of experiments. New York, NY: Hafner; 1951.
16. Heckerman D, Geiger D, Chickering DM. Learning Bayesian networks: the combination of knowledge and statistical data. Mach Learn. 1995;20(3):197–243.
17. Andrews B, Spirtes P, Cooper GF. On the completeness of causal discovery in the presence of latent confounding with tiered background knowledge. In: International conference on artificial intelligence and statistics. PMLR; 2020. p. 4002–11.
18. Rosenfeld A, Kraus S. Predicting human decision-making: from prediction to action. San Rafael, CA: Morgan & Claypool; 2018.
19. Dafoe A, Bachrach Y, Hadfield G, Horvitz E, Larson K, Graepel T. Cooperative AI: machines must learn to find common ground. Nature. 2021;593(7857):33–6.
20. Yu K-H, Beam AL, Kohane IS. Artificial intelligence in healthcare. Nat Biomed Eng. 2018;2(10):719–31.
21. Clarke MA, Belden JL, Koopman RJ, Steege LM, Moore JL, Canfield SM, Kim MS. Information needs and information-seeking behaviour analysis of primary care physicians and nurses: a literature review. Health Info Libr J. 2013;30(3):178–90.
22. Del Fiol G, Huser V, Strasberg HR, Maviglia SM, Curtis C, Cimino JJ. Implementations of the HL7 context-aware knowledge retrieval ("Infobutton") standard: challenges, strengths, limitations, and uptake. J Biomed Inform. 2012;45(4):726–35.
23. Gallego B, Walter SR, Day RO, Dunn AG, Sivaraman V, Shah N, Longhurst CA, Coiera E. Bringing cohort studies to the bedside: framework for a 'green button' to support clinical decision-making. J Comp Eff Res. 2015;4(3):191–7.
24. King AJ, Cooper GF, Clermont G, Hochheiser H, Hauskrecht M, Sittig DF, Visweswaran S. Using machine learning to selectively highlight patient information. J Biomed Inform. 2019;100:103327.
25. Qiu S, Joshi PS, Miller MI, Xue C, Zhou X, Karjadi C, Chang GH, Joshi AS, Dwyer B, Zhu S, Kaku M, Zhou Y, Alderazi YJ, Swaminathan A, Kedar S, Saint-Hilaire MH, Auerbach SH, Yuan J, Sartor EA, Au R, Kolachalama VB. Development and validation of an interpretable deep learning framework for Alzheimer's disease classification. Brain. 2020;143(6):1920–33.
26. Lundberg SM, Nair B, Vavilala MS, Horibe M, Eisses MJ, Adams T, Liston DE, Low DK, Newman SF, Kim J, Lee SI. Explainable machine-learning predictions for the prevention of hypoxaemia during surgery. Nat Biomed Eng. 2018;2(10):749–60.
27. Lakhani P, Sundaram B. Deep learning at chest radiography: automated classification of pulmonary tuberculosis by using convolutional neural networks. Radiology. 2017;284(2):574–82.
28. Rajpurkar P, Irvin J, Ball RL, Zhu K, Yang B, Mehta H, Duan T, Ding D, Bagul A, Langlotz CP, Patel BN, Yeom KW, Shpanskaya K, Blankenberg FG, Seekins J, Amrhein TJ, Mong DA, Halabi SS, Zucker EJ, Ng AY, Lungren MP. Deep learning for chest radiograph diagnosis: a retrospective comparison of the CheXNeXt algorithm to practicing radiologists. PLoS Med. 2018;15(11):e1002686.

29. Arevalo J, Gonzalez FA, Ramos-Pollan R, Oliveira JL, Guevara Lopez MA. Convolutional neural networks for mammography mass lesion classification. In: Annual International Conference of the IEEE Engineering in Medicine and Biology Society, vol. 2015; 2015. p. 797–800.
30. Esteva A, Kuprel B, Novoa RA, Ko J, Swetter SM, Blau HM, Thrun S. Dermatologist-level classification of skin cancer with deep neural networks. Nature. 2017;542(7639):115–8.
31. Gulshan V, Peng L, Coram M, Stumpe MC, Wu D, Narayanaswamy A, Venugopalan S, Widner K, Madams T, Cuadros J, Kim R, Raman R, Nelson PC, Mega JL, Webster DR. Development and validation of a deep learning algorithm for detection of diabetic retinopathy in retinal fundus photographs. JAMA. 2016;316(22):2402–10.
32. Bulten W, Pinckaers H, van Boven H, Vink R, de Bel T, van Ginneken B, van der Laak J, Hulsbergen-van de Kaa C, Litjens G. Automated deep-learning system for Gleason grading of prostate cancer using biopsies: a diagnostic study. Lancet Oncol. 2020;21(2):233–41.
33. Ström P, Kartasalo K, Olsson H, Solorzano L, Delahunt B, Berney DM, Bostwick DG, Evans AJ, Grignon DJ, Humphrey PA, Iczkowski KA, Kench JG, Kristiansen G, van der Kwast TH, Leite KRM, McKenney JK, Oxley J, Pan CC, Samaratunga H, Srigley JR, Takahashi H, Tsuzuki T, Varma M, Zhou M, Lindberg J, Lindskog C, Ruusuvuori P, Wählby C, Grönberg H, Rantalainen M, Egevad L, Eklund M. Artificial intelligence for diagnosis and grading of prostate cancer in biopsies: a population-based, diagnostic study. Lancet Oncol. 2020;21(2):222–32.
34. Liu Y, Kohlberger T, Norouzi M, Dahl GE, Smith JL, Mohtashamian A, Olson N, Peng LH, Hipp JD, Stumpe MC. Artificial intelligence-based breast cancer nodal metastasis detection: insights into the black box for pathologists. Arch Pathol Lab Med. 2019;143(7):859–68.
35. Zhang J, Gajjala S, Agrawal P, Tison GH, Hallock LA, Beussink-Nelson L, Lassen MH, Fan E, Aras MA, Jordan C, Fleischmann KE, Melisko M, Qasim A, Shah SJ, Bajcsy R, Deo RC. Fully automated echocardiogram interpretation in clinical practice. Circulation. 2018;138(16):1623–35.
36. Mori Y, Kudo SE, Misawa M, Saito Y, Ikematsu H, Hotta K, Ohtsuka K, Urushibara F, Kataoka S, Ogawa Y, Maeda Y, Takeda K, Nakamura H, Ichimasa K, Kudo T, Hayashi T, Wakamura K, Ishida F, Inoue H, Itoh H, Oda M, Mori K. Real-time use of artificial intelligence in identification of diminutive polyps during colonoscopy: a prospective study. Ann Intern Med. 2018;169(6):357–66.
37. Wang P, Xiao X, Glissen Brown JR, Berzin TM, Tu M, Xiong F, Hu X, Liu P, Song Y, Zhang D, Yang X, Li L, He J, Yi X, Liu J, Liu X. Development and validation of a deep-learning algorithm for the detection of polyps during colonoscopy. Nat Biomed Eng. 2018;2(10):741–8.
38. Center for Artificial Intelligence in Medicine & Imaging. RSNA 2017: Rads who use AI will replace rads who don't. 2021. https://aimi.stanford.edu/news/rsna-2017-rads-who-use-ai-will-replace-rads-who-don-t.
39. Shimabukuro DW, Barton CW, Feldman MD, Mataraso SJ, Das R. Effect of a machine learning-based severe sepsis prediction algorithm on patient survival and hospital length of stay: a randomised clinical trial. BMJ Open Respir Res. 2017;4(1):e000234.
40. Rajkomar A, Oren E, Chen K, Dai AM, Hajaj N, Hardt M, Liu PJ, Liu X, Marcus J, Sun M, Sundberg P, Yee H, Zhang K, Zhang Y, Flores G, Duggan GE, Irvine J, Le Q, Litsch K, Mossin A, Tansuwan J, Wang D, Wexler J, Wilson J, Ludwig D, Volchenboum SL, Chou K, Pearson M, Madabushi S, Shah NH, Butte AJ, Howell MD, Cui C, Corrado GS, Dean J. Scalable and accurate deep learning with electronic health records. NPJ Digit Med. 2018;1:18.
41. Cai X, Perez-Concha O, Coiera E, Martin-Sanchez F, Day R, Roffe D, Gallego B. Real-time prediction of mortality, readmission, and length of stay using electronic health record data. J Am Med Inform Assoc. 2016;23(3):553–61.
42. Ng T, Chew L, Yap CW. A clinical decision support tool to predict survival in cancer patients beyond 120 days after palliative chemotherapy. J Palliat Med. 2012;15(8):863–9.
43. Coroller TP, Agrawal V, Narayan V, Hou Y, Grossmann P, Lee SW, Mak RH, Aerts HJ. Radiomic phenotype features predict pathological response in non-small cell lung cancer. Radiother Oncol. 2016;119(3):480–6.

44. Pryor TA, Gardner RM, Clayton PD, Warner HR. The HELP system. J Med Syst. 1983;7(2):87–102.
45. FDA approves stroke-detecting AI software. Nat Biotechnol. 2018;36(4):290.
46. Hauskrecht M, Batal I, Hong C, Nguyen Q, Cooper GF, Visweswaran S, Clermont G. Outlier-based detection of unusual patient-management actions: an ICU study. J Biomed Inform. 2016;64:211–21.
47. Siddiqui MK, Morales-Menendez R, Huang X, Hussain N. A review of epileptic seizure detection using machine learning classifiers. Brain Inform. 2020;7(1):5.
48. Coiera E, Kocaballi B, Halamka J, Laranjo L. The digital scribe. NPJ Digit Med. 2018;1:58.
49. Zech JR, Badgeley MA, Liu M, Costa AB, Titano JJ, Oermann EK. Variable generalization performance of a deep learning model to detect pneumonia in chest radiographs: a cross-sectional study. PLoS Med. 2018;15(11):e1002683.
50. Larrazabal AJ, Nieto N, Peterson V, Milone DH, Ferrante E. Gender imbalance in medical imaging datasets produces biased classifiers for computer-aided diagnosis. Proc Natl Acad Sci U S A. 2020;117(23):12592–4.
51. Adamson AS, Smith A. Machine learning and health care disparities in dermatology. JAMA Dermatol. 2018;154(11):1247–8.
52. Kaushal A, Altman R, Langlotz C. Geographic distribution of US cohorts used to train deep learning algorithms. JAMA. 2020;324(12):1212–3.
53. Obermeyer Z, Powers B, Vogeli C, Mullainathan S. Dissecting racial bias in an algorithm used to manage the health of populations. Science. 2019;366(6464):447–53.
54. Panch T, Mattie H, Atun R. Artificial intelligence and algorithmic bias: implications for health systems. J Glob Health. 2019;9(2):010318.
55. Parasuraman R, Wickens CD. Humans: still vital after all these years of automation. Hum Factors. 2008;50(3):511–20.
56. Povyakalo AA, Alberdi E, Strigini L, Ayton P. How to discriminate between computer-aided and computer-hindered decisions: a case study in mammography. Med Decis Making. 2013;33(1):98–107.
57. Bond RR, Novotny T, Andrsova I, Koc L, Sisakova M, Finlay D, Guldenring D, McLaughlin J, Peace A, McGilligan V, Leslie SJ, Wang H, Malik M. Automation bias in medicine: the influence of automated diagnoses on interpreter accuracy and uncertainty when reading electrocardiograms. J Electrocardiol. 2018;51(6s):S6–s11.
58. Lyell D, Magrabi F, Raban MZ, Pont LG, Baysari MT, Day RO, Coiera E. Automation bias in electronic prescribing. BMC Med Inform Decis Mak. 2017;17(1):28.
59. Golchin K, Roudsari A. Study of the effects of clinical decision support system's incorrect advice and clinical case difficulty on users' decision making accuracy. Stud Health Technol Inform. 2011;164:13–6.
60. Buchanan BG, Shortliffe EH. Rule-based expert systems: the MYCIN experiments of the Stanford heuristic programming project. Addison-Wesley; 1985.
61. Ribeiro MT, Singh S, Guestrin C. "Why should I trust you?" explaining the predictions of any classifier. In: Proceedings of the 22nd ACM SIGKDD International conference on knowledge discovery and data mining; 2016. p. 1135–44.
62. Lundberg SM, Lee S-I. A unified approach to interpreting model predictions. Adv Neural Inf Proces Syst. 2017;30:4765–74.
63. FDA. Software as a Medical Device (SAMD): Clinical Evaluation 2017. https://www.fda.gov/media/100714/download.
64. Benjamens S, Dhunnoo P, Meskó B. The state of artificial intelligence-based FDA-approved medical devices and algorithms: an online database. NPJ Digit Med. 2020;3:118.
65. Angus DC. Optimizing the trade-off between learning and doing in a pandemic. JAMA. 2020;323(19):1895–6.
66. Angus DC. Fusing randomized trials with big data: the key to self-learning health care systems? JAMA. 2015;314(8):767–8.

Chapter 11
Predicting Medical Outcomes

Riccardo Bellazzi, Arianna Dagliati, and Giovanna Nicora

After reading this chapter, you should know the answers to these questions:
- How do different types of clinical outcomes map to machine learning problems?
- What are the main approaches to predict clinical outcomes?
- What are the best strategies to evaluate the performance of a predictive model in clinical medicine during the statistical validation phase?

Clinical Outcomes: An Enlarged Perspective

Clinical outcomes are measurable changes in health, function or quality of life that result from patients' care. In other words, they are the outputs of an input intervention (actions related to individual patient's care or change in patients' care organization) over a system (the patient, the health care system). Outcome research, a well-established field of public health, usually divides outcomes into two broad groups: patient-related outcomes and systems related ones. The presentation that follows mainly focuses on patient-related outcomes, even if the methodologies

R. Bellazzi (✉)
Department of Electrical, Computer and Biomedical Engineering, University of Pavia, Pavia, Italy

Laboratory of Informatics and Systems Engineering for Clinical Research, Istituti Clinici Scientifici Maugeri, Pavia, Italy
e-mail: riccardo.bellazzi@unipv.it

A. Dagliati · G. Nicora
Department of Electrical, Computer and Biomedical Engineering, University of Pavia, Pavia, Italy

T. A. Cohen et al. (eds.), *Intelligent Systems in Medicine and Health*, Cognitive Informatics in Biomedicine and Healthcare,
https://doi.org/10.1007/978-3-031-09108-7_11

it refers to can be extended to the system perspective. Focusing on patients' clinical outcomes, a variety of clinical outcomes can be considered, ranging from mortality and morbidity to patient satisfaction and engagement, i.e. including both events and individual perceptions.

Artificial Intelligence may provide a variety of approaches to predict clinical outcomes ranging from purely data-driven strategies to methods able to exploit formalized knowledge of the clinical domain of interest.

Forecasting can be based on one or more machine learning algorithms belonging to the wide class of supervised methods (see Chap. 6). Supervised methods assume a collection of past cases is available, in which some input variables, such as measurements or clinical decisions, are associated with an outcome.

It is important to mention that the goal of a prediction model is to forecast in a reliable manner the outcome, and not to describe what are the most important statistical correlations between the input variables and the outcomes.

Where medical outcome prediction is concerned, machine learning shares goals and methods with statistics and statistical modeling. As a matter of fact, machine learning refers to "the ability (of AI systems) to acquire their own knowledge, by extracting patterns from raw data" [1]. The subset of machine learning methods designed to predict outcomes are children of statistics, optimization, and operational research. If one wants to discern between statistics and machine learning, a possible distinction might be that statistics draws population inferences from a sample, while machine learning methods tend to find generalizable predictive patterns [2]. However, a perhaps more valuable way of characterizing these differences is to have an historical perspective of the fields.

In the following sections, the chapter concentrates on strategies that are nowadays widely accepted to be part of the machine learning realm, and in the section related to model assessment, the chapter concentrates on measures of the prediction performance rather than on statistical significance.

To approach the description of the different aspects involved in building a forecasting system, this section will introduce a suitable notation that will support the discussion. The outcome will be denoted with the letter y. If a database of retrospective cases is collected, the number of collected cases will be denoted with n.

The $n \times 1$ column vector containing the outcome related to the n cases will be denoted with the capital letter Y. The chapter also discusses situations in which the outcome is a temporal profile, i.e. a vector of t time points. In this case the outcome row vector $1 \times t$ will be denoted with the bold letter $\mathbf{y}$, and the $n \times t$ output matrix will be denoted with the capital bold letter $\mathbf{Y}$. It is assumed that it is possible to perform a prediction of the outcome based on m input variables, or attributes or features, that will be denoted, following the same notation, as a $1 \times m$ row vector $\mathbf{x}$, and the $n \times m$ input matrix $\mathbf{X}$ (Fig. 11.1). The forecasts will be denoted with $\hat{y}$ (single case), $\hat{\mathbf{y}}$ (temporal profile), $\hat{Y}$ (vector of all cases), and $\hat{\mathbf{Y}}$ (matrix of all cases profiles).

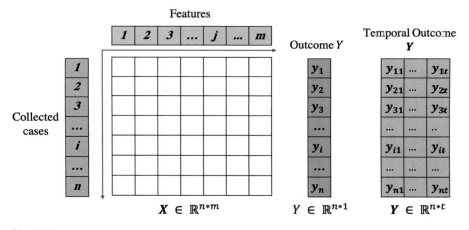

Fig. 11.1 Dataset notation for clinical outcome prediction

From a machine learning viewpoint, the type of outcome measurement determines the very nature of the prediction problem.

In many cases outcome prediction can be modeled as a *classification problem*. In these situations, the outcome is a discrete variable, such as death: *yes/no, morbidity*: yes/no, *cancer relapse at five years*: yes/no, or *covid-19 symptoms*: mild/moderate/severe. The prediction problem corresponds therefore to building a classification rule that associates the outcome value y with different configurations of the input vector $\mathbf{x}$. Very often, instead of providing a crisp classification, an AI system outputs the probability (or the score) of each different value of the outcome variable, thus providing a *risk profile P(y|x)*.

Many practical cases represent the outcome as a binary classification problem, even if more classes are possible. However, differently from what happens in diagnostic problems, when more classes are available, they are often associated with an *ordinal scale* of severity. In this case the problem can still be approached as a classification, or it is possible to resort to *ordinal regression* algorithms.

Regression analysis is performed when the outcome is a continuous variable, such as hemoglobin concentration after one week of erythropoietin treatment in cancer, or fasting blood glucose level after treatment with hypoglycemic drugs. In this case, a *regression function* is learned, in order to be able to forecast the outcome value y with different configurations of the input vector $\mathbf{x}$.

Clinical outcome prediction always needs to consider the temporal dimension. In both cases reported above, outcome is measured after a predefined amount of time: *relapse at five years* and *hemoglobin after one week* are outcome definitions that simplify the problem of outcome prediction treating time as a hidden variable that defines the modeling effort.

The explicit representation of time can be handled in outcome prediction following different strategies. The most widely used approach in biostatistics is *survival analysis*. In this case the time of occurrence of an event is recorded, so that for each patient a timestamp associated with the output variable is reported. This, of course, happens with time of death, time of relapse of a disease or time of occurrence of a morbidity event.

The complexity of the description of the clinical outcome may therefore encompass the entire temporal trajectory of a patient, described by one or more outcome variables. For example, the outcome of insulin treatment can be the daily blood glucose profile, or the outcome of a rehabilitation therapy can be the sequence of visits and procedures that the patient is undergoing together with the final quality of rehabilitation achieved. When the complexity of the outcome description increases, the vector/matrix representation can be insufficient, so that a univariate or multivariate sequence of time stamped events might be needed.

Rather interestingly, prediction of patients' outcomes can be performed also resorting to models of outcome dynamics, which can be deterministic or stochastic, and AI and machine learning (ML) approaches allow using a variety of modeling techniques, including **Monte Carlo simulations.**

Understanding the nature of the input matrix $\mathbf{X}$ is crucial to select the proper approaches for outcome prediction. In general one does not put constraints on the type of the input variables, so that each variable x_j can be either continuous (it can assume any numerical value, and it is usually the result of a measurement, such as a blood glucose measurement), categorical (it can assume a specific value in a finite set of elements, such as the treatment type) binary (categorical variable that can assume only two possible values), or finally ordinal (categorical variables with ordered values, such as levels of risk). In this latter case, some methods transform a categorical variable with s values into $s-1$ binary variables, called dummy variables. There are cases in which the variables that are related to the outcomes cannot be easily represented as a matrix or at least transformed into a matrix. In this chapter we will not consider those cases, but we will rather focus on the large number of practical applications that, after suitable preprocessing, will be amenable to being represented as an $\mathbf{X}, Y$ pair.

It is important to mention that subsequent parts of the chapter mainly focus on the problem of forecasting the outcome, assuming that it is a consequence of a treatment or decision taken at a certain time point. The chapter therefore does not address sequential decisions or policies, i.e. strategies that may lead to a sequence of outcome measurements. In particular, it does not cover the area of reinforcement learning, which recently gained attention as a means to optimize sequential decisions in clinical medicine [3].

The following section provides an overview the main approaches available in the literature spanning over these different outcome representations.

AI Approaches for Clinical Outcomes Prediction

Starting from the discussion about the different clinical outcomes presented in the previous section, a selection of different machine learning models is introduced in this section. Emphasis is on general concepts, such as the role of latent variables with some strategies to extract them, the problem of coupling supervised and unsupervised analysis, and the challenges posed by the prediction of clinical outcomes as a time course, which can be modeled by trajectory modeling approaches and advanced simulation strategies.

The following subsections are also included: aspects of preprocessing, including missing values imputation and features transformation; different outcome prediction problems, including classification, regression and survival analysis; and a subsection with a focus on temporal AI models, including temporal trajectories and Markov models.

Preprocessing: Missing Values, Features Transformation and Latent Variables Extraction

As previously introduced, in clinical studies, the unit of observation and analysis is almost always a patient. So, the first step to analyze clinical outcomes is to create a data matrix where each i-th row contains all the data for a single patient, each j-th column contains a different feature (Fig. 11.2).

Once the unit of observation and analysis (i.e. the patients' cohort) is defined, the first steps are to determine which features to extract from the data, thus what to do

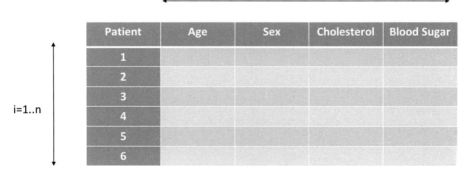

Fig. 11.2 An example of Data Matrix

if features are missing and to evaluate the impact of transformation methods on the clinical outcome predictions.

Missing Values

When a feature's element is missing, it is possible to assume that it should have been recorded but was not. However, while a data matrix is the by-product of clinical processes projected into a structured record, the mere existence of a feature, does not mean that it should be filled with a value.

Indeed, the absence of a feature value could mean different things: (i) the value should have existed but does not - this is the common meaning of missing data; (ii) the value absence is an artefact of adopting a specific view of the data. For example, if we have different columns, each one coding a disease, then most of the columns will have missing values; (iii) the value could have existed, but it was not required nor necessary to collect it. For example, a test measuring mid-term metabolic control in diabetes (i.e. Hba1c) could be listed as a feature when creating a data set for monitoring cardiovascular patients. However, some patients will have this value, and others will not. Those that do not, probably didn't need the test, meaning that the fact that the value is missing is an intentional choice related to the clinical process and it is informative in itself. Such missing values raise several issues for analysis: it is important to deal with how they are reported in the data and, more importantly, it is necessary to plan—considering that they are missing—how to impute them (Fig. 11.3).

Rubin classified missing data problems into three categories [4]. In his theory every data point has some likelihood of being missing. The process that governs these probabilities is called the missing data mechanism [5]:

- Missing Completely At Random (MCAR), when there is no relationship between missing data and observed or unobserved data. Thus, the causes of the missing data are unrelated to the data. Some typical examples of MCAR are when indi-

Patient	Age	Sex	Cholesterol	Blood Sugar	DX. CVD	DX. Diabetes	DX. Cancer
1	39	M	190	132	1	1	0
2	56	NA	165	NA	0	0	0
3	27	F	NA	110	0	0	0
4	NA	M	170	90	0	0	0
5	91	M	NA	NA	0	1	1
6	36	M	188	121	0	1	0
7	55	F	165	NA	0	0	0

Fig. 11.3 Data Matrix with missing data. In this example (i) Age and Sex should have been collected but haven't; (ii) Cholesterol and Blood Sugar might have been measured, but eventually were not required to be collected; (iii) value 0 in Diagnosis of CVD, Diabetes and Cancer is an artefact of adopting this specific data format

viduals have no measurement because the equipment to perform an analysis was broken or when an individual drops-out of a study for reasons not related to health-issues (e.g. moving to another city).

- Missing At Random (MAR), when there is a relationship between missing data and observed data, and the missingness depends on already observed information. Thus, the probability of being missing is the same within groups defined by the observed data. For example, data can be said to be MAR, given gender, if men are less likely than women to undergo follow-ups. Once gender is observed, the missingness does not depend on the stage of their disease.
- Missing Not At Random (MNAR), when there is a relationship between missing data and both observed and unobserved data. This means that the probability of being missing varies for reasons that are unknown. For example, when individuals with severe diabetes are more or less likely to undergo follow-ups: in this case missingness is directly related to the stage of their disease.

One could think about different strategies to deal with missing data. For example, removing patient rows with missing data values is a simple solution, however it might lead to biased results, especially if the feature was not measured because of a crucial patient characteristic (i.e. the inability to attend a visit). Another imputation method is column-mean imputation, which replaces the missing value with the average of the known values in the same column. This approach should also not be pursued. Indeed it assumes that the variable values in the other rows (i.e. from other patients) of that column have information about the missing value, which is not true in clinical research.

Multiple imputation is now accepted as the best general method to deal with incomplete data. It was developed by Rubin [4], who observed that imputing one value (single, column-mean imputation) for the missing value could not be correct in general and imputation should be performed through a model able to relate the unobserved data to the observed data and noted that even for a given model the imputed values could not be calculated with certainty. Thus, his solution was to create multiple imputations that reflect the uncertainty of the missing data.

The so-called "Rubin's Rule" is based on a model that accounts for the relationship between observed and missing data.

Let with ($j = 1,\ldots,p$) be one of p incomplete variables. The observed and missing parts of x_j are denoted by x_{obs} and x_{mis}, respectively. Let Q denote a quantity of scientific interest (e.g., a regression coefficient). In practice, Q is often a multivariate vector. The posterior distribution of quantity of interest Q given observed data only is provided by the following equation:

$$f\left(Q \mid x_{obs}\right) = \int f\left(Q \mid x_{obs}, x_{mis}\right) f\left(x_{mis} \mid x_{obs}\right) dx_{mis}$$

where $f(Q \mid X_{obs}, X_{mis})$ indicate the distribution of Q given complete data (outcome model), $f(X_{mis} \mid X_{obs})$ the distribution of missing data given observed data (missing data model), and the dx_{mis} the integration over the missing data distribution.

From a practical point of view, this imputation model is implemented within the multiple imputation workflow, within publicly available software packages such as the R package *mice* [6], where the algorithm starts with a random draw from the observed data and imputes the incomplete data in a variable-by-variable fashion.

Dimensionality Reduction and Feature Transformation

Very often clinical studies allow the extraction of hundreds or thousands of features. However, it is common to have constraints—linked both to computing resources or model clinical relevance and interpretability—which entail removing or transforming features that reduce the size of the data set.

Dimensionality reduction techniques can be defined as the process of transforming the original data matrix into a new one with fewer columns but including approximately the same information as the original one. Because this matrix is composed of a smaller number of features, it can be used more efficiently than the original matrix. Dimensionality reduction techniques are typically divided into feature selection and feature extraction methods. The main difference between them is that feature selection selects a subset of the original features, whereas feature extraction combines the original features to create a set of new features. Feature extraction transforms data from the original input space to a feature space with different dimensions. Starting from the initial data matrix, these methods build new features intended to be informative and non-redundant, facilitating the subsequent learning and generalization steps and, in some cases, leading to better interpretations (Figs. 11.4 and 11.5).

It is thus important to introduce how it is possible to use subtle information that is implicit in the data, which one can also define as non-observable or latent, to define and/or create features. These "hidden" features can be metadata, that is indicator variables that refer to other data. For example, the data gathered from two common actions: ordering a laboratory test and recording the measured value. In the former case, the data indicate that the test was carried out, whereas in the latter they capture the measured value as a continuous variable. If the goal is to determine whether the diabetic disease is stable, ideally one should look at the results of a test (i.e. *HbA1c* continuous values). However, it might also be possible to leverage the counts of ordering an *Hba1c* test, or the frequency of *Hba1c* tests, or changes in the patient's prescriptions to ascertain whether the disease is worsening.

Another common action when preprocessing a feature matrix is to standardize features and transform them into uniform numerical ranges. Feature standardization (or normalization) reduces the effect of values extremely large or small in comparison to other values in the feature matrix. Common approaches to normalize features are to rescale them into a [0–1] range, or to transform each j-th column so that it has a mean of 0 with a standard deviation of 1.

While latent features can be extracted or created through prior knowledge, it is also possible to learn them via computational methods, and a few such methods are illustrated at the end of this section. In the same way, when implementing an AI

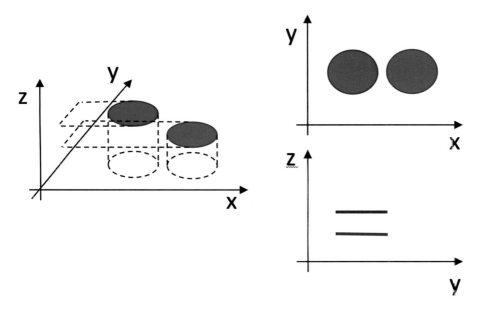

Fig. 11.4 A simple dimension reduction example where the 3-D space is split into two 2-D feature spaces, allowing a representation of the object in a lower dimensional space. The two discs, represented in 3-D in the left panel, are oriented such as their surface varies along the axes: the top right panel corresponds to a top-down view of the 3D space, looking down the Z axis, while the bottom right panel corresponds to a re-oriented view from the behind, looking along the X axis.

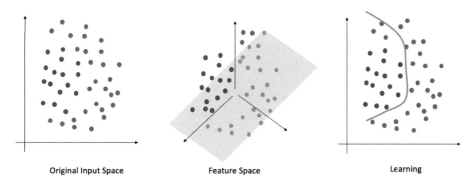

Fig. 11.5 Projection of the original input space into a novel feature space where the problem is linearly separable, thus allowing for accurate prediction, with the decision boundary (green curve) projected back to the original space

model to predict clinical outcomes, several methods can automatically remove features [7] that contribute the least to the accuracy of the final model.

While the general objective for reducing the number of features or transforming them is to improve the accuracy of the models, there are several specific and practical reasons for doing so. There may be features that have no utility for prediction (i.e. some phenotypic traits unrelated to the outcome of interest) or are missing for most patients. The latter case is usually referred to as data sparsity, indicating that many features are missing for a given patient or group of patients. Another reason to reduce the number of features is redundancy, that is when two or more features are highly correlated. It is also important to take into consideration that a large number of features will slow down the analysis, which could be a major constraint depending on the available computational resources.

Features that have the same values for all the patients or are nearly constant over time might be removed. Features missing for most patients and with very low prevalence should be removed as well.

As in all the steps to analyze clinical outcomes, knowledge of the context and the clinical problem plays a central role. An in-depth knowledge of the cohort of patients to analyze, including not only the pathophysiological aspects but also the clinical processes and the data gathering procedures, is the basis for knowing which features one should remove or transform.

Thus, one way to transform, and reduce features, is to select features using domain knowledge. Indeed, some features may indicate information too fine grained for the analysis. For example, indicating the brand of a drug rather than its active principles and molecules will make it difficult for models to learn ingredient-level drug effects. For these reasons it may be desirable to aggregate features into coarser categories. Even though this topic is not discussed in this chapter, it is important to highlight that this step requires accurate representations of domain knowledge, for example in the form of ontologies (see Chap. 4).

As already mentioned, it is also possible to use computational approaches able to detect and use latent features patterns. The benefit - but also the possible drawback—of using such techniques is that they are domain independent and do not require specific medical knowledge. Indeed, mathematically combining existing features might make derived features difficult for clinical interpretation. This loss of interpretability is something that one should always consider when preprocessing the feature matrix to build a model for clinical outcome prediction.

Several methods for feature extraction use linear algebra and are based on matrix factorization. Principal Component Analysis (PCA) [8, 9] is one of the most popular of these techniques. It works by finding new variables that are given by a linear combination of those in the original dataset, that can best summarize the original data distribution and that are uncorrelated with each other. Finding such new variables, called the principal components (PCs), reduces to solving an eigenvalue/eigenvector [10] problem. PCA can also be used for feature selection, as it is possible to rank the PCs with respect to the amount of variance in the data they represent, and select the most informative ones to be used in the following analysis.

Other approaches, such as t-distributed Stochastic Neighbor Embedding (t-SNE) [11], are nonlinear dimensionality reduction techniques well-suited for embedding high-dimensional data for visualization in a low-dimensional space. t-SNE is a graph-based nonlinear dimensionality reduction algorithm that works in two steps: it builds a weighted graph based on the top k nearest neighbors for each point, then it computes a low-dimensional graph, where the goal is to find the low-dimensional space that best preserves the nearest neighborhood structure of the original high-dimensional space. While this concerns a human information processing constraint rather than being an inherent property of the t-SNE algorithm, with reduction down to two or three dimensions it can be also applied for the purpose of visualization. In this case, it is possible to view each high-dimensional object as a two- or three-dimensional point in such a way that similar objects are modeled by nearby points and dissimilar objects are modeled by distant points with high probability.

Deep Learning

It is widely recognized that one of the most important technologies of modern AI is represented by novel artificial neural networks architectures collectively referred to as deep learning methods [12].Those methods jointly perform two tasks: variable transformation and prediction (in general any kind of input/output forecasting goal, including classification and regression). In the transformation step, variable values are transformed into a set of latent variables by a series, called layers, of non-linear transformations. These transformations can consider complex internal relationships between input variables, also looking at the data with different abstraction or zooming lenses. For this reason, deep learning has proven to be extremely effective in dealing with data that traditionally needed manually derived features, such as images, videos, signals, and texts. As previously mentioned, key components of deep learning architectures are a series of layers designed to deal with specific tasks. For example, a widely exploited layer, in particular in image processing, is the so-called Convolutional Neural Network layer [13] (see also Chap. 6), which computes the similarity of the input data with predefined templates based on specific kernel functions or filters. Other key components are layers able to deal with sequences, such as Recurrent Neural Networks (RNN) and their subtypes, Gated Recurrent Units (GRU), and Long short-term memory (LSTM) [14]. All those layers are designed to build latent features that incorporate nonlinear relationships between sequential inputs, as happens with time series or texts. Recently, in particular where natural language processing is concerned, the so-called transformers architectures, which are based on special units known as attention units, have become the model of choice [15]. Such architectures can process sequences and text looking at the entire set of input features along the sequence to be processed and then learning flexibly and in dependence of the context, such as the surrounding words, the best latent representation [16].

Deep learning models, though, are highly parameterized. One of the most popular deep learning models, Inception V.3 [17], published in 2015 to deal with the ImageNet Large Scale Visual Recognition Challenge[1] has 23 million parameters. BERT, currently the best architecture for many NLP tasks, has more than 110 million parameters, and BERTLarge more than 340 million [18]. This fact has three important implications. First, these architectures are very flexible, and can

---

[1] ImageNet is an image database that has been very important in advancing computer vision and deep learning research also by means of a number of large image recognition challenges.

memorize an extremely large number of relationships between input variables. Second, training these types of models requires an extremely large amount of data and wide computational resources. As a matter of fact, the most successful large architectures have been trained by big-tech companies or very large research consortia. Third, some of the tasks performed by these very large deep learning models can be considered as basic cognitive tasks, such as mapping images into a convenient latent space. For this reason, it is not always necessary to retrain the models from scratch in presence of new data, but it is rather possible to exploit such pretrained models as feature transformation mechanisms. The new features can be then used as input for prediction purposes in a machine learning pipeline. This is the goal of transfer learning, which looks to be a very promising direction for conveniently exploiting deep learning models, without getting trapped into overfitting due to poor parameter estimation.

Classification

As previously mentioned, the most common representation of an outcome prediction problem is the one of classification. In this case the outcome is a class with a finite, usually small, number of possible values and the prediction problem is solved by learning a classification rule that associates a class value y to any instance of the input vector x.

The first important aspect that needs to be defined is the mapping between the outcomes and the class. For example, if the outcome of interest is mortality, it is fundamental to clearly define a temporal scale of interest. In general, the knowledge of the clinical domain allows a time threshold to define the classes, such as *"dead during hospitalization (yes/no)"*. However arbitrary temporal thresholds, computed for example relying on the median time of death in the data set available, run the risk of adding biases in the analysis and poor reproducibility of the results. It is therefore very important to decide if classification is the right way of representing the problem, or if it is rather that survival analysis should be preferred to deal with outcome prediction.

A similar issue can be related to classes that are derived from discretization of a continuous variable or from grouping outcomes measured in an ordinal way. This step is related to an abstraction activity that is performed several times in the clinic, to synthesize outcomes observed, for example on scales, into coarser but more actionable measures. Sometimes, this is anchored to definitions coming from clinical guidelines, such as for example the *lower limit of normal hemoglobin* that is used to define anemia, but quite often discretization and grouping are performed to obtained *balanced class distributions*, i.e. almost the same proportion of examples in each class. Every time this latter situation happens the entire classification exercise is biased by the decisions taken and prone to derive classification systems that are hardly replicable in other settings, unless the amount of available data is a sample fully representative of the population distribution.

Perhaps the main reason to represent outcome prediction as a classification system, apart from the simplicity of results interpretations, is the availability of a very large number of classification algorithms and a wide variety of tools that implement them. The readers can refer to Chap. 6 of this book for an introduction to the most important machine learning strategies. In the area of outcome prediction, several interesting studies have shown the capability of machine and deep learning methods to outperform currently used prognostic systems. For example, machine learning approaches, including deep networks, have been effectively used to predict clinical outcomes in prognostic classification in emergency departments [19], in forecasting outcomes of colorectal cancer after primary resection [20] and in predicting breast cancer from mammography [21]. Examples of machine learning applied to the prognosis of COVID-19 and to predict Diabetes mellitus complications will be discussed in more detail in the section on "Case Studies and Examples".

It is important to mention that when a classification system provides a predicted class y, this usually provides the class associated to the largest value of a score function, which in probabilistic method corresponds to $P(y|x)$. However, choosing the class with the largest probability value is not necessarily what a clinician will do in an outcome prediction problem, in particular if consequential decisions are related to the classification, such as additional treatment, surgery, or hospital discharge. In fact, deciding the class is a decision analytic problem, which is related to the utility values of the decision maker. In this case, if one wants to approach the problem from a formal viewpoint, it would be possible to define the best decision threshold, i.e. the probability that a class of interest should have to classify that example as belonging to that class, by eliciting from the decision maker his or her costs and utilities. In binary classification, this means the cost of deciding that the class is negative when the true class is positive (the cost of false negatives), and the cost of deciding that the class is positive when the true class is negative (the cost of false positives). In this case it is easy to show that the threshold depends only on the ratio between the two costs, i.e. asking how many times one case is more dangerous than the other [22]. Researchers are devoting increasing interest to explicitly dealing with utility of decision makers, including patients' opinions [23, 24].

Regression

While in classification problems the outcome y is a discrete variable that assumes a predefined set of values, in regression problems y is a continuous variable. As pointed out in the previous section, a continuous clinical outcome can be discretized in order to manage a classification problem rather than a regression problem. For instance, in drug discovery and development, the problem of predicting how much of a particular drug is needed to inhibit a relevant biological process by 50% can be tackled using regression analysis or using classification. Regression aims at describing the relationships between the input vector $\mathbf{x}$, which contains the set of attributes, also called *covariates* in a regression problem, and the continuous outcome y. The outcome is often called the *dependent* or *response* variable, while the input vector **x** contains the *independent* or *predictor* variables. To predict the continuous values of the independent variables, the underlying assumption of regression analysis is that there is some mathematical function that can describe their relationship to the independent variables $y = f(x)$.

Based on the assumption made on $f(x)$, regression techniques can be non-parametric or parametric. Non-parametric approaches do not assume any form for $f(x)$, while parametric techniques assume a particular form of $f(x)$ that must fit the data. The most common form of parametric regression is linear regression, which assumes a linear relationship between the covariates and the continuous outcome of interest. Examples of non-parametric regressions include Generalized Additive Models (GAM), in which non-parametric functions of the predictors are estimated through splines [25]. Assumptions on the relationship between **x** and y can be empirical or may be supported by biological reasons [26].

By modeling the relationships among the dependent and the independent variables, regression analysis allows us (1) to describe a particular clinical problem, such as the influence of body weight and age on blood pressure, (2) to identify risk factors that influence the outcome, and (3) to forecast the values of the dependent variables from the observed values of the independent variables using mathematical equations.

Survival Analysis

In survival analysis, the objective is to model the ***time until an event occurs***, by using a collection of different statistical approaches. The "*event*" can be one or more medical outcomes of interest, such as disease onset, relapse from remission, or death. Time can be measured in days, weeks, months or even years from the beginning of follow-up until the event of interest occurs [27]. Therefore, survival analysis implicates monitoring, over a specific period, one or more cohorts of patients. One of the main challenges in the context of such longitudinal studies is the presence of instances (in our case, patients) that do not experience the event during the monitoring period or that become unobservable. This phenomenon is called censoring. The time to event of interest (which is the quantity we would like to model) is known only for those patients who experienced the event within the study period, while for the other patients we can only observe a censored time. Censored time can be either the time withdrawn from the study or the end of the study in case the patient did not have the event. In the presence of censored data, predictive algorithms coming from standard statistical and machine learning approaches are not suitable, and a subset of statistics, known as "survival analysis" has been developed specifically to handle this problem (Fig. 11.6).

As for the application of survival analysis in medicine, this approach has been widely employed to predict survival time of patients diagnosed with heart failure [28], or to compare the beneficial effect of different treatments on overall and

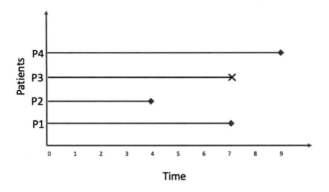

Fig. 11.6 Example of the survival analysis data. During a follow-up period of ten months, only patient P3 experienced the event (for instance, death). The observed time for P3 is therefore the event time. Patients P1 and P2 are censored due to withdrawal or being lost during follow-up, P4 is censored since he/she did not experience the event during the study period

disease-free survival in women diagnosed with breast cancer [29]. In public health, major applications of survival analysis include the identification of risk/prognostic factors, the estimation of survival distribution as well as testing the hypothesis of equal survival distribution between different groups.

A typical survival analysis involves the application of the Kaplan-Meier method and Cox's regression. The former is usually applied to estimate survival distribution at a given time step. This estimate is the product of a series of estimated conditional probabilities, where such conditional probabilities represent the proportion of patients surviving in each time interval, given that he/she survives in the previous time intervals (we refer the reader to [30] for a comprehensive explanation of statistical approaches). Thanks to data collected during longitudinal studies, survival curves can be estimated through the Kaplan-Meier curve for different groups of patients. Patients can be grouped according to their clinical or biological characteristics, such as their gender, their cancer type, or the presence of specific alterations along the genome. By comparing, through statistical tests, the estimated survival curves for each group, it is possible to understand whether patients with specific clinical/biological characteristics show a longer or shorter survival time. Patients can be categorized in different cohorts also based on the type of treatment they received. In this case, survival analysis is extremely useful in determining the potential benefit of a particular treatment over others.

To estimate whether a particular characteristic is related to the occurrence of a health-related event, Cox's regression model can be used. During longitudinal studies, many potential risk factors (such as family history, smoking, pre-existing conditions) are collected. Cox's regression allows us to identify the most significant risk factors among those collected.

Along with traditional statistical methods, approaches belonging to the machine learning literature have been adapted in the last years for survival analysis. While statistical methods for survival analysis focus more on characterizing the distributions of the event times and the statistical properties of the parameter estimation, machine learning methods focus more on the prediction of event occurrence at a given time point. This is usually achieved by combining traditional survival analysis methods with different machine learning techniques [31]. Machine learning methods can be preferred over traditional statistical methods for highly dimensional datasets, given their ability to transform the data into a lower dimensional space. Different machine learning algorithms have been adapted to handle censored data for predicting the event occurrence at each time step. Survival trees were implemented from **decision trees** (see Chap. 14) by modifying the splitting criteria used to partition the data. Also, **random forests** and **gradient boosting** have been adapted to the survival problem [31]. Cox models have been incorporated in Bayesian models and more recently have been incorporated in **artificial neural networks** and **deep networks** for survival analysis. Unlike the Cox model, which assumes that the log of the hazard function is a linear function of the covariates, the use of complex machine learning models, such as deep learning, allows for the modeling of non-linear interaction between risk factors, encoded in the dataset's attributes. Deep learning can be used for different purposes, from classification to feature engineering. In this latter case, deep networks can transform a highly dimensional and sparse dataset into a lower informative dimension that maintains important statistical properties of the initial dataset. Such data transformation allows for the integration of multi-omics data describing transcriptomics, proteomics and genomics status of each patient. The flexibility of the deep network architectures enables the implementation of feature transformation/integration followed by survival prediction. A specific type of network, named the Cox proportional hazards regression network, has been used to predict survival outcome in cancer patients after the integration of transcriptomics and clinical features [32]. Another recent approach built a two-layer neural network, with the output layer performing Cox regression, to predict prognosis of cancer patients from high-dimensional gene expression data [33].

Deep learning is also used to learn the distribution of survival time from data directly, without making any assumption about the stochastic processes that generate the data. In this case, the loss function of the network can be specifically designed to handle censored data [34, 35].

Compared with regression and classification problems, specific metrics for the evaluation of survival analysis need to be used to handle the problem of censored data. Such metrics usually consider the relative risk of an event for two different instances instead of the absolute survival time for each instance. An example is the concordance probability, also known as concordance index (C-index) [36], which computes the probability that a prediction value of an instance $\hat{y}_a$ is greater than the prediction value of a second instance $\hat{y}_b$, given that the observed value y_a is greater or equal to the observed value y_b. When the outcome value is binary, the C-index represents the Area Under the ROC curve (AUC). Finally, the Brier score [37] has been adapted to the survival analysis problem by weighting each individual contribution of the score using the censoring information.

The analysis of survival data is extremely useful in health-care problems. Yet, survival analysis involves the collection of data for (even long) periods of time. Data collection can be time consuming and costly, especially when collected features include -omics data. For this reason, cross sectional studies are more often available to the research community. Simulation of longitudinal data from cross sectional studies can allow for the application of survival analysis, as illustrated in the section on "Case studies and examples".

Time Lines and Trajectory Modeling

Another possible representation of clinical care data is with patient timelines, which explicitly capture when the i-th patient experienced a specific event and illustrate when the j-th feature has been measured k times. It is worth noting that temporal features can be modeled as continuous variables, when features are continuously represented through time (for example, measures taken from devices such as a continuous glucose monitor, which monitors blood glucose on a continual basis), or as discrete counts, when measurements are taken at specific time (for example HbA1c measurements taken at follow-up visits). The modeling decision to represent time in a continuous or discrete manner depends on measurement types, their availability, and by the chosen temporal granularity. The example in Fig. 11.7 illustrates two variables modeled in a discrete way.

Even if it brings several further challenges when analyzing data, capturing the temporal dimension of clinical data can enhance models and help in "making sense" of clinical data and outcomes. Indeed, examining the order in which events occur could be a useful tool to understand the correlation between exposures and outcomes. If A caused B, then one should expect to see some evidence of A in the patient's data before we see some evidence of B.

In general, timelines represent a useful tool to integrate the different sources and types (e.g. event-type data like diagnosis and continuous values like laboratory test results) of data for a patient. The timeline explicitly captures when the i-th patient experienced each event or shows a certain level of a measure.

The first step to apply methods for clinical outcome models from longitudinal data is to convert the patient timeline into a patient feature matrix. Thus, there are several decisions to be made about the useful timescales for answering the clinical question and the possible ways to represent time. As for cross-sectional data, a good knowledge of the feature set is fundamental in representing time. For example, it is important to understand the interval of time over which a feature is relevant, and to observe if data changes in systematic ways over the analysis timescale.

To represent longitudinal data, the patient-feature matrix can be coded into "long" and "wide" formats (Fig. 11.7). A wide dataset will have one record for each i-the patient. The j-th observations made at different k-th time points are coded as different columns. In the wide format every j-th measure that varies in time occupies a set of columns. In the long format there will be multiple records for each i-th individual. Some variables that do not vary in time are identical in each record, whereas other variables vary across the records.

Wide Format

Patient	Cholesterol @1	Blood Sugar @1	Cholesterol @2	Blood Sugar @2	Cholesterol @3	Blood Sugar @3	Cholesterol @4	Blood Sugar @4
1	190	132	165	121	165	110	NA	NA
2	170	90	170	100	188	121	165	134

Long Format

Patient	Time	Cholesterol	Blood Sugar
1	1	190	132
1	2	165	121
1	3	165	110
2	1	170	90
2	2	170	100
2	3	188	121
2	4	165	134

Fig. 11.7 Wide and long format example for longitudinal data

Several approaches that attempt to model life-course changes or disease progression simply extract features for use in standard regression approaches, for example, an Hba1c measure change over time. More sophisticated approaches take account of within-individual correlations and use of latent classes. One of the most popular techniques to represent clinical outcomes that vary over time is latent trajectory analysis, that is techniques to estimate membership of unobserved subgroups of individuals developing over time [38]. These techniques couple the idea of latent growth modeling—that all individuals are drawn from one population—with mixture modeling that assumes that growth parameters (i.e. intercept, slope) vary across a number of prespecified, unobserved subpopulations. This is accomplished using categorical latent variables, which allow for groups of individual growth trajectories and results in separate latent growth models for each latent group, each with its unique set of growth parameters [39]. For a given data matrix, it is possible to derive different models based on the number of clinical outcomes, how these outcomes are measured, the number of latent classes, model structure and trajectory property. Thus, one should follow a structured framework to construct and interpret latent class trajectory models [40] (Fig. 11.8).

Markov Models

As described in the previous sections, an area of great interest for outcome prediction is related to chronic diseases. Many such diseases are characterized by complex temporal behaviors, made of different **disease states**. Each state is characterized by some key pathophysiological variables, values, and specific symptoms. When such states are part of a sequence of deterioration steps are usually called **disease stages**. The rate of transition between states or stages may be dependent on different factors, including patient characteristics (sex, age,

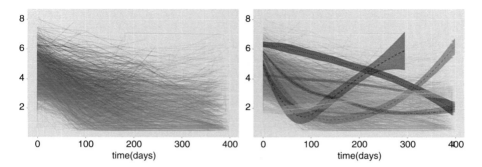

Fig. 11.8 Example of the application of trajectory analysis. On the left pane each line represents the measurements in time for single patients. On the right pane the trajectories discovered by the latent class trajectory modelling. (Figure from [41] (Dagliati, Plant, et al. 2020)) (This article was published in the Arthritis Rheumatol, Dagliati A, Plant D, Nair N, Jani M, Amico B, Peek N, Morgan AW, Isaacs J, Wilson AG, Hyrich KL, Geifman N, Barton A; BRAGGSS Study Group. "Latent Class Trajectory Modeling of 2-Component Disease Activity Score in 28 Joints Identifies Multiple Rheumatoid Arthritis Phenotypes of Response to Biologic Disease-Modifying Antirheumatic Drugs". Creative commons terms.)

genotypic background), medications, and health care conditions (frequency of visits, availability of healthcare resources). In this case, predicting the outcomes can be seen as forecasting the next state given the current one, or deriving the most probable future temporal trajectory, made of a sequence of disease states. In the AI literature the most popular methods to deal with this kind of prediction problem are represented by **Markov models, hidden Markov models** and **dynamic Bayesian networks**, using either discrete or continuous time. These approaches share a common theoretical framework. We suppose that at a given time point t the disease state can be described by a state vector $\boldsymbol{q}$ of k variables. The main assumption of this class of methods is the Markovian property, i.e. that the probability of a state in a future time point is only dependent on the value of the state at the current time, which in turn depends on the state at the previous time point and so forth [42].

In the discrete time case, the state is observed on a discrete time grid, so that $P(\boldsymbol{q}(t + 1)|\boldsymbol{q}(t), \boldsymbol{q}(t - 1), ..., \boldsymbol{q}(0)) = P(\boldsymbol{q}(t + 1)|\boldsymbol{q}(t))$.

The simplest form of model to describe the temporal trajectory of patients over time is represented by the case in which $k = 1$ and q is a discrete variable with s values. A Markov model describes the transitions over time with a transition probability matrix, that contains $P(q(t + 1) = j|q(t) = i)$, where i and j are one of the s values. Usually, these types of models assume that the transition probability matrix is time-independent. The machine learning task thus consists of learning the transition probabilities. Different modeling strategies can be taken when one wants to consider patients' individual characteristics.

A first strategy is to derive a model, that can be a *regression* model or a *survival* model, of the conditional probability given the attribute values of the patient, so that $P(q(t + 1)|q(t)) = f(\mathbf{x}(t))$, where $\mathbf{x}$ is the input vector.

Another strategy models the state variable as the vector of the m features measured on the patient. In this case $q = \mathbf{x}$, and $k = \mathbf{m}$. In this case the learning step stands in computing the conditional probabilities $P(\mathbf{x}(t + 1)|\mathbf{x}(t))$. A suitable strategy in this case is to resort to *dynamic Bayesian networks*, that allow one to conveniently parametrize the probability through a set of probability densities of smaller dimensions, exploiting local conditional independence between attributes.

A more complex situation occurs when the state cannot be observed, but rather we can measure only a set of output variables $\mathbf{y}(t)$. In this case, the dynamic system needs to be described with two sets of conditional probabilities, $P(\mathbf{q}(t + 1)|\mathbf{q}(t))$ and $P(\mathbf{y}(t)|\mathbf{q}(t))$. In this case, one needs to resort to the theory of hidden Markov models, since the Markov model that drives the dynamic is not observed [43].

Although not widely used in the literature due to the complexity of the learning algorithm and complexity in interpretation of results, it is also possible to exploit continuous time versions of the previously presented strategies [44]. Moreover, extensions with continuous states have been also published [45, 46].

Once a disease states model has been built from data, it is possible to only to look for the most probable next state or to derive the most probable trajectory, but also to perform **Monte Carlo simulations**. In this case, given a certain initial disease state, it is possible to generate many simulated cases by sampling from the conditional probability distributions. This is a powerful approach for outcome prediction, since it provides a distribution of trajectories that can show the variability of potential outcomes and may allow one to perform "what-if" and sensitivity analyses [42].

Performance Assessment

A crucial aspect of predicting clinical outcomes is related to the assessment of the quality of prediction models. Assessment can be performed considering several aspects. Different measures can be used to assess the quality of an outcome prediction model, although most of them are related to the capability of forecasting correctly the outcome itself: accuracy (and/or error), sensitivity and specificity, balanced accuracy, precision, and recall, Area Under the ROC Curve and the C-index, Area under the Precision-Recall Curve measures are used quite often to assess the discrimination capability of a model (see Chap. 6). Other measures, such as the Brier Score, jointly evaluate the discrimination and calibration properties, where calibration is the capability of estimating the correct probability of the outcome given the inputs.

For the benefit of the chapter, it is important however, to highlight what are the strategies to effectively compute the above-mentioned quantities from the training data. First, it is necessary to apply a proper experimental design when machine learning models are applied, to soundly estimate generalization error. Second, it is essential to evaluate the performance on independent data and to understand the issues related to the applicability of a model in health care settings different from the one(s) that generated the data. Third, there are important issues related to stability of the models, model drift and model update.

Experimental Design for Learning

Outcome prediction models based on machine learning techniques are fully dependent on the data available. Data are usually the result of a retrospective study, where suitable cases are selected and organized to extract the prediction model. A crucial step is therefore related to the selection of the examples, which should be performed with the goal of extracting a data set that is representative of the available population. This is crucial because the models will extract regularities that should generalize beyond the specific sample used for training the predictive model. Once this is done, the main goal of the experimental design is to properly assess the generalization performance of the machine learning model, i.e. to estimate how well the learned model will behave on unseen data. As already described in Chap. 6, it is common to resort to data set subdivision and resampling strategies. In an approach called **hold-out**, data are usually divided into two sets, the training set and the test set. While training is used to learn the classifiers, the test set should only be used to assess the generalization performance on unseen cases. In order to tune the algorithms' design parameters, the training set can be further divided into a learning and a validation set. **Repeated hold-out** allows one to derive an estimate of the stability of the prediction performances, even if, in this case, the set of performance measures obtained are strongly correlated, so that confidence intervals on the prediction cannot be reliably computed using standard statistics related to the properties of the sample mean. To lower the correlation between the repeated samples, a very popular approach is **k-fold cross-validation**, that divides the data set into k folds, which, in turn, allows training the model with k-1 fold and test on the remaining one. In this way the test data are always different from each other. As it has been recently shown, also this approach tends to underestimate the confidence intervals of the prediction, so that **nested k-fold cross-validation** can be used, to obtain a more reliable estimation of the confidence intervals of the accuracy [47]. Alternative strategies to obtain estimates of the generalization error are represented by **bootstrap** approaches, where several samples with replacement are obtained from the training set, thus generating a series of bootstrap samples of the same size of the original data set, where some data are left out due to the resampling mechanism (out of bag samples). Models are learned on each sample and tested on the out of bag data. Since the estimates of the performance obtained are biased and correlated, proper correction mechanisms are needed to derive reliable estimates of the generalization error as well as of its confidence intervals. Such confidence intervals can be obtained for example via non-parametric strategies, such as showing the sampling distributions of the bootstrap error.

Common Mistakes in the Design of Experimental Validation

Sampling strategies for assessing quality of outcome prediction are prone to subtle mistakes related to the preprocessing steps, such as imputation, feature selection, feature transformation and sometimes even normalization. As a matter of fact, *test set data should be kept separated from training data in all steps* [48]. It is essential to keep attention to all preprocessing steps that exploit, explicitly or implicitly, information about the class. The most common mistake made by students, but also in some published papers, is to perform feature selection before dividing training and test data. Since many approaches use ranking or shrinkage strategies that select the features that are more related to the class, feature selection becomes the first step of the learning algorithm, and thus should be performed on the training set only. This means, of course, that when running k-fold cross-validation, for example, feature selection should be performed k times, and the procedure may generate k models with (slightly) different features. Other cases with subtle overfitting mechanisms occur when the distribution of the data is changed before learning, for example when the training set is oversampled because one of the classes is underrepresented. If oversampling is performed on the entire data set, using for example resampling with replacement, or its variants that uses all data to generate the new samples, such as the Synthetic Minority Oversampling TEchnique (SMOTE) [49], it is important to keep the test data separated before oversampling, to avoid having copies or highly correlated samples in both training and test sets. Overfitting may be related to other preprocessing steps, one of the most common being class-aware discretization. In these approaches, the binning of the discrete values of a continuous variable are defined to maximize the class separation between the generated bins.

Experimental Design for Testing: External Validation

External validation is critical for establishing machine learning model quality. It involves the use of independently derived, external, data to validate the performance of a model trained on initial input data. External validation brings fundamental evidence for models' generalizability. For example, when a validation set comes from independent sources, any feature set that was wrongly selected for the input training data (e.g. due to sampling bias) would likely cause the model to fail [50].

Positive external validation performance is regarded as proof of generalizability: the idea is that if a good performance persistently replicates in independently sampled data, the learned model is more likely to be generalizable.

Data taken from completely separate sources (e.g. two cohorts coming from different studies) may capture useful domain-relevant aspects, and a well-trained model, which takes into account possible confounders and captures informative features, should continue to have good performances when repeatedly applied to new data. Furthermore, external validation should assure that these models are more domain-wise interpretable.

Checking Performance Stability, Model Drifts, Diagnostics, and Model Revision

After model development, validation and clinical impact evaluation, the AI model can be deployed in the clinical setting. When we deploy a model, we would expect that it will perform as well as in the validation phase. Yet, performance drift and reduced accuracy are often reported when the model is applied to new patients. Differences in performances can be due to substantial differences between the validation set and the patient population we are applying the model to. Healthcare environments are continuously evolving over time: demographic compositions, population ages and outcome incidence may change, differences between clinical settings and hospitals can be marked, clinical guidelines and scientific insights usually evolve over time. Dynamism and heterogeneity impact model performance over time or even instantly, from research to bedside. Therefore, performance monitoring should be mandatory when the model is applied in clinical practice [51].

First, we should assure that the deployed approach is being applied to a population as similar as possible to the training set: we have no guarantee that the model will perform as intended on patients that do not come from the same distribution as the training set. Much interest is currently devoted to include regulatory constraints in the design and application of AI-based tools[2] and to introduce the concept of algorithmovigilance, as discussed in Chap. 18. In terms of methods for performance monitoring, some pattern recognition models embed a rejection option in their classification, so that the classifier refuses (or labels as unreliable) the prediction on a particular instance that is somehow distant or different from the training set [52]. Reliability assessment of single prediction would represent a useful metric to monitor a model's performance and increase trust in the prediction. Pointwise reliability is a measure of confidence that the predicted class for a specific instance (i.e. patient) is equal to the true class of the instance. In deployment, we do not often hold the information about the true clinical outcome, yet reliability assessment can provide a measure of trust on that prediction. Two principles can be followed to compute a reliability measure. First, the prediction on an instance that is "not close" to the training set, is more likely to be unreliable, given that the model has not been trained on that area of the feature space. Second, the prediction of an instance will be more reliable if the model was accurate on similar instances of the training set [53]. Pointwise reliability may be a useful monitoring tool to (1) guarantee that the model is being applied at its "working point" (2) to detect possible underrepresented populations (3) to detect possible population shifts over time.

Monitoring the performance of our model over time involves: (1) monitoring the *discriminative performance* (i.e. the ability to predict the true class of an example), and (2) monitoring *calibration* (i.e. the ability to align predicted posterior

---

[2] https://www.fda.gov/medical-devices/software-medical-device-samd/artificial-intelligence-and-machine-learning-software-medical-device, with (accessed August 18, 2022).

probabilities to the true posterior probabilities). In some applications, a lower calibration can be tolerated, for instance when our aim is to stratify patients by risk. However, when the predicted probabilities are used to support personalized decision making, it is important to maintain good calibration. Moreover, it has been observed that calibration is more likely to deteriorate over time. When performance drift, either in discriminative or calibration performance, is diagnosed, different strategies can be adopted. The model can be re-estimated, i.e. re-trained on new data, without changing its form or variable definitions, while hyper-parameters are re-tuned if necessary. Alternatively, a completely different model can be trained on new data. These approaches should be performed in response to substantial dataset shift and/or new critical insights. In addition, different updating methods have been developed to retain and increase knowledge from the starting model [54].

Recently, model evaluation in terms of its explainability is gaining traction, leading to the development of so-called eXplainable AI (XAI). XAI investigates methods to interpret the internal logic and/or the prediction of AI black box models, and it has been boosted by recent regulations such as the European Union's General Data Protection Regulation [55]. The reader can refer to Chap. 8 for an overview of AI explainability.

Case Studies and Examples

This section will provide some case studies in the areas of diabetes, myelodysplastic diseases, and COVID-19.

Type 2 Diabetes

The prediction of clinical outcomes within type 2 diabetes poses several challenges. The pathology itself entails a few complications and comorbidities and managing type 2 diabetes patients is a complex task, such complexity being embodied in long clinical histories characterized by substantial variability in the type and frequency of clinical events. To build efficient pipelines to derive a set of predictive models of type 2 diabetes complications, it is necessary to follow several of the approaches described in this chapter.

For example, in a previous study, authors implemented a pipeline comprising clinical center profiling, predictive model targeting, predictive model construction and model validation [56]. After having dealt with missing data by multiple imputation and having applied suitable strategies to handle class imbalance, they used logistic regression with stepwise feature selection to predict the onset of retinopathy, neuropathy, or nephropathy, at different time scenarios. As small differences in terms of prediction accuracy were noticeable among the applied models (logistic regression, SVM, random forest and naive bayes), logistic regression was chosen, given its capability of visualizing results through nomograms and as the instrument to deliver the model predictions to users, in accordance with explainability paradigms.

Other applications aim at predicting type 2 Diabetes clinical outcomes leveraging modeling of patient trajectories. More recently, it has been shown that temporal models that capture disease progression can identify key features that underpin patients' trajectories and characterize their subtypes [57]. The authors identified multivariate disease trajectories with an approach based on **topological data analysis**, then pseudo time-series were used to infer a state space model characterized by transitions between hidden states that represent distinct trajectories. Each patient was associated with one of the identified trajectories, and this information was used as a predictor for the onset of type 2 diabetes microvascular complications. Outcomes were contrasted for subjects belonging to the discovered trajectories using a Kaplan-Meier visualization. Given the results obtained by the Kaplan-Meier analyses (Fig. 11.9), the authors investigated whether the mined patient groups were significant predictors of the onset of microvascular complications when also considering the available clinical variables in a statistical model. To this end, they carried out a multivariate survival analysis by using Cox-Regression to predict onset probabilities. Results indicate worst prognosis (i.e. higher risk of an earlier development of microvascular complications) in patients following the so-called trajectory A (in red in Fig. 11.9). When analyzed in a univariate way, patients following to the A trajectory show a higher and increasing level of HbA1c, a decreasing and then increasing trend of cholesterol, and an increasing trend of triglycerides.

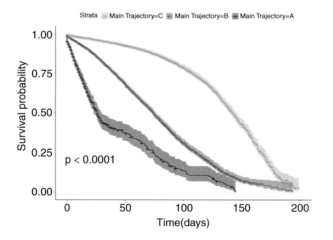

Fig. 11.9 Kaplan-Meier having the onset of micro vascular complication as endpoints for different groups of patients following the different mined trajectories. (Figure from [57] (Dagliati, Geifman, et al. 2020) (This article was published in Artificial Intelligence in Medicine, Dagliati A, Geifman N, Peek N, Holmes JH, Sacchi L, Bellazzi R, Sajjadi SE, Tucker A. "Using topological data analysis and pseudo time series to infer temporal phenotypes from electronic health records". Copyright Elsevier (2020))

Myelodysplastic Syndromes

The advent and development of high-throughput sequencing technologies provide novel insights into patients' individual genomics landscapes. Analytics integrating both genomics and clinical data are therefore needed to better support clinical decisions. As we have already mentioned, Cox models can inform understanding of individual patient characteristics that significantly impact on diagnosis, prognosis, or therapeutic response in cancers. Data collected over time (i.e. longitudinal data) from patients' cohorts could be useful to assess risk factors for disease progression and, through Markov approaches, to calculate probabilities of transition to subsequent stages. However, longitudinal analysis can be time- and cost-intensive. Therefore, many studies only cover a short time window within the disease progression.

For instance, cross-sectional data from patients in different disease stages were exploited to simulate probabilistic trajectories describing patient's possible disease progression pathways [58]. The approach exploits data transformation methods, in particular matrix factorization, and Monte Carlo simulation. The resulting simulated longitudinal dataset can be analyzed with Cox and Markov models.

This method was applied to study the dynamics of myelodysplastic syndromes (MDS), heterogeneous clonal hematopoietic disorders[3] associated with mutations and abnormalities in maturation and differentiation of hematopoietic cell lines. MDS patients are characterized by different risks of development of acute myeloid leukemia (AML), and genetic events are found to drive MDS progression towards AML. In clinical practice, patients are categorized into different levels of progression risk according to the International Prognostic Scoring System Revised (IPSSR). Based on clinical features, the IPSSR score categorizes patients into one of the following levels of risk: "Very Low", "Low", "Intermediate", "High", and "Very High" [59]. Yet, recent studies suggest that genomics characteristics may have an important role in driving disease progression.

To study disease progression and the influence of genomics characteristics, in a recent study authors developed a method to simulate longitudinal data from cross-sectional data, considering the similarity between patients [58]. Such similarity is calculated through a matrix trifactorization strategy that computes similarity using patient data and several knowledge sources, represented by relational matrices that associate clinical data, mutations, genes, and diseases. Each patient in a given stage has a probability of progression to the following stage defined by the mean survival probability in that stage. Moreover, it is possible to compute the similarity of this patient to every patient in the subsequent stage. Starting from each patient in the first stage, when running the simulation, he/she may evolve to the following stage, or he/she may remain in the same stage. If a patient evolves, he/she "becomes" one of the patients of the following stage with a probability proportional to their

---

[3] Hematopoietic disorders are heterogeneous diseases that can be caused by problems with red blood cells, white blood cells, platelets, bone marrow, lymph nodes, and the spleen.

similarity through a roulette wheel algorithm. Two patients linked by the simulation strategy become a single macro-patient. This procedure is applied again until all disease's stages are evaluated. Ten thousand Monte Carlo simulations were performed to select the longest most frequent trajectories. The result is a simulated longitudinal dataset which is exploited for Cox analysis and for Markov modeling to calculate transition probabilities between different stages of the disease or death.

Despite Cox and Markov models being built from simulated data, the former was able to reveal many significant covariates with support in the literature. For instance, the IDH2 gene encodes a protein that plays a role in intermediary metabolism and energy production. According to the results of the Cox model, mutations in this gene are associated with disease progression (Fig. 11.10), in accordance with previous studies that showed that IDH2 mutated patients have a significantly higher risk of developing AML and are associated with significantly worse overall survival. Survival curves obtained from the simulated analysis were consistent with survival curves observed in a previous study.

The COVID-19 Pandemic

The pandemic of coronavirus disease (COVID-19) caused by the severe acute respiratory syndrome coronavirus 2 (SARS-CoV-2) has boosted the application of AI methods for clinical purposes in a collaborative way. The Consortium for Clinical Characterization of COVID-19 by EHR (4 CE) is an international collaboration addressing COVID-19 with federated analyses of electronic health record (EHR) data. 4 CE involves more than 340 international hospitals jointly analyzing more than 30,000 COVID patients' data [60]. The initiative has been able to collect summary data on demographics, hospitalization time, diagnosis codes, lab values, drugs in a standardized way on data coming from six countries starting from spring 2020. Several studies have been carried out, focusing on different outcomes related to COVID-19, and different research projects have started leveraging this initiative [61].

One of the aims of the 4CE consortium was to develop and validate computable phenotypes for COVID-19 severity [62].

During the 4CE activities it became apparent that to properly analyze patient disease trajectories and investigate outcomes based on EHR data, it is essential to obtain reliable disease severity measures, such as ICU admission and in-hospital death. However, these measures were not always available in all collaborating centers. For this reason, it was necessary to develop a surrogate severity measure, based on data available on all EHRs, such as medications, diagnosis, and lab codes. Such surrogate measure is a *computable phenotype*.

Two different approaches have been followed. On the one hand an "expert-driven" 4CE severity phenotype has been derived. This algorithm was validated against the severity outcome "ICU admission and/or death" in the subset of the global 4CE consortium data in which this information was available. On the other

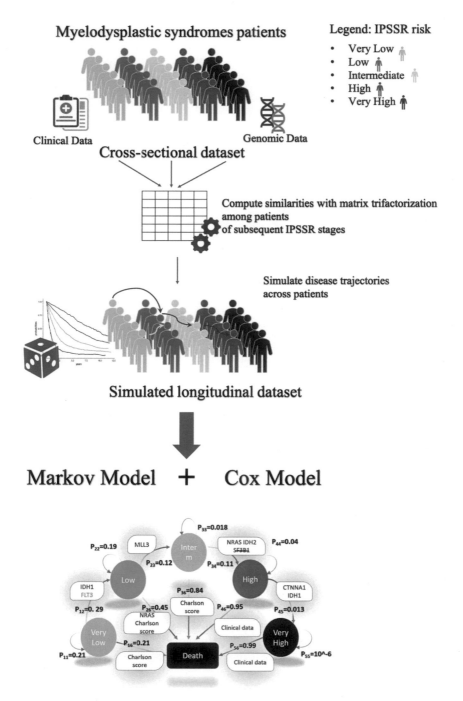

Fig. 11.10 Workflow to simulate and analyze longitudinal data from patients in different risk stages. (Figure from (Nicora et al. 2020)) (This article was published in the Journal of Biomedical Informatics, Volume 104, G.Nicora, F.Moretti, E.Sauta, M.Della Porta, L.Malcovati, M.Cazzola, S.Quaglini, R.Bellazzi, "A continuous-time Markov model approach for modeling myelodysplastic syndromes progression from cross-sectional data", Copyright Elsevier (2020))

hand, relying on data of one center only, a data-driven phenotype was learned using a classification algorithm, and its results have been compared with the "expert-driven" one.

The main goal of this step was to develop a clinical severity phenotype that was possible to compute at any site participating in the work, thus limiting the data to: demographics, diagnoses, labs, medications, and ICD procedure codes [63]. In particular, the following concepts were extracted from the data:

- Demographics:
  - Sex, Age
- Diagnoses:
  - ARDS, ventilator-associated pneumonia;
- Lab Tests:
  - $PaCO_2$ or PaO_2;
- Medications:
  - sedatives/anesthetics or treatment for shock;
- Procedures:
  - endotracheal tube insertion or invasive mechanical ventilation.

Since the concepts are related to different concepts in standard coding systems (see Chap. 3), the i2b2 (Informatics for Integrating Biology and the Bedside, https://www.i2b2.org/) ontology of the ATC (Anatomical Therapeutic Chemical) network [64] was used to extract a list of about 100 codes belonging to one of: International Classification of Diseases versions 9 and 10 (ICD-9 and ICD-10), Logical Observation Identifiers Names and Codes (LOINC) [65], and RxNorm format [66].

The "phenotyping" algorithm simply assigns a patient to the class "severe" if any of these codes is present in the EHR during a Covid hospitalization.

Resorting to the data coming from one of the centers involved in 4CE, Mass General Brigham (MGB), a computable phenotyping pipeline was applied to compare the expert-driven approach to a fully data-driven method.

The problem has been modeled as a supervised classification task, where the binary class is $y = \{severe, not\text{-}severe\}$. The feature set was either represented by the codes identified by the expert-driven approach (see above) or by all the codes from all possible data elements, generating the fully data-driven strategy. In the latter strategy the Minimize Sparsity Maximize Relevance (MSMR) dimensionality reduction algorithm [67] was used as a feature selection step. In both approaches, logistic regression coupled with component-wise functional gradient boosting was exploited to derive the final classification model. The model was tested on 3290 patients with a repeated hold-out approach, using an 80–20 train-test split and 9 iterations.

The expert-driven 4CE severity phenotype had pooled sensitivity of 0.73 and specificity 0.83. The comparison of the performance of the two strategies showed that expert-derived phenotypes had mean AUC 0.903 (95% CI: 0.886, 0.921), compared to AUC 0.956 (95% CI: 0.952, 0.959) for the data-driven approach. Rather interestingly, the best features selected by the MSMR-based algorithm were partly related to the 4CE definition, such as PaCO2, PaO2, ARDS, sedatives; added ICU related exams, such as d-dimer, immature granulocytes, albumin; and finally provided different insights, probably related to the peculiarities of the specific hospital, such as chlorhexidine, glycopyrrolate, palliative care encounter.

In conclusion, expert-driven phenotypes seem robust and can be applied in many international centers, and data-driven ones, although prone to overfitting, may reveal interesting novel relationships between variables and outcomes.

Conclusion

In this chapter we have discussed the application of AI strategies to deal with the problem of predicting clinical outcomes. Clinical outcomes are defined as measurable changes in health, function or quality of life that result from patients' care. The capability to predict such changes is of course of paramount importance in a variety of clinical contexts, in day-by-day clinical activities. In order to highlight the most important aspects of AI modeling to forecast clinical outcomes, we first provided an enlarged view about the different outcomes' evaluation measures, which are crucial to understand the different classes of AI methods that need to be exploited. Following this analysis, we then discussed the most important set of AI approaches that are needed for outcome prediction, namely pre-processing, including deep learning strategies, classification, regression, survival analysis, trajectory modeling and Markov models. Of utmost importance in medicine is model evaluation and performance assessment. For this reason, we devoted a section to presenting the most important aspects of experimental design in machine learning, highlighting common mistakes and pitfalls in biomedical machine learning studies. We introduced the topic of validating the model against external data sets, i.e. data collected in clinical centers different from the one(s) used to train the model, and finally we presented the problem of monitoring performance stability and revising the model while it is in operation. AI for outcome prediction can be seen as a biomedical engineering exercise, where the selection of the methodologies and the data analytics pipeline need to be coupled with the profound understanding of the clinical problem. To show practical examples of this approach, we reported three case studies of AI applied for clinical outcomes prediction, covering complications in type 2 Diabetes, prognosis in myelodysplastic syndrome, and finally severity modeling in COVID-19 patients.

While AI provides new ways for modeling patients' evolution after a clinical intervention, different sources of uncertainty make this problem extremely hard, and inherently prone to high variability. Such sources include individual responses to treatment that depend on unmodeled factors, like the environmental context, as well as operational differences between and within hospital institutions. For these reasons, it is crucial to remember that AI can be very beneficial to understand better data to formulate hypotheses about the future patient evolution, but all decisions related with these hypotheses need to be taken with human judgement and discernment.

Questions for Discussion

- Define some practical scenarios of use of prediction models in the clinic, answering the following questions related (1) to data collection: who collects the data. and when is it collected? (2) to deployment of the model: how should predictions be presented (e.g. apps, charts)? and finally (3) to the decision-making process (who takes decisions based on model predictions and what are the consequences of model errors?)
- What are some criteria for choosing the best strategy to deal with an outcome prediction problem? How would one go about selecting the type of outcome measure, identifying the number and nature of the features available for analysis and the amount of data available?
- What are the key components of experimental design to evaluate the results of outcome prediction models?
- What are the differences and relationships between prediction and causation? To what extent should explanation, prediction, and causality be jointly considered when starting a clinical machine learning project?

Further Reading

Trevor Hastie, Robert Tibshirani, Jerome Friedman, The Elements of Statistical Learning: Data Mining, Inference, and Prediction, Second Edition (Springer Series in Statistics) 2nd Edition.

- In this classic volume, authors provide an overview of statistical learning, from the methodologies (supervised and unsupervised machine learning approaches) to validation strategies.

Chunhua Weng, Nigam H. Shah, George Hripcsak: Deep phenotyping: Embracing complexity and temporality - Towards scalability, portability, and interoperability. J. Biomed. Informatics 105: 103433 (2020).

- This is a special issue that includes twenty original articles presenting novel methodologies for case ascertainment, patient stratification, disease subtyping and temporal phenotyping.

David Hand, Construction and Assessment of Classification Rules, Wiley 1997.

- This book outlines different approaches to construct classification rules. Emphasis is placed on comparison and evaluation of performance.

Charu C. Aggarwal, Neural Networks and Deep Learning, A Textbook, Springer, 2018.

- This volume contains a thorough examination of neural networks and deep learning approaches, from a theoretical and algorithmic point of view.

Ewout W Steyerberg, Clinical Prediction Models: A Practical Approach to Development, Validation, and Updating, Springer, 2009.

- This book provides practical illustration on how statistical and regression approaches are applied to predict diagnostic and prognostic outcomes.

References

1. Goodfellow IJ, Bengio Y, Courville A. Deep learning. Cambridge, MA: MIT Press; 2016.
2. Bzdok D, Altman N, Krzywinski M. Statistics versus machine learning. Nat Methods. 2018;15:233–4.
3. Tejedor M, Woldaregay AZ, Godtliebsen F. Reinforcement learning application in diabetes blood glucose control: a systematic review. Artif Intell Med. 2020;104:101836.
4. Rubin DB. Inference and missing data. Biometrika. 1976;63:581–92.
5. Pedersen AB, et al. Missing data and multiple imputation in clinical epidemiological research. Clin Epidemiol. 2017;9:157–66.
6. van Buuren S, Groothuis-Oudshoorn K. Mice: multivariate imputation by chained equations in R. J Stat Softw. 2011;45:1–67.
7. Chandrashekar G, Sahin F. A survey on feature selection methods. Comput Electr Eng. 2014;40:16–28.
8. Pearson KLIII. On lines and planes of closest fit to systems of points in space. Lond Edinb Dublin Philos Mag J Sci. 1901;2:559–72.
9. Hotelling H. Analysis of a complex of statistical variables into principal components. J Educ Psychol. 1933;24:417–41.
10. Jolliffe IT, Cadima J. Principal component analysis: a review and recent developments. Philos Trans R Soc A Math Phys Eng Sci. 2016;374:20150202.
11. van der Maaten L, Hinton G. Visualizing data using t-SNE. J Mach Learn Res. 2008;9:2579–605.
12. Wang F, Casalino LP, Khullar D. Deep learning in medicine-promise, progress, and challenges. JAMA Intern Med. 2019;179:293–4.
13. Xu X, Liang T, Zhu J, Zheng D, Sun T. Review of classical dimensionality reduction and sample selection methods for large-scale data processing. Neurocomputing. 2019;328:5–15.
14. Yu Y, Si X, Hu C, Zhang J. A review of recurrent neural networks: LSTM cells and network architectures. Neural Comput. 2019;31:1235–70.
15. Yang X, Bian J, Hogan WR, Wu Y. Clinical concept extraction using transformers. J Am Med Inform Assoc. 2020;27:1935–42.
16. Vaswani A, et al. Attention is all you need. arXiv. 2017:1706.03762 [cs].
17. Russakovsky O, et al. ImageNet large scale visual recognition challenge. arXiv. 2015:1409.0575 [cs].
18. Devlin J, Chang M-W, Lee K, Toutanova K. BERT: pre-training of deep bidirectional transformers for language understanding. arXiv. 2019:1810.04805 [cs].
19. Goto T, Camargo CA, Faridi MK, Freishtat RJ, Hasegawa K. Machine learning-based prediction of clinical outcomes for children during Emergency Department Triage. JAMA Netw Open. 2019;2:e186937.
20. Skrede O-J, et al. Deep learning for prediction of colorectal cancer outcome: a discovery and validation study. Lancet. 2020;395:350–60.
21. Yala A, Lehman C, Schuster T, Portnoi T, Barzilay R. A deep learning mammography-based model for improved breast cancer risk prediction. Radiology. 2019;292:60–6.
22. Ling CX, Sheng VS. Cost-sensitive learning. In: Sammut C, Webb GI, editors. Encyclopedia of machine learning. New York: Springer; 2010. p. 231–5. https://doi.org/10.1007/978-0-387-30164-8_181.

23. Bayati M, et al. Data-driven decisions for reducing readmissions for heart failure: general methodology and case study. PLoS One. 2014;9:e109264.
24. Salvi E, Parimbelli E, Quaglini S, Sacchi L. Eliciting and exploiting utility coefficients in an integrated environment for shared decision-making. Methods Inf Med. 2019;58:24–30.
25. Hastie T, Tibshirani R. Generalized additive models. Stat Sci. 1986;1:297–310.
26. Schneider A, Hommel G, Blettner M. Linear Regression Analysis. Dtsch Arztebl Int. 2010;107:776–82.
27. Kleinbaum DG, Klein M. Survival analysis: a self-learning text. 3rd ed. New York: Springer-Verlag; 2012. https://doi.org/10.1007/978-1-4419-6646-9.
28. Giolo SR, Krieger JE, Mansur AJ, Pereira AC. Survival analysis of patients with heart failure: implications of time-varying regression effects in modeling mortality. PLoS One. 2012;7:e37392.
29. Goldhirsch A, Gelber RD, Simes RJ, Glasziou P, Coates AS. Costs and benefits of adjuvant therapy in breast cancer: a quality-adjusted survival analysis. J Clin Oncol. 1989;7:36–44.
30. Lee ET, Go OT. Survival Analysis in Public Health Research. Annu Rev Public Health. 1997;18:105–34.
31. Wang P, Li Y, Reddy CK. Machine learning for survival analysis: a survey. ACM Comput Surv. 2019;51:110.
32. Huang Z, et al. SALMON: Survival Analysis Learning With Multi-Omics Neural Networks on Breast Cancer. Front Genet. 2019;10:166.
33. Ching T, Zhu X, Garmire LX. Cox-nnet: An artificial neural network method for prognosis prediction of high-throughput omics data. PLoS Comput Biol. 2018;14:e1006076.
34. Lee, C., Zame, W., Yoon, J. & van der Schaar, M. DeepHit: A deep learning approach to survival analysis with competing risks. AAAI 32, (2018).
35. Lee C, Yoon J, van der Schaar M. Dynamic-DeepHit: a deep learning approach for dynamic survival analysis with competing risks based on longitudinal data. IEEE Trans Biomed Eng. 2020;67:122–33.
36. Harrell FE, Califf RM, Pryor DB, Lee KL, Rosati RA. Evaluating the yield of medical tests. JAMA. 1982;247:2543–6.
37. Brier GW. Verification of forecasts expressed in terms of probability. Mon Wea Rev. 1950;78:1–3.
38. Muthén B, Muthén LK. Integrating person-centered and variable-centered analyses: growth mixture modeling with latent trajectory classes. Alcohol Clin Exp Res. 2000;24:882–91.
39. van der Schoot R, Sijbrandij M, Winter SD, Depaoli S, Vermunt JK. The GRoLTS-Checklist: guidelines for reporting on latent trajectory studies. Struct Equ Model Multidiscip J. 2017;24:451–67.
40. Lennon H, et al. Framework to construct and interpret latent class trajectory modelling. BMJ Open. 2018;8:e020683.
41. Dagliati A, et al. Latent class trajectory modeling of 2-component disease activity score in 28 joints identifies multiple rheumatoid arthritis phenotypes of response to biologic disease-modifying antirheumatic drugs. Arthritis Rheumatol. 2020;72:1632–42.
42. Komorowski M, Raffa J. Markov models and cost effectiveness analysis: applications in medical research. In: Secondary Analysis of Electronic Health Records (ed. MIT Critical Data). New York: Springer International Publishing; 2016. p. 351–67. https://doi.org/10.1007/978-3-319-43742-2_24.
43. Mor B, Garhwal S, Kumar A. A systematic review of hidden markov models and their applications. Arch Computat Methods Eng. 2021;28:1429–48.
44. Liu M, et al. A comparison between discrete and continuous time Bayesian networks in learning from clinical time series data with irregularity. Artif Intell Med. 2019;95:104–17.
45. Ferrazzi F, Sebastiani P, Ramoni MF, Bellazzi R. Bayesian approaches to reverse engineer cellular systems: a simulation study on nonlinear Gaussian networks. BMC Bioinformatics. 2007;8:S2.

46. Chen R, Zheng Y, Nixon E, Herskovits EH. Dynamic network model with continuous valued nodes for longitudinal brain morphometry. NeuroImage. 2017;155:605–11.
47. Bates S, Hastie T, Tibshirani R. Cross-validation: what does it estimate and how well does it do it? arXiv. 2021:2104.00673 [math, stat].
48. Cabitza F, Campagner A. The need to separate the wheat from the chaff in medical informatics: Introducing a comprehensive checklist for the (self)-assessment of medical AI studies. Int J Med Inform. 2021;153:104510. https://doi.org/10.1016/j.ijmedinf.2021.104510.
49. Chawla NV, Bowyer KW, Hall LO, Kegelmeyer WP. SMOTE: Synthetic minority over-sampling technique. J Artif Intell Res. 2002;16:321–57.
50. Ho SY, Phua K, Wong L, Bin Goh WW. Extensions of the external validation for checking learned model interpretability and generalizability. Patterns. 2020;1:100129.
51. Toll DB, Janssen KJM, Vergouwe Y, Moons KGM. Validation, updating and impact of clinical prediction rules: a review. J Clin Epidemiol. 2008;61:1085–94.
52. Mesquita DPP, Rocha LS, Gomes JPP, Rocha Neto AR. Classification with reject option for software defect prediction. Appl Soft Comput. 2016;49:1085–93.
53. Saria S, Subbaswamy A. Tutorial: safe and reliable machine learning. 2019. Preprint at https://arxiv.org/abs/1904.07204.
54. Moons KGM, et al. Risk prediction models: II. External validation, model updating, and impact assessment. Heart. 2012;98:691–8.
55. Caruana R, Lundberg S, Ribeiro MT, Nori H, Jenkins S. Intelligible and Explainable Machine Learning: Best Practices and Practical Challenges. In: Proceedings of the 26th ACM SIGKDD International Conference on Knowledge Discovery & Data Mining 3511–3512. New York: Association for Computing Machinery; 2020. https://doi.org/10.1145/3394486.3406707.
56. Dagliati A, et al. Machine learning methods to predict diabetes complications. J Diabetes Sci Technol. 2018;12:295–302.
57. Dagliati A, Geifman N, et al. Using topological data analysis and pseudo time series to infer temporal phenotypes from electronic health records. Artif Intell Med. 2020;108:101930. https://doi.org/10.1016/j.artmed.2020.101930.
58. Nicora G, et al. A continuous-time Markov model approach for modeling myelodysplastic syndromes progression from cross-sectional data. J Biomed Inform. 2020;104:103398.
59. Greenberg PL, et al. Revised international prognostic scoring system for myelodysplastic syndromes. Blood. 2012;120:2454–65.
60. Brat GA, et al. International electronic health record-derived COVID-19 clinical course profiles: the 4CE consortium. NPJ Digital Medicine. 2020;3:109.
61. Weber GM, et al. International Comparisons of Harmonized Laboratory Value Trajectories to Predict Severe COVID-19: Leveraging the 4CE Collaborative Across 342 Hospitals and 6 Countries: A Retrospective Cohort Study. medRxiv. 2021:2020.12.16.20247684. https://doi.org/10.1101/2020.12.16.20247684.
62. Klann JG, et al. Validation of an internationally derived patient severity phenotype to support COVID-19 analytics from electronic health record data. J Am Med Inform Assoc. 2021;28(7):1411–20. https://doi.org/10.1093/jamia/ocab018.
63. World Health Organization. International statistical classification of diseases and related health problems. World Health Organization; 2015.
64. WHO Expert Committee on the Selection and Use of Essential Medicines, World Health Organization. The selection and use of essential medicines. In: Report of the WHO expert committee, 2005 (including the 14th model list of essential medicines), 2006.
65. Huff SM, et al. Development of the Logical Observation Identifier Names and Codes (LOINC) Vocabulary. J Am Med Inform Assoc. 1998;5:276–92.
66. Liu S, Ma W, Moore R, Ganesan V, Nelson S. RxNorm: prescription for electronic drug information exchange. IT Professional. 2005;7:17–23.
67. Estiri H, Strasser ZH, Klann JG, McCoy TH Jr., Wagholikar KB, Vasey S, Castro VM, Murphy ME, Murphy SN. Transitive sequencing medical records for mining predictive and interpretable temporal representations. Patterns 2020.

Chapter 12
Interpreting Medical Images

Zongwei Zhou, Michael B. Gotway, and Jianming Liang

After reading this chapter, you should know the answers to these questions:
- What are medical images, and how are they different from photographic images?
- How are medical images used in clinical medical practice?
- What are the challenges and opportunities for interpreting medical images?
- What are the promising approaches and directions for AI in medical imaging?

Overview

Modern imaging systems generate enormous volumes of data, far exceeding the human capacity for interpretation—a manifestation of **big data** in medical imaging. However, it is not the images themselves but rather the clinically relevant information contained within them that is of importance. **Computer-aided diagnosis** (CAD) empowered by **artificial intelligence** (AI) and **deep learning** (DL, see Chap. 6) has led to radical progress in automatically interpreting medical images.

Z. Zhou
Johns Hopkins University, Baltimore, MD, USA
e-mail: zzhou82@jh.edu

M. B. Gotway
Mayo Clinic, Scottsdale, AZ, USA
e-mail: Gotway.Michael@mayo.edu

J. Liang (✉)
Arizona State University, Phoenix, AZ, USA
e-mail: jianming.liang@asu.edu

© The Author(s), under exclusive license to Springer Nature   343
Switzerland AG 2022
T. A. Cohen et al. (eds.), *Intelligent Systems in Medicine and Health*, Cognitive
Informatics in Biomedicine and Healthcare,
https://doi.org/10.1007/978-3-031-09108-7_12

There is no doubt that the impact of AI/DL on medical imaging will be tremendous. In the future, many medical images will reach a physician along with an interpretation provided by a computer. Although this chapter is largely focused on the role of AI/DL in medical imaging, we start with some background information on medical imaging itself, which will help you to understand the later discussions regarding AI's role in image interpretation.

Introduction to Medical Images

"Medical imaging" is a broad term that encompasses a wide variety of techniques used to create images of the human body. Worldwide, the most commonly employed imaging technique is conventional radiography—the use of X-ray radiation to create images of human anatomy non-invasively. Conventional radiography is performed by directing a focused X-ray beam toward a patient and using a specialized detector placed against the patient to record the relative amount of X-ray absorption by the irradiated tissues. In essence, conventional radiography creates an image akin to a "shadow" that reflects relative tissue density—denser tissues, such as bone, absorb relatively more X-ray photons than less dense tissues, such as soft tissues and fat. The summation of this process of differential absorption produces a medical image. Figure 12.1a displays the first X-ray (probably the first medical image in history) produced by Wilhelm Roentgen in 1895. Conventional radiography is widely employed in a number of situations, particularly for musculoskeletal and chest disorders; for example, "X-rays" of the extremities and bones are routinely performed for patients with a traumatic injury. Also, chest X-rays (conventional radiography of the chest) are performed for numerous conditions affecting the thorax, including for patients presenting with chest pain, shortness of breath, suspected pneumonia, and other heart or lung conditions.

Despite the widespread use of conventional radiography, this technique suffers from significant limitations. In particular, conventional radiography is a summation technique—the created images are two-dimensional representations of three-dimensional human anatomy. This situation results in anatomic structures overlapping one another, which can obscure important diagnoses. Furthermore, since the X-rays used for conventional radiography create a density map of a patient's tissues, tissues with similar density may not be seen as distinct structures. This physical limitation is profound—most soft tissues in the human body (e.g., liver, heart, blood, and muscle among others) have similar density, and hence the ability of conventional radiography to depict these structures adequately is quite limited.

Recognition of the limitations of conventional radiography has led to advanced medical imaging techniques, notably **Ultrasound**, **Magnetic Resonance Imaging (MRI)**, and **Computed Tomography (CT)**. These imaging modalities are

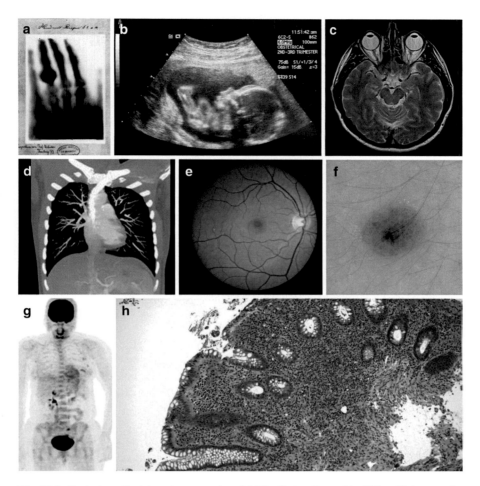

Fig. 12.1 Typical medical imaging examples. (**a**) The first radiographic ("X-ray") image of a woman's hand (source: https://en.wikipedia.org/wiki/X-ray, accessed Aug 19, 2022). (**b**) Ultrasound image of a fetus. (**c**) Magnetic resonance imaging (MRI) of the brain. (**d**) Computed tomography (CT) of the thorax. (**e**) Ophthalmologic image of the retina. (**f**) Dermoscopic image of the skin lesion. (**g**) PET image of the human body. (**h**) Pathology image of the tissue

commonly referred to as **cross sectional imaging** techniques because they create two-dimensional, thin section, "slice-like" images of the human body that can be summed to create exquisite three-dimensional anatomic images (Fig. 12.1b–d). Their introduction occurred during the last half of the twentieth century:

- *Ultrasound was developed in the 1960s.* Ultrasound creates images using high-frequency sound waves, which are directed into a patient and differentially transmitted or reflected by the various issues encountered. When a transducer is placed on the skin in a particular area of the patient, sound beams are directed into the patient's tissues and either absorbed or reflected back to the transducer according to the various properties of the tissues and interfaces encountered, allowing the creation of a medical image. Ultrasound imaging has wide applications in medicine, including assessment of cardiac function, patency of blood vessels, detection of neoplasms, and assessment of acute abdominal and pelvic pain, among numerous other uses. In particular, ultrasound examinations can often be performed portably and therefore are widely employed at the point of medical care.

- *MRI was invented in 1970.* MRI creates images of human anatomy in an entirely different manner from ultrasound. MRI uses a radiofrequency energy pulse directed into human tissue, which excites hydrogen atoms in that tissue. Because the hydrogen atoms in the imaged tissue exposed to the radiofrequency pulse are at a higher energy state, when the radiofrequency energy pulse is turned off, the hydrogen atoms return to their resting state by emitting an energy signal, doing so in a manner unique to their local environment. Hence this signal, or echo, returned from tissue exposed to the radiofrequency pulse, can be sampled and used to create an image of the examined tissue. MRI has been widely applied to differentiate between white matter and grey matter in the brain and can also be used to diagnose aneurysms and tumors.

- *CT was created in 1972.* As with conventional radiography, CT uses X-rays to create density maps of human tissue, but unlike conventional radiography, CT is not a summation technique; instead, CT is a projection technique in which X-ray photons are directed from various angles through a patient and X-ray absorption (referred to as attenuation) is recorded along the photon paths. In this manner, tissues of similar density can be differentiated, and an image of internal human anatomy is generated. CT has wide applications in medicine, e.g., showing internal injuries and bleeding; locating a tumor, blood clot, excess fluid, or infection; detecting cancer, heart disease, emphysema, or liver masses; guiding biopsies, surgeries, and radiation therapy.

Characteristics of Medical Images

Medical images possess unique characteristics compared with photographic images, providing unique opportunities for applying computer-aided techniques to assist in medical diagnosis. These characteristics provide the basis for imaging research advances that have subsequently been translated into clinically usable products. This section summarizes some of the unique characteristics of medical images that can be exploited by AI techniques to advance computer-aided diagnosis in medical imaging.

- *Medical images are created by modalities.* Photographic images typically consist of 3-channel (red, green, and blue) images within the visible light spectrum, whereas there are many modalities to create medical images, including CT, MRI, positron emission tomography (PET), mammography, ultrasound, radiography, and many more. Each modality uses a portion of the non-visible electromagnetic spectrum (except for ultrasound, which employs sound waves for image creation) to create images for visualizing and identifying certain medical disorders and procedural complications. Certain medical imaging modalities are more conducive to the evaluation of particular disorders than to others. For example, abnormalities such as acute active hemorrhage are more readily diagnosable by intravenous contrast-enhanced CT than by MRI, whereas small or subtle lesions such as prostate cancer, uterine cancer, and metastases to the bone and brain may be better shown by MRI. Also, although they may often require the use of ionizing radiation or intravenous contrast administration, cross sectional techniques (e.g., CT and MRI) are capable of producing images with substantially richer details than is conventional radiography (often colloquially referred to as "X-ray" imaging).

- *Medical images possess high dimensionality.* Cross sectional imaging techniques, such as CT and MRI, produce three-dimensional images, and when **dynamic imaging** is performed, a fourth dimension—time—is added. While the world around us is three-dimensional, human eyesight is essentially a two-dimensional process. Although various reconstruction algorithms effectively "simulate" the 3D world from multiple 2D views, human eyesight nevertheless relies on two-dimensional spatial information processing. When reading a volumetric cross sectional imaging examination, radiologists must scroll through a stack of images to mentally "reconstruct" the underlying anatomy in three dimensions. This procedure is cumbersome and time-consuming, especially when one is searching for small lesions, which are only seen on a few images within a large volumetric image stack, and particularly when an abnormality is similar in appearance to normal anatomies, such as a small lung nodule (which can closely resemble a normal pulmonary vessel). To avoid overlooking potentially significant abnormalities, radiologists must scrutinize all aspects of each image contained within a large **volumetric stack**; nevertheless, it has been well-established through eye-tracking perceptual research that even trained observers fail to visually scan all parts of a medical image [1]. In contrast, computer algorithms can interpret high-dimensional images the same way as 2D images by directly harnessing spatial and temporal information.

- *Medical images vary in quality.* Owing to substantial differences among medical imaging manufacturers as well as variable proprietary hardware and software platforms, medical images may vary in quality and content among various institutions as well as within a given institution. Furthermore, acquisition protocol parameters (of which numerous considerations must be addressed for a given application) vary considerably among institutions, even for a given manufacturer and application. Such variability often results in "domain gaps" in terms of image quality and technical display. These domain gaps are significant obstacles to developing robust AI/DL methods—a situation often referred to as "domain shift" or "distribution drift." For example, CT scans performed using 5 mm slice thickness can handicap a model trained using CT scans performed using a 0.75 mm thickness, resulting in AI/DL interpretations that have limited clinical value. While the domain shift problem can be addressed by a universally applied configuration for acquiring medical images across hospitals, such a requirement does not currently exist and is unlikely to be adopted. Approaches such as semi-supervised learning, domain adaptation, domain generalization, and federal learning have been explored to address the "domain shift" problem [2, 3].

• *Medical images convey physical meaning.* The color information in photographic images does not usually carry a taxonomic meaning of the object. For instance, a shirt is a shirt, no matter what color it is. In contrast, the exact or relative pixel intensity value in a given medical image corresponds to a specific constituent within the human body, particularly for cross sectional imaging modalities such as CT and MRI. CT images are created by directing ionizing radiation through a body part and counting the relative number of photons absorbed by the tissue traversed by the X-ray beam—a greater number of photons absorbed occurs with denser tissue, such as bone, whereas a greater number of photons transmitted (not absorbed and thus reaching the detector) occurs with less dense tissue, such as lung **parenchyma**. The commonly used scale representing the relative amount of X-ray photon absorption at CT is the Hounsfield Units (HU) and reflects tissue density. By convention, an attenuation coefficient of 0 HU is equivalent to the density of water (1 gm/cm^3). Air or gas, as may be encountered within the large airways and bowel, has an attenuation coefficient of -1000 HU, whereas bone, a very dense structure, has an attenuation coefficient of approximately 1000 HU. Other tissues within the human body have attenuation coefficients between these values. For example, fat has a value between -80 and -30 HU, whereas muscle has an attenuation coefficient ranging between 35 and 55 HU. This ability to directly measure the density of human tissue enables human experts and computer algorithms to identify normal human anatomy and potential abnormalities. More importantly, the semantics derived from pixel intensity offer a weak annotation that can be harnessed to facilitate the model learning the appearance of anatomic structures without extensive manual annotation [4].

• *Medical images encode relative location and orientation.* When identifying objects in photographic images, their locations are generally not important—a cat is a cat no matter if it appears in the left or right of the image. In contrast, in medical imaging, the relative location and orientation of a structure and the intrinsic consistency of anatomical relationships are important characteristics that allow recognition of normal anatomy and pathological conditions. Thus, the regular and predictable location of various structures in the human body is valuable for developing AI/DL methods. Furthermore, since medical imaging protocols assess patients in fairly consistent and reproducible orientations, these methods generate images with great similarity across various patients, equipment manufacturers, and facility locations. Therefore, recognizing the stereotypical position and orientation information of human anatomy provides an opportunity to reduce the **false-positive rate** and to improve the accuracy of disease detection and segmentation. Several investigations have demonstrated the value of this embedded prior knowledge by adding location features, modifying objective functions, and constraining coordinates relative to landmarks in images [5–8]. For instance, when employing ultrasound to measure **carotid arterial intimal-medial thickness** for cardiovascular risk stratification, the measurement could be performed at any point along the longitudinal aspect of the vessel, and such variability could adversely affect results and reproducibility [9]. However, it is standard practice to perform this measurement 1 cm beyond a recognizable anatomic landmark—the carotid bulb [10]. As a result, the anatomically recognizable carotid bulb provides a contextual constraint for developing AI/DL methods.

- *Medical images encode both scale and distance.* The uncertain distance between camera and object limits precise size measurements in photographic images; in contrast, the physical size of a structure is preserved in medical images. Therefore, scale is one of several quantitative attributes of standard imaging formats. The size of a pixel in CT, as an example, is often specified in the **metadata of Digital Imaging and Communications in Medicine (DICOM)**.[1] By obtaining the number of pixels belonging to an object and the pixel scale from the header, the physical scale and distance between normal structures and lesions in the image can easily be computed. This information is a critical feature in the assessment of disease, both by human interpretation and computer-aided diagnosis because the physical size of a lesion influences disease stage, treatment options, and prognosis. Moreover, the meta-information associated with images (e.g., pixel spacing, slice thickness, and image position) can be used to estimate the domain gaps among datasets collected from different equipment manufacturers, facilities, and regions. This allows the creation of more robust models and enhances the ability to extrapolate computer-aided diagnosis across various medical practices.

- *Medical images have sparse and noisy labels.* Unlike photographic imaging datasets, it is impractical to annotate millions of medical images with a systematic label hierarchy. Most medical imaging datasets focus on particular anatomic regions and only provide annotation for the object of interest [11]. For example, the KiTS dataset[2] provides annotation only for the kidney, the LiTS dataset[3] for the liver, and the NIH Pancreas-CT dataset[4] for the pancreas. There is no publicly available dataset that provides systematic annotation for all visible structures in a medical imaging dataset; existing annotated datasets are either partially annotated or only annotated only on a small scale. Moreover, medical images are often associated with noise labels due to interobserver and

---

[1] https://www.dicomstandard.org/ (accessed August 19, 2022)

[2] https://kits19.grand-challenge.org/ (accessed August 19, 2022)

[3] https://competitions.codalab.org/competitions/17094 (accessed August 19, 2022)

[4] https://wiki.cancerimagingarchive.net/display/Public/Pancreas-CT (accessed August 19, 2022)

intraobserver variability [12]. That is, different human experts can provide conflicting opinions regarding a given lesion, reflecting interobserver variability. Furthermore, the same expert is likely to outline the contour of the same lesion very differently over multiple attempts separated in time, reflecting intraobserver variability [13]. Additionally, more severely noisy labels occur if the abnormality has indistinct boundaries, such as in the case of diffuse lung diseases. The partial and imperfect annotation compromises model training and results in ambiguous and unreliable results when AI/DL methods undergo testing.

In summary, medical images contain quantitative imaging characteristics—the intensity value and physical size of pixels—that can be used as additional information to enhance AI/DL performance. Medical images also present qualitative imaging characteristics—consistent and predictable anatomical structures with great dimensional details—that can provide an opportunity for comprehensive model training. Nevertheless, several characteristics unique to medical images create new challenges, such as isolated, discrepant data and partial, noisy labels, that must be addressed through additional investigation.

Historical Perspectives

Pioneer CAD Systems

Radiologists' daily workflow consists of image acquisition and interpretation with the provision of a radiologic diagnosis in the form of a written report. The development of increasingly sophisticated imaging methods has allowed a more explicit depiction of the anatomical structure of the human body and has translated to substantial improvements in diagnostic accuracy. However, such improvements have come at the cost of large increases in data acquisition; these large datasets require greater levels of both time and effort on the part of radiologists for interpretation. Furthermore, in addition to the increasing data requirements for individual radiologic examinations, the total number of examinations has also increased. The burgeoning workload demands and the increasing sophistication of computer technology in medicine, as well as a growing interest in applying the quantitative methodology to medical diagnosis and treatment, have all brought about enormous interest in the development of AI methods to assist in medical imaging interpretation. In the early 1980s, large-scale and systematic investigation and development of CAD systems began at the Kurt Rossmann Laboratories for Radiologic Image Research at the University of Chicago [14]. This period witnessed a fundamental shift in the utilization of computer outputs from *automated computer diagnosis* (the 1960s) to *computer-aided diagnosis* (the 1980s). Automated computer diagnosis assumes that computers could replace physicians for detecting abnormalities and the assessment of this notion focuses on pitting radiologists against the computer.

On the other hand, computer-aided diagnosis is not developed to replace physicians but rather enhance their capabilities through computer-physician interaction and synergy; therefore, the evaluation of computer-aided diagnosis focused on comparing radiologists' diagnostic performance alone versus radiologists' performance supplemented by the computer. The concept of CAD has since spread quickly and widely in clinical imaging practice due to the synergistic effect obtained by combining the radiologist's competence and the computer's capability. More recently, CAD applications have broadened from detection of abnormalities in medical images to determining disease treatment and prognosis through improved measurement accuracy.

Numerous CAD studies have been published since the 1980s, primarily concentrating on three major diseases, cardiovascular diseases, lung cancer, and breast cancer; but other organs such as brain, liver, and skeletal and vascular systems have also been the subject to CAD research [14]. The development of pioneer CAD systems was mainly composed of two stages:

1. *Feature extraction* computes quantitative features from images through signal analysis and statistical modeling. Features are a numerical vector with a lower dimensionality than images and show necessary invariances and covariances to intensity or scale changes. A number of algorithms were proposed to capture local correlation and disentangle frequency components spanning **Fourier transform** to the more advanced **Gabor filters, Scale-Invariant Feature Transform (SIFT), Gray-Level Co-occurrence Matrices (GLCM)**, etc. To further reduce feature dimensionality, **Principal Component Analysis** [15] was utilized to project the features onto a few principal component directions without losing too much information about the image. The study of Radiomics—an endeavor that employs computer extraction of quantitative features from medical images to assist in disease characterization and to define prognosis and direct treatment—has evolved from this effort [16, 17].

2. *Decision making* integrates the features extracted from the image and outputs the decision for a classification or regression task. **Machine learning** algorithms have been proposed for this purpose using statistical, data-driven rules that are automatically derived from a large set of examples. The mainstream of machine learning algorithms includes **Random Forest, Support Vector Machines (SVM), Adaptive Boosting (AdaBoost)**, and **Artificial Neural Network (ANN)**. Random Forests [18] employ an ensemble of decision trees, whereby each tree is trained on different training examples, improving the robustness of the overall classifier. SVM [19] determine the model parameters by solving a convex optimization problem, so the solution could always reach the global optimum. AdaBoost [20] forms a strong classifier using a boosting approach from multiple weak classifiers. We refer the readers to Marsland's textbook [21] for a detailed introduction of the classical machine learning methods (see also Chap. 6).

Despite being fast and customized, these pioneer CAD systems required significant effort and expertise for identifying the proper image features; the resulting features were explicitly specified by human experts and tailored to medical conditions and thus were fragile to alternative medical specialties. There is a wealth of literature on medical image analysis using machine learning, but their performance lags behind the recent advances in deep learning [22]—a significant extension of ANN algorithm (Chap. 6). In contrast with traditional machine learning, deep learning represents an important paradigm shift, which takes over the stages of *feature extraction* and *decision making*, optimizing the learning process simultaneously in an end-to-end fashion.

Recent Successes in Deep Learning

This section focuses on deep learning methods for medical imaging, highlighting several milestones and breakthroughs occurring since 2012. The tremendous progress in neural architectures, large-scale imaging benchmarks, and high-performance computational power resurrected deep learning in image recognition, and in turn, fostered further investments towards more possibilities. However, applying deep learning to medical imaging faces unique challenges—one of the most crucial obstacles is the lack of annotated datasets. Unlike the task of annotating photographic images (e.g., identifying different breeds of dogs and cats), annotating medical images is not only tedious and time-consuming, but it also requires limited, costly, specialty-oriented knowledge and skills. The remarkable success of deep learning and the unique technical barriers of medical image interpretation (elaborated in the Section on "Technical Barriers") launched a debate regarding the applicability of deep learning to medical imaging. In essence, the question was, *"how can we reproduce the remarkable success of deep learning in the medical imaging field, where large-scale, well-annotated datasets are difficult to obtain?"*

A breakthrough occurred in 2016 when transfer learning was first utilized to mitigate the data requirements. The idea was to transfer the knowledge from a source domain (with a large-scale image dataset) to a target domain (where only limited images are available). Transfer learning was proven to accelerate training, improve performance, and reduce annotation costs [23, 24]. Pre-training a deep learning model using the large-scale **ImageNet**[5] and then fine-tuning it on various target tasks was a *de facto* practice across many medical specialties. Applications in medical imaging (e.g., radiology) would be expected to process higher-resolution and volumetric images, for which the ImageNet pre-trained models may not be optimal. In 2019, Zhou et al. [4] developed generic pre-trained models, enabling models to learn visual features directly from 3D volumetric medical images (rather than 2D photographic images) without any human annotation. Generic, autodidactic methods could potentially recognize intricate patterns in medical images and

---

[5] https://www.image-net.org/update-mar-11-2021.php (accessed August 19, 2022)

potentially allow for transfer learning across diseases, organs, datasets, and modalities.

Another critical development was data augmentation, which amplified an image into multiple copies with minor or major modifications. From the outset, some simple strategies were considered, such as image translation, rotation, flipping, color distortion, etc. These augmentations did not fundamentally modify the content of images and, therefore, were limited to increasing data variation. Tumors remain tumors if they are rotated, scaled, or translated. More advanced augmentation strategies were devised thanks to the development of **Generative Adversarial Networks** (GAN) [25], yielding an improved performance by synthesizing more examples. For example, by learning many tumor examples, GAN can generate realistic tumors that do not exist in the real world.

With transfer learning, data augmentation, and continued advancements in computer vision, many studies in deep learning have raised enthusiasm and hopes for automating specific diagnostic tasks spanning dermatology, radiology, ophthalmology, and pathology. While most of the AI/DL applications remain on systems that aid the physicians in viewing and manipulating medical images, there is an increasingly growing body of work towards an automated computer diagnosis, some rivaling a human-level precision, particularly for disease localization and detection [26–29]. The field of medical image analysis is increasingly interdisciplinary, driven forward by international competitions, enhanced collaborations among physicians and computer scientists, and substantial funding from industry, universities, and government agencies.

Clinical Needs and Existing Challenges

Clinical Needs

Imaging data account for about 90% of all healthcare data and hence are among the most important sources of evidence for clinical decision support [30]. The primary uses of images are for detecting medical abnormalities, assessing the severity of those abnormalities, and guiding therapeutic interventions. This section describes interpretation tasks in medical imaging and offers an overview of how these tasks meet clinical needs. Some of the tasks can be quite challenging and time-consuming, e.g., disease detection and segmentation, where physicians' performance may be decreased due to the limitations of human perception and fatiguability. Therefore, with the aid from AI/DL methods, the breadth of clinical needs for these systems has grown rapidly in recent decades.

- *Medical image classification* refers to classifying what type of lesion is contained in an image. Such classification may be binary (e.g., benign or malignant) or multi-class (various types of lesions). The approach to annotation for classification tasks is to assign one or a few labels to an image or a study. Image classification is used for computer-aided diagnosis to determine the disease type in the image. An example of a classification task is The National Institute of Health (NIH) Chest X-ray dataset,[6] wherein 14 chest diseases in 112,120 X-ray images are annotated.

- *Disease localization and detection* refer to identifying the location of specific lesions. This distinction is subtle: localization aims to locate a single lesion, whereas detection seeks to find all lesions in the image. The annotation for detection and localization provides both the specific location and the scale of the lesion within a bounding box. The Lung Image Database Consortium image collection (LIDC-IDRI)[7] is a representative dataset for the task of detecting lung nodules, which provides lung nodule locations for a total of 1308 studies.

- *Medical image segmentation* refers to determining the outline around an object of interest in the image. Segmentation facilitates analysis by measuring more accurate and desirable imaging biomarkers. The annotation for segmentation tasks aims to assign every pixel in an image to at least one class. Medical Segmentation Decathlon[8] is a typical benchmark for segmentation, providing ten tasks that cover different organs, diseases, and modalities.

- *Medical image registration* refers to aligning the spatial coordinates of one or more images into a standard coordinate system. Image registration plays a vital role in assessing disease prognosis by establishing correspondence among multiple scans performed at different time points. Image registration is an important task for subsequent landmark detection. A common dataset for registration is Benchmark on Image Registration methods with Landmark validations (BIRL),[9] in which image pairs of related sections (mainly, consecutive cuts) are provided.

- *Medical image reconstruction* refers to producing images suitable for human interpretation from raw data obtained by imaging devices like CT or MRI scanners. Fast and high-quality radiological image reconstruction can reduce radiation exposure and intravenous contrast material doses.

- *Medical image enhancement* refers to adjusting the intensity of an image for better visualization or subsequent processing. Such enhancement includes denoising, super-resolution, histogram equalization, artifact removal, MR bias field correction, and image harmonization. These techniques increase local contrast and enhance the visibility of fine-detail structures.

- Other related tasks include *landmark detection*, *image or view recognition*, and *automatic report generation*.

---

[6] https://www.kaggle.com/nih-chest-xrays/data (accessed August 19, 2022)

[7] https://wiki.cancerimagingarchive.net/display/Public/LIDC-IDRI (accessed August 19, 2022)

[8] http://medicaldecathlon.com/ (accessed August 19, 2022)

[9] https://borda.github.io/BIRL/ (accessed August 19, 2022)

Medical Applications

The introduction of AI/DL methods into clinical medicine, particularly diagnostic imaging, has greatly transformed medical practice. These applications focus on a number of aspects ranging from patient and workflow management to image production and interpretation, including *imaging management*, such as coordination of patient scheduling and workflow; *imaging processing*, such as the automated selection of standard imaging planes for cardiac imaging or segmenting anatomic models; and *imaging interpretation* at the physician's level, functioning as a "second reader" for image interpretation. The surest indicator of the success of AI/DL methods applied to clinical medicine would be the daily use of CAD in routine clinical work at many hospitals worldwide. As is summarized in Table 12.1, numerous AI/DL applications are already available commercially to assist physicians with imaging interpretation for a wide variety of disorders affecting diverse organ systems. These applications promise to improve accuracy through enhanced detection and specificity using the "second reader" paradigm. Furthermore, AI/DL offers expertise for imaging examination interpretation where subspecialty interpretation expertise is lacking and also mitigates the increasing workloads experienced by physicians due to the rise of advanced imaging techniques. We describe two representative tools that have been used at the Mayo Clinic for pulmonary nodule and embolism detection.

- *CAD of pulmonary embolism.* The application of AI/DL for pulmonary embolism detection provides an illustrative example of how these methods have been integrated into clinical image interpretation. Pulmonary embolism (PE) is a condition in which a thrombus (often colloquially referred to as a "blood clot") travels to the lungs, often from a lower extremity venous source, producing a blockage of the pulmonary arteries within the lungs. Pulmonary emboli represent the third most common cause of cardiovascular death after myocardial infarction ("heart attack") and stroke [31]. They are responsible for 100,000–200,000 deaths annually in the United States [32]. Pulmonary emboli are typically treated with anticoagulation ("blood thinners"), a treatment that may be effective but is associated with significant bleeding risk. Therefore, early and accurate PE diagnosis is critical. Computed tomography pulmonary angiography (CTPA) is the primary modality used to detect PE, which appears as "filling defects" within enhanced pulmonary arteries following the administration of intravenous contrast (Fig. 12.2). Since the number of CTPA examinations performed far exceeds the availability of subspecialty trained cardiopulmonary radiologists, most CTPA examinations are interpreted by general radiologists. Moreover, accurately interpreting CTPA examinations requires significant training and experience, so the discordance (level of disagreement) of CTPA interpretations may exceed 25% between cardiopulmonary radiologists and general radiologists [33]. Due to inaccurate interpretations, including false-negative studies (failure to detect emboli) and false-positive studies (diagnosing emboli that are not present, or "overdiagnosis"), there is a significant risk of morbidity

Table 12.1 Examples of AI-based systems employed for clinical imaging interpretation

Organ system	Applications	Manufacturer[a]
Breast	Detection of cancer, breast density assessment	Hologic iCAD Zebra-Med Koios Medical
Neurologic	Detection of hemorrhagic brain contusion, communicating hydrocephalus, cerebrospinal fluid flow quantification, white matter lesion tracking in multiple sclerosis, atherosclerotic plaque quantification in the carotid arteries, tumor identification	Icometrix AIDOC MaxQ Zebra-Med
Pulmonary	Lung nodule detection Pulmonary embolism detection Pneumothorax detection Pneumonia detection Chronic Obstructive Pulmonary Disease Quantification	Siemens Medical Systems, Corelinesoft, Riverrain AIDOC GE Siemens Medical Siemens Medical Systems, Corelinesoft Arterys
Cardiac	Coronary calcium detection and quantification Aortic measurements	Siemens Medical Systems Zebra-Med
Musculoskeletal	Rib fracture detection Compression fracture detection Vertebral body level labeling	AIDOC Zebra-Med Siemens Medical Systems GE Medical Systems
Abdominal	Colonic polyp detection	Siemens Medical Systems Phillips Medical Systems
Head	Triaging of intracranial hemorrhage Interpretation of CT and MRI brain images	MaxIQ AI Icometrix

[a] A number of commercially available, proprietary, and research platforms exist; this list is necessarily abbreviated

and mortality. AI/DL applications have been developed to assist radiologists with the task of PE detection and exclusion [34]. One particular system, developed by AIDOC medical (Tel Aviv, Israel), has recently been adopted by the Mayo Clinic. Once a CTPA examination is transferred from the CT scanner to radiologists for interpretation, the system will perform embolism detection and exclusion. This system runs "silently" in the background and delivers results as either negative or positive for PE. If positive, a pop-up window will localize the embolus for radiologist confirmation (Fig. 12.2c). In a study by Weikert et al. [34], the AIDOC algorithm showed a sensitivity of 92.7% on a per-patient basis with a false

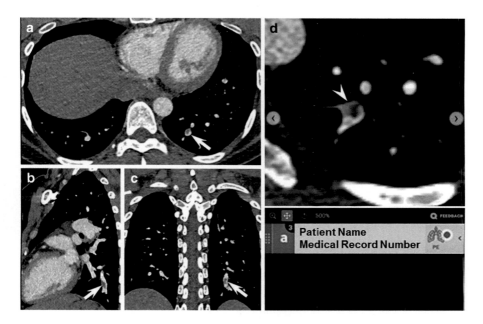

Fig. 12.2 Pulmonary embolism detection using an AI/DL model. (**a**) axial; (**b**) sagittal (as if viewing the patient from the side; front of the body is to the left of the image); and (**c**) coronal (as if looking at someone from the "front" patient right side is to the image left and head is at the image "top") enhanced CT images show a "filling defect" (arrows) within a left lower lobe pulmonary artery, appearing as a "dark" structure surrounded by a brightly enhanced pulmonary blood pool. (**d**) The output of the automated PE detection by the AIDOC medical system shows detection of the same pulmonary embolism (arrowhead) noted by the interpreting radiologist. The system flags the examination as positive for pulmonary embolism by displaying an orange circle (●) in the left lower lobe aspect of the lung diagram; examinations negative for pulmonary embolism are denoted by ∅

positive rate of 3.8%, or 0.12 false-positive results/detection (Fig. 12.3). Most notably, the average processing time for the algorithm was 152 s, but typically this processing occurred while the data were being transferred from the CT scanner to the **Picture Archiving Communication System (PACS)**, during which time the images are not completely available for radiologists to review anyway. An additional 25 seconds is required for the case uploading [34]. In practice, the AIDOC system analysis is either complete and ready for review when the study is opened by the radiologist, or the case is being actively processed and the algorithm results provided before the radiologist completes the review of the study.

- *CAD of pulmonary nodules.* Pulmonary nodules are commonly encountered using chest imaging. Many are innocuous, often resulting from a pulmonary infection. However, pulmonary malignancy, both primary pulmonary malignancy and malignancy spread from elsewhere, may present on chest imaging studies as one or more lung nodules. Therefore, the detection and characterization of lung nodules have become a major focus for AI/DL, particularly since the early detection of lung cancer from chest CT images has been shown to reduce

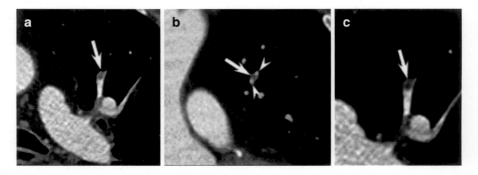

Fig. 12.3 False-positive pulmonary embolism detection by an AI/DL model. (**a**) Axial enhanced CT image shows a "filling defect" (arrow) immediately adjacent to a left upper lobe pulmonary artery, closely resembling PE. (**b**) Coronal CT image (orientation of this image as if the observer is facing directly at someone) shows the apparent filling defect (arrow) is positioned between two pulmonary arteries (arrowheads)- this location and appearance are typical of lymph node tissue. (**c**) The output of the automated PE detection by the AIDOC medical system shows that the finding was flagged by the system as PE, representing a false-positive diagnosis

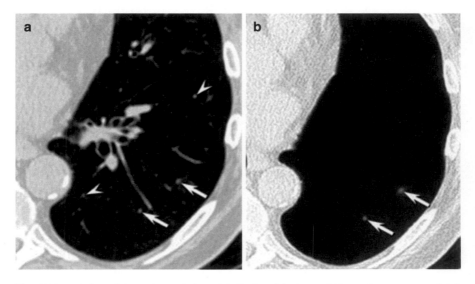

Fig. 12.4 (**a**) The axial unenhanced chest CT displayed in lung windows shows two small left lower lobe pulmonary nodules (arrows). Note how these small nodules very closely resemble pulmonary vessels (arrowheads); this close resemblance can easily result in diagnostic errors, particularly inadvertently overlooking small nodules that could reflect potentially precancerous or cancerous lesions. (**b**) The output from AI/ML algorithm (ClearRead CT, Riverain Technologies, Miamisburg, OH) shows that the normal pulmonary vessels have been "suppressed" and are no longer visible, which clearly exposes the two small pulmonary nodules (arrowheads)

cancer-related and all-cause mortality in properly selected individuals [35]. Further research has shown that lung cancer mortality is reduced when nodules are detected at smaller sizes. AI/DL for lung nodule assessment has focused on three major efforts: (*i*) nodule detection (separating nodules from a background of similar appearing pulmonary vessels, Fig. 12.4); (*ii*) nodule morphology assessment, particularly the nodule border characteristics since certain border characteristics are associated with the presence of malignancy; and (*iii*) accurate assessment of nodule growth. The detection of nodule growth is important because many benign lesions show no, or little, growth over time, whereas malignant lung nodules frequently grow within a recognized time frame. AI/DL models have the ability to calculate the nodule size using volumetry, as opposed to the manual placement of two-dimensional electronic calipers (the traditional standard). Nodule volume has been suggested to be a more accurate means for determining size thresholds for nodule intervention in addition to the assessment of growth. The latter is often regarded as a surrogate for the aggressive potential for a given nodule and is thus often used as an endpoint for nodule intervention.

Technical Barriers

Deep learning is intensely data-hungry in nature, requiring large, high-quality annotated datasets—more so than other algorithms. **Annotation** is the process of assigning labels to raw data in preparation for training the computer on the pairs of data and labels; the computer predicts labels for many new data. For the development of deep learning algorithms, supervised learning (in which the annotation is used to guide model learning and error propagation) is the most prominent learning paradigm. Therefore, annotating datasets is an indispensable stage for data processing in the deep learning era. For most image analysis tasks, data are collected from numerous photos from social media, and annotation is often provided by non-experts through crowdsourcing. Annotating medical images, however, demands costly, specialty-oriented knowledge and skills, which are not readily accessible. Therefore, medical image annotation is performed primarily by human experts, who manually annotate the existence, appearance, and severity of diseases in each medical image using appropriate software tools, such as Pair, Lionbridge AI, ITK-SNAP, Cogito, Labelbox, 3D Slicer, etc. For some abnormalities that experts may not immediately recognize from images, the results of tissue sampling procedures can also be used to supplement the experts' annotation. Figure 12.5 illustrates different types of annotation in medical imaging.

Recent advances in AI/DL methods suggest that to match a physician's diagnostic precision, deep learning algorithms require 42,290 radiologist-annotated CT images for lung cancer diagnosis [27], 137,291 radiologist-annotated mammographic images for breast cancer identification [29], 129,450 dermatologist-annotated images for skin cancer classification [26], and 128,175 ophthalmologist-annotated retinal images for diabetic retinopathy detection [28]. It is therefore clear that adopting deep learning for medical imaging requires a curation process for data collection to reliably train, validate, and test algorithms. Without such large, annotated datasets, deep learning often results in algorithms that perform poorly and lack generalizability for new data. However, such perfectly-sized and carefully-annotated datasets are rarely available for training deep learning models, particularly for applications in medical imaging, where both images and

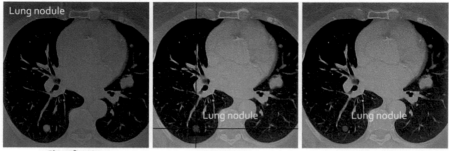

| Classification | Detection | Segmentation |
| Lung nodule image | Lung nodule location | Lung nodule boundary |

Fig. 12.5 When approaching the use of large-scaled annotated datasets in medical imaging, the critical question is "what annotation should be collected?" There are several types of annotation, depending on the task requirements in clinical practice. Different types of annotation are associated with different costs. For example, to annotate lung nodules for the tasks of classification, detection, and segmentation, human experts must consider different types of annotation—labeling the existence of the nodule, indicating its location, and defining its boundary, respectively. These three types of annotation are anticipated to span manual annotation efforts from easy to labor-intensive, annotation qualities from coarse to precise, and the annotation time commitment from short to long

annotations are expensive to acquire. This requirement becomes more challenging in situations where one can collect only limited annotated data or when scaling up to include rare diseases where it is impractical to collect large quantities of annotated data [36]. Therefore, one of the chief obstacles to the development and clinical implementation of AI/DL imaging systems is the availability of sufficiently large, curated datasets with human expert annotation. To this end, several efforts have been made to create large datasets of annotated medical images, such as the Cancer Imaging Archive,[10] Kaggle,[11] and Grand Challenge sets.[12]

There are additional barriers that AI/DL methods face when applied to medical imaging. The limitations of AI/DL include the generalizability and robustness of methods [37], the interpretability of results (see Chap. 8), the lack of clinical context other than images, and the non-standardized acquisition of images and annotations across hospitals. From a practical perspective, although several CAD systems based on AI/DL methods have already gained traction in clinical imaging, a number of serious limitations remain before more widespread implementation of these algorithms can take place.

- *Reliability.* A major target for a CAD system is lesion detection; once detected, it is essential to precisely measure the lesion because many disorders are allocated into risk categories for intervention based on lesion size. Furthermore, many detected lesions will be followed with serial imaging surveillance, with changes in size providing the endpoint for determining therapeutic success. In

---

[10] https://www.cancerimagingarchive.net/ (accessed August 19, 2022)

[11] https://www.kaggle.com/ (accessed August 19, 2022)

[12] https://grand-challenge.org/ (accessed August 19, 2022)

the example of nodule detection and assessment, AI/DL can provide accurate and reproducible measurement for solid nodules and subsolid nodules (nodules with a more "hazy" appearance in chest CT); pulmonary malignancies often present with the latter morphology [38]. However, for patients with subsolid nodule morphologies, the variable and inaccurate measurements provided by AI/DL have been shown to be insufficient for patient management or determination of prognosis. Additionally, measurements using different software programs may show substantial inter-platform variability, resulting in inaccurate serial assessment.

- *Usability.* CAD systems must also be integrated into radiologists' workflow (see Chap. 5), which requires such programs to run silently and quickly in the background and to present timely and accurate results that can be readily integrated into the radiologist's product—the **radiology report**. Therefore, the outcome predictions of AI/DL must be presented in an understandable format to radiologists within the radiology report and perhaps to patients within their **electronic health record**. The proper presentation of AI/DL predictions could be in an image format that all examinations can be retrieved from the patient's medical record, and in a chart format that provides a user-friendly display for growth trends for lesions undergoing serial evaluation.
- *Affordability.* The adoption and ongoing maintenance of CAD systems in medical practice will generate costs to healthcare systems that must be addressed Therefore, widespread adoption of these systems will necessitate approval of reimbursement from third-party payers, which is a process that is slow, cumbersome, and difficult in the context of ongoing efforts for healthcare cost containment.

Opportunities and Emerging Techniques

This section presents three unique opportunities that AI/DL and medical imaging can offer to overcome the significant barrier—annotation sparsity. Several emerging techniques that tackle this barrier by harnessing the unique opportunities are surveyed.

Acquiring Annotation from Human Experts

Opportunity 1: The continual learning capability of AI/DL incrementally improves the algorithm through fine-tuning. With millions of new image data generated every day, it is impractical to store all the data and repeatedly develop CAD systems from scratch once new data become available. Instead, the aim is to leverage prior knowledge obtained from existing data and to continuously accommodate new data in a fashion analogous to human learning. The notion of **continual learning** is based on the observation that learners adaptively use new data to update their knowledge sets.

The continual learning capability is one of the unique benefits of deep learning because deep learning models can be fine-tuned on top of previously learned ones, which often store the knowledge learned from old data. Specifically, we can employ a set of trained parameters to initialize the model. The continual learning capability is much more appreciable in the scenario of the **human-in-the-loop** procedure, whereby physicians interact with computers to promote the development of CAD systems using a continuous stream of data. An efficient "human-in-the-loop" procedure helps physicians quickly dismiss data redundancy, thereby dramatically reducing the annotation burden. Moreover, an instant online feedback process encourages data, annotation, and model re-use, making it possible for CAD systems to self-improve via continual learning.

A typical strategy in the human-in-the-loop procedure is called **active learning**. Rather than randomly sampling, active learning aims to find the most representative data and annotate them first. Intuitively, focusing on these representative data can quickly elevate the AI/DL performance while demanding less annotation. In active learning, the key is to develop effective selecting criteria that can estimate the potential "worthiness" of annotating a data point. *Uncertainty* and *diversity* are the most popular active selecting criteria, which appraise the worthiness of annotating a data point from two different aspects. Uncertainty-based criteria are based on the notion that the more uncertain a prediction is, the more value will be added when including that annotation of that data point into the training set. As a result, sampling with the least confidence, large entropy, and margins of the prediction has been a more successful approach than random sampling for training models with sparse annotation. A major limitation of uncertainty-based selecting criteria is that some of the selected data are prone to redundancy and outliers and may not be representative enough for the data distribution as a whole. Alternatively, diversity-based criteria have the advantage of selecting a set of highly representative data, with respect to the annotated data, from the remainder of the unannotated set. The underlying concept is that it is unnecessary to annotate similar data repeatedly. Although alleviating redundancy and outliers, a serious hurdle to the success of diversity-based criteria is the computational complexity required to address a large pool of unannotated samples. To exploit the benefits and potentials of both uncertainty- and diversity-based criteria, recent studies employed a "mixture strategy" by combing uncertainty and diversity explicitly. For example, Zhou et al. [39] devised an annotation query procedure to integrate uncertainty and diversity into a single framework, reducing the manual annotation cost by at least a half.

Utilizing Annotation by Advanced Models

Opportunity 2: The representation learning capability of AI/DL alleviates exhaustive feature engineering for specific medical conditions. **Feature engineering** manually designs features based on the texture and shape present in images, which is easier to describe and troubleshoot, allowing humans to manipulate features on their own. However, crafting such features demands a great deal of patience, diligence, and expertise. Most hand-crafted features focus on specific medical conditions, thereby greatly limiting the discriminative powers and depreciating the capacity to generalize to other medical conditions. For instance, **Radiomics features** at radiologic imaging have been shown to predict outcomes for various medical disorders, but they are not adaptable to other areas of medical practice, such as dermatology, histopathology, and ophthalmology. Deep learning has supplanted previous hand-crafted features, proving that deep neural networks can solve diverse tasks by extracting image features at multiple levels of abstraction. In networks, each layer projects the image into a particular feature space—the deeper layer generates a higher level of abstraction by extracting more complex features built on top of simpler ones. The unique aspect of deep learning is that humans do not have to design the varying feature levels manually. As such, deep learning is often referred to as "representation learning," a procedure that automatically learns visual features to represent an image. Representation learning is more efficient and repeatable than exhaustive feature engineering, saving tremendous amounts of manual work. Compared with hand-crafted features, deep features offer four advantages: (*i*) deep features can be dynamically computed by models during training and test stages; (*ii*) deep features present a hierarchic image representation, varying from layer to layer; (*iii*) deep features can be used for not only classification but also registration, localization, and segmentation; (*iv*) deep features can be fine-tuned and adapted to different tasks and domains. Many studies have reaffirmed that representation learning can produce more generalizable image features than hand-crafted features. Developing high-performance deep neural networks concentrates mainly on *crafting network architectures* and *optimizing training recipes*.

The success of **AlexNet** for image classification on the ImageNet Large Scale Visual Recognition Challenge (ILSVRC) [40] signaled the importance of network architecture design. Following AlexNet, most neural networks are built upon several key components, such as **Convolution**, **Activation**, and **Pooling**. This prefigured compositionality and differentiability gave rise to an astonishing variety of network architectures that are deeper and wider. Additionally, the introduction of deep residual learning [41] demonstrated the importance of connectivity within the architecture, other than simply piling up layers on top of one other. In general, there are several aspects to consider to craft architectures with greater learning capacity, such as depth, width, and connectivity. However, manually designed architectures rely heavily on computer experts' choice, requiring hands-on experience and task-specific consideration. It is safe to say that no single architecture is optimal for every imaging task. This leads to the emerging technique called "**Neural Architecture Search**" [42], which automatically searches for an optimal architecture for a specific task, eliminating extensive hand-crafted designing efforts.

Another promising direction for advancing deep neural networks is to optimize the training recipe. For example, U-Net is a widely used architecture for medical image segmentation [43], which consists of an **encoder** and a **decoder**, with **skip connections** in between. Its success is largely attributed to the skip connections, which combine deep, semantic, coarse-grained feature maps from the decoder with shallow, low-level, fine-grained feature maps from the encoder and have proven effective for recovering fine-grained details within the target objects. Numerous architectural innovations have been developed based on the original U-Net architecture, suggesting the benefit from redesigned encoder, decoder, and skip connections [44–47]. On the other hand, a study by Isensee et al. [48] discovered that a well-designed training recipe, including preprocessing, data augmentation, network architecture, training, and post-processing, can also substantially improve performance.

Extracting Features from Unannotated Images

Opportunity 3: The consistent and recurrent anatomy embedded in medical images empowers AI/DL with a generic visual representation. Human anatomy is intrinsically structured, exhibiting consistency in appearance, position, and layout. Medical imaging protocols focus on particular body parts, often generating images of great similarity and yielding an abundance of sophisticated anatomical patterns across patients. These patterns are naturally associated with comprehensive knowledge about human anatomy. Therefore, consistent and recurrent anatomy facilitates the analysis of numerous critical problems and should be considered a significant advantage for medical imaging. Due to the consistency of anatomy, the same body parts in different images express similar visual patterns and, therefore, can be retrieved by what is known as "**Nearest Neighbor Search.**" As a result, given a single annotated medical image, similar anatomical patterns can be found in many other images, which enables physicians to track disease progress with landmark detection and lesion matching. In addition to correspondence matching, the recurrent anatomical structures in medical images are associated with rich knowledge about the human body and intrinsic structural coherence, offering great benefit and potential to foster generalizable image representation [49, 50]. Consequently, **one-shot learning** in various medical applications may eventually be achieved.

Self-supervised learning enables AI/DL to learn image representation directly from unannotated images. This learning paradigm has existed for some time, but its power historically lagged behind state-of-the-art **supervised learning**. However, the recent pace of progress in self-supervised learning has increased dramatically and led to image representation that matches and even surpasses the representation learned from supervised learning. In self-supervised learning, the AI/DL model learns by studying the properties of real-world images. There are two major research approaches in self-supervision: (i) learning a discriminative model to distinguish multiple views and (ii) learning a predictive model to fill in the blank. First, the AI/DL model is expected to distinguish objects from each other. The discriminative model compares images that have undergone data augmentation to learn image representation, which is resilient to various view changes. The early attempts included MoCo [51], SimCLR [52], BYOL [53], and recently several improved methods have been applied to medical imaging [54]. Second, the AI/DL model should develop meaningful expectations about the world, developing a hypothesis and then verifying it. As a result, the predictive model predicts some hidden information (e.g., color, future events, or contexts of an image) to identify prior knowledge and physical properties in nature, such as the sky being blue or a running beast approaching you. For example, image restoration has been shown as an effective proxy task [4, 55, 56]—first deforming an image and then training the model to restore the original image; Zhu et al. [57, 58] trained a model to recover the rearranged and rotated Rubik's cube puzzle.

Conclusion

This chapter has introduced computer-aided diagnosis in medical imaging, centering its discussion on a historical review, the motivating clinical needs, technical barriers, opportunities, and current frontiers of technology. Computer-aided diagnosis aims to develop automated algorithms for gleaning clinically useful information from images to support clinical decision-making and to facilitate precision medicine, predominantly covering the fields of radiology [59], cardiology [60], and pathology [61]. An increasing shortage of qualified physicians to interpret complex medical images suggests a clear need for reliable CAD systems to alleviate the growing burden on healthcare practitioners. Thus, we anticipate that CAD systems could significantly influence health care in the future, particularly on two prevailing tasks. *First*, the tasks that physicians must do but do not really want to do, which are often of low value or are repetitive. These tasks are tedious, laborious, and time-consuming, such as outlining the contours of the tumors and at-risk organs. *Second*, the tasks that physicians really want to do but cannot do very well, owing to the lack of knowledge, skill, or relevant experience, or the limitations of human perception. Examples include determining the presence of malignancy within a lesion prior to tissue sampling or surgery, predicting the tumor response to radiation/chemotherapy, etc. Physicians should become familiar with the principles and potential applications of AI/DL methods, using the output from CAD systems as a "second opinion"; yet it is the physicians who eventually must make the final decisions.

Questions for Discussion

- How might you determine whether an AI/DL system, developed for a specific application, demonstrates clinically acceptable performance?
- Where can AI/DL have the greatest influence in the healthcare environment? What roles may computer-aided diagnosis systems play for physicians? For patients?
- What is the difference between computer-aided diagnosis and automated computer diagnosis? Do you have a preference for one approach? If so, why?
- How might you measure the diagnostic performance of human experts? What constitutes reliable evidence that computers outperform humans in specific applications? Do you think that a CAD system can eliminate the need for a radiologist?

- Distinguish among the common medical imaging modalities (CT, MRI, Ultrasound, PET, and optical imaging) and explain their advantages and suitable clinical applications for their use.

Further Reading

Doi, K. (2007). Computer-aided Diagnosis in Medical Imaging: Historical Review, Current Status and Future Potential. *Computerized Medical Imaging and Graphics*, 31(4-5), 198-211.

- This paper describes the state of the medical imaging field in the early 2000s, the time before the wide adoption of deep learning. The two concepts—computer aided diagnosis and automated computer diagnosis—are clearly defined and clarified in this paper. In addition, the paper provides both insightful views of the early development of CAD and an introduction of existing challenges concerning the incorporation of CAD systems into daily clinical work.

Zhou, S. K., Greenspan, H., Davatzikos, C., Duncan, J. S., van Ginneken, B., Madabhushi, A., ... & Summers, R. M. (2021). A Review of Deep Learning in Medical Imaging: Imaging Traits, Technology Trends, Case Studies with Progress Highlights, and Future Promises. *Proceedings of the IEEE*.

- This paper describes the state of the medical imaging field approaching the year 2020. The paper overviews the emerging trends in deep learning, covering the topics of network architecture, sparse and noisy labels, federated learning, interpretability, uncertainty quantification, etc. The paper also presents several case studies that are commonly found in clinical practice, including digital pathology, and chest, brain, cardiovascular, and abdominal imaging.

Erickson, B. J. (2021). Imaging Systems in Radiology. Ch. 22 in EH Shortliffe and JJ Cimino, eds, *Biomedical Informatics: Computer Applications in Health Care and Biomedicine* (pp. 733-753). Springer, Cham.

- This chapter discusses the important role of imaging in biomedicine, with a special focus on image management and integration in radiology systems with an account of illustrative examples. Specifically, the chapter includes how medical images are acquired from imaging equipment, stored, transmitted, and presented for interpretation.

Rubin, D. L., Greenspan, H., & Hoogi, A. (2021). Biomedical Imaging Informatics. Ch. 10 in EH Shortliffe and JJ Cimino, eds, *Biomedical Informatics: Computer Applications in Health Care and Biomedicine* (pp. 299-362). Springer, Cham.

- This chapter reviews the frontier techniques for computational representation and for processing images in biomedicine. Apart from radiology, the chapter also introduces imaging techniques that have been applied for diverse medical domains, such as microscopy, pathology, ophthalmology, and dermatology.

Chartrand, G., Cheng, P. M., Vorontsov, E., Drozdzal, M., Turcotte, S., Pal, C. J., ... & Tang, A. (2017). Deep learning: A Primer for Radiologists. *Radiographics*, 37(7), 2113-2131.

- This paper reviews the key concepts of deep learning for clinical radiologists, discusses technical requirements, describes emerging applications in clinical radiology, and outlines limitations and future directions in this field.

Tajbakhsh, N., Shin, J. Y., Gurudu, S. R., Hurst, R. T., Kendall, C. B., Gotway, M. B., & Liang, J. (2016). Convolutional Neural Networks for Medical Image Analysis: Full training or fine tuning? *IEEE Transactions on Medical Imaging*, 35(5), 1299-1312.

- This paper systematically demonstrates the capability of transfer learning from natural images to medical images across diseases, imaging modalities, and medical specialties for the first time. It concludes that ImageNet pre-trained models offer significant performance gain compared with learning from scratch and varying handcrafted approaches.

Zhou, Z., Sodha, V., Pang, J., Gotway, M. B., & Liang, J. (2021). Models Genesis. *Medical Image Analysis*, 67, 101,840.

- This paper presents the first general-purpose source models for 3D medical image analysis. It surveys and benchmarks existing 3D transfer learning techniques, examining their capability across diseases, organs, datasets, and modalities. The medical applications in this paper include the tasks of disease classification and segmentation, as well as an account of typical imaging modalities, such as CT, MRI, X-ray, and Ultrasound. Both datasets and software are publicly available, which may serve as a primary source of 3D medical imaging studies.

References

1. Rubin GD, Roos JE, Tall M, Harrawood B, Bag S, Ly DL, et al. Characterizing search, recognition, and decision in the detection of lung nodules on CT scans: Elucidation with eye tracking. Radiology. 2015;274(1):276–86. Available from: https://pubmed.ncbi.nlm.nih.gov/25325324/
2. Tajbakhsh N, Jeyaseelan L, Li Q, Chiang JN, Wu Z, Ding X. Embracing imperfect datasets: A review of deep learning solutions for medical image segmentation. Med Image Anal. 2020;63:101693.
3. Rieke N, Hancox J, Li W, Milletarì F, Roth HR, Albarqouni S, et al. The future of digital health with federated learning. NPJ Digit Med. 2020;3(1):1–7. Available from: https://doi.org/10.1038/s41746-020-00323-1
4. Zhou Z, Sodha V, Pang J, Gotway MB, Liang J. Models Genesis. Med Image Anal. 2021;67:101840.
5. Iglesias JE, Sabuncu MR. Multi-atlas segmentation of biomedical images: A survey. Med Image Anal. 2015;24(1):205–19. Available from: https://pubmed.ncbi.nlm.nih.gov/26201875/

6. Smoger LM, Fitzpatrick CK, Clary CW, Cyr AJ, Maletsky LP, Rullkoetter PJ, Laz PJ. Statistical modeling to characterize relationships between knee anatomy and kinematics. J Orthop Res. 2015;33(11):1620–30. Available from: https://pubmed.ncbi.nlm.nih.gov/25991502/

7. Anas EMA, Rasoulian A, Seitel A, Darras K, Wilson D, John PS, et al. Automatic Segmentation of Wrist Bones in CT Using a Statistical Wrist Shape + Pose Model. IEEE Trans Med Imaging. 2016;35(8):1789–801. Available from: https://pubmed.ncbi.nlm.nih.gov/26890640/

8. Mirikharaji Z, Hamarneh G. Star Shape Prior in Fully Convolutional Networks for Skin Lesion Segmentation. Lect Notes Comput Sci. 2018;11073 LNCS:737–45. Available from: https://link.springer.com/chapter/10.1007/978-3-030-00937-3_84

9. Zhou Z, Shin J, Feng R, Hurst RT, Kendall CB, Liang J. Integrating active learning and transfer learning for carotid intima-media thickness video interpretation. J Digit Imaging. 2019;32(2):290–9. https://doi.org/10.1007/s10278-018-0143-2.

10. Stein JH, Korcarz CE, Hurst RT, Lonn E, Kendall CB, Mohler ER, et al. Use of Carotid Ultrasound to Identify Subclinical Vascular Disease and Evaluate Cardiovascular Disease Risk: A Consensus Statement from the American Society of Echocardiography Carotid Intima-Media Thickness Task Force Endorsed by the Society for Vascular Medicine. J Am Soc Echocardiogr. 2008;21:93–111. Available from: https://pubmed.ncbi.nlm.nih.gov/18261694/

11. Kang M, Lu Y, Yuille AL, Zhou Z. Data, Assemble: Leveraging Multiple Datasets with Heterogeneous and Partial Labels. 2021. Available from: https://arxiv.org/abs/2109.12265.

12. Karimi D, Dou H, Warfield SK, Gholipour A. Deep learning with noisy labels: Exploring techniques and remedies in medical image analysis. Med Image Anal. 2020;65:101759.

13. Bridge P, Fielding A, Rowntree P, Pullar A. Intraobserver variability: should we worry? J Med Imaging Radiat Sci. 2016;47(3):217–20. Available from: http://www.jmirs.org/article/S1939865416300479/fulltext

14. Doi K. Computer-aided diagnosis in medical imaging: Historical review, current status and future potential. Comput Med Imaging Graph. 2007;31(4–5):198–211. Available from: /pmc/articles/PMC1955762/

15. Ghosh-Dastidar S, Adeli H, Dadmehr N. Principal component analysis-enhanced cosine radial basis function neural network for robust epilepsy and seizure detection. IEEE Trans Biomed Eng. 2008;55(2):512–8.

16. Chu LC, Park S, Kawamoto S, Fouladi DF, Shayesteh S, Zinreich ES, et al. Utility of CT radiomics features in differentiation of pancreatic ductal adenocarcinoma from normal pancreatic tissue. Am J Roentgenol. 2019;213(2):349–57. Available from: https://pubmed.ncbi.nlm.nih.gov/31012758/

17. Chu LC, Park S, Kawamoto S, Yuille AL, Hruban RH, Fishman EK. Pancreatic cancer imaging: a new look at an old problem. Curr Probl Diagn Radiol. 2021;50(4):540–50.

18. Criminisi A, Shotton J, Konukoglu E, Criminisi A, Shotton J, Konukoglu E. Decision Forests: A Unified Framework for Classification, Regression, Density Estimation, Manifold Learning and Semi-Supervised Learning. Found Trends R Comput Graph Vis. 2012;7(3):81–227. Available from: https://www.microsoft.com/en-us/research/publication/decision-forests-a-unified-framework-for-classification-regression-density-estimation-manifold-learning-and-semi-supervised-learning/

19. Schölkopf B. SVMs - A practical consequence of learning theory. IEEE Intell Syst Their Appl. 1998;13(4):18–21.

20. Freund Y, Schapire RE. A Short Introduction to Boosting. J Jpn Soc Artif Intell. 1999;14(5):771–80. Available from: www.research.att.com/

21. Marsland S. Machine learning: An algorithmic perspective. 2nd ed. Boca Raton, Florida: CRC Press; 2014. p. 1–452.

22. Lecun Y, Bengio Y, Hinton G. Deep learning. Nature. 2015;521:436–44. Available from: https://www.nature.com/articles/nature14539

23. Tajbakhsh N, Shin JY, Gurudu SR, Hurst RT, Kendall CB, Gotway MB, et al. Convolutional neural networks for medical image analysis: full training or fine tuning? IEEE Trans Med Imaging. 2016;35(5):1299–312.

24. Shin HC, Roth HR, Gao M, Lu L, Xu Z, Nogues I, et al. Deep convolutional neural networks for computer-aided detection: cnn architectures, dataset characteristics and transfer learning. IEEE Trans Med Imaging. 2016;35(5):1285–98.
25. Goodfellow IJ, Pouget-Abadie J, Mirza M, Xu B, Warde-Farley D, Ozair S, et al. Generative adversarial nets. Adv Neural Inform Proce Syst. 2014;27. Available from: http://www.github.com/goodfeli/adversarial
26. Esteva A, Kuprel B, Novoa RA, Ko J, Swetter SM, Blau HM, et al. Dermatologist-level classification of skin cancer with deep neural networks. Nature. 2017;542(7639):115–8. Available from: https://licensing.eri.ed.ac.uk/i/
27. Ardila D, Kiraly AP, Bharadwaj S, Choi B, Reicher JJ, Peng L, et al. End-to-end lung cancer screening with three-dimensional deep learning on low-dose chest computed tomography. Nat Med. 2019;25(6):954–61. https://doi.org/10.1038/s41591-019-0447-x.
28. Gulshan V, Peng L, Coram M, Stumpe MC, Wu D, Narayanaswamy A, et al. Development and validation of a deep learning algorithm for detection of diabetic retinopathy in retinal fundus photographs. J Am Med Assoc. 2016;316(22):2402–10. Available from: https://jama-network.com/
29. McKinney SM, Sieniek M, Godbole V, Godwin J, Antropova N, Ashrafian H, et al. International evaluation of an AI system for breast cancer screening. Nature. 2020;577(7788):89–94. https://doi.org/10.1038/s41586-019-1799-6.
30. Zhou SK, Greenspan H, Davatzikos C, Duncan JS, Van Ginneken B, Madabhushi A, et al. A review of deep learning in medical imaging: imaging traits, technology trends, case studies with progress highlights, and future promises. Proc IEEE. 2021;109(5):820–38. Available from: https://ieeexplore.ieee.org/abstract/document/9363915
31. Martin KA, Molsberry R, Cuttica MJ, Desai KR, Schimmel DR, Khan SS. Time Trends in Pulmonary Embolism Mortality Rates in the United States, 1999 to 2018. J Am Heart Assoc. 2020;9(17):e016784. Available from: https://www.ahajo
32. Pauley E, Orgel R, Rossi JS, Strassle PD. Age-stratified national trends in pulmonary embolism admissions. Chest. 2019;156(4):733–42. Available from: https://pubmed.ncbi.nlm.nih.gov/31233745/
33. Hutchinson BD, Navin P, Marom EM, Truong MT, Bruzzi JF. Overdiagnosis of pulmonary embolism by pulmonary CT angiography. Am J Roentgenol. 2015;205(2):271–7. Available from: https://pubmed.ncbi.nlm.nih.gov/26204274/
34. Weikert T, Winkel DJ, Bremerich J, Stieltjes B, Parmar V, Sauter AW, et al. Automated detection of pulmonary embolism in CT pulmonary angiograms using an AI-powered algorithm. Eur Radiol. 2020;30(12):6545–53. Available from: https://pubmed.ncbi.nlm.nih.gov/32621243/
35. National Lung Screening Trial Research Team. Reduced Lung-Cancer Mortality with Low-Dose Computed Tomographic Screening. N Engl J Med. 2011;365(5):395–409. https://doi.org/10.1056/NEJMoa1102873.
36. Zhou Z. Towards Annotation-efficient deep learning for computer-aided diagnosis. Arizona State University; 2021.
37. Yuille AL, Liu C. Deep Nets: What have They Ever Done for Vision? Int J Comput Vis. 2020;129(3):781–802. https://doi.org/10.1007/s11263-020-01405-z.
38. Chelala L, Hossain R, Kazerooni EA, Christensen JD, Dyer DS, White CS. Lung-RADS Version 1.1: Challenges and a Look Ahead, From the AJR Special Series on Radiology Reporting and Data Systems. Am J Roentgenol. 2021;216(6):1411–22.
39. Zhou Z, Shin JY, Gurudu SR, Gotway MB, Liang J. Active, continual fine tuning of convolutional neural networks for reducing annotation efforts. Med Image Anal. 2021;71:101997.
40. Krizhevsky A, Sutskever I, Hinton GE. ImageNet Classification with Deep Convolutional Neural Networks. Adv Neural Inform Process Syst. 2012;25. Available from: http://code.google.com/p/cuda-convnet/
41. He K, Zhang X, Ren S, Sun J. Deep residual learning for image recognition. In: Proceedings of the IEEE Computer Society Conference on Computer Vision and Pattern Recognition. London: IEEE Computer Society; 2016. p. 770–8.

42. Liu C, Zoph B, Neumann M, Shlens J, Hua W, Li LJ, et al. Progressive Neural Architecture Search. In: Lecture Notes in Computer Science (including subseries Lecture Notes in Artificial Intelligence and Lecture Notes in Bioinformatics). New York: Springer Verlag; 2018. p. 19–35. https://doi.org/10.1007/978-3-030-01246-5_2.

43. Ronneberger O, Fischer P, Brox T. U-net: Convolutional networks for biomedical image segmentation. In: Lecture Notes in Computer Science (including subseries Lecture Notes in Artificial Intelligence and Lecture Notes in Bioinformatics). New York: Springer Verlag; 2015. p. 234–41. Available from: http://lmb.informatik.uni-freiburg.de/http://lmb.informatik.uni-freiburg.de/people/ronneber/u-net.

44. Zhou Z, Siddiquee MMR, Tajbakhsh N, Liang J. UNet++: redesigning skip connections to exploit multiscale features in image segmentation. IEEE Trans Med Imaging. 2020;39(6):1856–67.

45. Alom MZ, Hasan M, Yakopcic C, Taha TM, Asari VK. Recurrent Residual Convolutional Neural Network based on U-Net (R2U-Net) for Medical Image Segmentation. 2018. Available from: https://arxiv.org/abs/1802.06955v5

46. Oktay O, Schlemper J, Folgoc L Le, Lee M, Heinrich M, Misawa K, et al. Attention U-Net: Learning Where to Look for the Pancreas. 2018 . Available from: https://arxiv.org/abs/1804.03999v3

47. Li X, Chen H, Qi X, Dou Q, Fu CW, Heng PA. H-DenseUNet: Hybrid Densely Connected UNet for Liver and Tumor Segmentation from CT Volumes. IEEE Trans Med Imaging. 2018;37(12):2663–74.

48. Isensee F, Jaeger PF, Kohl SAA, Petersen J. Maier-Hein KH. nnU-Net: a self-configuring method for deep learning-based biomedical image segmentation. Nat Methods. 2021;18(2):203–11. https://doi.org/10.1038/s41592-020-01008-z.

49. Haghighi F, Taher MRH, Zhou Z, Gotway MB, Liang J. Transferable visual words: exploiting the semantics of anatomical patterns for self-supervised learning. IEEE Trans Med Imaging. 2021;40(10):2857–68.

50. Haghighi F, Hosseinzadeh Taher MR, Zhou Z, Gotway MB, Liang J. Learning semantics-enriched representation via self-discovery, self-classification, and self-restoration. In: Lecture Notes in Computer Science (including subseries Lecture Notes in Artificial Intelligence and Lecture Notes in Bioinformatics). Cham: Springer; 2020. p. 137–47. https://doi.org/10.100 7/978-3-030-59710-8_14.

51. He K, Fan H, Wu Y, Xie S, Girshick R. Momentum Contrast for Unsupervised Visual Representation Learning. In: Proceedings of the IEEE Computer Society Conference on Computer Vision and Pattern Recognition; 2020. p. 9726–35. Available from: https://github.com/facebookresearch/moco.

52. Chen T, Kornblith S, Norouzi M, Hinton G. A simple framework for contrastive learning of visual representations. In: 37th International Conference on Machine Learning, ICML 2020. International Machine Learning Society (IMLS); 2020. p. 1575–85. Available from: http://arxiv.org/abs/2002.05709.

53. Grill J-B, Strub F, Altché F, Tallec C, Richemond PH, Buchatskaya E, et al. Bootstrap your own latent a new approach to self-supervised learning. Adv Neural Inform Proce Syst. 2020;33. Available from: https://github.com/deepmind/deepmind-research/tree/master/byol

54. Azizi S, Mustafa B, Ryan F, Beaver Z, Freyberg J, Deaton J, et al. Big Self-Supervised Models Advance Medical Image Classification. 2021. Available from: https://arxiv.org/abs/2101.05224v2

55. Zhou Z, Sodha V, Siddiquee MMR, Feng R, Tajbakhsh N, Gotway MB, et al. Models Genesis: Generic Autodidactic Models for 3D Medical Image Analysis. Lect Notes Comput Sci. 2019;11767 LNCS:384–93. Available from: http://arxiv.org/abs/1908.06912

56. Feng R, Zhou Z, Gotway MB, Liang J. Parts2Whole: Self-supervised Contrastive Learning via Reconstruction. Lect Notes Comput Sci. 2020;12444 LNCS:85–95.

57. Zhu J, Li Y, Hu Y, Ma K, Zhou SK, Zheng Y. Rubik's Cube+: A self-supervised feature learning framework for 3D medical image analysis. Med Image Anal. 2020;64:101746.

58. Tao X, Li Y, Zhou W, Ma K, Zheng Y. Revisiting Rubik's Cube: Self-supervised Learning with Volume-Wise Transformation for 3D Medical Image Segmentation. In: Lecture Notes in Computer Science (including subseries Lecture Notes in Artificial Intelligence and Lecture Notes in Bioinformatics). Cham: Springer; 2020. p. 238–48. Available from: https://link.springer.com/chapter/10.1007/978-3-030-59719-1_24.

59. Giger ML, Chan HP, Boone J. Anniversary paper: History and status of CAD and quantitative image analysis: The role of Medical Physics and AAPM. Med Phys. 2008;35:5799–820. Available from: https://aapm.onlinelibrary.wiley.com/doi/full/10.1118/1.3013555

60. Willems JL, Abreu-Lima C, Arnaud P, van Bemmel JH, Brohet C, Degani R, Denis B, Gehring J, Graham I, van Herpen G, et al. The diagnostic performance of computer programs for the interpretation of electrocardiograms. N Engl J Med. 1991;325(25):1767–73. Available from: https://pubmed.ncbi.nlm.nih.gov/1834940/

61. Xing F, Yang L. Robust nucleus/cell detection and segmentation in digital pathology and microscopy images: A comprehensive review. IEEE Rev Biomed Eng. 2016;9:234–63. Available from: https://pubmed.ncbi.nlm.nih.gov/26742143/

Chapter 13
Public Health Applications

David L. Buckeridge

After reading this chapter, you should know the answers to these questions:
- What aspects of public health functions have determined if they are amenable to the application of AI? What are the functions that have been the most transformed?
- How have public health surveillance systems used AI methods to detect infectious disease outbreaks? What are some example systems?
- What biases should be considered when using AI to develop prediction models in population and public health?
- Which public health functions have the greatest potential to be transformed by AI applications in the future?

Public Health and AI

Public Health, Essential Public Health Functions, and Public Health Informatics

Public health is the science and the art of preventing disease, prolonging life, and promoting health through organized community efforts [1]. With a focus on health promotion and disease prevention in populations, public health is complementary to clinical medicine, which is focused on diagnosis and treatment of disease in individual patients. Although they have distinct perspectives, public health and clinical systems should act in a coordinated manner to advance individual and population

D. L. Buckeridge (✉)
McGill University, Montreal, QC, Canada
e-mail: david.buckeridge@mcgill.ca

© The Author(s), under exclusive license to Springer Nature
Switzerland AG 2022
T. A. Cohen et al. (eds.), *Intelligent Systems in Medicine and Health*, Cognitive
Informatics in Biomedicine and Healthcare,
https://doi.org/10.1007/978-3-031-09108-7_13

health. Ideally, this coordination should occur at both strategic and operational levels, ensuring, for example, the exchange of data about reportable diseases and **social determinants of health**.

The systematic application of information and computer science and technology to public health practice, research, and learning is the domain of **public health informatics** (see Box 13.1 for definitions) [2], which was first identified as a subdiscipline of biomedical informatics in 1995 [3]. A public health informatics perspective is critical for the effective application of AI in public health for at least two reasons. First, AI methods are generally implemented within software and introduced into public health settings in the same manner as other digital tools and interventions. For these tools to be effective, careful consideration must be given to the context in which they will be used and public health informatics takes a comprehensive view of this challenge. In addition to the information technology and data management aspects of this context, evidence has shown that cognitive [4] and organizational aspects [5] are important determinants of adoption and effective use. Second, AI-based software tools in public health often depend on data and knowledge contained in systems outside of public health. AI-based tools must therefore be implemented with careful consideration of data standards and **interoperability** to ensure the availability and quality of these inputs. For example, during the COVID-19 pandemic, the most common barrier to hospitals sharing electronic data with public health departments in the US was the lack of capacity within public health agencies to electronically receive data [6].

From an applied perspective, the essential public health functions describe the nature and scope of activities in public health [7]. Consequently, these functions also determine the information requirements of public health practitioners [8]. The essential functions, which were most recently updated in a US context in 2020, can be grouped under the three themes of assessment, policy development, and assurance (Box 13.2). These functions are not performed by a single monolithic system, but rather through a system of systems [9], with different public health entities operating at local, regional, national and international levels. These different systems interact with one another and systems outside of public health (e.g., clinical care, social services, urban planning) through a variety of formal and informal mechanisms.

Box 13.1: Public Health and Public Health Informatics

- *"Public Health is the science and the art of preventing disease, prolonging life, and promoting physical health and efficiency through organized community efforts"* [1]
- *"Public health informatics is the systematic application of information and computer science and technology to public health practice, research, and learning"* [2]

The Nature of Essential Public Health Functions and the Application of AI

Each of the ten essential public health functions has unique objectives, approaches, and available resources, including information systems, data and knowledge. Consequently, AI methods are more or less applicable to the different public health functions. In this chapter, the main AI methods considered are knowledge-based systems (Chap. 4), machine learning (ML, see Chap. 6), and natural language processing (NLP, see Chap. 7). The potential applicability of these AI methods to public health is considered below and examples of the application of these methods to specific public health functions are presented later in this chapter (see the section on "Examples of AI Applications to Public Health Functions").

Assessment functions, such as public health surveillance, rely extensively on the collection and analysis of data to monitor population health status and to manage population health hazards. These data are increasingly accessed from information systems used primarily in social and clinical settings and then transferred to public health organizations for secondary use. As such, the data available for assessment often have a volume sufficient for the application of machine learning methods. In primary or source systems, such as in electronic health records, many data are captured as free text, so natural language processing methods are used to extract from the free text structured data of relevance to public health (e.g., smoking status, occupation).

Functions under the *policy development* theme include communication, advocacy and coordination with stakeholders. These activities do not tend to be driven by quantitative data analysis to the same extent as the assessment functions. Consequently, data-intensive methods such as machine learning have not been used extensively to support these functions, but knowledge-based systems have been used to support the organization and application of evidence to these functions (e.g., evidence to guide implementation of chronic disease prevention programs). One exception to this general trend is the communication function, where machine learning and natural language processing methods have been used with digital media platforms to support the delivery and evaluation of public health communication campaigns.

Assurance functions are heterogenous, including public health training, research, and the evaluation of public health services. Training to enable the effective implementation and use of AI-based tools is limited in many public health programs, as is the opportunity for training in public health informatics more generally [10]. In research, there has been considerable activity to explore applications of machine learning, natural language processing, and knowledge-based systems in public health, but the translation of research on AI methods to public health practice has been challenging.

Finally, many models of essential public health functions include at their core the concept of **equity**. Consideration of equity follows naturally from a population perspective, where the distributions of health determinants and outcomes are a primary focus and often revealing of inequities. While AI methods can potentially help to identify and address inequities, there is also concern that such methods, and particularly machine learning, could reinforce or worsen inequities through mechanisms such as differential access and algorithmic bias [11].

A Vision for AI in Public Health

To realize the full potential of AI in public health, it is helpful to apply the perspective of **digital transformation** [12] to essential public health functions. Digital transformation draws upon user-centered design to re-imagine how essential functions can be improved by exploiting AI methods and other digital technologies. The goal is to move beyond the use of AI methods to automate manual data processing towards the use of AI to support effective decision-making in public health. In this context, a truly AI-enabled public health system is one where the data needed to perform essential functions are available and processes are optimized, through the appropriate use of AI methods, with the goal of supporting the effective and efficient delivery of essential public health services.

Box 13.2: Essential Public Health Functions [7]

Assessment
1. *Assess and monitor population health status, factors that influence health, and community needs and assets*
2. *Investigate, diagnose, and address health problems and hazards affecting the population*

Policy Development
1. *Communicate effectively to inform and educate people about health, factors that influence it, and how to improve it*
2. *Strengthen, support, and mobilize communities and partnerships to improve health*
3. *Create, champion, and implement policies, plans, and laws that impact health*
4. *Utilize legal and regulatory actions designed to improve and protect the public's health*

Assurance
1. *Assure an effective system that enables equitable access to the individual services and care needed to be healthy*

> 2. *Build and support a diverse and skilled public health workforce*
> 3. *Improve and innovate public health functions through ongoing evaluation, research, and continuous quality improvement*
> 4. *Build and maintain a strong organizational infrastructure for public health*

Applications of AI in Public Health

As discussed in the section on "The Nature of Essential Public Health Functions and the Application of AI", AI methods are more easily applied to some public health functions than others due to differences in the nature of each function. In this section, specific examples of how AI has been applied to different functions are presented and barriers and risks to the application of AI methods in public health are discussed.

Examples of AI Applications to Public Health Functions

In this section, examples of applications of AI to public health functions are presented considering both the public health functions (Box 13.2) and the AI approaches used (i.e., knowledge-based, machine learning, natural language processing). The intent is to illustrate different types of applications and not to provide a systematic or comprehensive review of all applications of AI methods to public health functions.

Assessment

The theme of assessment includes two essential public health functions, monitoring population health and surveillance of health hazards. Population health is a complex construct, which can be measured in terms of sentiment, attitudes, beliefs, and health outcomes. It is also influenced by a wide range of social, behavioral and physical determinants. Similarly, health hazards are diverse, including environmental conditions, workplace environments, and infectious diseases. The multidimensional nature of assessment lends itself well to AI methods such as machine learning and knowledge representation, which have both been applied to distill large amounts of data and information in this context. Many sources of data are unstructured and NLP has the potential to extract structured data from these sources for further analysis. While monitoring population health tends to have a longer-term focus to guide policy, surveillance can require rapid decision-making and action to control health threats.

Population health monitoring systematically collects data on health status, usually to inform longer-term planning and evaluation of programs. ML methods have been used in population health monitoring to analyze data from wearable devices, social media [13] and other high-dimensional data sources such as electronic health records [14] to predict population health. Researchers have also demonstrated the use of ML to measure associations between the built environment and health [15]. More broadly, these uses of ML methods in public health practice reflect their broader adoption in epidemiology and health outcomes research [16]. NLP has been used to monitor aspects of population health through analysis of posts and discussions in online digital media, such as identifying neighborhood characteristics associated with discussions of food on Twitter [17]. Knowledge-based systems have also been applied to exploit knowledge of causal relationships between the determinants of health to help users make sense of epidemiological indicators of chronic disease determinants and outcomes [18].

Public health surveillance is the systematic, ongoing collection and analysis of data to detect and guide actions to control hazards such as infectious disease outbreaks. It includes indicator-based surveillance (IBS) and event-based surveillance (EBS). IBS entails the systematic collection, analysis and interpretation of data about individuals, such as infectious disease reports, while EBS routinely analyzes online media to detect events of public health interest, such as disease outbreaks (Fig. 13.1). NLP methods have been applied in IBS to extract information from medical charts for case detection in areas such as syndromic surveillance [19], communicable disease surveillance [20], and occupational health surveillance [21]. To facilitate this type of surveillance, researchers have developed automated systems such as RiskScape [22] for public health surveillance using electronic health records. Machine learning methods have also been used to forecast the incidence of infectious disease [23] and to detect aberrations in epidemiological indicators [24]. Knowledge-based methods have been used to develop systems for syndromic surveillance, such as BioSTORM [25], and have also been used to develop a Population Health Record [26] for integrating indicators of chronic disease using knowledge of the determinants of health [18].

While IBS can be facilitated by AI methods, EBS is critically dependent on AI methods, in particular NLP methods for recognizing and extracting entities from large amounts of online media [27]. Notable systems in this space include the ontology-based BioCaster [28], HealthMap [29], which uses ML to automate many tasks, and GPHIN [30, 31], which uses AI methods to support human analysts. Related approaches, such as probabilistic topic modelling, have also been used in EBS to monitor diseases [32] and interventions [33]. Finally, given the wide range of relevant knowledge (i.e., spatial, temporal, and semantic aspects of disease outbreaks and other public health events) and the small number of global events detected by EBS, knowledge-based systems have also been applied to interpret the information extracted by NLP from online media [28].

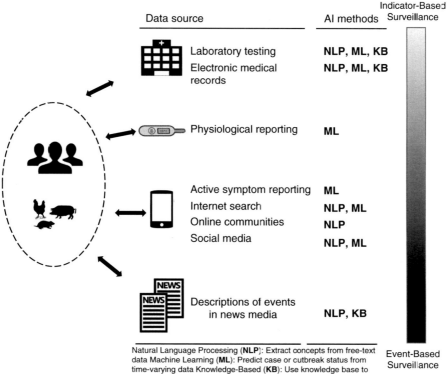

Fig. 13.1 Applications of artificial intelligence methods to infectious disease surveillance. Human and animal populations can be monitored for infectious disease outbreaks using a range of data sources. Data such as laboratory results and electronic medical records allow measurement of cases of disease (i.e., indicator-based surveillance), while other sources, such as news media allow detection of events, without measuring individual cases (i.e., event-based surveillance). Regardless of the data source, many approaches to surveillance rely on artificial intelligence methods to extract concepts from free-text, predict cases or outbreaks from time-varying data, or to reason about data using existing knowledge

Policy Development

The theme of policy development includes the functions of communication, mobilizing communities and partnerships to improve health, creating and implementing policy, and taking legal and regulatory actions to protect health. A task common to many of the functions in this theme is the extraction and synthesis of evidence from the literature about public health interventions. Machine learning and NLP methods have been used for this task in biomedicine [34], but adaptations are necessary for application in public health. For example, existing approaches to representing knowledge about interventions require adaptation [35] to accommodate the different nature of interventions in public health, where individuals and populations are targeted through a range of mechanisms [36]. Another example is the need to consider different types of evidence as randomized controlled trials are not possible for many types of public health interventions [37].

Public health communication provides information to individuals and communities with the aim of improving health outcomes [36]. In targeting communication to individuals, the incorporation of AI into health communication tools can make the communication more engaging, increasing immediacy [38]. There have been many applications of ML and NLP methods to detect changes in health status and to gather information and provide guidance for self-management or additional support of mental and physical health, but the evidence for their effectiveness is limited [39]. A related application of AI methods is the widespread use of social media and machine translation to target communities. For example, NLP methods have been applied to social media content to detect and analyze discourse on topics such as vaccine hesitancy [40], misinformation [41], and foodborne illness [42, 43]. This type of analysis can help to develop targeted messaging campaigns, such as those that apply AI methods to social media platforms to prevent foodborne illness due to restaurant dining (Fig. 13.2).

The application of AI and informatics more generally to policy creation and program planning in public health has led to proposals to update the determinants of health model to account for how information technologies can be used to influence

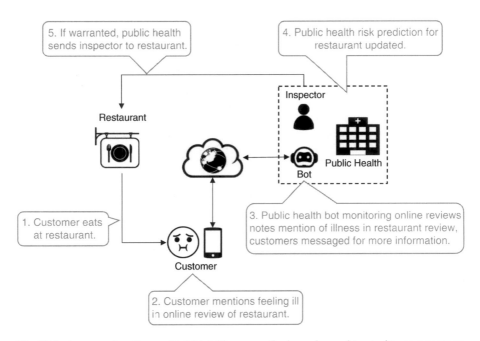

Fig. 13.2 An example of how artificial intelligence methods can be used to monitor comments on social media and generate information to guide public health interventions. Here, a bot developed by a public health organization detects a comment that may indicate foodborne illness due to a restaurant meal. This information is used to update the risk assessment of the restaurant and possibly trigger an in-person inspection (See [43] for more information)

health [36]. Precision public health provides another perspective on the use of AI for program planning [44]. As with precision medicine, the intent is to precisely match interventions to subjects, but in public health the subject is a population, not an individual. Measurement in the public health context entails high-resolution surveillance data for a population [45] and matching interventions requires transferring evidence from studies in other settings to that population in a causal reasoning framework [35, 46]. However, this application of AI has raised concerns about the effect on equity of employing targeted interventions at the expense of efforts to address the broader determinants of health [47], such as social position, which can be challenging to measure accurately [48].

Assurance

The theme of assurance groups together functions that assure equity, a diverse and skilled workforce, research and continuous quality improvement, and a strong organizational infrastructure. The application of AI methods to assurance functions has been more limited than in other themes. An exception is public health research, which has seen the exploration of AI methods to support many public health functions, as noted throughout this section and particularly for monitoring and surveillance.

There is a recognized need to educate the public health workforce about AI methods to enable the development and use of effective AI-enabled tools [12]. As discussed earlier, it would be ideal if pedagogical content about AI could be incorporated into public health informatics training, thereby providing practitioners with an appreciation of AI methods within the broader context of data and information management and analysis in public health. However, despite the widely recognized importance of training in public health informatics, and examples of effective programs [49], significant gaps in data and informatics skills persist in the public health workforce [10]. While there are likely many reasons for this continued lack of capacity, it may be attributable in part to the underinvestment in public health more generally and the challenges of applying computer-based innovations in this context

The public health system is recognized as being critical for a nation's health [50] and measurement and optimization of the operations of public health systems is one area where AI methods have considerable potential [51]. However, progress in the application of AI methods has been limited by challenges in conceptualizing [52] and measuring public health activities and interventions [53].

Barriers and Risks to AI Applications in Public Health

The previous section highlighted how the current state of AI applications in public health has been shaped to a large extent by the availability of novel data sources and innovations in algorithms. In addition to demonstrating the potential of AI, the research and practice efforts to date have also identified barriers and risks to

implementing AI in public health. To enable the future application of AI, it is helpful to consider the barriers and risks to applying AI methods in public health and
how they might be addressed.

Barriers to implementing AI in public health include a limited understanding
among public health professions of the applications to which AI methods are best
suited, a limited capacity for implementing and using AI in many public health settings, and a lack of data and knowledge in some contexts [54]. A limited understanding of AI among public health professionals can be addressed through training,
including continuing education. (Chap. 16) As noted in the previous section, however, challenges in enhancing training in public health informatics more generally
suggest that this barrier may take time to address. The limited capacity for implementing and using AI results from the lack of skilled human and information technology resources in many public health settings, which has been noted as a barrier
to digital transformation in public health more generally [12].

Risks to implementing AI in public health include algorithmic biases that may
disadvantage specific groups [44] (see Chap. 18), the potential to exacerbate health
inequalities by limiting access to interventions such as language-based models [55],
and unrealistic expectations that may make it difficult to scale-up translational
research. As an example of a bias, a widely used algorithm for making referrals to a
chronic disease management programs was found to be biased against Black patients
[56]. The bias was introduced through the problem formulation, because the model
was developed to predict costs, which reflect barriers to accessing health care. A
solution in this case would be to use another outcome, such as a measure of illness.
Table 13.1 presents different types of bias that should be considered when using
machine learning to develop prediction models in population and public health.

While the barriers and risks are real, they can be addressed through measures
such as guidelines [59] and enhanced training opportunities targeting different
stages of the public health career trajectory. For example, recognizing and avoiding
bias in training and applying ML algorithms can be taught within MPH programs
and continuing education programs can support practitioners in developing a realistic assessment of the potential contributions of AI in public health.

Table 13.1 Types of biases to be considered when developing machine learning models for
prediction in population and public health. For further discussion of these biases, see [44]

Type of Bias	Description
Sampling Bias	The proportion of subjects or records sampled differs systematically across subpopulations. For example, a model is trained with input from mainly adult, but intended to be applied to people of all ages
Information Bias	The quality or amount of data differs systematically by subpopulations. For example, electronic health records tend to provide a more complete history of people with higher as opposed to lower socioeconomic status ([57]; [58])
Random Error	The number of subjects or records for a subpopulation is too small to achieve an acceptable precision when making predictions
Objective Specification	The outcome of the prediction model is misaligned with its intended use and may reinforce existing inequities. For example, developing a chronic disease program referral model based on health care costs as opposed to illness [56]

Future Applications of AI in Public Health

The previous sections have considered the potential for AI methods to be applied to public health functions and have highlighted examples of current AI applications in public health. In this section, progress towards the vision presented earlier (see the section on "A Vision for AI in Public Health") is considered, and the potential for AI methods to transform public health in the future is examined.

Progress Towards the Vision

While in many respects the breadth of application of AI methods to public health functions is impressive, the examples reviewed in the section on "The Nature of Essential Public Health Functions and the Application of AI" suggest that it will take time to reach the vision presented. Notably, many applications of AI in public health have focused on automating manual tasks related to the functions of population health monitoring, surveillance, and communication. Moreover, many research advances, such as in the application of ML methods to aberration detection [24], have seen a slow and uneven translation into practice.

The reasons for the limited progress include the lack of high-quality evidence supporting the use of AI methods along with the barriers identified earlier, namely limitations in training, resources, and data access in some public health settings. The lack of high-quality evidence reflects in part the challenge in evaluating public health interventions more generally, but there is also a similar lack of high-quality evidence supporting the application of AI methods in clinical domains [60]. Minimal reporting guidelines have been developed for clinical applications of AI [61] and similar guidelines should be advanced in public health.

Training in public health informatics and the application of AI methods more specifically are critical for progress towards the vision presented. Many efforts are underway in this regard, but the current situation remains one where awareness and knowledge of AI methods is limited in public health. Coordinated efforts by multiple stakeholders, including public health agencies, professional associations, and educational institutions are required to update public health competencies and make training available through a variety of mechanisms.

Future Applications

To close this chapter, it is helpful to consider future applications of AI that have the potential to advance the vision of AI in public health. In general, given the reliance of ML and NLP methods on large amounts of data, many future applications would be enabled by ensuring that the necessary data are generated and available for analysis (Chaps. 6, 7). For example, as discussed previously, there is great potential for ML to support the monitoring and optimization of public health services. However, data about public health activities are not currently generated and represented in a consistent manner. If public health organizations were to systematically track activities, such as the delivery of interventions, ML and other AI methods could be used to support decisions about the effective use of interventions in specific communities. This type of data generation and analysis about actions occurs routinely in clinical domains and would provide an essential foundation for a learning public health system [62].

Another foundational advance that would enable broader application of AI in public health is improved integration of individual-level and public health data. For example, tighter integration of individual-level public health data with records for clinical care and social services, such as housing support, would enable the use of machine learning to search for opportunities to improve essential services across sectors. These opportunities could emerge from the ability to better coordinate clinical and public health interventions, allowing a "person-centered" approach that integrates health promotion, disease prevention, and clinical services.

Finally, a view to the future should consider how applications of AI methods in public health are related to broader public health goals such as digital transformation and the Sustainable Development Goals [63]. Preparing public health systems for digital transformation requires attention to ensuring that enabling information technology and human resources are in place [12, 64]. This foundation can enable a broader re-imagination of how AI methods can transform public health services to achieve goals within communities, for nations, and globally.

Questions for Discussion

- What characteristics of public health functions make them amenable to the application of AI methods? Are some AI methods better suited to some public health functions than others? Explain.
- Machine learning (ML) methods have been applied in surveillance to detect individual cases and to detect outbreaks. How is the application of ML methods different for these two purposes? Are there any common challenges to applying ML methods in both contexts?
- Given what you know about knowledge-based systems, explain how they can be used most effectively in public health.
- What is the most important barrier to the application of AI in public health? Justify your choice and propose potential solutions.
- What is a risk of applying AI in public health? Explain.
- In your opinion, what future application of AI could have the greatest impact on public health?

Further Readings

Lavigne M, Mussa F, Creatore MI, Hoffman SJ, and Buckeridge DL. A population health perspective on artificial intelligence. *Healthcare Management Forum* 2019;32(4):173–177.

- This paper provides an overview of artificial intelligence in the context of population health. The field of AI and major sub-fields are introduced with examples of their application in population and public health.

Buckeridge DL. Precision, Equity, and Public Health and Epidemiology Informatics – A Scoping Review. *IMIA Yearbook of Medical Informatics* 2020;29(1):226–230.

- This paper summarizes recently published literature on two topics of central relevance to the application of AI in public health, namely precision public health (PPH) and equity in the development of prediction models. Applications of PPH are presented and debates about the concept of PPH are explored. Guidelines and barriers to promoting equity in prediction modelling are presented and discussed.

Yasnoff WA, O'Carroll PW, Koo D, Linkins RW, Kilbourne EM. Public Health Informatics: Improving and Transforming Public Health in the Information Age. *Journal of Public Health Management and Practice* 2000;6(6):67–75.

- This paper introduces the discipline of public health informatics, describing its role and the challenges it sought to address at its inception. Although not about AI directly, it provides an important context regarding the state of informatics within the domain of public health.

Hosny A, Aerts H. Artificial intelligence for global health. *Science* 2019;366(6468):955–956.

- This paper presents a framework with examples of applications of AI in resource-poor health care settings. Applications in population health are considered along with portable diagnostics and clinical decision support.

Rodriguez-Gonzalez A, Zanin M, Menasalvas-Ruiz E. Can Artificial Intelligence Help Future Global Challenges? An Overview of Antimicrobial Resistance and Impact of Climate Change in Disease Epidemiology. *IMIA Yearbook of Medical Informatics* 2019;28(1):224–231.

- This paper presents a review of AI applications in two areas of global public health importance—antimicrobial resistance and health effects of climate change. The authors summarize the recent literature highlighting where AI methods have been applied, the results, and what has been learned to guide future applications.

References

1. Winslow CE. The untilled fields of public health. Science. 1920;51(1306):23–33. Available from: http://eutils.ncbi.nlm.nih.gov/entrez/eutils/elink.fcgi?dbfrom=pubmed&id=17838891&retmode=ref&cmd=prlinks
2. Yasnoff WA, O'Carroll PW, Koo D, Linkins RW, Kilbourne EM. Public health informatics improving and transforming public health in the information age. J Public Health Manag Pract 2000;6(6):67–75. Available from: http://content.wkhealth.com/linkback/openurl?sid=WKPTLP:landingpage&an=00124784-200006060-00010
3. Friede A, Blum HL, McDonald M. Public health informatics: how information-age technology can strengthen public health. Annual review of public health [Internet]. 1995;16(1):239–52 Available from: http://www.annualreviews.org/doi/10.1146/annurev.pu.16.050195.001323

4. Kushniruk AW, Patel VL. Cognitive and usability engineering methods for the evaluation of clinical information systems. J Biomed Inform. 2004;37(1):56–76. Available from: https://linkinghub.elsevier.com/retrieve/pii/S1532046404000206

5. Lorenzi NM, Riley RT, Blyth AJ, Southon G, Dixon BJ. People and organizational aspects of medical informatics. Stud Health Technol Inform. 1998;52(Pt 2):1197–200. Available from: http://eutils.ncbi.nlm.nih.gov/entrez/eutils/elink.fcgi?dbfrom=pubmed&id=10384649&retmode=ref&cmd=prlinks

6. Holmgren AJ, Apathy NC, Adler-Milstein J. Barriers to hospital electronic public health reporting and implications for the COVID-19 pandemic. J Am Med Inform Assoc. 2020;27(8):1306–9. Available from: http://eutils.ncbi.nlm.nih.gov/entrez/eutils/elink.fcgi?dbfrom=pubmed&id=32442266&retmode=ref&cmd=prlinks

7. Castrucci BC. The "10 Essential Public Health Services" Is the Common Framework Needed to Communicate About Public Health. Am J Public Health. 2021;111(4):598–9. Available from: http://eutils.ncbi.nlm.nih.gov/entrez/eutils/elink.fcgi?dbfrom=pubmed&id=33689415&retmode=ref&cmd=prlinks

8. Revere D, Turner AM, Madhavan A, Rambo N, Bugni PF, Kimball A, et al. Understanding the information needs of public health practitioners: a literature review to inform design of an interactive digital knowledge management system. J Biomed Inform. 2007;40(4):410–21. Available from: https://linkinghub.elsevier.com/retrieve/pii/S1532046407000020

9. Keating C, Rogers R, Unal R, Dryer D, Sousa-Poza A, Safford R, et al. System of systems engineering. Eng Manag J. 2003;15(3):36–45. Available from: https://www.tandfonline.com/doi/abs/10.1080/10429247.2003.11415214

10. McFarlane TD, Dixon BE, Grannis SJ, Gibson PJ. Public Health Informatics in Local and State Health Agencies: An Update From the Public Health Workforce Interests and Needs Survey. J Public Health Man. 2019;25(2):S67–77.

11. Smith MJ, Axler R, Bean S, Rudzicz F, Shaw J. Four equity considerations for the use of artificial intelligence in public health. Bull World Health Organ. 2020;98(4):290–2. Available from: http://www.who.int/entity/bulletin/volumes/98/4/19-237503.pdf

12. Ricciardi W, Barros PP, Bourek A, Brouwer W, Kelsey T, Lehtonen L, et al. How to govern the digital transformation of health services. Eur J Public Health. 2019;29(Supplement_3):7–12. Available from: http://eutils.ncbi.nlm.nih.gov/entrez/eutils/elink.fcgi?dbfrom=pubmed&id=31738442&retmode=ref&cmd=prlinks

13. Nguyen H, Nguyen T, Nguyen DT. An empirical study on prediction of population health through social media. J Biomed Inform. 2019;99(4):103277. Available from: https://linkinghub.elsevier.com/retrieve/pii/S1532046419301960

14. Morgenstern JD, Buajitti E, O'Neill M, Piggott T, Goel V, Fridman D, et al. Predicting population health with machine learning: a scoping review. BMJ Open. 2020;10(10):e037860. Available from: https://bmjopen.bmj.com/lookup/doi/10.1136/bmjopen-2020-037860

15. Keralis JM, Javanmardi M, Khanna S, Dwivedi P, Huang D, Tasdizen T, et al. Health and the built environment in United States cities: measuring associations using Google Street View-derived indicators of the built environment. BMC Public Health. 2020;20(1):215–0. Available from: https://bmcpublichealth.biomedcentral.com/articles/10.1186/s12889-020-8300-1

16. Wiemken TL, Kelley RR. Machine learning in epidemiology and health outcomes research. Annu Rev Public Health. 2020;41(1):21–36. Available from: https://www.annualreviews.org/doi/10.1146/annurev-publhealth-040119-094437

17. Vydiswaran VGV, Romero DM, Zhao X, Yu D, Gomez-Lopez I, Lu JX, et al. Uncovering the relationship between food-related discussion on Twitter and neighborhood characteristics. J Am Med Inform Assoc. 2020;27(2):254–64. Available from: https://academic.oup.com/jamia/article/27/2/254/5601669

18. Shaban-Nejad A, Adam NR, Lavigne M, Okhmatovskaia A, Buckeridge DL. PopHR: a knowledge-based platform to support integration, analysis, and visualization of population health data. Ann N Y Acad Sci. 2016;1387(1):44–53. Available from: http://doi.wiley.com/10.1111/nyas.13271

19. Conway M, Dowling JN, Chapman WW. Using chief complaints for syndromic surveillance: A review of chief complaint based classifiers in North America. J Biomed Inform. 2013;46(4):734–43. Available from: https://linkinghub.elsevier.com/retrieve/pii/S1532046413000464

20. Dexter GP, Grannis SJ, Dixon BE, Kasthurirathne SN. Generalization of Machine Learning Approaches to Identify Notifiable Conditions from a Statewide Health Information Exchange. AMIA Jt Summits Transl Sci Proc. 2020;2020:152–61. Available from: http://eutils.ncbi.nlm.nih.gov/entrez/eutils/elink.fcgi?dbfrom=pubmed&id=32477634&retmode=ref&cmd=prlinks

21. Burstyn I, Slutsky A, Lee DG, Singer AB, An Y, Michael YL. Beyond Crosswalks: Reliability of Exposure Assessment Following Automated Coding of Free-Text Job Descriptions for Occupational Epidemiology. Ann Occup Hyg. 2014;58(4):482–92.

22. Cocoros NM, Kirby C, Zambarano B, Ochoa A, Eberhardt K, et al. RiskScape: A Data Visualization and Aggregation Platform for Public Health Surveillance Using Routine Electronic Health Record Data. Am J Public Health. 2021;111(2):269–76.

23. Berke O, Trotz-Williams L, de Montagne S. Good times bad times: Automated forecasting of seasonal cryptosporidiosis in Ontario using machine learning. Can Commun Dis Rep. 2020;46(6):192–7. Available from: https://www.canada.ca/content/dam/phac-aspc/documents/services/reports-publications/canada-communicable-disease-report-ccdr/monthly-issue/2020-46/issue-6-june-4-2020/ccdrv46i06a07-eng.pdf

24. Yuan M, Boston-Fisher N, Luo Y, Verma A, Buckeridge DL. A systematic review of aberration detection algorithms used in public health surveillance. J Biomed Inform. 2019;94:103181. Available from: https://linkinghub.elsevier.com/retrieve/pii/S1532046419300991

25. O'Connor M, Buckeridge DL, Choy M, Crubezy M, Pincus Z, Musen MA. BioSTORM: a system for automated surveillance of diverse data sources. AMIA. In: Annual Symposium proceedings/AMIA Symposium AMIA Symposium; 2003. p. 1071. Available from: http://eutils.ncbi.nlm.nih.gov/entrez/eutils/elink.fcgi?dbfrom=pubmed&id=14728574&retmode=ref&cmd=prlinks.

26. Friedman DJ, Parrish RG. The population health record: concepts, definition, design, and implementation. J Am Med Inform Assoc. 2010;17(4):359–66. Available from: https://academic.oup.com/jamia/article-lookup/doi/10.1136/jamia.2009.001578

27. Brownstein JS, Freifeld CC, Madoff LC. Digital disease detection--harnessing the Web for public health surveillance. N Engl J Med. 2009;360(21):2153–7. Available from: http://www.nejm.org/doi/abs/10.1056/NEJMp0900702

28. Collier N, Doan S, Kawazoe A, Goodwin RM, Conway M, Tateno Y, et al. BioCaster: detecting public health rumors with a Web-based text mining system. Bioinformatics. 2008;24(24):2940–1.

29. Freifeld CC, Mandl KD, Reis BY, Brownstein JS. HealthMap: global infectious disease monitoring through automated classification and visualization of Internet media reports. J Am Med Inform Assoc. 2008;15(2):150–7. Available from: https://academic.oup.com/jamia/article-lookup/doi/10.1197/jamia.M2544

30. Baclic O, Tunis M, Young K, Doan C, Swerdfeger H, Schonfeld J. Challenges and opportunities for public health made possible by advances in natural language processing. Can Commun Dis Rep. 2020;46(6):161–8. Available from: https://www.canada.ca/content/dam/phac-aspc/documents/services/reports-publications/canada-communicable-disease-report-ccdr/monthly-issue/2020-46/issue-6-june-4-2020/ccdrv46i06a02-eng.pdf

31. Mykhalovskiy E, Weir L. The Global Public Health Intelligence Network and early warning outbreak detection: a Canadian contribution to global public health. Can J Public Health. 2006;97(1):42–4. Available from: http://link.springer.com/10.1007/BF03405213

32. Ghosh S, Chakraborty P, Nsoesie EO, Cohn E, Mekaru SR, Brownstein JS, et al. Temporal Topic Modeling to Assess Associations between News Trends and Infectious Disease Outbreaks. Sci Rep. 2017;7(1):40841.

33. Li Y, Nair P, Wen Z, Chafi I, Okhmatovskaia A, Powell G, et al. Global Surveillance of COVID-19 by mining news media using a multi-source dynamic embedded topic model. In: Proc 11th Acm Int Conf Bioinform Comput Biology Heal Informatics; 2020. p. 1–14.

34. Marshall IJ, Wallace BC. Toward systematic review automation: a practical guide to using machine learning tools in research synthesis. Syst Rev. 2019;8(1):163–10. Available from: https://systematicreviewsjournal.biomedcentral.com/articles/10.1186/s13643-019-1074-9

35. Okhmatovskaia A, Buckeridge DL. Intelligent Tools for Precision Public Health. Stud Health Technol Inform. 2020;270:858–63. Available from: http://eutils.ncbi.nlm.nih.gov/entrez/eutils/elink.fcgi?dbfrom=pubmed&id=32570504&retmode=ref&cmd=prlinks

36. Rice L, Sara R. Updating the determinants of health model in the Information Age. Health Promot Int. 2019;34(6):1241–9. Available from: http://eutils.ncbi.nlm.nih.gov/entrez/eutils/elink.fcgi?dbfrom=pubmed&id=30212852&retmode=ref&cmd=prlinks

37. Sanson-Fisher RW, Bonevski B, Green LW, D'Este C. Limitations of the randomized controlled trial in evaluating population-based health interventions. Am J Prev Med. 2007;33(2):155–61.

38. Kreps GL, Neuhauser L. Artificial intelligence and immediacy: designing health communication to personally engage consumers and providers. Patient Educ Couns. 2013;92(2):205–10. Available from: http://eutils.ncbi.nlm.nih.gov/entrez/eutils/elink.fcgi?dbfrom=pubmed&id=23683341&retmode=ref&cmd=prlinks

39. Milne-Ives M, de Cock C, Lim E, Shehadeh MH, de Pennington N, Mole G, et al. The effectiveness of artificial intelligence conversational agents in health care: systematic review. J Med Internet Res. 2020;22(10):e20346.

40. Gunaratne K, Coomes EA, Haghbayan H. Temporal trends in anti-vaccine discourse on Twitter. Vaccine. 2019;37(35):4867–71.

41. Smith ST, Kao EK, Mackin ED, Shah DC, Simek O, Rubin DB. Automatic detection of influential actors in disinformation networks. Proc Natl Acad Sci U S A. 2021;118(4):e2011216118.

42. Margetts H, Dorobantu C. Rethink government with AI. Nature. 2019;568(7751):163–5.

43. Oldroyd RA, Morris MA, Birkin M. Identifying Methods for Monitoring Foodborne Illness: Review of Existing Public Health Surveillance Techniques. JMIR Public Health Surveill. 2018;4(2):e57.

44. Buckeridge DL. Precision, Equity, and Public Health and Epidemiology Informatics - A Scoping Review. Yearb Med Inform. 2020;29(1):226–30. Available from: http://www.thieme-connect.de/DOI/DOI?10.1055/s-0040-1701989

45. Dwyer-Lindgren L, Cork MA, Sligar A, Steuben KM, Wilson KF, Provost NR, et al. Mapping HIV prevalence in sub-Saharan Africa between 2000 and 2017. Nature. 2019;570(7760):189–93. Available from: http://www.nature.com/articles/s41586-019-1200-9

46. Bareinboim E, Pearl J. Causal inference and the data-fusion problem. Proc Natl Acad Sci U S A. 2016;113(27):7345–52. Available from: http://www.pnas.org/lookup/doi/10.1073/pnas.1510507113

47. Kenney M, Mamo L. The imaginary of precision public health. Med Humanit. 2019;46(3):192–203. Available from: http://mh.bmj.com/lookup/doi/10.1136/medhum-2018-011597

48. Olstad DL, McIntyre L. Reconceptualising precision public health. BMJ Open. 2019;9(9):e030279. Available from: http://bmjopen.bmj.com/lookup/doi/10.1136/bmjopen-2019-030279

49. Schwartz DG, McGrath SP, Monsen KA, FAMIA, Dixon BE. Current Approaches and Trends in Graduate Public Health Informatics Education in the United States: Four Case Studies from the Field. Online J Public Health inform. 2020;12(1):e7. Available from: http://eutils.ncbi.nlm.nih.gov/entrez/eutils/elink.fcgi?dbfrom=pubmed&id=32742557&retmode=ref&cmd=prlinks

50. Baker EL, Potter MA, Jones DL, Mercer SL, Cioffi JP, Green LW, et al. The public health infrastructure and our nation's health. Ann Rev Public Health. 2005;26(1):303–18. Available from: http://www.annualreviews.org/doi/10.1146/annurev.publhealth.26.021304.144647

51. Institute of Medicine. For the Public's Health: The Role of Measurement in Action and Accountability. Washington, D.C.: The National Academies Press; 2011.

52. Bekemeier B, Park S. Development of the PHAST model: generating standard public health services data and evidence for decision-making. J Am Med Inform Assoc. 2018;25(4):428–34.

Available from: http://eutils.ncbi.nlm.nih.gov/entrez/eutils/elink.fcgi?dbfrom=pubmed&id=29106585&retmode=ref&cmd=prlinks

53. Litvak E, Dufour R, Leblanc É, Kaiser D, Mercure S-A, Nguyen CT, et al. Making sense of what exactly public health does: a typology of public health interventions. Can J Public Health. 2019:1–7. Available from: http://link.springer.com/10.17269/s41997-019-00268-3

54. Morgenstern JD, Rosella LC, Daley MJ, Goel V, Schünemann HJ, Piggott T. "AI's gonna have an impact on everything in society, so it has to have an impact on public health": a fundamental qualitative descriptive study of the implications of artificial intelligence for public health. BMC Public Health. 2021;21(1):40–14. Available from: https://bmcpublichealth.biomedcentral.com/articles/10.1186/s12889-020-10030-x

55. Straw I, Callison-Burch C. Artificial Intelligence in mental health and the biases of language based models. PLoS One. 2020;15(12):e0240376. Available from: http://eutils.ncbi.nlm.nih.gov/entrez/eutils/elink.fcgi?dbfrom=pubmed&id=33332380&retmode=ref&cmd=prlinks

56. Obermeyer Z, Powers B, Vogeli C, Mullainathan S. Dissecting racial bias in an algorithm used to manage the health of populations. Science. 2019;366(6464):447–53. Available from: http://www.sciencemag.org/lookup/doi/10.1126/science.aax2342

57. Chien AT, Newhouse JP, Iezzoni LI, Petty CR, Normand S-LT, Schuster MA. Socioeconomic Background and Commercial Health Plan Spending. Pediatrics. 2017;140(5):e20171640. Available from: http://pediatrics.aappublications.org/lookup/doi/10.1542/peds.2017-1640

58. Gianfrancesco MA, Tamang S, Yazdany J, Schmajuk G. Potential biases in machine learning algorithms using electronic health record data. JAMA Intern Med 2018;178(11):1544–7. Available from: http://archinte.jamanetwork.com/article aspx?doi=10.1001/jamainternmed.2018.3763

59. Wiens J, Saria S, Sendak M, Ghassemi M, Liu VX, Doshi-Velez F, et al. Do no harm: a roadmap for responsible machine learning for health care. Nat Med. 2019;25(9):1337–40. Available from: http://www.nature.com/articles/s41591-019-0548-6

60. Wynants L, Calster BV, Collins GS, Riley RD, Heinze G, Schuit E, et al. Prediction models for diagnosis and prognosis of covid-19: systematic review and critical appraisal. BMJ. 2020;369:m1328.

61. Norgeot B, Quer G, Beaulieu-Jones BK, Torkamani A, Dias R, Gianfrancesco M, et al. Minimum information about clinical artificial intelligence modeling: the MI-CLAIM checklist. Nat Med. 2020;26(9):1320–4. Available from: http://www.nature.com/articles/s41591-020-1041-y

62. Friedman CP, Rubin JC, Sullivan KJ. Toward an Information Infrastructure for Global Health Improvement. Yearbook of medical informatics [Internet]. 2017;26(1):16–23. Available from: http://www.thieme-connect.de/DOI/DOI?10.15265/IY-2017-004

63. Colglazier W. Sustainable development agenda: 2030. Science. 2015;349(6252):1048–50.

64. Topol E. The Topol review: preparing the healthcare workforce to deliver the digital future. 2019. Available from: https://topol.hee.nhs.uk/

Chapter 14
AI in Translational Bioinformatics and Precision Medicine

Thanh M. Nguyen and Jake Y. Chen

After reading this chapter, you should know the answers to these questions:
- Which key translational bioinformatics problem are AI methods positioned to solve?
- What principles would guide your choice of which AI techniques and tools to apply to a translational bioinformatics problem?
- What are some important "-omic" databases that can be used to interpret and validate translational bioinformatics related machine learning results from the biomedical perspective?

Introduction and Concepts

The field of **translational bioinformatics** is concerned with the development of *storage, analytic, and interpretive* methods to optimize the transformation of increasingly voluminous *biomedical data and genomic data* into proactive, predictive, preventive, and participatory health. Translational bioinformatics includes research on the development of novel techniques for the integration of biological and clinical data and the evolution of clinical informatics methodology to encompass biological observations. The end product of translational

T. M. Nguyen · J. Y. Chen (✉)
Informatics Institute, University of Alabama at Birmingham, Birmingham, AL, USA
e-mail: jakechen@uab.edu

© The Author(s), under exclusive license to Springer Nature
Switzerland AG 2022
T. A. Cohen et al. (eds.), *Intelligent Systems in Medicine and Health*, Cognitive
Informatics in Biomedicine and Healthcare,
https://doi.org/10.1007/978-3-031-09108-7_14

bioinformatics is newly found knowledge from these integrative efforts that can be disseminated to various stakeholders, including biomedical scientists, clinicians, and patients [1].

Voluminous data, which are often understood as data volume of a few gigabytes and beyond, can be due to:

- A *large proportion of irrelevant information* in the data. For example, bulk RNA sequencing data for just one sample is more than ten gigabytes before compression and a few gigabytes after compression [2]. However, the ratio of **exon** reads, which are used in later analysis, over **intron** reads, which are not used, is small (it is expected to be 1/24 [3]).
- A *large number of samples*, also called datapoints (each of which may represent a subject), in the data. For example, the Nationwide Emergency Department Sample data [4] contains more than 30 million subjects. In this dataset, there are just over 100 features only.
- A *large number of features*. For example, **human gene expression** data have 20,412 protein-encoding **genes**, 14,600 **pseudogenes**, 14,727 long **non-coding RNAs**, and 5037 small non-coding RNAs. Some datasets may have large numbers of both samples and features. For example, single-cell RNA sequencing data may contain data from hundreds of thousands of cells [5], capturing the whole **genome**.

A Brief History of Translational Bioinformatics

Translational bioinformatics is a relatively young field. According to Ouzounis [6], translational bioinformatics started in 1996. In the beginning, the field primarily researched how to organize biomedical data and build an ontology system improving the interpretation and searching of biomedical research. After the first version of the human genome project in 2003 [7], genomic analysis was added to translational bioinformatics and continued growing to be a key area in the field. Since 2005 in Europe and 2009 in the United States, programs to widely adopt **electronic medical record**s in patient care and research have been launched [8]. Consequently, large amounts of past clinical data stored in electronic format could readily be used in translational research. This enabled the development of the biomedical informatics component of translational bioinformatics. As translational bioinformatic techniques mature in the areas of genomics and biomedical informatics, they are further adapted to carry out research on other biomedical data, such as microbiome, chemical informatics, and metabolomics data. Today, translational bioinformatics is a multidisciplinary field, extending from the molecular level (genes, proteins, and other molecular entities below the cell) to the population level (collections of living subjects).

Concepts of AI in Translational Bioinformatics

AI in translational bioinformatics covers a broader range of problems than it does in other clinical fields. In clinical practice, the main goal of applying AI is often to complete tasks that used to require manual labor. Some AI applications, such as predicting patient readmission, may perform tasks not typically conducted by human beings. However, producing new knowledge is not required. In translational bioinformatics, besides supporting manual labor, an important goal when using AI is to infer new knowledge, with typical applications including:

- Association Studies: mining for novel relationships among different biomedical entities.
- Subtyping and clustering: dividing patients and samples into different groups such that each group may explicitly represent a sub-clinical outcome or a sub-phenotype.
- Modeling and knowledge representation: mathematically representing the associations and cause-effect relations among different biomedical entities. The representation, in this case, is often in a system of differential equations.
- Simulation: mathematically representing the changes observed in biomedical subjects by a system of dynamic equations. The system has the general form $\mathbf{x}(t + 1) = F(\mathbf{x}(t), \mathbf{u}(t))$. Here, $\mathbf{x}(t)$ represents the subject at timepoint t, $\mathbf{u}(t)$ represents the interference at timepoint t, and $\mathbf{x}(t + 1)$ represents the subject at the next timepoint.
- Spatial visualization: visualizing biomedical datapoints in 2D or 3D space.

Primary Data Categories in Translational Bioinformatics

Genomic Data

This chapter broadly refers to all types of data involving genes, proteins, **miRNAs**, metabolites, proteins, and biological reactions as genomic data, which includes data in both genomic and functional genomic subcategories.

Genomic and other -omic data, as introduced in Chap. 3, refer to the measure, characteristic, and annotation of genes. The original definition of genomics only referred to the study of genes or the DNA sequences and their related information [9]. However, the data and research scope in bioinformatics also covers other molecular entities involved in the transcription and translation processes. Therefore, -omic data include:

- **Proteomics** is the study of proteins [10].
- **Metabolomics** studies the chemicals participating in dynamic metabolic processes [11].

– **Transcriptomics** studies the transcription process [12], which focuses on RNAs and other transcription-regulator molecular functions.

In some literature [13, 14], the word "genomics" (or gene) is used interchangeably with "transcriptomics" (RNA) and "proteomics" (protein).

When analyzing translational bioinformatics data, it is important to recognize and categorize the data by *measure* and *resolution*. *Measure* refers to the type of molecular entities that are collected, counted, or observed. The technical terms **microarray** [15], **copy-number variation** [16], and mutation only refer to DNA. The technical terms **RNA sequencing** and **transcript count** only refer to RNA [17, 18]. The terms **western blotting** [19], multi-level structure, and protein-protein **binding affinity** [20] refer only to protein. Each measure and molecular type has its unique physical characteristics; therefore, applying a method built for one measure to another should be very carefully considered. *Resolution* refers to whether the measures are collected from the tissue (bulk) sample, which is a collection of cells, at the single-cell level, or at the sub-cellular molecular level (i.e., isolated proteins). While bulk and single-cell samples can have the same measures (e.g., transcript count in bulk RNA and single-cell RNA), their numerical characteristics are very different.

The results from analyzing -omic data by researchers from multiple fields are carefully curated and organized into *annotated catalogs*. The Gene Ontology catalog [21, 22] identifies which genes participate in specific biological processes, belong to specific cellular components, or share a specific molecular function. Pathway catalogs, such as the Kyoto Encyclopedia of Genes and Genomes (KEGG) [23] and Reactome [24], annotate how groups of genes interact with each other and activate in specific orders to regulate cellular phenotypes and processes in response to external stimuli. Protein catalogs, such as UniProt [25], Protein Data Bank [26], and STRING [27], collect and organize protein structures and interactions. These catalogs are important to interpret the new omic analytic results, highlighting the molecular features that differentiate two or more phenotypes.

Clinomic Data

Clinomic data, which is also called the "**clinotype**"[28], refers to the measures and characteristics of the living subject, which are useful for medical research and interventions [28, 29]. The major biomedical data categories are diagnosis-related data, laboratory test results, medication data, and medical imaging data [30]. Diagnosis-related data refer to the time, stage, and survivability of a disease or disorder in a subject. Laboratory test results, which are also called biomeasures [31], refer to a subject's quantifiable observations and the biological material concerned (i.e., blood and urine samples). Because laboratory test results are quantifiable, we can systematically define thresholds and criteria to determine whether the result indi-cates particular diseases or disorders. Medication data refer to the time and types of interventions, or treatments, received by a subject. Medical imaging data, such as X-rays and functional magnetic resonance images, can be understood as observa-tions from a subject that are not directly quantified. Therefore, interpretation cf medical images in research and clinical practice often occurs on a case-by-case basis and depends on physicians' and researchers' training experience. Besides, biomedical data may contain other types of data that are specifically collected for particular research and clinical practice scenarios, such as smoking history [32, 33], diet type [34], exercise frequency [35], and drug side-effect history. Also, clinomic data may include genomic data when a subjects' genetic data is used to diagnose and help decide a treatment [36–38].

Phenotypic Data

In translational bioinformatics, the basic phenotype definition refers to the diseases and abnormalities affecting each subject, such as breast cancer and diabetes. In the broader context, phenotype refers to the subjects' categorization and definition as assigned by biomedical experts. In this context, a phenotype definition, such as 'cell proliferation' and 'chemotherapy resistance', is specific to each research project or clinical trial. To differentiate phenotypic data from clinomic data, we may under-stand that phenotypic data are directly derived from clinomic observations.

Categorizing AI Applications in Translational Bioinformatics

In treating complex diseases and **precision medicine**, linking omics and biomedical data is expected to improve the quality of care [39, 40] from the current practice, which primarily relies only on clinomic data or phenomic data (which is also referred as biomedical data) alone. Biomedical data will still be essential to detect and monitor disease progression, tasks for which single-type omics data has not yet shown superiority [39]. Meanwhile, omics data is essential to find driver mutations and their functionalities, prerequisites to understanding their roles in causing a dis-ease. Besides, even when the major causes of a disease are not exclusively genetic, such as with hypertension, knowing the patients' omics data may still improve treat-ment precision [41, 42].

Linking of -omics, clinotype, and phenotype data opens new questions that require advanced AI, machine learning, and data mining techniques to resolve. *Clinotype-to-clinotype* (C2C) association discovery, similar to "omic association" [43, 44], finds the clinotypes that co-occur in subjects' data and determines whether

Fig. 14.1 Categorizing AI
Translational
Bioinformatics

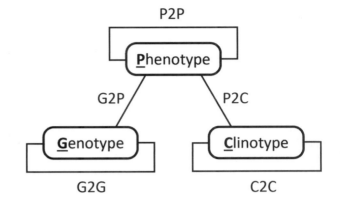

one clinotype occurrence is likely to precede those of other clinotypes. Discovery of novel *clinotype-to-phenotype* associations may advance risk assessment beyond current disease:lab-test markers toward finding sets of simpler, more cost-effective risk markers. This would allow patients and physicians to take early and preventive actions [45].

From a knowledge discovery perspective, Fig. 14.1 summarizes AI applications in translational bioinformatics according to the data categories we have introduced. Here, three data categories yield six possible types of association. In this figure, *genomic-to-clinomic* association has not been well-defined (and is therefore not illustrated). The other five types of association are as follows.

G2G (Genomic to Genomic)

G2G refers to applications involving finding gene-gene associations using AI techniques. G2G has many sub-problems, which are defined by the gene-gene mechanisms of interaction concerned. Sub-problems that are foci of current research include estimation of protein-protein binding affinity [46], and prediction of the targets of transcription factors [47].

G2P (Genomic to Phenotypic): Genome-Wide Association Studies (GWAS)

The main purpose of GWAS is to find the genetic variants associated with a specific disease or phenotype. According to the GWAS catalog in 2019 [48], there have been 5687 GWAS studies, which list 71,673 variant-phenotype associations computed using statistical methods. AI methods can improve GWAS results by enhancing the statistical power of associations, improving **polygenic risk scoring**, and ranking gene variants that are strongly associated to a genetic disease [49]. In most AI applications in GWAS, the key step is to build classification models using variant features to differentiate the phenotype, such as disease vs. normal.

From an AI perspective, the GWAS data has the following characteristics:

- Statistical feature selection is generally applied before using AI methods to analyze the data. However, the statistical methods select the features one by one; thus, they may not address important dependencies among the features.
- The data is often represented by a binary matrix, which represents whether or not a patient's genome has a specific variant.

In analyzing GWAS, linear models such as regularized regression and support vector machines (Chap. 6) are widely applied (see for example [50–53]). Here, model scores, such as the predicted probabilities, can serve as risk scoring, and model coefficients can be used to rank the features. Random forest [54] models can also support these two tasks (see for example [55, 56]). Meanwhile, some research [57, 58] shows that **artificial neural network** models may have the advantage in risk scoring/classification performance; however, the model architecture is less conducive to feature ranking than other more straightforward approaches such as regression models.

P2P (Phenotypic to Phenotypic): Identify Disease Genomic Subtypes

Subtyping of complex genomic disease, such as glioblastoma multiforme (GBM) [59], can answer key questions in both pre-clinical studies and clinical practice. These diseases are caused by multiple genetic anomalies and signaling pathway disruptions; therefore, a combination of therapeutic strategies is required to treat them. The purpose of subtyping in this context is to partition the disease into multiple subgroups, and find the explicitly disrupted signaling pathways in each of them. This may allow for customizing the treatment for each group according to the affected pathways. Solving this problem requires clustering and feature selection algorithms in AI. The clustering results reduce the subtyping problem into classification (which imputed subtype does this patient belong to?) and feature selection (which signaling pathways are affected in this imputed subtype?) problems for follow-up analyses. For example, in the TCGA-GBM dataset [59], the clustering was followed by GWAS analysis in each patient group. Here, GWAS mutations defined four GBM subtypes: classical, mesenchymal, proneural, and neural, and 29 subtype-related prognostic markers.

P2C (Phenotypic to Clinomic)

The protocol to diagnose a disease, which often consists of a pre-defined set of laboratory tests, is the most commonly used type of phenotype-clinotype association. Other phenotype-clinotype associations, once discovered by AI techniques, are considered novel. For example, in work on the identification of hypertension risk [45], the patients' future hypertension could be predicted by using non-blood-pressure affordable lab tests and AI.

C2C (Clinomic to Clinomic)

From a narrow perspective, clinotype-clinotype association refers to the correlation among laboratory test results. In the broader perspective, this type of association refers to how a specific clinotype result might change, or be predicted, given other clinotype results. For example, in work seeking to derive links between the primary translational informatics data categories [28], a linear model was constructed in which all other clinotypes become input features, to predict clinotype values. Here, the model coefficients were used to quantify clinotype-clinotype association.

Informatics Challenges in Translational Bioinformatics

Big Data Characteristics

An understanding of big data characteristics is required to apply AI in translational bioinformatics. This section reviews the characteristics of big data and how each characteristic can impact AI performance.

Volume of Data

Large data size constrains AI performance in translational bioinformatics in two ways. First, on account of associated logistic challenges, large data size may make solving some AI problems impractical without sufficient computer storage and specialized hardware. For example, Quang et al. [60] show an example of a motif discovery problem that may take a few weeks for a computer to complete without a big-data-specific GPU. Second, on account of the "curse of dimensionality" challenge, the very large number of features in big data can decrease the predictive performance, which is known as the Hughes phenomenon [61]. While dimension reduction may help relieve the curse of dimensionality, it also reduces the interpretability of the AI results (because the components of a reduced-dimensional representation may not map back to individual features). In other words, it leads to inferring less powerful hypotheses from the input feature to the predicted output variable.

Veracity of Data

Veracity refers to data quality, and conversely, noise. Noise detection and filtering is a challenge in analyzing data from many fields. However, in translational bioinformatics, differentiating between noise and meaningful but as-yet-unverified novel information makes this challenge more difficult. In biomedical research, the data often contain yet-to-be-discovered information. This information may only appear in a very small percentage of the data; therefore, statistically, it has similar characteristics to the noise. For example, single-cell expression data [62] usually show small cell clusters, which consist of less than 5% of the cell population. These clusters may correspond to "**doublets**"[63], a technical error (real noise), or stem/progenitor cells (which would constitute critical and novel information). Tackling this challenge requires reasonable noise assumptions and novel hypotheses to emerge from a strong collaboration between the AI analyst and the biomedical experts concerned.

Variability of Data

Data heterogeneity, or variability, has always been among the most difficult challenges in translational bioinformatics [64]. There are many aspects of data heterogeneity. First, the data are of many types, including omics data subtypes and biomedical data subtypes. In this aspect, the data integration strategy and integrative analysis are the keys to overcome the challenge. Second, the same data type may have significant variability due to the methods and platforms of collection, such as the batch effect [65] when single-cell sequencing the same tissue using **10X** and **ICell8** RNA-seq platforms [66]. In this aspect, computational mapping across the platforms is critical to the analysis. Third, results with the same data type and the same collection method can still be interpreted differently by different healthcare providers. For example, the Hematocrit percentage test normal range can be 35–40% or 40–50%, depending on specific patients and physicians who analyze the test result [28]. In this aspect, accurate and comprehensive biomedical domain knowledge is required.

Velocity of Data

Velocity refers to how quickly the data must be processed and analyzed, and how quickly results must be produced. In general translational bioinformatics research, velocity is not a major challenge. However, requirements to deliver results on time must be considered when building online tools and clinical decision support. The principle requirement to tackle this challenge is to understand the data management system and hardware infrastructure from which the AI tools are to be deployed (see the section on "Applications of AI in Translational Bioinformatics").

Social-Economic Bias

Unlike pre-clinical research, clinical translational bioinformatics research uses patients' clinical information. In this setting, incorporating socioeconomic factors into analyses may be unavoidable. However, predictive models based on such factors raise concerns about algorithmic fairness with the potential to exacerbate existing socioeconomic disparities (see Chap. 18). Thus, in the data processing pipeline, strongly associated features to the socioeconomic factors should be removed.

Domain Knowledge Representation and Interpretability

Using *domain knowledge collections to validate findings* can improve the interpretability of AI results, which is desirable before making clinical decisions on the basis of these findings. In bioinformatics, the common practice is to use feature extraction methods or infer model-explicit features (biomarkers) that differentiate the sample classes. These features are then forwarded to pathway, gene set, and gene ontology analysis to reveal which biological mechanisms are involved. The closeness between the highlighted mechanisms and the biomedical samples justifies the quality of the analysis. For example, when analyzing the fetal mouse heart proliferation data [67], the proliferative pathways and gene ontologies, such as cell cycle and cell differentiation, are expected to be enriched. If the proliferative pathways and ontologies are not enriched, while the 'hypertrophy' ones are, then the analytic quality could be questionable.

Model Robustness and Quality Control

Sample imbalance is usually the first issue impacting model quality in AI applications in translational bioinformatics. In the pre-clinical setting, the proportion of *negativ*e samples, such as healthy or disease-free samples, is often much smaller. In the clinical setting, we often see a very small proportion of *positive* samples. Here, we expect that the number of patients will be small compared to the population size. Extremely imbalanced data may seriously impair AI models, which are often optimized for accuracy. For example, when the positive sample proportion is only 5%, a naïve "all negative" prediction model yields an accuracy of 95% (very high). However, this model cannot predict positive samples; thus, it has no clinical value. To tackle imbalance, oversampling or undersampling can be applied to create a training dataset with a positive/negative sample ratio that is more balanced than it is in the whole dataset. In *oversampling*, a rare-class sample may randomly appear more than once in the training set, such as in the Synthetic Minority Over-sampling Technique (SMOTE) [68]. Here, the sample may be slightly permuted if it is selected more than once, using techniques of data augmentation [69, 70] analogous to those applied to images when training models for computer vision, such as rotations and reflections [71]. Alternatively, in *undersampling,* only a subset of popular-class samples are randomly selected for inclusion into the training set.

The optimization criteria in training AI models should be carefully decided case by case. This involves two choices. The first is the choice or definition of the loss function (see Chap. 6), with commonly applied examples including the mean-square error, L1 loss, hinge loss, or cross-entropy loss. The second is the choice of metric to focus on: maximizing accuracy, AUC, positive-predictive value, or negative-predictive value.

Statistical tests for model robustness. Many AI methods are model-based, and assume the data have certain characteristics and follow particular distributions. Therefore, these assumptions need to be verified before applying the AI methods. The Kolmogorov–Smirnov test (KS test) [72] addresses whether a set of numbers follows a pre-defined distribution, and to what degree two sets of numbers are drawn from the same distribution. Thus, in principle, the KS test and another similarly-purposed test should be applied to examine the data before deciding the AI method. On the other hand, the model result depends on its **hyperparameters** [73], which must be set before applying the AI algorithm. Choosing the hyperparameter is beyond the scope of the optimizations that can be achieved by the AI algorithm itself. Therefore, post-hoc analyses, such as the Wald test [74] and other model-fitness tests, should be used to test for fitness of the computed parameters (which are also commonly called the *model parameters*). To conduct these tests, the null model parameters need to be pre-defined; usually, a null model parameter is set as 0, which implies that the parameter plays no role in the model. If the test result is insignificant, which means the computed model parameters are very similar to the null parameters, then the model parameter may not be robust. This means that one should choose other algorithm hyperparameters to recompute the model.

Translational Bioinformatics Tools & Infrastructure

The big data characteristics described in the section on "Concepts of AI in Translational Bioinformatics" necessitate efficient, scalable tools and infrastructure components. In this section we will describe some of the key tools and components required to conduct translational bioinformatics analyses.

Extended Data Management Systems

While improving translational bioinformatics data storage may not be the primary research objective of AI in medicine, the developers of AI tools should consider the existing data facilities in order to improve their runtime performance in practice.

First, the **object-relational database** is still the primary translational bioinformatics data structure, with prominent examples including the Mayo Clinic database [75], STRING (a database of protein-protein interactions) [27], and the US National Inpatient Sample database [76]. The relational structure has the advantage of supporting the transformation of the data into any customized data structure used by AI applications. Meanwhile, to improve data retrieval performance, some translational bioinformatics data warehouses choose a non-relational structure for specific data types. Second, when the data has a hierarchy and/or primarily association among different entities, the non-relational database is adopted. For example, the Reactome biological pathway repository [24] is built upon the Neo4j [77] **graph database** engine, and Gene Ontology [22] organizes data based on the hierarchical Extensible Markup Language (XML) files [78]. Some other systems may adopt a hybrid structure when the data are extremely large and the data should be kept in multiple formats; for example, *cBioPortal* for cancer genomics [79] uses a relational table structure for patient clinical data and a file data system for patient omic data. Third, hybrid and distributed data warehouses implement both relational and non-relational infrastructure, such as in CloudBurst [80], BiobankCloud [81], and Hydra [82].

Data Preprocessing Pipelines

Pipelines to Build the Data Matrix

AI techniques view data in matrix format. However, before processing, biomedical data, such as high-throughput sequencing data, are not in this format. Therefore, data-type specific pipelines are required to convert the raw biomedical data to a matrix format. Table 14.1 summarizes the well-known pipelines in translational bioinformatics.

Table 14.1 Popular standard pipelines used in translational bioinformatics

Name	Data type	Input Data	Output Data	References
RAMPAGE (Encode project)	Bulk RNA sequencing	Fastq file: data and reference genome	– gene alignment – gene quantification (*matrix*)	[83]
miRNA-seq (Encode project)	microRNA sequencing	Fastq files	– miRNA quantification	[84]
CellRanger	Single-cell RNA sequencing	Fast1 files	– gene-cell expression *matrix* – simple analysis of single-cell data	[85]
Stanford CoreNLP	Medical text	Medical text collection	– medical term quantification (*matrix*)	[86]

Enhancing the Data Matrix

After formatting the data as a matrix, the matrix must be further processed to remove bias and noise. Choosing which method to use in this step is an ad-hoc decision and is made on a case-by-case basis. Well-known problems and techniques in data processing are:

- *Dimension reduction*: typically used methods include **principal component analysis** [87] and **canonical correlation analysis** [88].
- *Data scaling and normalization*. For example, gene expression data is assumed to follow the negative binomial distribution [89]. Gene expression analysis packages, such as DeSeq2 [90] and SAGE [91] implement negative binomial scaling before applying the main statistical analysis.
- *Batch effect correction* [92] is applied when the same type of dataset is generated at different rounds of experiments. Variance due to uncontrolled and random technical issues may appear in the data.
- *Embedded data visualization*, such as **TSNE** [93] and **UMAP** [94].

Supervised and Unsupervised Learning

Supervised machine learning (see Chap. 6), also called supervised analysis, involves finding a function that reproduces an output from an input. Here, "reproduce" implies that the correct output is already available without using the machine learning function. In biomedicine, supervised analysis often involves creating and fine-tuning computer algorithms and software that can substitute for a human performing a task. Examples of supervised analysis in biomedicine are:

- Automated detection of a tumor region and estimation of tumor size from a radiological image [95, 96] (see Chap. 12).
- Identifying cell type from single-cell gene expression data [97].
- Detecting patients' chronic disease diagnoses from their general health checkup records [28].

The main purpose of such supervised analysis is to automate and speed up manual tasks. Supervised learning can be implemented by digitizing rules and human knowledge, which is also called rule-based learning [98, 99], or through computation exclusively without such rules or knowledge. Support vector machines [100], linear regression [101], random forests [54], and deep learning methods [102] are well-known fully computational techniques that neither encode nor require human rules and knowledge. Although inferring novel knowledge may be achieved with supervised analysis (for example, by making predictions of drug effects beyond the scope of the training data), this is not usually the main goal when conducting supervised analysis in translational bioinformatics.

Unsupervised learning still finds a function from input to output, but the correct output has not been determined in advance. The main purpose of unsupervised learning in translational bioinformatics is to generate new biomedical knowledge that can be tested and verified in follow-up studies. Some examples of unsupervised learning are:

- Identifying new disease subtypes from *genomic data* [28], such as identifying genetic mutations that potentially indicate subtypes of glioblastoma [103].
- *Drug repurposing* [104], or finding ways of applying an old drug to treat a new disease. For example, the disease-drug and drug-drug associations could be represented by a graph [105]. Clustering this graph, which is an unsupervised learning problem, results in many clusters. Each cluster consists of multiple diseases and drugs to be further examined for repurposing.
- Identify and characterize *new cell subtypes* in single-cell omics data.

Some popular unsupervised machine learning problems are **clustering** [106], **expectation-maximization methods** [107], and **non-negative matrix factorization** [108].

Popular Algorithms in Translational Bioinformatics

Extending the discussion of algorithms and tools in Chap. 6, this section provides additional details for popular AI algorithms in translational bioinformatics.

Classification Algorithms

Random forest [54] is a well-known example of an ensemble classification algorithm. A random forest consists of many **decision trees** (Fig. 14.1). Each tree is a discrete classification model, which consists of multiple classification rules. Each tree is constructed by applying the decision tree algorithm [109] to a random subset, including randomly selected samples and features, of the training data. Then, to classify a sample, random forest combines all trees' classification results, using majority rule voting or some other aggregation procedure.

Figure 14.2 illustrates a random forest. Here, the classification has 4 features. Three decision trees are randomly constructed: tree 1 only uses x_1 and x_2, tree 2 only uses x_3 and x_4, tree 3 uses x_1, x_2, and x_4. Each tree is a classification model, which consists of multiple if-then rules. For example, tree 1 has three rules: $x_1 \leq 5 \rightarrow$ Class: No, $x_1 > 5$ & $x_2 \leq 50 \rightarrow$ Class: No, $x_1 > 5$ & $x_2 > 50 \rightarrow$ Class: Yes. When classifying the sample (2, 68, 342, 6899), each tree finds the decision branch according to the sample feature (grey-shaded hexagon). Then, all trees' results (2 No, 1 Yes) are combined using a majority rule vote to make the final decision (Class: No).

To measure how important a feature x is in each tree, the algorithm compares the classification accuracies where x is included and removed from the tree [110]. The more accuracy decreases when removing x, the more important x is in the tree. The

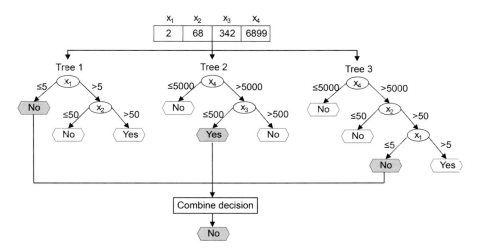

Fig. 14.2 Illustration of a random forest

random forest combines x's feature importance scores for all tree into x feature importance score in the forest. The random forest feature importance can be used as a metric for feature ranking.

Naïve Bayesian classifier. Given a datapoint $\mathbf{x} = (x_1 = a_1, x_2 = a_2, ..., x_n = a_n)$ in n dimensions; here, we denote $x_1, x_2, ..., x_n$ as the attributes, and $a_1, a_2, ..., a_n$ as the values. The objective is to predict which class C_i $\mathbf{x}$ belongs to among k classes. According to Bayes' rule, the *posterior probability* that $\mathbf{x}$ belongs to class C_i is:

$$p\left(C_i|\mathbf{x}\right) = \frac{p\left(\mathbf{x} = \left(a_1, a_2, ..., a_n\right)|C_i\right) \times p\left(C_i\right)}{p\left(\mathbf{x} = \left(a_1, a_2, ..., a_n\right)\right)}. \tag{14.1}$$

In Eq. (14.1), the denominator is negligible because it is the same for all k classes. Thus, the classification is decided by which class has the largest $p(\mathbf{x} = (a_1, a_2, ..., a_n)| C_i) \times p(C_i)$. Here, the *prior* $p(C_i)$ is the frequency of class i appearing in the population. The likelihood $p(\mathbf{x} = (a_1, a_2, ..., a_n)| C_i)$ is the probability of observing a sample $\mathbf{x} = (a_1, a_2, ..., a_n)$ in class C_i. In the naïve scenario, we assume that all attributes $x_1, x_2, ..., x_n$ are independent from the other. Therefore:

$$p\left(\mathbf{x} = \left(a_1, a_2, ..., a_n\right)|C_i\right) = p\left(x_1 = a_1|C_i\right) \times p\left(x_2 = a_2|C_i\right) \times ... p\left(x_n = a_n|C_i\right). \tag{14.2}$$

In discrete data, all elements in Eqs. (14.1) and (14.2) are computed by counting. In continuous data, the probabilities $p(x_j = a_j| C_i)$ are the probabilistic mass function of class C_i. This requires advanced probabilistic modeling. Also, when the attributes are not completely independent, the naïve Bayesian algorithm is extended to the **Bayesian Network**. The audience can freely practice these advanced cases using open source and freely available machine learning libraries such as Weka [111].

Clustering Algorithms

Expectation-maximization clustering [112], briefly, is a repeated process to identify the distribution parameters of the data. In each iteration, the datapoints are allocated to a distribution component; then, all component parameters are re-calculated according to the datapoint allocation. The process repeats until the component parameters converge.

K-mean clustering [113] is a popular clustering algorithm. In this problem, the goal is to partition the datapoints into k clusters. The defining parameter for each cluster is its centroid, which is the average of all datapoints assigned to it. A specific datapoint is allocated to the cluster with the closest cluster centroid. Clusters are initially assigned randomly, and the process of centroid estimation and cluster assignment is repeated iteratively until the centroids converge. Figure 14.3 illustrates k-means clustering using a toy example (n = 10 datapoints, $k = 3$).

Consensus clustering. In the GBM case study (introduced in the section on "Phenotypic Data"14.1.3.3) [59], *consensus clustering* was applied to divide the TCGA-GBM patients into $k = 4$ groups (subtypes). *Consensus clustering* is an iterative clustering procedure. The process starts by choosing the number of expected clusters (k) in the dataset. The core clustering algorithm, which was **hierarchical clustering** in TCGA-GBM [59], executes multiple runs with the same k parameter in the dataset. Then the results of these runs are aggregated and evaluated for clustering quality. The core clustering algorithm repeats the same process with other choices of k; here, larger k often yields higher clustering quality. After experimenting with many choices of k, the final k is chosen by balancing the preference for a smaller k against the desire for better clustering quality. Silhouette index [114] is a well-known metric for clustering quality.

Matrix factorization. In machine learning, briefly, matrix factorization is the decomposition of a data matrix $\mathbf{M}$ (m datapoints $\times n$ attributes) into the product $\mathbf{PQ} \approx \mathbf{M}$. Here, $\mathbf{P}$ is a $m \times k$ matrix, Q is a $k \times n$ matrix, and k is a pre-defined number determining the dimensions of the latent feature space. Each row in $\mathbf{P}$ represents a data point in the latent space, and each column in $\mathbf{Q}$ represents an attribute in the latent space (although such latent attributes may be derived from multiple input features in $\mathbf{M}$, and thus relatively difficult to interpret, as discussed in the section on "Volume of Data"). In matrix-factorization clustering, the latent space is defined by the number of clusters. Then, each row in $\mathbf{P}$ represents which clusters the corresponding datapoints may belong to; and each column in $\mathbf{Q}$ represents in which clusters the corresponding attribute is enriched.

Mathematically, matrix factorization is an optimization problem (for an introduction to solving optimization problems using gradient descent, see Chap. 6): find $\mathbf{P}$ and $\mathbf{Q}$ to minimize

$$F = \mathbf{M} - \mathbf{PQ}^2 + \alpha \mathbf{P}^2 + \beta \mathbf{Q}^2. \tag{14.3}$$

Iteration 1
Initialize (random) centroids
C1 = 4, C2 = 7, C3 = 9

Input

	Value	Cluster
x_1	1.8	
x_2	5.3	
x_3	2.1	
x_4	8.6	
x_5	9.3	
x_6	2.4	
x_7	2.2	
x_8	4.9	
x_9	4.7	
x_{10}	8.9	

Assign points to cluster

	Value	C1	C2	C3	Cluster
x_1	1.8	2.2	5.2	7.2	1
x_2	5.3	1.3	1.7	3.7	1
x_3	2.1	1.9	4.9	6.9	1
x_4	8.6	4.6	1.6	0.4	3
x_5	9.3	5.3	2.3	0.3	3
x_6	2.4	1.6	4.6	6.6	1
x_7	2.2	1.8	4.8	6.8	1
x_8	4.9	0.9	2.1	4.1	1
x_9	4.7	0.7	2.3	4.3	1
x_{10}	8.9	4.9	1.9	0.1	3

Update centroids
C1 = average (x_1,x_2,x_3,x_6,x_7, x_8,x_9) = 3.34
C2=7
C3= average(x_4,x_5,x_{10}) = 8.93

Iteration 2
Previous centroids
C1 = 3.34, C2 = 7, C3 = 8.93

Assign points to cluster

	Value	C1	C2	C3	Cluster
x_1	1.8	1.54	5.2	7.13	1
x_2	5.3	1.96	1.7	3.63	2
x_3	2.1	1.24	4.9	6.83	1
x_4	8.6	5.26	1.6	0.33	3
x_5	9.3	5.96	2.3	0.37	3
x_6	2.4	0.94	4.6	6.53	1
x_7	2.2	1.14	4.8	6.73	1
x_8	4.9	1.56	2.1	4.03	1
x_9	4.7	1.36	2.3	4.23	1
x_{10}	8.9	6.87	1.9	0.03	3

Update centroids
C1= average(x_1,x_3,x_6,x_7,x_8, x_9)= 3.01
C2= average(x_2) = 5.3
C3= average(x_4,x_5,x_{10}) = 8.93

Iteration 3
Previous centroids
C1 = 3.01, C2 = 5.3, C3 = 8.93

Assign points to cluster

	Value	C1	C2	C3	Cluster
x_1	1.8	1.21	3.5	7.13	1
x_2	5.3	2.29	0.0	3.63	2
x_3	2.1	0.91	3.2	6.83	1
x_4	8.6	5.59	3.3	0.33	3
x_5	9.3	6.29	4.0	0.37	3
x_6	2.4	0.61	2.9	6.53	1
x_7	2.2	0.81	3.1	6.73	1
x_8	4.9	1.89	0.4	4.03	2
x_9	4.7	1.69	0.6	4.23	2
x_{10}	8.9	5.89	3.6	0.03	3

Update centroids
C1= average(x_1,x_3,x_6,x_7)
   = 2.13
C2= average(x_2,x_8,x_9) = 4.97
C3= average(x_4,x_5,x_{10}) = 8.93

Iteration 4
Previous centroids
C1 = 2.13, C2 = 4.97, C3 = 8.93

Assign points to cluster

	Value	C1	C2	C3	Cluster
x_1	1.8	0.33	3.17	7.13	1
x_2	5.3	3.17	0.33	3.63	2
x_3	2.1	0.03	2.87	6.83	1
x_4	8.6	6.47	3.63	0.33	3
x_5	9.3	7.17	4.33	0.37	3
x_6	2.4	0.27	2.57	6.53	1
x_7	2.2	0.07	2.77	6.73	1
x_8	4.9	2.77	0.07	4.03	2
x_9	4.7	2.57	0.27	4.23	1
x_{10}	3.9	6.77	3.93	0.03	3

Update centroids
C1= average(x_1,x_3,x_6,x_7)
   = 2.13
C2= average(x_2,x_8,x_9) = 4.97
C3= average(x_4,x_5,x_{10}) = 8.93

Thecentroidsconverge.
Algorithm terminates.

Fig. 14.3 An illustrative example of the k-means clustering algorithm

In this formula, α and $\beta > 0$ are pre-selected regularization parameters. The popular approaches to solve (1) are based on gradient descent theory [115]. Computing the partial derivative of F over $\mathbf{P}$ and $\mathbf{Q}$, we have

$$\frac{\partial F}{\partial \mathbf{P}} = \frac{\partial \left(\mathbf{M} - \mathbf{PQ}^2 \right)}{\partial \mathbf{P}} + 2\alpha \mathbf{P}. \tag{14.4}$$

The first term in Eq. (14.4) can be computed by analyzing each entry (i, j) in $\mathbf{M}$. We have, by matrix multiplication:

$$m_{i,j} \approx \sum_{l=1}^{k} p_{i,l} q_{l,j}. \tag{14.5}$$

In Eq. (14.5), $m_{i,j}$ is the entry at i^{th} row and j^{th} column in $\mathbf{M}$, $p_{i,l}$ is the entry at i^{th} row and l^{th} column in $\mathbf{P}$, and $q_{l,j}$ is the entry at l^{th} row and j^{th} column in $\mathbf{Q}$. To minimize $\mathbf{M} - \mathbf{PQ}^2 = \sum\sum\left(m_{i,j} - \sum_{l=1}^{k} p_{i,l} q_{l,j} \right)^2$, we have partial derivative:

$$\frac{\partial\left(m_{i,j} - \sum_{l=1}^{k} p_{i,l} q_{l,j} \right)^2}{\partial p_{i,l}} = -2q_{l,j}\left(m_{i,j} - \sum_{l=1}^{k} p_{i,l} q_{l,j} \right). \tag{14.6}$$

This allows update each entry $p_{i,l}$ with a very small learning rate σ :

$$
\begin{aligned}
p_{i,l} &= p_{i,l} + \sigma\left(\sum_{j=1}^{n} \frac{\partial\left(m_{i,j} - \sum_{l=1}^{k} p_{i,l} q_{l,j} \right)^2}{\partial p_{i,l}} + 2\alpha p_{i,l} \right) \\
&= p_{i,l} + \sigma\left(\sum_{j=1}^{n}\left(-2q_{l,j}\left(m_{i,j} - \sum_{l=1}^{k} p_{i,l} q_{l,j} \right) \right) + 2\alpha p_{i,l} \right).
\end{aligned} \tag{14.7}
$$

The theory to update $q_{l,j}$ is similar and is left as an exercise. Formulae (14.6) and (14.7) are used in many iterations until $\mathbf{P}$ and $\mathbf{Q}$ converge.

Dimension Reduction Algorithms

Embedding, briefly, is a *non-affine* method to reduce the data dimensionality. By non-affine, we mean that a high-dimensional datapoint $\mathbf{x}$ is mapped to a lower, usually in 2D, dimensional datapoint $\mathbf{y}$ such that the inverse mapping from $\mathbf{y} \to \mathbf{x}$ does not have a precise formula. Embedding optimizes and preserves the original relative similarity between any datapoint $(\mathbf{x}_i, \mathbf{x}_j)$ pair in the embedded space $(\mathbf{y}_i, \mathbf{y}_j)$. In t-distributed Stochastic Neighbor Embedding (tSNE) [93], the pairwise similarity $(\mathbf{x}_i, \mathbf{x}_j)$ in the high-dimensional data space is defined as

$$p_{j|i} = \frac{\exp\left(-\mathbf{x}_i - \mathbf{x}_j^2 / 2\sigma_i^2\right)}{\sum_{\forall k \neq i} \exp\left(-\mathbf{x}_i - \mathbf{x}_k^2 / 2\sigma_i^2\right)}. \tag{14.8}$$

And the pairwise similarity space $(\mathbf{y}_i, \mathbf{y}_j)$ in the embedded data space is defined as

$$q_{j i} = \frac{\left(1+\|\mathbf{y}_i - \mathbf{y}_j\|^2\right)^{-1}}{\sum_k \sum_{l \neq k}\left(1+\|\mathbf{y}_k - \mathbf{y}_l\|^2\right)^{-1}}. \qquad (14.9)$$

Upon defining these similarities, tSNE minimize the Kullback–Leibler divergence

$$KL(P \ Q) = \sum_{i \neq j} p_{j i} \times \log\left(\frac{p_{j i}}{q_{j i}}\right). \qquad (14.10)$$

Then, tSNE finds the embedded datapoints y using the gradient descent approach, and computing the partial derivative $\partial KL / \partial \mathbf{y}_i$.

Association Mining Algorithms

In translational bioinformatics, mining associations among features depends on defining an association metric. Some popular choices are:

- Pearson's correlation. Briefly, Pearson's correlation is the ratio between the covariance of two features and the product of their standard deviations. This metric requires the features to be in numeric format, and only measures how the two features linearly correlate. If the two features have a non-linear association, Pearson's correlation may not detect the association.
- Mutual information metrics [116]. Mutual information measures the dependency between two features. For example, consider two Boolean features A and B. In a dataset, A and B are independent if the frequency of 'A is true' is approximately the same as the frequency of 'A is true given B is true'.
- The Jaccard index [117]. Given two Boolean features A and B. In a dataset, the Jaccard index is the ratio between the number of samples such that 'both A and B are true' (also called the intersection) and the number of samples such that 'A or B is true' (also called the union).

Security, Privacy, and Ethical Considerations (see also Chap. 18)

In practice, the AI scientist must consider the following ethical points, according to Safdar et al. [118]:

- *Population bias.* This happens when the sociodemographic group proportion in a research and training dataset does not reflect the study population. Rare demographics and ethnicities are often under-sampled.

- *Data ownership.* Translational bioinformatics data is often derived from human subjects. Therefore, consent from study participants, which allows using their data for research and tool development, must be obtained.
- *Privacy protection.* Human subject identifiable information must be removed before analyzing and publicly releasing the data for research.

Team Data Science Infrastructure

AI researchers in translational bioinformatics use publicly available big data and analytics infrastructures to accelerate their research. These infrastructures not only support scaling to large data sets, but also installation of popular analytic tools. Some examples are as follows:

- UAB UBRITE (https://ubrite.org/) integrates many machine learning programming libraries, which can be activated in R/Python scripts.
- Google Colab (https://colab.research.google.com/notebooks/) has a free collection of pre-built machine learning Jupyter notebooks [119] available for reuse. Community users may slightly modify these notebooks for specific projects, and freely run a notebook for up to 12 hours using Google Cloud computing resources.

Applications of AI in Translational Bioinformatics

Improving Translational Bioinformatics Data Infrastructure

Experimental validation and manual curation, which are the most reliable approaches to construct translational bioinformatics databases, are time-consuming and resource-costly. Therefore, AI methods are utilized to infer novel information and enrich these databases. For example, in the STRING database [27], text mining is the most significant channel contributing to broad coverage. Here, the number of protein-protein interactions (PPI) for human proteins in STRING is approximately 2.9 million [13] (though some of these may be inaccurate on account of natural language processing errors); meanwhile, BioGRID [120], which is among the largest experimentally-validated and manually-curated PPI collections, only has approximately 268,599 PPIs. As another example, JASPAR [121] uses a hidden Markov model [122, 123] to predict 337 (over 1964) transcription factor – target interactions.

Inferring Pairwise Molecular Regulation

Many biological research areas require understanding and predicting regulatory net-works to provide clear insight into living cells' cellular processes [124]. For exam-ple, in injury response, regulation from G Protein-coupled receptors and their interactees is crucial to DNA damage response [125]. In another example, the tran-scription factor c-JUN promotes and maintains the expression level of CCND1, which is required in cell cycle progression [126]. Thus, discovering the gene regula-tory network can enrich the translational bioinformatics database (see section on "Improving translational bioinformatics data infrastructure"), and inform the design of targeted therapies [127]. On the other hand, the number of possible regu-latory pairs is too large to be fully validated by biological experiments, and many have not yet been discovered. This explains why predictive methods to infer molec-ular regulation, especially transcription factor—target and ligand—receptor pairs, are still an active research area.

Transcription factors are a set of DNA-binding proteins, and the genes at the DNA location where the transcription factors bind to are their targets [128]. The expression of the genes encoded around the binding sites is significantly up or down-regulated by the transcription factor. Therefore, the focus of AI in predicting transcription factor—target relationships is to identify the binding sites, which may number in the tens of thousands [128], of a transcription factor. Furthermore, the prediction must be filtered due to two types of occurrences: one binding event may control multiple target genes, and one gene may be targeted by multiple bindings AI tools use **Chromatin immunoprecipitation** followed by sequencing (ChiP-seq) data and the expression data as inputs for prediction. IM-PET [129], RIPPLE [130] and PETModule [131] predict transcription-factor targets using the random forest algorithm. Here, the Chip-seq data is processed to obtain the distance between the binding/enhancer sites and the targets' DNA coding regions. Besides, deep learning based tools, such as DeepTFactor [132], TBiNet [133], and scFAN [134] focus on precisely predicting transcription factor binding sites. Their output can be provided to other AI methods to infer the targets.

A *ligand* is a substance that forms a complex with a cell surface protein (called a receptor) and then triggers a series of cellular signaling events [135]. These signal-ing events respond to the stimulus that produces the ligand. For example, in natural skin wounds, the fibroblast releases the WNT5A ligand; this ligand binds to FZD1/2 receptors on the skin cell and activates the WNT signaling pathway [136] and the pathway promotes skin cell proliferation and helps heal the wound [137]. In drug discovery, after selecting which signaling pathways and related receptors to acti-vate, the next task is designing an artificial ligand that can bind to the receptor. Computing the ligand-receptor affinity is an important task before testing the artifi-cial ligand. Recently, machine-learning-based models have been shown to outper-form other methods that do not apply machine learning on this task [138, 139].

Table 14.2 summarizes the popularly used AI tools described in this section

Table 14.2 Summary of AI tools used in inferring pairwise molecular regulation

Tool name & reference	Major AI algorithm	Clustering	Classification	Simulation	Data type (C, P, G)
IM-PET [129]	Random Forest		x		G
RIPPLE [130]	Random Forest		x		G
PETModule [131]	Random Forest		x		G
DeepTFactor [132]	Deep learning		x	x	G
TBiNet [133]	Deep learning		x		G
Pafnucy [138, 139]	Deep learning		x		G

Inferring and Characterizing Cellular Signaling Mechanism that Determines the Cellular Response

Identifying and characterizing signaling mechanisms is essential in complex phenotype research because the disease outcomes concerned involve many genes interacting and responding to each other in response to an external stimulus [140]. In each phenotype, the highly expressed genes and interactions are found in the in-vitro experiments and annotated as a "pathway". According to KEGG [23], at the time of this writing, 543 pathways have been well defined and annotated across all species included in the database. Adding species-specific pathways, Reactome [24] reports that the number may rise to 999. Extending from pathways, Gene Ontology [22] groups and characterizes 44,945 ontology terms, where each ontology term concerns a set of genes that participate in a biological process, are located in the same cellular location, and/or share the same molecular profile. Among this large number of pathways and ontologies, the most frequently investigated ones often regulate cell proliferation, cell apoptosis, and cell differentiation. Understanding the mechanisms regulating these processes helps to explain the progression and infer potential treatments for diseases with some of the highest mortality rates: cardiovascular diseases and cancers.

AI can support this research area by answering three basic questions. The first question concerns how to identify which pathways are involved in disease progression. Here, feature selection methods [141, 142] can identify highly differentiated genes between healthy controls and subjects with a disease of interest (identified genes can be considered as **biomarkers**). Then, applying pathway analysis techniques [143] to the biomarkers can yield a list of pathways involved in the disease. The second question concerns how to identify the "master regulator", or the "origin" of the perturbed signaling mechanisms. Here, in highly interconnected genes, many perturbed gene signals are just the responses to other genes. The third question concerns how to find a therapeutic target: interfering with genes such that the genes are targetable and yield the highest reduction in disease progression. These three questions can be answered using AI-based system simulations.

Before deep learning, the state-of-the-art approaches in this area focused on representing the interactive network among the pathway genes with a mathematical equation system, and then solving the system by either **logic programming** or

dynamic differential equations [144, 145]. In logic programming, the interaction between two (or more) genes is represented by a combination of logic gates. Since the logic gate is finite and deterministic, the simulation is straightforward. A limitation of the logic gate is that it cannot represent feedback loops or two-way gene-gene interactions. The feedback loops are critical to maintaining a stable environment inside a living subject. For example, in wound healing, after the initial platelets respond to the wound, these platelets release adenosine diphosphate (ADP); this ADP binds to P2Y1 and P2Y12 genes to activate more platelets; more platelets produces more ADP to continue this activation loop until the wound surface is completely covered and prevents further blood loss [146]. Dynamic differential equations can overcome this limitation. In principle, the dynamic differential equations discretize the system into multiple time points, define the dynamic equation for each gene expression at each timepoint, and calculate gene expression over a sequence of time points.

Below are some simple examples of how to simulate a 2-gene and a 3-gene system using dynamic equations. The system has two proteins (*objects*), denoted PA and PB. These proteins have the *initial values* $S_0 = (-1, 0)$ for PA (strongly inhibited) and PB (normal), correspondingly. PA up-regulates PB while PB down-regulates PA in a negative-feedback loop [147], as in Fig. 14.4. These interactions can be represented by *system matrix* $\mathbf{M} = \begin{bmatrix} 0 & 1 \\ -1 & 0 \end{bmatrix}$. Suppose the discrete *dynamic*

equation, which takes both the *initial values* and the *system matrix*, is as follows (this equation is related to the equation underlying the PageRank algorithm [148]):

Fig. 14.4 The system (top) and simulation result when M = [0 1;-1 0]

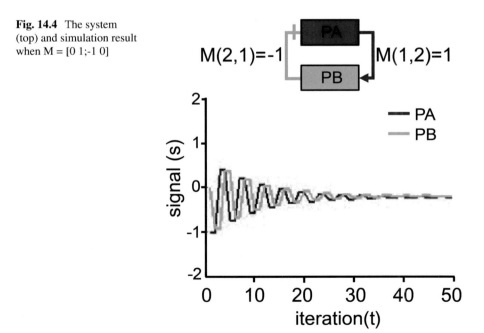

$$S_t = 0.15 \times S_0 + 0.85 \times \mathbf{M}^T S_{t-1}$$

The following Matlab code shows how to implement this system:

```
S0 = [-1; 0]; % initial S0
S = zeros(2, 200); % store all S
from t = 0 to t = 200
M = [0 1; -1 0];
S(:, 1) = S0;
for i = 2 : 200 % for iterations
from t = 0 to 200
    % iteratively apply the dynamic
equation
    S(:, i) = 0.25*S0 + 0.85*M'*S(:,
i-1);
end
```

The result in Fig. 14.5 shows that over tim e, PA and PB converge to (−0.15, −0.13), respectively. This system is closely balanced ($S_\alpha \approx 0$), suggesting that the initial inhibition of A can balance the system. Figure 14.4 shows that the system results are completely different if we make a slight change to the model parameters by setting $\mathbf{M} = \begin{bmatrix} 0 & -1 \\ 1 & 0 \end{bmatrix}$, such that PA downregulates PB, while PB upregulates PA.

Fig. 14.5 The system (top) and simulation result when M = [0 1;-1 0]

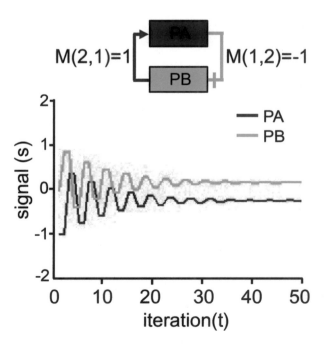

Table 14.3 Summary of AI tools for inferring and characterizing cellular signaling mechanisms

Tool name & reference	Major AI algorithm	Clustering	Classification	Simulation	Data type (C, P, G)
COPASI [144]	Logic gate			x	G
DCell [149]	Deep learning		x	x	G
MWSLE [150]	Differential equation			x	G

With deep learning approaches, signaling interactions can be used to construct and train a deep learning architecture. For example, Ma et al. describe a deep learning approach to simulate cell proliferation, in which the learning architecture is organized according to the proliferation-related gene ontology hierarchy instead of a conventional convolutional structure [149].

The AI tools described in this section are summarized in Table 14.3.

Identifying and Characterizing New Cell Types and Subtypes

Single-cell transcriptomics technologies enable measuring genetic information at the individual cell resolution [151], which is the "building-block" level of all living organisms. Single-cell transcriptomic data also present new questions, and require new analytic techniques that are not available in bulk transcriptomics. First, does the data present novel cell populations that have not been studied due to the limitations of bulk technologies, especially of the stem and progenitor cell types? Second, for signaling pathways that function differently in different cells of the same cell type and in the same tissue, how might we quantify the signaling activity within each cell? AI techniques are essential to answer these questions.

To answer the first question, state-of-the-art single-cell analytic tools [152, 153] apply clustering algorithms to partition the entire cell dataset. In each cell cluster, genes explicitly expressed in the cluster are queried in the cell-type canonical marker literature, such as the CellMarker database [154], to determine which cell type the cluster corresponds to. For the clustering step, density-based clustering [155] and Louvian clustering [156] are the most popular methods. Also, embedding methods, such as tSNE [93] and UMAP [157], are often used to visualize the cell clusters. In many single-cell datasets [158–160], small clusters that highly express canonical markers from more than one cell type appear. These small clusters need careful examination because they could either be technical errors, such as doublets [161], or may indeed represent a new cell population.

To answer the second question, the major challenge is the potential for missing values in single-cell data, which is called the *dropout effect* [162]. The best contemporary single-cell transcriptomic techniques may achieve 6500 genes per cell [163], which only covers 25–30% of the human genome. Consequently, single-cell gene expression data often have a high proportion of zero values. Here, a zero can either mean the gene does not express in the cell, or that the gene does express, but the sequencing step did not capture this expression. To tackle the dropout effect, single-cell pathway analysis may employ machine learning to quantify pathway activity. This requires choosing "positive" cells, in which the pathway is known to function, and "negative" cells in which it is known not to function or to express at a very low level. For example, fetal and adult cardiomyocytes are excellent "positive" and "negative" cells for cell cycle signaling pathways. The pathway genes can be used as features to build a classifier distinguishing between the "positive" and the "negative" cells. Here, the "positive" cells should have a high model score and vice versa. Then, the model can be applied to analyze the pathway activity in other cells.

The AI tools in this section are summarized in Table 14.4.

Drug Repurposing

Drug repurposing, briefly, is applying an approved or investigational drug to treat a new disease [104]. In principle, drug repurposing can be conducted by calculating similarity. If two drugs A and B are highly similar, and A is approved to treat disease C, then B may also be used to treat C. Similarly, if two proteins D and E are highly similar, and A targets D, then A may also target E. Thus, drug repurposing includes many sub-problems for which machine learning techniques can be promising solutions.

Generating and mining a drug-drug similarity network. In this problem, each drug is represented by a vector. The drug vector represents structural chemical information, known drug-protein interactions, and information about the drug's side effect [164]. The drug-drug pairwise similarity matrix, or network, is computed from a matrix containing vectors for all the drugs under consideration. Then,

Table 14.4 Summary of AI tools used for identifying and characterizing new cell types and subtypes. C, P and G indicate Clinotypic, Phenotypic and Genotypic data respectively

Tool name & reference	Major AI algorithm	Clustering	Classification	Simulation	Data type (C, P, G)
Seurat [152]	Canonical analysis, regression, Louvian clustering	x	x		G
density-based clustering [155]		x			G, also in P and C
Louvian clustering [156]		x			G, also in P and C
DoubletFinder [161]	Louvian, Support vector machine	x	x	x	G

applying matrix factorization [165–167] results in drug clusters. Here, drugs sharing the same cluster are more likely to be repurposed for each other's diseases.

Mining target-target a similarity network. Similarly to mining the drug-drug similarity network, machine learning techniques can be applied to cluster the target-target network [168, 169]. Then, a drug targeting one gene may be repurposed to target the other genes in the same cluster.

Mining a bi-partite drug-target network. Here, the drug-drug similarity, target-target interaction, and drug-target networks are co-factorized [170, 171].

Model-based simulation. This approach utilizes dynamic modeling, as discussed in sect. 14.4.3. The approach requires the following definition. First, the initial disease condition is represented by a non-zero vector of gene expression values (S_0). The computational goal is to get $S_\infty = 0$, which represents the non-disease state. Second, the treatment is also characterized by a vector **u**. Usually, **u** has the same dimension as S; and the dimensions in **u** and S correspond to each other. Third, the gene-gene interaction and signaling mechanisms dynamically change the expression vector, yielding the equation $S_t = F(S_{t-1})$ or $S_t = F(S_{t-1}, \mathbf{u})$. Then, there are two options to score the repurposing candidate. First, all drug treatments can be computed and ranked in the recursive system $S_t = F(S_{t-1}) \mid S_t = F(S_{t-1}, \mathbf{u})$. Second, applying the system control approach [172] yields a "hypothetical treatment", which optimally returns $S_\infty = 0$. The hypothetical treatment can be used as a template to match with real drug treatments to select the repurposing candidates.

The AI tools discussed in this section are presented in Table 14.5.

Supporting Clinical Decisions with Bioinformatics Analysis

In genetic diseases caused by a single genetic disorder [174], mutation-analysis protocols can be used for diagnosis directly. Meanwhile, in complex diseases, bioinformatics analysis is used case by case. For example, in work by Kim et al. [36], the single-cell transcriptomic analysis, which used AI methods for clustering, detected that a JAK-STAT signaling pathway disruption was the cause of severe hypersensitivity syndrome/drug reaction in a patient. Therefore, tofacitinib, a JAK-STAT inhibitor, was selected and successfully treated the patient, although the drug is not indicated to treat hypersensitivity syndrome or drug reactions in general.

Table 14.5 Summary of AI tools in drug repurposing

Tool name & reference	Major AI algorithm	Clustering	Classification	Simulation	Data type (C, P, G)
MRMF [165]	Matrix factorization	x			G, P
PREDICT [173]	Logistic regression		x		G, P
DeCost [172]	System control			x	G, P

In cancer, the **patient-derived xenograft** (PDX) [175] platform is another direction for bioinformatics protocols to support clinical decision-making. Briefly, PDX is a technique to host a patient tumor biosample in a mouse. Cancer researchers can perform many mouse interventions and observe the mouse clinical outcomes, such as survival and speed of tumor growth. Given a sufficiently large amount of PDX samples with experimental results, called a *PDX catalog*, a new patient tumor biosample can be mapped to the PDX catalog. Here, the most closely mapped PDX samples' experimental outcomes can be used to infer the patient's likely clinical outcome under different treatment decisions, and fulfill the role of clinical decision support. Due to the heterogeneity of biomedical samples, designing the mapping algorithm for this application is a significant challenge that may require advanced AI techniques [176].

Predicting side effects is another clinical application where AI-based translational bioinformatics methods are potentially helpful. In pre-clinical applications, similarly to drug repurposing, predicting side-effects relies on mining drug-drug similarity [177, 178]. In the clinical setting, the principle involves mining past side effects recorded in a patients' medical records. Thus, the side-effect analysis is provider-specific and customized according to the medical record data infrastructure, such as in the work of Sohn et al. [179]. Here, itemset (drug – side effect) mining and rule-mining are standard AI methods used to predict the drugs' side effects.

Predicting Complex Biochemical Structures

After finding the target gene and other genetic causes for a disease, the next cornerstones in drug discovery are (i) to represent the physical structures of the target protein (the protein encoded by the target gene); (ii) to represent the physical structures of the chemical.

Representing **protein physical structure** involves reconstructing the 3D arrangement of atoms, or each amino acid, given the sequential order of the amino acids on the protein polypeptide chain [180]. The sequential order of the amino acids, also called the protein primary structure [177], identifies the protein, is always the first step in studying a protein, and can easily be found using today's protein sequencing techniques [181]. Meanwhile, the protein functionalities and its interaction with other proteins and chemicals are primarily determined by its higher-level 3D structures. How to infer the protein 3D structure from the primary structure has been a grand challenge for decades [182]. Before deep learning, machine learning techniques were used to solve some protein structure subproblems, such as predicting pairwise distances among the amino acids in 3D [179] and predicting the 3D structure class [183]. The recent deep-learning-based methods can predict the 3D position of the protein atoms, which is a more challenging problem. For example, most recently, AlphaFold directly predicts the 3D coordinates of all heavy atoms for a given protein using the primary amino acid sequence [184]. AlphaFold shows significantly superior performance over other methods in the Critical Assessment of

Techniques for Protein Structure Prediction 14th Challenge [185], which indicates a major breakthrough of AI in solving one of the cornerstones of chemical biology.

Representing **chemical structure**, also called ligand structure or drug structure, is somewhat a reverse-engineering problem compared to representing protein physical structure. In this problem, given a 3D physical structure, the objective is to find the arrangement, or order, of atoms that can create the 3D structure [186]. Here, the chemical 3D structure is defined such that the chemical structure can bind to the targeted protein 3D structure [187]. This problem is manually solved by chemical engineering experts, which often take years to complete [188]. Recently, it has been shown that deep learning can significantly accelerate this process. For example, GENTRL [189] designed new chemicals binding to DDR1 within just 23 days. Here, GENTRL applied deep-learning **autoencoder** [190], which is a technique to synthesize new datapoints from the existing (original) datapoints such that the AI classifier could not easily differentiate the synthetic ones from the original ones. The GENTRL deep autoencoder was trained on more than 200 million 3D chemical structures in the ZINC v.15 database [191]. Then, to find new chemicals binding to DDR1, GENTRL took the existing DDR1 inhibitors, which could be found in the ChEMBL database [192], as the input, then synthesized 'similar' compounds using the autoencoder.

Trends and Outlook

In pre-clinical research, future translational bioinformatics research will likely pivot around the current and forthcoming breakthroughs in biotechnology. By the time this chapter is published, single-cell -omics, which measure the molecular environment inside cells, and the patient-derived xenograft, which allows hosting a patient's biosample in living organisms, will be the major platforms for new AI translational bioinformatics techniques. Key problems that require new and further technical development are:

- *Identifying and characterizing small but novel cell types from single-cell omics data*. In this problem, stem, progenitor, and high-capacity proliferative cells are often the main focus because they are the key to treating the commonly fatal diseases: cardiovascular diseases and cancer. In cardiovascular disease, which is often due to the cardiac tissue's low regenerative capacity, the goal is to promote cell proliferation [193]. Meanwhile, in cancer, the goal is to restrain the proliferative cells.
- *Characterizing the tissue microenvironment*, which significantly contributes to the growth and survivability of the tissue. Single-cell data allows observing and separating the main tissue cell types, such as neural cells in brain cancers, and environmental cell types, such as immune cells and fibroblast cells. Cancer immunotherapies [194] are examples of how the microenvironment can impact the tissues. Here, key questions concern which molecular and signaling mecha-

nism the microenvironment can stimulate tissue cell types, and which signaling pathways the tissue cells activate in response to the stimulus.
- *Characterizing cell differentiation* explains tissue regeneration and tumor recurrence. Analyzing time-series single-cell data is the key to approach this problem.

Meanwhile, utilizing deep-learning-based models, especially autoencoders, will be the main focus in virtual docking, molecular design, and system biology simulation. In this area, the keys to successful AI applications include reducing overfitting, enlarging the molecular dataset, and setting up a gold-standard validation Scheme [195].

To make a higher impact in clinical applications, AI translational bioinformatics still requires substantial effort to build multi-omics, clinome, and phenotype integrative data infrastructure. In this aspect, the All of Us research program [196] is a pioneering project. While preparing for these infrastructures to emerge, AI researchers can solve smaller-scale research problems, such as predicting patients' risk from clinome data, and linking omics and clinome data via text mining. Also, as shown in the work of Jensen et al. [27], AI can already play a significant role in clinical decision support under clinical experts' guidance in specific cases.

Questions for Discussion

- What are three types of translational bioinformatics data?
- Clinotype-genotype association has not been well-explored in translational bioinformatics. Sketch a research strategy to mine this type of association using Natural Language Processing (NLP - Chap. 7),

  Hint: find a catalog of clinotype terms; apply NLP tools using the Pubmed collection of abstracts.
- In the section on "Clustering Algorithms", matrix factorization, derive the formula for $\dfrac{\partial F}{\partial \mathbf{Q}}$ using the method in Eqs. (14.2)–(14.6).
- The section on "Inferring and Characterizing Cellular Signaling Mechanism that Determines the Cellular Response" shows that when the system has negative feedback, the signal oscillates. This is a well-known phenomenon in system biology modeling. Show that phenomenon again in the following system $\mathbf{M} = \begin{bmatrix} -1 & 1 \\ 0 & 0 \end{bmatrix}$, $S_t = 0.15 \times S_0 + 0.85 \times \mathbf{M}^T S_{t-1}$, $S_0 = (-1, 0)$. Draw the system diagram and PA, PB signals as in Figs. 14.3 and 14.4. How about with $S_0 = (1, 0)$?
- In the section on "Supporting Clinical Decision with Bioinformatics Analysis", mapping new patients' tumor expression (NPT) data to existing patients' tumor (EPT) expression data may help predicting clinical outcomes. Two data processing methods are proposed to map the NPT to EPT. One way to select the better method is to plot the combined NPT-EPT embedding after processing the data. Recall, embedding preserves the pairwise similarity from the original data space in the embedded space. The embedding visualization is in Fig. 14.6 (below). Which processing method is better, and why?

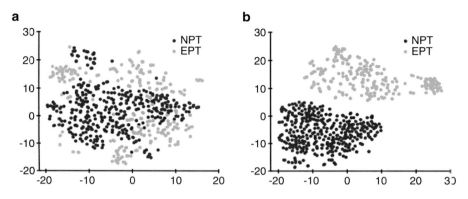

Fig. 14.6 (for question 3). NPT-RPT-combined embedding visualization with two data processing methods. (**a**) Method 1. (**b**) Method 2

Further Reading

Russell, S., & Norvig, P. (2009). *Artificial intelligence: a modern approach*, 3rd edition. Prentice Hall, ISBN 0-13-604,259-7.

- This book comprehensively covers AI theories, principles, algorithms, and techniques. This is considered a leading AI textbook. The student may find and read the 2nd edition as well.

Wei, D. Q., Ma, Y., Cho, W. C., Xu, Q., & Zhou, F. (Eds.). (2017). *Translational Bioinformatics and Its Application*. Springer.

- This is the most up-to-date and comprehensive textbook about translational bioinformatics.

Tenenbaum, J. D. (2016). Translational bioinformatics: past, present, and future *Genomics, proteomics & bioinformatics*, 14(1), 31–41.

- This review summarizes the most prominent roles of translational bioinformatics, and provides a perspective of how the field may further improve health care.

Larranaga, P., Calvo, B., Santana, R., Bielza, C., Galdiano, J., Inza, I., ... & Robles, V. (2006). Machine learning in bioinformatics. *Briefings in bioinformatics*, 7(1), 86–112.

- This review describes the most popular AI algorithms in bioinformatics at the turn of the century.

Ciaburro, G. (2017). *MATLAB for machine learning*. Packt Publishing Ltd.

- Licensing cost notwithstanding (Matlab is a commercial product), Matlab is without a doubt one of the most learner-friendly and easy-to-learn platform to learn, practice, and implement AI in many fields.

Lantz, B. (2013). *Machine learning with R*. Packt publishing ltd.

• For open-source programming, R is a good platform to practice AI. Compared to Matlab, it provides a trade-off between convenience and programming speed and cost. Many translational bioinformatics algorithms have publicly available R implementation.

Raschka, S. (2015*). Python machine learning*. Packt publishing ltd.

• For open-source programming, Python is a good platform to practice AI, and provides ready integration with a range of powerful publicly available machine learning libraries.

References

1. Informatics Areas Translational Bioinformatics 2020; Available from: https://www.amia.org/applications-informatics/translational-bioinformatics.
2. Zhang E, et al. Identifying the key regulators that promote cell-cycle activity in the hearts of early neonatal pigs after myocardial injury. PLoS One. 2020;15(7):e0232963.
3. Venter JC, et al. The sequence of the human genome. Science. 2001;291(5507):1304–51.
4. Overview of the Nationwide Emergency Department Sample (NEDS). 2020. Available from: https://www.hcup-us.ahrq.gov/nedsoverview.jsp.
5. Cui M, et al. Dynamic Transcriptional Responses to Injury of Regenerative and Non-regenerative Cardiomyocytes Revealed by Single-Nucleus RNA Sequencing. Dev Cell. 2020;53(1):102–116 e8.
6. Ouzounis CA. Rise and demise of bioinformatics? Promise and progress. PLoS Comput Biol. 2012;8(4):e1002487.
7. Human Genome Project FAQ. 2020. Available from: https://www.genome.gov/human-genome-project/Completion-FAQ.
8. Evans RS. Electronic Health Records: Then, Now, and in the Future. Yearb Med Inform. 2016;Suppl 1:S48–61.
9. Organization WH. Genomics and world health: Report of the Advisory Committee on Health Research. 2002: World Health Organization.
10. Anderson NL, Anderson NG. Proteome and proteomics: new technologies, new concepts, and new words. Electrophoresis. 1998;19(11):1853–61.
11. Idle JR, Gonzalez FJ. Metabolomics. Cell Metab. 2007;6(5):348–51.
12. Lowe R, et al. Transcriptomics technologies. PLoS Comput Biol. 2017;13(5):e1005457.
13. Chen JY, Pandey R, Nguyen TM. HAPPI-2: a Comprehensive and High-quality Map of Human Annotated and Predicted Protein Interactions. BMC Genomics. 2017;18(1):182.
14. Hu T, et al. Characterizing genetic interactions in human disease association studies using statistical epistasis networks. BMC Bioinformatics. 2011;12:364.
15. Hardiman G. Microarray technologies 2003—an overview. Pharmacogenomics. 2003;4(3):251–6.
16. McCarroll SA, Altshuler DM. Copy-number variation and association studies of human disease. Nat Genet. 2007;39(7 Suppl):S37–42.
17. Chu Y, Corey DR. RNA sequencing: platform selection, experimental design, and data interpretation. Nucleic Acid Ther. 2012;22(4):271–4.
18. Wang Z, Gerstein M, Snyder M. RNA-Seq: a revolutionary tool for transcriptomics. Nat Rev Genet. 2009;10(1):57–63.
19. Moritz CP. 40 years Western blotting: A scientific birthday toast. J Proteome. 2020;212:103575.

20. Gromiha MM, Yugandhar K, Jemimah S. Protein-protein interactions: scoring schemes and binding affinity. Curr Opin Struct Biol. 2017;44:31–8.
21. Huntley RP, et al. The GOA database: gene Ontology annotation updates for 2015. Nucleic Acids Res. 2015;43(Database issue):D1057–63.
22. The Gene Ontology Consortium. The Gene Ontology Resource: 20 years and still GOing strong. Nucleic Acids Res. 2019;47(D1):D330–8.
23. Kanehisa M, et al. KEGG: new perspectives on genomes, pathways, diseases and drugs. Nucleic Acids Res. 2017;45(D1):D353–61.
24. Jassal B, et al. The reactome pathway knowledgebase. Nucleic Acids Res. 2020;48(D1):D498–503.
25. UniProt C. UniProt: a worldwide hub of protein knowledge. Nucleic Acids Res. 2019;47(D1):D506–15.
26. Burley SK, et al. Protein Data Bank (PDB): The Single Global Macromolecular Structure Archive. Methods Mol Biol. 2017;1607:627–41.
27. Szklarczyk D, et al. STRING v11: protein-protein association networks with increased coverage, supporting functional discovery in genome-wide experimental datasets. Nucleic Acids Res. 2019;47(D1):D607–13.
28. Nguyen T, et al. Linking Clinotypes to Phenotypes and Genotypes from Laboratory Test Results in Comprehensive Physical Exams. BMC Med Inform Decis Mak. 21(3):1–12.
29. Bernstam EV, Smith JW, Johnson TR. What is biomedical informatics? J Biomed Inform. 2010;43(1):104–10.
30. Jensen PB, Jensen LJ, Brunak S. Mining electronic health records: towards better research applications and clinical care. Nat Rev Genet. 2012;13(6):395–405.
31. Sakshaug JW, et al. The collection of biospecimens in health surveys. In: Handbook of health survey methods; 2015. p. 383–419.
32. Chen DL, Li QY, Tan QY. Smoking history and the efficacy of immune checkpoint inhibitors in patients with advanced non-small cell lung cancer: a systematic review and meta-analysis. J Thorac Dis. 2021;13(1):220–31.
33. Stokes PR, et al. History of cigarette smoking is associated with higher limbic GABAA receptor availability. NeuroImage. 2013;69:70–7.
34. Ahnen RT, Jonnalagadda SS, Slavin JL. Role of plant protein in nutrition, wellness, and health. Nutr Rev. 2019;77(11):735–47.
35. Nielsen TT, et al. Improved metabolic fitness, but no cardiovascular health effects, of a low-frequency short-term combined exercise programme in 50-70-year-olds with low fitness: A randomized controlled trial. Eur J Sport Sci. 2021:1–14.
36. Kim D, et al. Targeted therapy guided by single-cell transcriptomic analysis in drug-induced hypersensitivity syndrome: a case report. Nat Med. 2020;26(2):236–43.
37. Green RF, et al. Evaluating the role of public health in implementation of genomics-related recommendations: a case study of hereditary cancers using the CDC Science Impact Framework. Genet Med. 2019;21(1):28–37.
38. Bauer DC, et al. Supporting pandemic response using genomics and bioinformatics: A case study on the emergent SARS-CoV-2 outbreak. Transbound Emerg Dis. 2020;67(4):1453–62.
39. Karczewski KJ, Snyder MP. Integrative omics for health and disease. Nat Rev Genet. 2018;19(5):299–310.
40. Toga AW, et al. Big biomedical data as the key resource for discovery science. J Am Med Inform Assoc. 2015;22(6):1126–31.
41. Arnett DK, Claas SA. Omics of Blood Pressure and Hypertension. Circ Res 2018;122(10):1409–19.
42. Cooper-DeHoff RM, Johnson JA. Hypertension pharmacogenomics: in search of personalized treatment approaches. Nat Rev Nephrol. 2016;12(2):110–22.
43. Cordell HJ. Detecting gene-gene interactions that underlie human diseases. Nat Rev Genet. 2009;10(6):392–404.
44. Miryala SK, Anbarasu A, Ramaiah S. Discerning molecular interactions: A comprehensive review on biomolecular interaction databases and network analysis tools. Gene. 2018;642:84–94.

45. Nguyen T, et al. Abstract P108: Identify Hypertension Risk from Health Exam Results. Hypertension. 2019;74(Suppl_1):AP108.
46. Ballester PJ, Mitchell JB. A machine learning approach to predicting protein-ligand binding affinity with applications to molecular docking. Bioinformatics. 2010;26(9):1169–75.
47. Honkela A, et al. Model-based method for transcription factor target identification with limited data. Proc Natl Acad Sci U S A. 2010;107(17):7793–8.
48. Buniello A, et al. The NHGRI-EBI GWAS Catalog of published genome-wide association studies, targeted arrays and summary statistics 2019. Nucleic Acids Res. 2019;47(D1):D1005–12.
49. Nicholls HL, et al. Reaching the End-Game for GWAS: Machine Learning Approaches for the Prioritization of Complex Disease Loci. Front Genet. 2020;11:350.
50. Isakov O, Dotan I, Ben-Shachar S. Machine Learning-Based Gene Prioritization Identifies Novel Candidate Risk Genes for Inflammatory Bowel Disease. Inflamm Bowel Dis. 2017;23(9):1516–23.
51. Hoffman GE, Logsdon BA, Mezey JG. PUMA: a unified framework for penalized multiple regression analysis of GWAS data. PLoS Comput Biol. 2013;9(6):e1003101.
52. Wang S, et al. HEALER: homomorphic computation of ExAct Logistic rEgRession for secure rare disease variants analysis in GWAS. Bioinformatics. 2016;32(2):211–8.
53. Ban HJ, et al. Identification of type 2 diabetes-associated combination of SNPs using support vector machine. BMC Genet. 2010;11:26.
54. Breiman L. Random forests. Mach Learn. 2001;45(1):5–32.
55. Chen W, et al. Risk of GWAS-identified genetic variants for breast cancer in a Chinese population: a multiple interaction analysis. Breast Cancer Res Treat. 2013;142(3):637–44.
56. Chuang LC, Kuo PH. Building a genetic risk model for bipolar disorder from genome-wide association data with random forest algorithm. Sci Rep. 2017;7:39943.
57. Liang Z, et al. DL-ADR: a novel deep learning model for classifying genomic variants into adverse drug reactions. BMC Med Genet. 2016;9(Suppl 2):48.
58. Kim SH, et al. Prediction of Alzheimer's disease-specific phospholipase c gamma-1 SNV by deep learning-based approach for high-throughput screening. Proc Natl Acad Sci U S A. 2021;118(3):e2011250118.
59. Verhaak RG, et al. Integrated genomic analysis identifies clinically relevant subtypes of glioblastoma characterized by abnormalities in PDGFRA, IDH1, EGFR, and NF1. Cancer Cell. 2010;17(1):98–110.
60. Quang D, Guan Y, Parker SCJ. YAMDA: thousandfold speedup of EM-based motif discovery using deep learning libraries and GPU. Bioinformatics. 2018;34(20):3578–80.
61. Shahshahani BM, Landgrebe DA. The effect of unlabeled samples in reducing the small sample size problem and mitigating the Hughes phenomenon. IEEE Trans Geosci Remote Sens. 1994;32(5):1087–95.
62. Pellin D, et al. A comprehensive single cell transcriptional landscape of human hematopoietic progenitors. Nat Commun. 2019;10(1):2395.
63. McGinnis CS, et al. MULTI-seq: sample multiplexing for single-cell RNA sequencing using lipid-tagged indices. Nat Methods. 2019;16(7):619–26.
64. Sarkar IN, et al. Translational bioinformatics: linking knowledge across biological and clinical realms. J Am Med Inform Assoc. 2011;18(4):354–7.
65. Tung PY, Blischak JD, Hsiao CJ, Knowles DA, Burnett JE, Pritchard JK, Gilad Y. Batch effects and the effective design of single-cell gene expression studies. Scientific reports. 2017;7(1): pp. 1–15.
66. Chen W, et al. A multicenter study benchmarking single-cell RNA sequencing technologies using reference samples. Nat Biotechnol. 2021;39(9):1103–14.
67. Wang Y, et al. Single-cell analysis of murine fibroblasts identifies neonatal to adult switching that regulates cardiomyocyte maturation. Nat Commun. 2020;11(1):2585.
68. Chawla NV, et al. SMOTE: synthetic minority over-sampling technique. J Artif Intell Res. 2002;16:321–57.
69. Lu X, et al. Enhancing text categorization with semantic-enriched representation and training data augmentation. J Am Med Inform Assoc. 2006;13(5):526–35.

70. Sayyari E, Kawas B, Mirarab S. TADA: phylogenetic augmentation of microbiome samples enhances phenotype classification. Bioinformatics. 2019;35(14):i31–40.
71. Shorten C, Khoshgoftaar TM. A survey on image data augmentation for deep learning. J Big Data. 2019;6(1):1–48.
72. Massey FJ Jr. The Kolmogorov-Smirnov test for goodness of fit. J Am Stat Assoc. 1951;46(253):68–78.
73. Bergstra J, Bengio Y. Random search for hyper-parameter optimization. J Mach Learn Res. 2012;13(2):281–305.
74. Hauck WW Jr, Donner A. Wald's test as applied to hypotheses in logit analysis. J Am Stat Assoc. 1977;72(360a):851–3.
75. Chute CG, et al. The Enterprise Data Trust at Mayo Clinic: a semantically integrated warehouse of biomedical data. J Am Med Inform Assoc. 2010;17(2):131–5.
76. NIS Database Documentation. 2020. Available from: https://www.hcup-us.ahrq.gov/db/nation/nis/nisdbdocumentation.jsp.
77. Stothers JAM, Nguyen A. Can Neo4j Replace PostgreSQL in Healthcare? AMIA Jt Summits Transl Sci Proc. 2020;2020:646–53.
78. Boley H. The rule markup language: RDF-XML data model, XML schema hierarchy, and XSL transformations. In: International conference on Applications of Prolog. New York: Springer; 2001.
79. Gao J, et al. Integrative analysis of complex cancer genomics and clinical profiles using the cBioPortal. Sci Signal. 2013;6(269):l1.
80. Schatz MC. CloudBurst: highly sensitive read mapping with MapReduce. Bioinformatics. 2009;25(11):1363–9.
81. Bessani A, et al. BiobankCloud: a platform for the secure storage, sharing, and processing of large biomedical data sets. In: Biomedical data management and graph online querying. New York: Springer; 2015. p. 89–105.
82. Lewis S, et al. Hydra: a scalable proteomic search engine which utilizes the Hadoop distributed computing framework. BMC Bioinformatics. 2012;13:324.
83. The ENCODE Project Consortium n.d.. https://www.encodeproject.org/pipelines/ENCPL122WIM/
84. The ENCODE Project Consortium n.d.. https://www.encodeproject.org/pipelines/ENCPL444CYA/
85. 10x Genomics n.d.. https://support.10xgenomics.com/single-cell-gene-expression/software/pipelines/latest/what-is-cell-ranger
86. Manning CD, et al. The Stanford CoreNLP natural language processing toolkit. In: Proceedings of 52nd annual meeting of the association for computational linguistics: system demonstrations; 2014.
87. Ringner M. What is principal component analysis? Nat Biotechnol. 2008;26(3):303–4.
88. Jendoubi T, Strimmer K. A whitening approach to probabilistic canonical correlation analysis for omics data integration. BMC Bioinformatics. 2019;20(1):15.
89. Di Y, et al. The NBP negative binomial model for assessing differential gene expression from RNA-Seq. Stat Appl Genet Mol Biol. 2011;10(1)
90. Love MI, Huber W, Anders S. Moderated estimation of fold change and dispersion for RNA-seq data with DESeq2. Genome Biol. 2014;15(12):550.
91. Robinson MD, Smyth GK. Small-sample estimation of negative binomial dispersion, with applications to SAGE data. Biostatistics. 2008;9(2):321–32.
92. Tran HTN, et al. A benchmark of batch-effect correction methods for single-cell RNA sequencing data. Genome Biol. 2020;21(1):12.
93. van de Maaten L, Hinton G. Visualizing data using t-SNE. J Mach Learn Res. 2008;9(Nov):2579–605.
94. Becht E, McInnes L, Healy J, Dutertre CA, Kwok IW, Ng LG, Ginhoux F. and Newell EW. Dimensionality reduction for visualizing single-cell data using UMAP. Nature biotechnology. 2019;37(1): pp. 38–44.
95. Zhou M, et al. Radiomics in Brain Tumor: Image Assessment, Quantitative Feature Descriptors, and Machine-Learning Approaches. AJNR Am J Neuroradiol. 2018;39(2):208–16.

96. Bi WL, et al. Artificial intelligence in cancer imaging: Clinical challenges and applications. CA Cancer J Clin. 2019;69(2):127–57.
97. Hu J, et al. Iterative transfer learning with neural network for clustering and cell type classification in single-cell RNA-seq analysis. Nat Mach Intell. 2020;2(10):607–18.
98. Glaab E, et al. Using rule-based machine learning for candidate disease gene prioritization and sample classification of cancer gene expression data. PLoS One. 2012;7(7):e39932.
99. Mykowiecka A, Marciniak M, Kupsc A. Rule-based information extraction from patients' clinical data. J Biomed Inform. 2009;42(5):923–36.
100. Cortes C, Vapnik V. Support vector machine. Mach Learn. 1995;20(3):273–97.
101. Marill KA. Advanced statistics: linear regression, part II: multiple linear regression. Acad Emerg Med. 2004;11(1):94–102.
102. LeCun Y, Bengio Y, Hinton G. Deep learning. Nature. 2015;521(7553):436–44.
103. Young JD, Cai C, Lu X. Unsupervised deep learning reveals prognostically relevant subtypes of glioblastoma. BMC Bioinformatics. 2017;18(Suppl 11):381.
104. Pushpakom S, et al. Drug repurposing: progress, challenges and recommendations. Nat Rev Drug Discov. 2019;18(1):41–58.
105. Udrescu L, et al. Clustering drug-drug interaction networks with energy model layouts: community analysis and drug repurposing. Sci Rep. 2016;6:32745.
106. McLachlan GJ, Bean RW, Ng SK. Clustering. Methods Mol Biol. 2017;1526:345–62.
107. Do CB, Batzoglou S. What is the expectation maximization algorithm? Nat Biotechnol. 2008;26(8):897–9.
108. Cai D, et al. Non-negative matrix factorization on manifold. In: 2008 Eighth IEEE International Conference on Data Mining. London: IEEE; 2008.
109. Utgoff PE. Incremental induction of decision trees. Mach Learn. 1989;4(2):161–86.
110. Qi Y. Random forest for bioinformatics. In: Ensemble machine learning. Springer; 2012. p. 307–23.
111. Bouckaert RR. Bayesian network classifiers in weka. 2004. https://researchcommons. waikato.ac.nz/bitstream/handle/10289/85/content.pdf.
112. Dempster AP, Laird NM, Rubin DB. Maximum Likelihood from Incomplete Data via the EM Algorithm. J R Stat Soc Ser B Methodol. 1977;39(1)
113. Lloyd S. Least squares quantization in PCM. IEEE Trans Inf Theory. 1982;28(2):129–37.
114. Rousseeuw PJ. Silhouettes: a graphical aid to the interpretation and validation of cluster analysis. J Comput Appl Math. 1987;20:53–65.
115. Koren Y, Bell R, Volinsky C. Matrix factorization techniques for recommender systems. Computer. 2009;42(8):30–7.
116. Haussler D, Opper M. Mutual information, metric entropy and cumulative relative entropy risk. Ann Stat. 1997;25(6):2451–92.
117. Jaccard P. The distribution of the flora in the alpine zone. 1. New Phytol. 1912;11(2):37–50.
118. Safdar NM, Banja JD, Meltzer CC. Ethical considerations in artificial intelligence. Eur J Radiol. 2020;122:108768.
119. Kluyver T, et al. Jupyter Notebooks-a publishing format for reproducible computational workflows. In: Fernando, Birgit S, editors. Positioning and Power in Academic Publishing: Players, Agents and Agendas. Amsterdam: IOS Press; 2016. p. 87–90.
120. Chatr-Aryamontri A, et al. The BioGRID interaction database: 2013 update. Nucleic Acids Res. 2013;41(Database issue):D816–23.
121. Fornes O, et al. JASPAR 2020: update of the open-access database of transcription factor binding profiles. Nucleic Acids Res. 2020;48(D1):D87–92.
122. Mathelier A, Wasserman WW. The next generation of transcription factor binding site prediction. PLoS Comput Biol. 2013;9(9):e1003214.
123. Eddy SR. What is a hidden Markov model? Nat Biotechnol. 2004;22(10):1315–6.
124. Chai LE, et al. A review on the computational approaches for gene regulatory network construction. Comput Biol Med. 2014;48:55–65.
125. Leysen H, et al. G Protein-Coupled Receptor Systems as Crucial Regulators of DNA Damage Response Processes. Int J Mol Sci. 2018;19(10)

126. Wisdom R, Johnson RS, Moore C. c-Jun regulates cell cycle progression and apoptosis by distinct mechanisms. EMBO J. 1999;18(1):188–97.
127. Villate-Beitia I, et al. Gene delivery to the lungs: pulmonary gene therapy for cystic fibrosis. Drug Dev Ind Pharm. 2017;43(7):1071–81.
128. Essebier A, et al. Bioinformatics approaches to predict target genes from transcription factor binding data. Methods. 2017;131:111–9.
129. He B, et al. Global view of enhancer-promoter interactome in human cells. Proc Natl Acad Sci U S A. 2014;111(21):E2191–9.
130. Roy S, et al. A predictive modeling approach for cell line-specific long-range regulatory interactions. Nucleic Acids Res. 2015;43(18):8694–712.
131. Zhao C, Li X, Hu H. PETModule: a motif module based approach for enhancer target gene prediction. Sci Rep. 2016;6:30043.
132. Kim, G.B., et al., DeepTFactor: A deep learning-based tool for the prediction of transcription factors. Proc Natl Acad Sci U S A, 2021. 118(2).
133. Park S, et al. Enhancing the interpretability of transcription factor binding site prediction using attention mechanism. Sci Rep. 2020;10(1):13413.
134. Fu L, et al. Predicting transcription factor binding in single cells through deep learning. Sci Adv. 2020;6(51)
135. Guryanov I, Fiorucci S, Tennikova T. Receptor-ligand interactions: Advanced biomedical applications. Mater Sci Eng C Mater Biol Appl. 2016;68:890–903.
136. Jin, S., et al., Inference and analysis of cell-cell communication using CellChat. Nat Commun, 2021. 12(1): p. 1088.
137. Fathke C, et al. Wnt signaling induces epithelial differentiation during cutaneous wound healing. BMC Cell Biol. 2006;7:4.
138. Stepniewska-Dziubinska MM, Zielenkiewicz P, Siedlecki P. Development and evaluation of a deep learning model for protein-ligand binding affinity prediction. Bioinformatics 2018;34(21):3666–74.
139. Wu J, et al. WDL-RF: predicting bioactivities of ligand molecules acting with G protein-coupled receptors by combining weighted deep learning and random forest. Bioinformatics 2018;34(13):2271–82.
140. Creixell P, et al. Pathway and network analysis of cancer genomes. Nat Methods. 2015;12(7):615–21.
141. Abeel T, et al. Robust biomarker identification for cancer diagnosis with ensemble feature selection methods. Bioinformatics. 2010;26(3):392–8.
142. Xiong M, Fang X, Zhao J. Biomarker identification by feature wrappers. Genome Res. 2001;11(11):1878–87.
143. Garcia-Campos MA, Espinal-Enriquez J, Hernandez-Lemus E. Pathway Analysis: State of the Art. Front Physiol. 2015;6:383.
144. Hoops S, et al. COPASI--a COmplex PAthway SImulator. Bioinformatics. 2006;22(24):3067–74.
145. Karplus M, Petsko GA. Molecular dynamics simulations in biology. Nature. 1990;347(6294):631–9.
146. Saad J, Asuka E, Schoenberger L. Physiology, Platelet Activation, in StatPearls. Treasure Island (FL); 2021.
147. Tsai TY, et al. Robust, tunable biological oscillations from interlinked positive and negative feedback loops. Science. 2008;321(5885):126–9.
148. Bianchini M, Gori M, Scarselli F. Inside pagerank. ACM Trans Internet Technol. 2005;5(1):92–128.
149. Ma J, et al. Using deep learning to model the hierarchical structure and function of a cell. Nat Methods. 2018;15(4):290–8.
150. Chen T, He HL, Church GM. Modeling gene expression with differential equations. In: Biocomputing'99. Singapore: World Scientific; 1999. p. 29–40.
151. Kanter I, Kalisky T. Single cell transcriptomics: methods and applications. Front Oncol. 2015;5:53.

152. Butler A, et al. Integrating single-cell transcriptomic data across different conditions, technologies, and species. Nat Biotechnol. 2018;36(5):411–20.
153. Trapnell C, et al. The dynamics and regulators of cell fate decisions are revealed by pseudotemporal ordering of single cells. Nat Biotechnol. 2014;32(4):381–6.
154. Zhang, X., et al., CellMarker: a manually curated resource of cell markers in human and mouse. Nucleic Acids Res, 2019. 47(D1): p. D721-D728.
155. Ester M, et al. A density-based algorithm for discovering clusters in large spatial databases with noise. In: KDD'96: Proceedings of the Second International Conference on Knowledge Discovery and Data Mining; 1996. p. 226–31.
156. Blondel VD, et al. Fast unfolding of communities in large networks. J Stat Mech. 2008;2008(10):P10008.
157. McInnes, L., J. Healy, and J. Melville, UMAP: Uniform Manifold Approximation and Projection for Dimension Reduction, C. University, Editor. 2018, arXiv.
158. Nakada Y, et al. Single nucleus transcriptomics: Apical resection in newborn pigs extends the time-window of cardiomyocyte proliferation and myocardial regeneration. Circulation. 2022;145(23):1744–7.
159. Litvinukova M, et al. Cells of the adult human heart. Nature. 2020;588(7838):466–72.
160. McKenzie AT, et al. Brain Cell Type Specific Gene Expression and Co-expression Network Architectures. Sci Rep. 2018;8(1):8868.
161. McGinnis CS, Murrow LM, Gartner ZJ. DoubletFinder: Doublet Detection in Single-Cell RNA Sequencing Data Using Artificial Nearest Neighbors. Cell Syst. 2019;8(4):329–337 e4.
162. Qiu P. Embracing the dropouts in single-cell RNA-seq analysis. Nat Commun. 2020;11(1):1169.
163. What is sequencing saturation? Available from: https://kb.10xgenomics.com/hc/en-us/articles/115005062366-What-is-sequencing-saturation-.
164. Ding H, et al. Similarity-based machine learning methods for predicting drug-target interactions: a brief review. Brief Bioinform. 2014;15(5):734–47.
165. Zhang W, et al. Manifold regularized matrix factorization for drug-drug interaction prediction. J Biomed Inform. 2018;88:90–7.
166. Yu H, et al. Predicting and understanding comprehensive drug-drug interactions via semi-nonnegative matrix factorization. BMC Syst Biol. 2018;12(Suppl 1):14.
167. Shi JY, et al. TMFUF: a triple matrix factorization-based unified framework for predicting comprehensive drug-drug interactions of new drugs. BMC Bioinformatics. 2018;19(Suppl 14):411.
168. Greene D, et al. Ensemble non-negative matrix factorization methods for clustering protein-protein interactions. Bioinformatics. 2008;24(15):1722–8.
169. Zheng X, et al. Collaborative matrix factorization with multiple similarities for predicting drug-target interactions. In: Proceedings of the 19th ACM SIGKDD international conference on Knowledge discovery and data mining; 2013.
170. Cobanoglu MC, et al. Predicting drug-target interactions using probabilistic matrix factorization. J Chem Inf Model. 2013;53(12):3399–409.
171. Yang J, et al. Drug-disease association and drug-repositioning predictions in complex diseases using causal inference-probabilistic matrix factorization. J Chem Inf Model. 2014;54(9):2562–9.
172. Nguyen TM, et al. DeCoST: A New Approach in Drug Repurposing From Control System Theory. Front Pharmacol. 2018;9:583.
173. Gottlieb A, et al. PREDICT: a method for inferring novel drug indications with application to personalized medicine. Mol Syst Biol. 2011;7:496.
174. Alliance, G., Understanding genetics: a district of Columbia guide for patients and health professionals. 2010.
175. Lai Y, et al. Current status and perspectives of patient-derived xenograft models in cancer research. J Hematol Oncol. 2017;10(1):106.
176. Couturier CP, et al. Single-cell RNA-seq reveals that glioblastoma recapitulates a normal neurodevelopmental hierarchy. Nat Commun. 2020;11(1):3406.

177. Pauwels E, Stoven V, Yamanishi Y. Predicting drug side-effect profiles: a chemical fragment-based approach. BMC Bioinformatics. 2011;12:169.
178. Zhou M, Chen Y, Xu R. A Drug-Side Effect Context-Sensitive Network approach for drug target prediction. Bioinformatics. 2019;35(12):2100–7.
179. Sohn S, et al. Drug side effect extraction from clinical narratives of psychiatry and psychology patients. J Am Med Inform Assoc. 2011;18(Suppl 1):i144–9.
180. Karplus K, et al. Predicting protein structure using only sequence information. Proteins. 1999;Suppl 3:121–5.
181. Gevaert K, Vandekerckhove J. Protein identification methods in proteomics. Electrophoresis. 2000;21(6):1145–54.
182. Zhang Y. Progress and challenges in protein structure prediction. Curr Opin Struct Biol. 2008;18(3):342–8.
183. Jain P, Garibaldi JM, Hirst JD. Supervised machine learning algorithms for protein structure classification. Comput Biol Chem. 2009;33(3):216–23.
184. Jumper J, et al. Highly accurate protein structure prediction with AlphaFold. Nature. 2021:1–11.
185. 14th Community Wide Experiment on the Critical Assessment of Techniques for Protein Structure Prediction 2020. Available from: https://predictioncenter.org/casp14/results.cgi.
186. Merz KM Jr, Ringe D, Reynolds CH. Drug design: structure-and ligand-based approaches. Cambridge: Cambridge University Press; 2010.
187. Anderson AC. The process of structure-based drug design. Chem Biol. 2003;10(9):787–97.
188. Hughes JP, et al. Principles of early drug discovery. Br J Pharmacol. 2011;162(6):1239–49.
189. Zhavoronkov A, et al. Deep learning enables rapid identification of potent DDR1 kinase inhibitors. Nat Biotechnol. 2019;37(9):1038–40.
190. Kingma DP, Welling M. An introduction to variational autoencoders. arXiv preprint arXiv. 2019:1906.02691.
191. Sterling, T. and J.J. Irwin, ZINC 15--Ligand Discovery for Everyone. J Chem Inf Model. 2015. 55(11): p. 2324–2337.
192. Gaulton A, et al. The ChEMBL database in 2017. Nucleic Acids Res. 2017;45(D1):D945–54.
193. Sadek H, Olson EN. Toward the Goal of Human Heart Regeneration. Cell Stem Cell. 2020;26(1):7–16.
194. Hegde PS, Chen DS. Top 10 Challenges in Cancer Immunotherapy. Immunity. 2020;52(1):17–35.
195. Brown N, et al. Artificial intelligence in chemistry and drug design. J Comput Aided Mol Des. 2020;34(7):709–15.
196. Fox K. The Illusion of Inclusion—The "All of Us" Research Program and Indigenous Peoples' DNA. N Engl J Med. 2020;383(5):411–3.

Chapter 15
Health Systems Management

Adam B. Wilcox and Bethene D. Britt

After reading this chapter, you should know the answers to these questions:
- How has artificial intelligence (AI) been used in health systems management? What are the primary areas where it has been applied? What have been the benefits of AI for health systems?
- What factors should be considered when applying AI algorithms for health systems management? How can the choice of data affect their use?
- What are the challenges in matching the cognitive tasks of interpreting data with the capabilities of AI algorithms? How can the modeling of data and the framing of the decision task affect the ability to discover insights, either through human cognition or AI application?
- How can governance be applied effectively in the adoption and application of AI algorithms?

Promise of AI in Health Systems

Health care is both complex and information-intensive. Multiple disciplines are combined to care for patients, with each having a specific role with specific information needed to support that role. Coordination across roles also involves active

A. B. Wilcox (✉)
Washington University in St. Louis School of Medicine, St. Louis, MO, USA
e-mail: a.wilcox@wustl.edu

B. D. Britt
UW Medicine, University of Washington, Seattle, WA, USA
e-mail: betbritt@uw.edu

© The Author(s), under exclusive license to Springer Nature
Switzerland AG 2022
T. A. Cohen et al. (eds.), *Intelligent Systems in Medicine and Health*, Cognitive
Informatics in Biomedicine and Healthcare,
https://doi.org/10.1007/978-3-031-09108-7_15

use of information, for assessment, interpretation, comparison and communication. Care must be coordinated both for the individual patient but also for the healthcare delivery system, which increases the complexity substantially as it must consider the interaction of multiple individual patients. This complexity is reflected in various tasks where healthcare professionals must coordinate multiple sources of information and make decisions or predictions based on this information. For example, a nurse manager needs to consider the expected complexity of cases and patient volume for a unit when determining how many nurses need to be scheduled for a shift. Managers of operating rooms also need to make estimations of case complexity and time when considering scheduling for surgery to optimize resources. Clinics may over-schedule appointments based on a predicted or estimated no-show rate to optimize the total number of patients seen. These are all examples of prediction activities in the management of health systems that may benefit from the use of AI methods to quickly organize and interpret information, and are in addition to how AI can be used to make interpretations for recommended care with an individual patient.

There have been specific examples of successful adoption of various methods of AI for health systems management, ranging from resource allocation, demand and use prediction, and scheduling optimization. A review of clinical literature identifies the following published examples, which are representative of many more unpublished experiences of others in applying AI for health systems management:

- Aktas et al. reported on the development of a decision support system to improve resource allocation to be applied in a radiology department [1]. Using a **Bayesian belief network** to represent conditional dependencies, they were able to analyze the relationships of key variables affecting system efficiency for resource allocation.
- Gartner and Padman developed a **Naive Bayes classifier** to assist in early diagnosis group determination that can improve resource allocation decisions [2].
- Dennis et al. demonstrated that **artificial neural networks** were effective at predicting trauma volume and acuity within emergency departments, based on seasonality-related measures such as time of year, day of week, temperature and precipitation levels [3]. These results were consistent with heuristics related to trauma prediction, but were more precise in predicting "trauma seasons" across multiple centers.
- Lee et al. used information collected from electronic health records for emergency department patients to predict disposition decisions with logistic regression and machine learning algorithms [4]. These predictions can be used to reduce boarding delays by prompting the initiation of admission processes where needed.
- McCoy et al. demonstrated that **time-series machine learning** methods could be applied to date, census and discharge data to predict daily discharge volumes [5]. Prediction errors outside 1 standard deviation occurred only about 5% of days,

indicating the AI methods could help in predicting volumes and matching resources to volumes.

- Vermeulen et al. developed adaptive rules for scheduling computer tomography scanning that adjusts to multiple patient and system features [6]. These rules showed an ability to better adjust to variations in volume according to different resource levels.
- Kontio et al. used machine learning algorithms to predict patient acuity levels that could support resource allocation [7]. They extracted information directly from demographic data, admission information, and concepts from radiology and pathology notes from previous days to classify patients with heart problems in five different acuity categories for the current day.

In some areas of health systems management, enough examples have been published to perform systematic reviews to identify both the breadth and patterns of success:

- Bellini et al. performed a systematic review of AI applications in operating room optimization [8]. They identified successful studies in predicting procedure duration; in coordinating post-acute care unit availability; and in cancellation prediction. All of these areas can improve surgery scheduling efficiency.

However, with all of these examples and studies, widespread, consistent and successful adoption of AI in health systems management remains elusive. A review of different risk prediction models performed by Wehbe et al. noted their modest performance, infrequent use, lack of evidence for improvement and barriers to implementation. They recommended that improved approaches to machine learning adoption be determined to overcome performance barriers and allow local customization of rules, which are a recognized challenge [9].

Understanding the cognitive aspects of applied AI in health systems management may provide a path forward for more successful adoption. There are numerous examples demonstrating that successful use of AI for improvement in these areas is possible; the challenge now is to identify the features that are prerequisites for success, and to demonstrate that the success can be reproduced.

One way to achieve this goal is to improve the understanding of the actual process of AI application in health systems management. Effective application of information in health systems practice is complex, giving rise to a whole field of clinical and health informatics focused on improving the use of information in the area. As that field moved from demonstration of success to broader adoption, a deeper understanding of the interrelationships among information sources, technology, and human users has demanded different methods focused on deeper understanding of interactions [10, 11]. These lessons from clinical informatics, and specifically in decision support (which arguably includes the application of AI to health systems management), become increasingly important. The balance of this chapter therefore focuses on providing that deeper understanding through a description of two applications of information to health systems management. We also include a discussion of governance approaches that can be used to ensure guided application of AI capabilities; this also matches the pattern of recommendations for adoption for clinical decision support by Wright et al. [12].

The first example relates to predicting no-shows for outpatient scheduling, with qualitative insights gathered from discussions with one of the authors who was a developer of the system. The second example relates to an analysis of testing approaches for monitoring devices and outcomes in heart failure patients.

Example: Outpatient Scheduling

The first example relates to an algorithm developed for predicting whether patients would arrive at clinics for scheduled appointments, in order to help staff appropriately schedule other patients to improve operational efficiency. This work was done at Massachusetts General Hospital in Boston, as described by Patrick Cronin who was working on process improvement with the Department of Medical Dermatology [13]. A critical management issue for the department was a patient rate for missed appointments that had reached 20%, which is significant and in line with general estimates nationally [14]. This meant that in a daily schedule that may include 100 appointments, 20 of those patients would not arrive as scheduled. The patients would either not arrive for the appointment (~12% "no-show" rate), or would cancel the appointment on the same day (same-day cancellation). This created important problems for the division because each no-show represented a point in the schedule with only costs but no revenue. While some same-day cancellation appointments could be filled with same-day appointment scheduling, the no-show appointments were unanticipated and therefore could not be refilled with other patients at the last minute.

Institutions have tried various methods to address the challenge of missed appointments and no-shows. One approach has been to remind patients of their appointment at least a day in advance, which can both prompt patients to attend or identify cancellations in advance. However, this approach generally requires additional staff to implement by contacting each patient beforehand, and studies have been mixed in showing differences due to reminders [14]. Another approach is to schedule additional overlapping appointments in the place of no-show appointments if they can be anticipated. This has obvious challenges if the prediction is wrong, however. If the patient does show up for the appointment, the clinic staff would then need to adapt the schedule for the rest of the day or until another gap in the schedule occurs to fit in the extra patient.

The approach applied in this example ("Smart Booking") was to create a prediction algorithm to predict patients who were most likely to miss appointments, and allow schedulers to create overlapping appointments for that day to fill the schedule. The prediction first involved identifying factors that may be related to no-shows and were available as data for predictions. These could be based on factors about the patient (e.g., age; insurance type) or the appointment itself (appointment type; days between appointment scheduling and appointment). Also available from the longitudinal database was a 15-year history of appointment scheduling data. This allowed a patient's history of no-shows and arrivals also to be included in the prediction model, and these variables were shown to be the most significant predictors.

The result was a Smart Booking algorithm that provided a daily recommendation for available overbookings to schedulers that were used to increase appointment bookings. It was initially implemented as a randomized controlled trial (randomized by clinic session) that measured both the number of arrived patients per clinic session and the perception by physicians of how busy the clinical session was (measured by a simple scale between "too slow" and "too busy"). The results were that the Smart Booking algorithm increased the number of patients booked for appointments by an average of 0.5 arrived patients per session, with physician perception of busyness being similar between the sessions with Smart Booking (and thus more patients) and without.

The success of this project led to other related AI-enabled interventions that varied in approach, clinical domain, outcome measures, and prediction goal. These included targeted reminder phone calls or patient navigation to decrease no-shows in other clinical departments [15–17], as well as prediction rule development for hospital readmissions [18, 19].

Discussions with the author of the main study have offered important lessons learned and insights that are important in understanding the overall reproducibility and sustainability of the approach. First, the data were seen as far more important than the algorithm that was used. That is, there was a greater impact in using the prior history of visits and the appointment types than in using more complicated algorithms like neural networks instead of logistic regression. The simplest algorithm performed similarly to more complicated AI algorithms, and had the benefit of being explainable to the clinic staff who interacted with the intervention (see Chap. 8). The actual implementation was more simple than robust, with the main algorithm running on a single desktop computer of the developer, at least for the studied version of the implementation. This was in part possible due to an internal development approach leveraging the electronic health record (EHR) at the institution at the time, which allowed for a more flexible but less sustainable approach. With the later implementation of a commercial EHR at the institution, the developed algorithm was removed. The commercial EHR provides its own predictive models that could be applied, but there have been challenges in the product's implementation and outcomes when studied [20]. In this study, the customized components of the AI implementation (choice of predictor data, flexibility in implementation) were critical to success, but this approach made it difficult to both replicate and sustain. This suggests an important factor explaining why consistent and successful adoption of AI in health systems management is challenging, because the maintenance effort to keep AI effective is often expensive.

Example: Device Monitoring

The second example is not an actual application of AI in health systems management, but rather a deep analysis of data related to outcomes for a high-risk patient population. However, the understanding of how these data were analyzed is important to recognize how data and cognitive aspects of data and information must be appropriately considered in applications of AI. This analysis was performed by one of the authors (AW) and Dr. Claudius Mahr at the University of Washington Medical Center in Seattle, WA.

In this example, a discordance in laboratory tests for monitoring **intravenous unfractionated heparin (IV-UFH)** was identified by clinicians performing a quality improvement review of a series of cases with negative outcomes [21, 22]. The laboratory tests were measuring activated **partial thromboplastin time (PTT)** and **anti-factor Xa (anti-Xa)**, both of which by measuring IV-UFH can help guide anticoagulation therapy to prevent bleeding and clotting complications. This is critical for patients who have received mechanical circulatory support, such as **left-ventricular assist device (LVAD)** implantation.

For individuals with end stage heart failure, assistive technologies are needed to improve cardiac function. A common device used is a left ventricular assist device (LVAD), which is a battery-operated mechanical pump that is surgically placed in the heart, in the left ventricle or main pumping chamber. The LVAD helps the left ventricle pump blood to the rest of the body. It is often used either temporarily until a patient receives a heart transplant, or as a long-term treatment for heart failure.

Because the device is surgically implanted in the circulatory system, it can lead to clotting of the blood which can then lead to severe outcomes such as strokes or myocardial infarctions when the blood clot moves into arteries and restricts blood flow to vital organs. To prevent this, patients are given medicine such as heparin, which helps prevent the blood from clotting. However, too much heparin can lead to other complications such as internal bleeding. As a result, it is important to balance the heparin dosing and amount of heparin in the blood at a level where both clots and internal bleeding are avoided. Maintaining this balance is challenging, and involves regular laboratory measures.

A study at one institution of 200 patients over 8 years with end stage heart failure who had received LVADs showed the challenges in managing treatment [23]. The survival rate for all patients was below 50% after 4 years, indicating the severe health problems of those receiving the treatment. The most common cause of death was stroke, with 32% of deaths. Three of the five most common adverse events were internal bleeding, stroke, and re-exploration for bleeding. This indicates the importance of managing clotting and bleeding among LVAD patients, as the most common causes of death and adverse events were related to it.

PTT is a laboratory test of blood that measures the time it takes for a blood clot to form. A common therapeutic range for PTT is 60–100 s for clotting. Anti-Xa is a test that measures the amount of heparin in the blood by measuring its inhibition of factor Xa activity, which is part of the clotting process. A common therapeutic range for anti-Xa is 0.3–0.7 IU/mL. Historically, PTT has been the more common test for clotting risk, but anti-Xa has become used increasingly. It is expected that PTT and anti-Xa would be concordant, or that when one shows a high clotting risk by a value above the therapeutic range, the other would as well. However, this is not always the case, and when there is a difference in measure it is important to know clinically which to respond to [21].

In a review of a series of patients with complications after LVAD implantation, clinicians at UW were concerned that this lack of concordance between PTT and anti-Xa could be important in patient management, and wanted an analysis of test values along with bleeding events among patients over a period of time. Over 6500 paired PTT and anti-Xa measures were identified among a patient population, and matched to bleeding events that occurred. Initially we looked at concordance measures directly as a matrix, within and above the therapeutic range for each test (Fig. 15.1). We also plotted the individual tests in a scatter plot to identify broader trends (Fig. 15.2).

To identify whether either PTT or anti-Xa were able to separate the bleeding and non-bleeding population, we plotted frequency curves for each of the measures, but

PTT

	<60	60 ≤ x ≤ 100	>100
>0.7	16 11 **0.2%** 5 (31%)	39 30 **1%** 9 (23%)	896 704 **14%** 192 (21%)
0.3 ≤ x ≤ 0.7	48 43 **1%** 5 (10%)	809 714 **12%** 95 (12%)	3143 2825 **47%** 318 (10%)
<0.3	659 520 **10%** 139 (21%)	699 573 **11%** 126 (18%)	308 259 **5%** 49 (16%)

Anti Xa (row label, left of matrix)

Fig. 15.1 Concordance matrix for PTT and anti-Xa measures. The blue central percentage listed in each cell gives the percent of all tests in the matrix in that cell. For example, the bottom left cell indicates that 10% of all paired measures had both an Anti Xa value of <0.3 and PTT values of 0.6. The upper left number in each cell represents the total tests in the cell, with the non-bleed count in the upper right, and the bleed count and rate at the bottom. If the tests were concordant, you would expect to see most of the test in the lower left, middle, or upper right cells, indicating the tests are low, within range, or high at the same time. In this matrix, however, the largest number of tests in the middle right cell indicates a discordance with anti-Xa in the therapeutic range (0.3–0.7 IU/mL) and PTT values above the therapeutic range (>100 s)

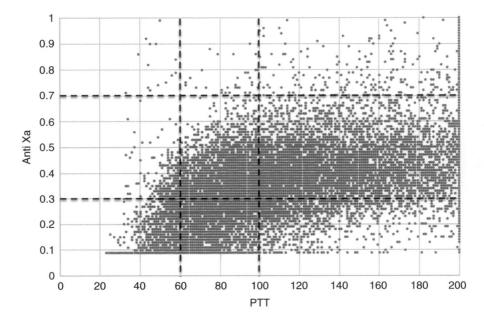

Fig. 15.2 Discordance scatter plot, which shows overall trends of PTT values being skewed above the therapeutic range, and anti-Xa values skewing below the therapeutic range. Lab tests for PTT values above 200 s had values of ">200" and were plotted as 201; anti-Xa values less than 0.1 IU/mL had values of "<0.1" and were plotted as 0.09

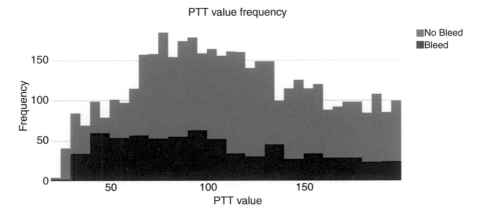

Fig. 15.3 PTT value frequency. There was no clear difference among the frequency curves that would show PTT as discriminating between bleeding risks

these showed nothing significant (Figs. 15.3 and 15.4). We also plotted PTT and anti-Xa values identifying bleeding events and calculated regression lines between the two populations (Fig. 15.5); while this showed a measurable difference, it was not convincing enough to warrant a different approach in monitoring.

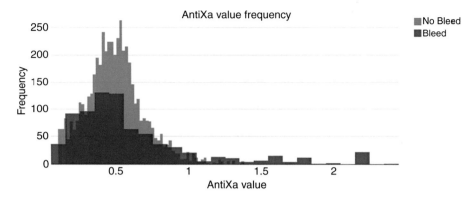

Fig. 15.4 Anti-Xa value frequency. Similar to PTT values, there was no clear discriminating di-ference for bleeding risks among anti-Xa values

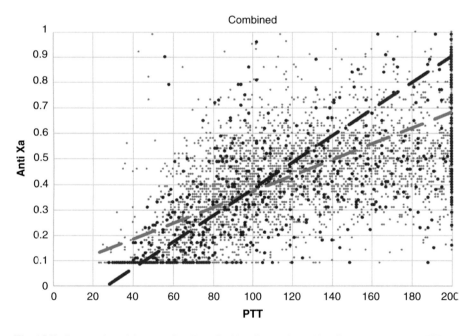

Fig. 15.5 Scatter plot with regression lines for bleeding and non-bleeding events among PTT and anti-Xa measures. The regression lines showed a measurable but unconvincing difference

Finally, we modeled the values in terms of *how they would be used in clinical decision-making*, rather than individually as values. That is, a PTT or anti-Xa result is used in making a decision to adjust therapy when it is above a threshold value that indicates a bleeding risk and need for the adjustment. To model this, we considered each value along the range of values the measure as a potential threshold point, and calculated the *bleed rate* as the proportion of bleeding events for measures at or

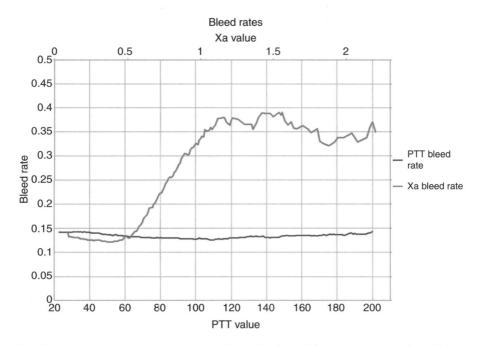

Fig. 15.6 Bleed rates calculated at varying threshold values. This approach modeled the clinical decisions by calculating the bleed rate above a threshold value, and then computing this rate for each PTT and anti-Xa value. The PTT threshold values were not helpful in discriminating bleed risks, while the anti-Xa values showed a differentiation as the values moved from the therapeutic range to high. At the highest values, there were fewer and fewer events to calculate the bleeding rate, and the rates became more variable

above that value. Modeling this threshold determination rate showed effectively how the measures would perform at different threshold value choices. As shown in Fig. 15.6, there was clear separation in the performance of anti-Xa in comparison to PTT for predicting bleeding as the threshold moved from the higher therapeutic range to the high ranges (around 0.7 for anti-Xa and 100 for PTT). Identifying this difference was important for determining the clinical approach in using anti-Xa for monitoring bleeding risk rather than PTT at the institution.

While this example did not directly use AI in creating a model, it is instructive regarding the challenges of using AI models for three primary reasons. First, there was a clear difference in the two tests and how they could be used clinically, but this wasn't apparent from many of the standard comparison approaches that are often used to evaluate AI algorithms. Rule-based approaches would be similar to a concordance matrix in their calculation approach, and regression or statistical models would be similar to the frequency distributions or regression lines. It took careful consideration of the clinical decision-making process to identify the trend. This could be identified by AI algorithms but likely only if the variable of the threshold bleed rate were determined a priori.

The second challenge relates to the actual data. These data were in many ways simpler than data that may often be used in EHR mining, in that they were numeric laboratory values. However, it took expert understanding to realize that the non-numeric values in the database of ">200" for PTT and "<0.1" for anti-Xa should be included. We did not perform a separate analysis that excluded these values, so we cannot for certain say that they needed to be included, but they contained meaning as if they were numeric values, specifically that they were above or below the therapeutic range. If nothing else, decision rules that may use the numeric values should be able to interpret how the non-numeric comparatives should be applied in the rules.

The third challenge is more subtle but also more important. This relates to how the analytic solution was reached. In the end, the analysis did not reveal something as a new hypothesis, that there was a difference in the PTT and anti-Xa values that could be important for predicting bleeding. The data analysis only verified a pattern that had been seen when experts reviewed data from a series of cases with adverse events. The pattern identification from experts was much more efficient than the complicated data analysis that verified the pattern. The verification was important, but the initial hypothesis drawn from a smaller set of examples was more important in identifying the hypothesis in the first place. Often such hypotheses are developed after observing a trend in the data that seems to indicate a significant issue. For example, if the adverse event rate was near 50% (high but not extreme for LVADs), the probability of seeing 8 patients with adverse events in a row would be 1/256 (2^{-8}), or <0.4%. This is similar to having 8 coin flips all end up "heads", which is remarkable. However, when considered among many events as a run of 8, the probability is much higher. In terms of coin flips, a run of 8 heads in a row among 200 coin flips is not nearly as rare, with a not-so-remarkable 32% probability of occurring at least once. This suggests that similar random sequences that appear rare may lead experts to perform a deeper analysis of an issue in a way that identifies underlying patterns that were not seen before. In comparing cognitive capabilities of human beings to AI methods, people may be better at identifying patterns in complex data, and worse at interpreting sequences that occur amid data reflecting random variation.

These two examples highlight important challenges when using AI in health systems management, which may be indicated by the challenges of demonstrating consistent and successful adoption of AI approaches. The second example demonstrates how the underlying data or hypothesis development can be challenging for AI development. The first example demonstrates how even when successfully implemented, AI solutions can require significant additional management and monitoring to be sustained. Other examples in AI show similar challenges [24]. Often the focus on AI is about algorithm performance, which is understandable since the algorithm is what makes it work. However, once the algorithms have been demonstrated as correct in output (which many algorithms in health systems management have), the primary challenge becomes implementation and sustainable maintenance. As a result, **governance** of resources to manage AI should be a major focus. This migration of focus from performance to governance is similar for rule-based clinical decision support (CDS) as mentioned above. Governance is critical for managing AI solutions in health systems.

Governance

Implementing AI in health systems requires practical interaction with the many systems necessary to get any technology in production. There are three main areas of governance that intersect in order to manage an AI model effectively: *Corporate Governance*, *IT Governance* and *Data Governance*.

- *Corporate Governance* provides the overall clinical and operational strategy and ethical framework for implementing AI models.
- *IT Governance* provides for the prioritization of technology investments, including the work necessary for predictive models, as well as for clinical or operational ownership and stewardship of the models.
- *Data Governance* provides governance over the underlying data that is critical for the initial development and ongoing management of the predictive models.

All three areas are necessary and must be integrated in order for AI models to be successfully able to meet the overall intended goals of the health system. (NOTE: Both IT and Data Governance are considered to be elements of Corporate Governance. We'll discuss each in turn below.)

Corporate Governance In our current environment, it is crucial that organizations develop and communicate a point of view regarding the ethical use of AI models. Fortunately, health care has a lot of experience with ethical risk management, and the Harvard Business Review offered up this long history as a model for other industries as they consider the application of AI models.

> Leaders should take inspiration from health care, an industry that has been systematically focused on ethical risk mitigation since at least the 1970s. Key concerns about what constitutes privacy, self-determination, and informed consent, for example, have been explored deeply by medical ethicists, health care practitioners, regulators, and lawyers [25].

The opportunity here is to take advantage of (hopefully) existing corporate structures and committees within a health system that are already engaged with ethical decision-making, and to ensure that AI models are brought under this same governance. These structures need to weigh in and provide overall direction and guardrails that the other two areas of governance can follow. For example, clinical committees that already consider decision support systems, including ways to minimize alert fatigue, should be engaged in discussions about clinical AI models. Similarly, committees currently addressing issues of access to care and equity should be engaged in discussions and provide direction on how to evaluate models for bias.

IT Governance IT Governance is a framework for making decisions about what technology investments will be made, how those technologies will be managed, and ultimately to ensure the delivery of value to the organization. AI models should be brought under IT governance and control and identified key stakeholders should be able to establish conditions for the ethical and appropriate use of models that meet the Corporate Governance directives. At the same time, health systems are being pressured to be agile from innovators and researchers who are discovering new opportunities to improve patient care and delivery.

Organizations like Mayo Clinic ("Mayo") and UW Medicine ("UWM") have been working on governance models for AI. Mayo Clinic recently shared their governance model that includes integrating the EHR AI governance with an existing Clinical Decision Support Subcommittee. They described the role of this committee as overseeing the overall implementation and priorities, but specify that "Specialty Practice Committee approval needed for both phases and will be governing body for ongoing use/maintenance." The development phases are described below:

Phase I:
- Configure model, migrate and activate in production
- Run in background several months to localize/train
- Validate to check performance against expected results

Phase II:
- Operationalize by building tools (e.g., BPAs, dashboards)
- Develop workflows, communicate and train practice
- Maintain, annually evaluate performance and relevance

This approach has many parallels with the governance model developed at UW Medicine. A new subcommittee was formed with clinical and technical membership, named the Predictive Analytics Oversight Committee. This committee is integrated into the IT Governance committee structure, but is responsible for oversight of the overall AI implementation process and strategy. Each model has a requirement that it be "clinically/operationally led and managed," and the appropriate committee and leadership must be engaged as sponsors. The phases for the work have a similar path, outlined below (Fig. 15.7):

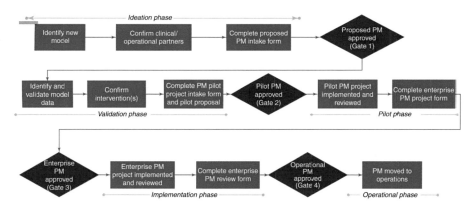

Fig. 15.7 Predictive analytics review phases. This pathway was created to assist governance of an organization's predictive analytics implementation products. *PM* predictive model

Models are independently evaluated at multiple steps in this process, including specific evaluations for patient outcomes, bias and impact to provider experience. Given the limited resources to implement models, the evaluation also factors into prioritization and schedules for implementing a specific model. Similar to the Mayo approach, the Operational Phase requires ongoing regular evaluation of the models to confirm the model is still relevant and performant.

Data Governance Most current AI approaches have been around for decades but it took large datasets and fast processors for them to find the levels of adoption seen recently (see Chap. 2). An early tenet of predictive analytics was that large data sets could overcome issues with data quality, but there are recent examples where that has been disproven [20]. AI models need high quality and timely data, and healthcare data requires appropriate data security. Healthcare data suffers from many data quality, currency and security issues:

- data collection by EHR's has been focused on the data necessary for billing purposes
- data are mostly collected and captured from busy human beings under stress
- much of the truly valuable data is captured in unstructured notes and resistant to easy feature engineering
- healthcare systems are still investing in the level of automated data entry and integration that other industries take for granted
- many organizations have defaulted to data silos in order to address data security requirements

The Data Management Book of Knowledge (DMBOK) describes Data Governance as "the exercise of authority and control over the management of data assets" [26]. A successful predictive model program in health care is dependent on maturing data governance and management to ensure optimal quality data, that is available to the right audience, with the appropriate performance and security controls.

Data pipelines will need to be architected, developed and managed in order to meet the timing needs of AI models. Critical data used by predictive models needs to be identified and real time data quality controls and alerts may be needed to monitor and manage these data over time. This monitoring can serve as an early warning that a predictive model's performance will degrade. Finally, the development of predictive models can be scaled and accelerated with the widespread adoption of meta-data management technologies, such as data dictionaries, data lineage, report catalogs, data quality dashboards, etc. This self-service infrastructure for using data assets enables a much larger range of users to identify and leverage data to develop new AI models in their own domain areas. The development of **citizen data scientists** is a significant enablement function that can have a high reward.

Operations and Maintenance As stated above, the final step in the AI implementation process is a formal transition to an operational state. The step prior to moving a model to an operational state calls for a final evaluation of the model, and the completion of an operational intake form. This step collects information about the dependent data fields, the clinical/operational owners, an agreed upon cadence for regularly reviewing and updating the model, and ensures that the model and its descriptive information is added to a published portfolio. The dependent data fields are identified as critical fields within the data governance process so that they can be specifically reviewed for changes, and the impact of broader changes that affect data can be appropriately managed in the affected models.

While the application of governance to AI in health systems management is complex due to the complexity of the algorithms and the data, much of the governance is similar to clinical decision support governance, which has been more established. Wright et al. reviewed governance structures across multiple institutions in managing clinical decision support applications [12]. They identified six recommended practices for CDS governance, which while named differently, map closely to the governance stages described here. These practices include considering and monitoring impact, assessing changes, and ongoing monitoring. Due to the deep data dependency of AI models, the monitoring must extend more deeply into the data rather than just changes to the rules as recommended for CDS, but otherwise the practices are similar.

Concluding Remarks

In this chapter, we have discussed the use of AI or predictive analytics in health systems management. We identified studies showing that they can be successfully implemented, but contrasted that with reviews that showed challenges in broader adoption. To elucidate these challenges, we gave two detailed examples that explained the challenges both in terms of understanding data complexity and implementation. We have argued the importance of governance due to these challenges, and documented a verified governance approach for implementing and maintaining AI applications. Our primary conclusion is that successful use of intelligent systems in health systems management has been demonstrated and is possible, but it requires appropriate management of its use. As institutions were applying clinical decision support applications that had been demonstrated at individual organizations, Kawamoto et al. studied factors related to the success of CDS implementations [27]. They found that factors related to implementation were significant in determining whether they were successful or not. As demonstrated by these examples and governance recommendations, the success factors are similar; it is less about what is being implemented, and more about how it is applied.

Questions for Discussion

- What is an example of an application of AI in health systems management? What is the beneficial effect of that application on the health system?
- How are the terms "artificial intelligence" and "predictive analytics" similar? What are some differences in meaning between them?

- What are some of the challenges that may be faced when implementing a predictive analytics solution for resource management in a health system? How might these challenges be different from implementing a standard rule-based clinical decision support application?
- What are the different phases of governance for AI implementation? For each phase, what might be the consequences if the phase is not used correctly?

Further Reading

Wehbe RM, Khan SS, Shah SJ, Ahmad FS. Predicting high-risk patients and high-risk outcomes in heart failure. Heart Fail Clin. 2020;16(4):387–407.

- This paper reviews different applications of AI to health systems management and identifies some of the challenges. These challenges are important to be addressed by governance.

Bellini V, Guzzon M, Bigliardi B, Mordonini M, Filippelli S, Bignami E. Artificial Intelligence: a new tool in operating room management. Role of machine learning models in operating room optimization. J Med Syst. 2019;44(1):20.

- This paper reviews different applications of AI in operating room optimization, which is a common area for AI application in health systems management. The review covers various areas of the operating room workflow where AI has been applied.

Wright A, Sittig DF, Ash JS, Bates DW, Feblowitz J, Fraser G, Maviglia SM, McMullen C, Nichol WP, Pang JE, Starmer J, Middleton B. Governance for clinical decision support: case studies and recommended practices from leading institutions. J Am Med Inform Assoc. 2011;18(2):187–94.

- This review of decision support implementations gives specific recommendations for governance, which are similar to the governance recommendations here.

Blackman R. A Practical guide to building ethical AI. Harv Bus Rev. 2020; https://hbr.org/2020/10/a-practical-guide-to-building-ethical-ai.

- This article describes steps that companies, including those in healthcare, can take to ensure AI is implemented in a way that addresses ethical risks of using AI.

References

1. Aktas E, Ulengin F, Önsel Ş. A decision support system to improve the efficiency of resource allocation in healthcare management. Socio Econ Plan Sci. 2007;41:130–46.
2. Gartner D, Padman R. Improving hospital-wide early resource allocation through machine learning. Stud Health Technol Inform. 2015;216:315–9.
3. Dennis BM, Stonko DP, Callcut RA, Sidwell RA, Stassen NA, Cohen MJ, et al. Artificial neural networks can predict trauma volume and acuity regardless of center size and geography: a multicenter study. J Trauma Acute Care Surg. 2019;87(1):181–7.

4. Lee S-Y, Chinnam RB, Dalkiran E, Krupp S, Nauss M. Prediction of emergency department patient disposition decision for proactive resource allocation for admission. Health Care Manag Sci. 2020;23(3):339–59.
5. McCoy TH, Pellegrini AM, Perlis RH. Assessment of time-series machine learning methods for forecasting hospital discharge volume. JAMA Netw Open. 2018;1(7):e184087.
6. Vermeulen IB, Bohte SM, Elkhuizen SG, Lameris H, Bakker PJM, La Poutré H. Adaptive resource allocation for efficient patient scheduling. Artif Intell Med. 2009;46(1):67–80.
7. Kontio E, Airola A, Pahikkala T, Lundgren-Laine H, Junttila K, Korvenranta H, et al. Predicting patient acuity from electronic patient records. J Biomed Inform. 2014;51:35–40.
8. Bellini V, Guzzon M, Bigliardi B, Mordonini M, Filippelli S, Bignami E. Artificial intelligence: a new tool in operating room management. role of machine learning models in operating room optimization. J Med Syst. 2019;44(1):20.
9. Wehbe RM, Khan SS, Shah SJ, Ahmad FS. Predicting high-risk patients and high-risk outcomes in heart failure. Heart Fail Clin. 2020;16(4):387–407.
10. Kaplan B. Evaluating informatics applications--some alternative approaches: theory, social interactionism, and call for methodological pluralism. Int J Med Inform. 2001;64(1):39–56.
11. Sittig DF, Wright A, Osheroff JA, Middleton B, Teich JM, Ash JS, et al. Grand challenges in clinical decision support. J Biomed Inform. 2008;41(2):387–92.
12. Wright A, Sittig DF, Ash JS, Bates DW, Feblowitz J, Fraser G, et al. Governance for clinical decision support: case studies and recommended practices from leading institutions. J Am Med Inform Assoc JAMIA. 2011;18(2):187–94.
13. Cronin PR, Kimball AB. Success of automated algorithmic scheduling in an outpatient setting. Am J Manag Care. 2014;20(7):570–6.
14. Kheirkhah P, Feng Q, Travis LM, Tavakoli-Tabasi S, Sharafkhaneh A. Prevalence, predictors and economic consequences of no-shows. BMC Health Serv Res. 2016;16:13.
15. Shah SJ, Cronin P, Hong CS, Hwang AS, Ashburner JM, Bearnot BI, et al. Targeted reminder phone calls to patients at high risk of no-show for primary care appointment: a randomized trial. J Gen Intern Med. 2016;31(12):1460–6.
16. Percac-Lima S, Cronin PR, Ryan DP, Chabner BA, Daly EA, Kimball AB. Patient navigation based on predictive modeling decreases no-show rates in cancer care. Cancer. 2015;121(10):1662–70.
17. Hwang AS, Atlas SJ, Cronin P, Ashburner JM, Shah SJ, He W, et al. Appointment "no-shows" are an independent predictor of subsequent quality of care and resource utilization outcomes. J Gen Intern Med. 2015;30(10):1426–33.
18. Cronin PR, Greenwald JL, Crevensten GC, Chueh HC, Zai AH. Development and implementation of a real-time 30-day readmission predictive model. AMIA Annu Symp Proc AMIA Symp. 2014;2014:424–31.
19. Greenwald JL, Cronin PR, Carballo V, Danaei G, Choy G. A novel model for predicting rehospitalization risk incorporating physical function, cognitive status, and psychosocial support using natural language processing. Med Care. 2017;55(3):261–6.
20. Wong A, Otles E, Donnelly JP, Krumm A, McCullough J, DeTroyer-Cooley O, et al. External validation of a widely implemented proprietary sepsis prediction model in hospitalized patients. JAMA Intern Med. 2021;181(8):1065–70.
21. Saifee N, Mahr C, Garcia D, Estergreen J, Sabath D. PTT and anti-Xa activity in adult mechanical circulatory support patients at a large academic medical center. Am J Clin Pathol. 2018;149(suppl_1):S174–5.
22. Adatya S, Uriel N, Yarmohammadi H, Holley CT, Feng A, Roy SS, et al. Anti-factor Xa and activated partial thromboplastin time measurements for heparin monitoring in mechanical circulatory support. JACC Heart Fail. 2015;3(4):314–22.
23. Tsiouris A, Paone G, Nemeh HW, Borgi J, Williams CT, Lanfear DE, et al. Short and long term outcomes of 200 patients supported by continuous-flow left ventricular assist devices. World J Cardiol. 2015;7(11):792–800.

24. STAT. Once billed as a revolution in medicine, IBM's Watson Health is sold off in parts. STAT. 2022. https://www.statnews.com/2022/01/21/ibm-watson-health-sale-equity/. Accessed 1 Feb 2022.
25. Blackman R. A practical guide to building ethical AI. Harv Bus Rev. 2020. https://hbr.org/2020/10/a-practical-guide-to-building-ethical-ai.
26. International D. DAMA-DMBOK: data management body of knowledge. 2nd ed. Basking Ridge, NJ: Technics Publications; 2017. 590 p.
27. Kawamoto K, Houlihan CA, Balas EA, Lobach DF. Improving clinical practice using clinical decision support systems: a systematic review of trials to identify features critical to success. BMJ. 2005;330(7494):765.

Chapter 16
Intelligent Systems in Learning and Education

Vimla L. Patel and Parvati Dev

After reading this chapter, you should know the answers to these questions:
- How has intelligent system-based medical education evolved from the days of Sir William Osler?
- What kinds of intelligent educational tools currently exist to support health professionals' education and training?
- What is the nature of mapping between learning with intelligent system tools and applying this learning in clinical practice?
- What are some of the challenges of using artificial intelligence tools for health professional education as we move to the future?

Introduction

Artificial Intelligence (AI) use is increasing rapidly in all fields, and it will have a significant impact on the way the doctors' practice medicine. However, the training that students and medical residents receive, about the importance of AI for their clinical practices, is woefully inadequate [1]. At the same time, the potential of using AI in the learning process has also not been completely realized in healthcare.

V. L. Patel (✉)
New York Academy of Medicine, New York, NY, USA
e-mail: vpatel@nyam.org

P. Dev
SimTabs LLC, Los Altos Hills, CA, USA
e-mail: parvati@parvatidev.org

© The Author(s), under exclusive license to Springer Nature Switzerland AG 2022
T. A. Cohen et al. (eds.), *Intelligent Systems in Medicine and Health*, Cognitive Informatics in Biomedicine and Healthcare,
https://doi.org/10.1007/978-3-031-09108-7_16

AI-based systems, such as intelligent tutoring systems [ITS], can change mass education to personalized education, helping each learner to proceed at his/her own pace, with a curriculum that is dynamically sequenced to achieve the individual learning goals.

The amount of medical knowledge has long exceeded the organizing capability of the human brain. Yet the curricula remain information-based, prioritizing memorization over reasoning and managing information. The underlying assumption is that physicians should be the major source of medical information. However, this assumption is untenable given the vast, publicly available, online sources of medical information. For example, AI-based personalized medicine will require the new practicing physician to be able to understand the basis of this personalization and to explain this, along with the resulting treatment options, to their patients. Consequently, the skills taught to a new generation of physicians must move from remembering or acquiring information to collaborating with AI applications that gather data from multiple sensors, search vast quantities of information, generate diagnoses, suggest treatments, and offer confidence ratings for their suggestions [2, 3] (Chap. 19). These abilities must also be complemented by the development of physicians' higher-order judgment and decision-making skills to evaluate the quality of information generated to be useful in clinical practice. In this context, in the best of two worlds, physicians learn new ways to work in their practices, and AI systems gain from a better understanding of human context.

This chapter will examine how medical education systems have evolved over time, and their potential to incorporate AI-based systems for the learner, the teacher, and the education enterprise. The chapter will review the status of intelligent learning tools in medical education and examine to what extent and within what limits such learning systems map to real world practices. Finally, the chapter will take a longer view and will look at the future profiles of physicians' practices in 10 years, given the recent pandemic-driven trend to remote learning and telehealth. What knowledge and skills will be required for the practicing physicians in the next decade?

Historical Evolution of Medical Education: Philosophical Perspectives and Related Educational Strategies

Healthcare delivery has changed dramatically since Osler established the first modern residency training system at the Johns Hopkins Hospital in 1889 [4, 5]. He was the first to bring medical students out of the lecture hall for hands-on bedside clinical training, where he encouraged medical residents to learn through observing, talking, listening, and touching the patient. As medical and scientific knowledge was expanding at an unprecedented rate, Osler's philosophy continued to be recognized in the basic structure of medical education, with its mix of classroom-based teaching and experiential learning through activities such as bedside rounds and clinical services. As our healthcare system began to evolve further, our training of the next generation of physicians also changed. US medical schools began to use diverse education systems, resulting in more informal training with no specific standards. In 1910, a commissioned report by Abraham Flexner to evaluate medical education programs in the US had a huge impact and shaped modern medical education [6]. To provide a scientific basis to medical education and training, the medical curriculum was divided into basic science and an applied clinical component, separating science from practice. In response to the pure biomedical education and training model, alternative curricula began to spring up around North America.

Our medical education system is still evolving over 100 years after the Flexner report. Current programs reflect a more hybrid model, with Flexnerian-based scientifically grounded clinicians, who are clinically skilled at the bedside, as advocated by Osler. Although intelligent technology has revolutionized medical training [7]. Osler and Flexner's fundamental principles of science and medicine have not changed with similar issues confronting us today.

Acquisition of Clinical Competence

The primary goal of clinical education is the acquisition of competencies that are integral to the functioning of clinicians. Medical trainees must develop competence in several clinical skills (performance-oriented) and competence in understanding domain concepts necessary for supporting clinical problem solving and interpersonal skills. In addition, competence needs to be demonstrated in applying and transferring knowledge and skills from training situations to the "real-world" clinical environment. The use of intelligent systems introduces a layer of complexity, where training with these systems, in simulation contexts, mimics the challenges in transfer to real-world practice.

The assessment of clinical competence is typically based on Bloom's taxonomy of educational objectives. Although his original 1956 taxonomy [8] included the cognitive domain, these categories were ordered based on complexity and abstraction. The taxonomy was considered hierarchical in that a simpler category would need to be mastered before mastery of a more complex one. A revised Bloom's taxonomy [9, 10] moved from a one-dimensional (*Knowledge*) to a two-dimensional (*Knowledge* and *Cognitive Processes*) framework. Cognitive research uncovered aspects of learning that were not reflected in the original taxonomy. Studies have shown that in a complex domain such as medicine, people do not work in a linear fashion, but follow a non-linear pattern of activity, yet decision support systems, such as those embedded in electronic health records [EHRs] are designed and standardized for a linear workflow [11, 12]. Bloom's revised taxonomy suggests how more linear learning objectives can be supplemented with non-linear learning to reflect how people work and learn in complex environments. A digital taxonomy was created based on Bloom's taxonomy, which is restricted to the cognitive domain [13], containing cognitive elements, methods, and tools. The digital taxonomy is about the effective use of technology to facilitate learning.

Cognitive Approaches to Learning and Instruction

A National Research Council report [14] on advancing scientific research in education reports a lack of rigorous research in designing education programs, recommending the development of tools for education and training to consider a scientific foundation for learning and instruction. Theoretical and methodological advances in the cognitive and learning sciences have greatly influenced curriculum, instruction, and learning in biomedicine [15]. Empirical studies on the role of memory, knowledge organization, and reasoning as well as studies of problem-solving and decision-making in the medical domain led to a more informed curriculum about how people think and learn, and more specifically, how clinical expertise is developed [16].

There are two major cognitive learning theories: one focuses on individual structured learning (**ACT-R**, [17]; **Cognitive Load Theory**, [18, 19]), and the other on constructivist learning theories (Situative theory, [20]; Cognitive Flexibility Theory, [21]), which focus on complex learning within interacting systems. Although they often appear to be conflicting, researchers have argued [22, 24], both perspectives are essential in learning and instruction. Ultimately, both perspectives provide significant and valuable insights into how effective performance and learning occur (see Table 16.1). Research in both these programs has resulted in necessary knowledge about human learning that can inform the designs of effective learning environments and instructional methods.

Table 16.1 Cognitive theories of learning relevant to medical education and training, showing basic concepts, conceptual differences, and diverse emphases (Published with permission from [23])

Theory	Basic concepts	Most applicable	Example
Adaptive Character of Thought-Rational (ACT-R)	Declarative and procedural knowledge, production rules	Well-structured domains, formal knowledge acquisition	Learning of anatomy, basic biochemistry using cognitive tutors
Cognitive Load Theory (CLT	Cognitive load, working memory, memory limitations	Well-structured domains and somewhat ill-structured domains; formal knowledge	Learning of basic clinical medicine in classroom situations; design of instructional materials
Situativity Theory	Situation, context, activity system, social interaction, collaboration	Ill-structured domains, apprenticeship	Learning in residency training involving interactions with clinical teams; acquisition of tacit knowledge
Cognitive Flexibility Theory (CFT)	Advanced learning, conceptual understanding involving abstract concepts	Formal learning of complex concepts, conceptual structures	Learning of advanced physiology, genetics, and clinical medicine during specialization

The situative theorists propose that cognition does not always involve the manipulation of symbols, but rather that agents in activity are involved in many cognitive processes by directly using aspects of the world around them without the mediation of symbols. The learning of surgery, for instance, is an example of **situated learning** in that the surgery apprentice learns to perform different tasks without having to represent symbolically the procedures involved in such tasks. Much of clinical performance, especially in routine situations, involves non-deliberative aspects, where **deliberation** would result in considerable inefficiency in performance. For example, in the diagnostic tasks in perceptual domains, such as dermatology and radiology, a significant degree of skilled performance relies on pattern recognition rather than deliberative reasoning. Furthermore, numerous clinical problems require rapid responses, such as in emergencies, where **deliberative reasoning** is not possible. In such cases, the situated approach can be used to characterize cognition as a process of directly using resources in the environment, rather than using **reflective thinking** to arrive at conclusions [20, 25]. The notion of a direct connection with one's environment is prominent in cognitive engineering [26], and human-computer interaction research [27]. Here, well-designed artifacts can be closely adapted to human needs and capabilities through the appropriate use of invariant features (e.g., panels on a screen display) [28]. Well-designed technologies provide "**affordances**" that are perceptually obvious to the user, making human interactions with objects virtually effortless [29]. Affordances refer to attributes of objects that enable individuals to know how to use them (e.g., a door handle affords turning or pushing downward to open a door).

One situated approach emerged from the investigation and development of intelligent systems that support performance in complex "dynamic real-world environment." Severe time constraints characterize such systems and continuously changing conditions in emergency departments, surgical operating rooms, or intensive care units [30].

The well-documented problem of implementing intelligent systems in training mirrors the gap between theories of learning and their application to medical practice. The notion of learning in context is one of the most important messages for education and even more critical with more sophisticated and intelligent systems. Well-designed, theory-based education and training programs are needed for the future healthcare workforce, where the development of these systems needs to be more user-centered, augmenting human intelligence. This argument begs for a careful evaluation of AI education systems before they are disseminated widely for use in education and training programs (Chap. 17). This allows us to reexamine and redefine the current technology design by considering these intelligent systems' different roles for various functions.

In summary, how does history enlighten us about the current education system in the digital age? Earlier, the medical education curriculum reflected the philosophy of William Osler, who famously stated, "Listen to your patient, he is telling you the diagnosis". Reconsidered from a complexity stance, Osler's suggestion hints at the insights clinicians may gain by viewing the patient as an embodiment of embedded complex systems (through biological and disease mechanisms), and as an individual whose health and the embeddedness of other complex systems shapes healthcare

Flexner's report, which followed, had a distinctive feature of the thoroughness with which theoretical and scientific knowledge were combined with what experience teaches in the practical responsibility of taking care of a patient. The revision of Bloom's Taxonomy reorganized the learning taxonomy into a higher-order cognitive hierarchy. Connecting Bloom's Revised Taxonomy characteristics was necessary for creating online learning activities according to students' needs. Bloom's **Digital Taxonomy** guides us to navigate various digital tools to match learning experiences for specific groups of students. Selecting the most appropriate digital activity depends on the level of difficulty associated with the cognitive levels stated within Bloom's Revised Taxonomy.

Approaches to Artificial Intelligence in Education and Training

AI has applications in learning, teaching and education management. However, much of today's technology in education is a one-way transmission of information, often using engaging methods of graphics, animation, and interaction. Feedback, if provided, is not personalized to the learner's level of knowledge or progress. A learning system is considered to be intelligent if it customizes its content and delivery, in real-time, based on learner performance, errors, misconceptions, needs and affect, and based on principles of cognitive and learning sciences. Underlying intelligent systems are a panoply of AI tools and methods, as well as a range of methods to represent data so that they can be operated on by AI tools, to move a learner along a path to an end-state of knowledge, skills and behavior competence (Fig. 16.1).

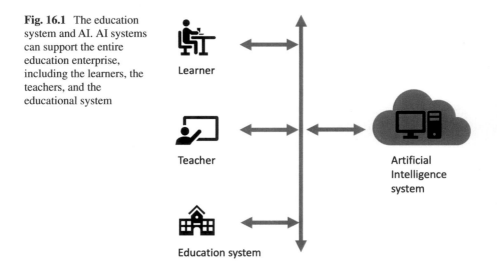

Fig. 16.1 The education system and AI. AI systems can support the entire education enterprise, including the learners, the teachers, and the educational system

Learner

Teacher

Artificial Intelligence system

Education system

AI tools can be applied to the individual learner, the teacher, as well as to the education enterprise. For the individual learner, the greatest promise is in personalizing learning and learning materials. AI systems can adapt pedagogic practices to individual learners and can allow learners to learn at their own pace. Such systems have been most successful in well-defined knowledge areas, such as school-level mathematics [31]. AI-based instructional systems are not yet widely available in healthcare, nor is continuous AI-augmented evaluation of learner or education program performance.

The next section will describe technology and studies on intelligent systems for educating the individual learner, followed by a description of the possible uses of AI methods in analyzing and improving the education enterprise.

Artificial Intelligence Systems and the Individual Learner

AI has the potential to curate and deliver knowledge at the point of need. At the same time, it is essential for the practitioner to understand the AI technology underlying new healthcare services such as imaging diagnostics, identification of biomarkers, and population health recommendations. Introductory courses are being designed to address the understanding of AI technology in healthcare practice [32]. However, AI-based learning systems, to support optimal knowledge delivery, are not in wide use yet.

The next section will examine the various components of AI systems for use in individual learning in medical education.

Computable Representations

For an AI system to function, it requires a formal, **computable representation** of the knowledge (content), skills (tasks, actions, or behaviors) and strategies (reasoning and decision-making underlying the use of specific knowledge or skills) that an expert may be expected to know. It may also contain the misconceptions, incorrect skills, and mistaken strategies that may be common when learning this domain. The data structure must be a formal, computable representation, so that learning objectives can be defined, such as a state in feature space, and a learner's progress can be assessed by movement towards a desired state. Inevitably, a domain model represents a subset of the actual domain. It may simplify the actual content, may leave out non-essential components, or may be unable to represent ill-defined areas. Further, any representation of a domain may be implementable in different data structures, for example as a graph, an ontology, or a feature vector space.

Fig. 16.2 The components
in an Intelligent Tutoring
System

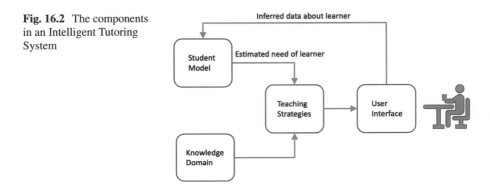

Intelligent Tutoring Systems

An Intelligent Tutoring System (ITS) models the learning process so as to provide personalized instruction or feedback to learners, without requiring intervention from a human teacher. It usually has the following four components: The Domain model, the Learner model, the Pedagogy model, and the Interface model (Fig. 16.2).

The **domain model** contains a formal, computable representation of the knowledge, skills and strategies, as described above. It also includes misconceptions, incorrect skills, and mistaken strategies. The learning objectives are defined as states in domain space, and a learner's progress is assessed by movement towards a desired state.

The **learner model** represents the learner's current state in the domain space, and is updated in real-time as the learner progresses through the learning exercises. For example, the learner model can be a record of the knowledge states that have been mastered within a domain model with a much larger set of possible knowledge states. The learner model and the domain model are compared, using tools such as Bayesian statistics, to select the next problem which will correct a misconception or fill in a deficit. The learner model may also include the affective and motivational state of the learner as a guide to the tutoring process.

The **pedagogical model** represents and selects effective approaches to teaching. These approaches include typical human pedagogic approaches such as providing new knowledge, assessing the student's knowledge to give hints, guidance or feedback, and allowing the student to explore and make mistakes (productive failure) before guiding them back to the correct path. The pedagogic model uses the domain and student models as input to select the instructional strategy to move the learner's state closer to a desired state in the domain model. Because there must be a correspondence between computational methods in the pedagogy model and representations in the learner model, they must be designed in tandem. For example, ITSs that teach using conversational dialog will use computational techniques that match words, phrases, and sentences in the learner's answer to recommended sentence-based preferred answers in the domain model, by using content matching, latent sematic analysis or other statistical methods based on features present in conversation. The pedagogical model moves learning forward by generating the next instructional step but can also respond to learner questions or requests for help.

The **interface model** enables the dialog between the ITS and the learner. While the interface model is not directly a component of pedagogy, its structure is important in how information is exchanged between the learner and the ITS. The learner receives information from the ITS through text and multimedia on the screen, through audio and, increasingly, through viewing simulations in immersive three-dimensional (3D) virtual worlds. The learner then responds through available devices such as keyboard, text, voice, and gestural or haptic devices. For ITS systems that include detection and use of affective states, the interface may include sensors for eye-tracking, facial expression detection, or neural state tracking.

Kulik and Fletcher [33] reviewed the effectiveness of ITSs, based on published studies, and found that students who received intelligent tutoring outperformed control students on posttests in 46 (or 92%) of the 50 studies included in the meta-analysis. Successes were particularly evident in systems where the domain knowledge could be formally represented and where the assessment method was based on the same representation as the digital content. Examples are the DARPA Digital Tutor for teaching information technology systems to Navy personnel [34], the Geometry Tutor for high school geometry [35], and iTutor for engineering mechanics [36]. Similarly, Ma et al. [37] showed that the only learning environment which out-performed the use of ITS was the small group learning environment.

Dialog Systems and Natural Language Processing

Bickmore and Wallace (Chap. 7) have provided an in-depth review of issues underlying current dialog systems. While there are many healthcare simulations and games that include or require dialog between the learner and a character in the simulation, only a few use AI to generate any part of the conversation. Commercial technologies such as Amazon's Alexa, Apple's Siri, or Google Home, or customized software from Recourse Medical or SimConverse, can generate conversation between a virtual patient and a learner. However, they do not apply the principles of Intelligent Tutoring to guide and coach the learner. AutoTutor is an example of a dialog or tri-alog based ITS.

AutoTutor is an ITS augmented with Natural Language Processing (NLP) that has been applied in numerous subject areas [38]. It simulates the conversation patterns of human tutors, based on analysis of human-to-human tutoring sessions and theoretically-grounded tutoring strategies based on cognitive learning principles [39]. AutoTutor's dialogues are system-driven and are organized around difficult questions and problems that require reasoning and explanations in the answers. The

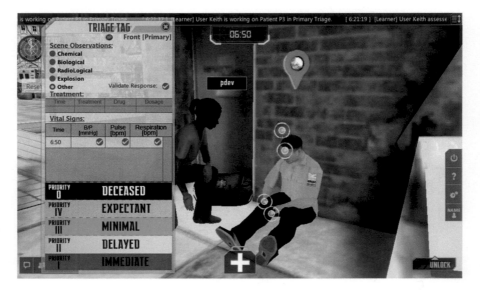

Fig. 16.3 The Virtual Civilian Aeromedical Evacuation Sustainment Training Program (V-CAEST) teaches triage processes for mass casualty

major components of AutoTutor include an animated conversational agent who initiates the dialog, dialogue management, speech act classification, a curriculum script, semantic evaluation of student contributions, and digital resources, such as a textbook or a procedure manual.

A medically relevant example is the Virtual Civilian Aeromedical Evacuation Sustainment Training program (V-CAEST), a learning simulation for teaching mass-casualty triage and aero-evacuation during an emergency [40, 41], that uses a web-based version of AutoTutor, AutoTutor Lite (Fig. 16.3). In V-CAEST, a team of learners enter the virtual environment, an earthquake disaster site, and search for injured casualties in the debris-covered streets. The learning task is to triage these victims correctly, assessing their need for medical intervention and air evacuation. The intelligent tutoring system intervenes if errors are made, and a digital tutor character walks the learner through the triage process, asking questions focused on the errors.

AutoTutor Lite uses natural language processing to analyze the learner's typed answers and matches the concepts against stored concepts of the ideal answer using **Latent Semantic Analysis**. With each answer, it updates its model of the learner's knowledge of that topic. Through hints and additional questions, the tutor prompts the learner to articulate a well-elaborated, detailed answer. When its model of the learner's knowledge is sufficiently like the stored model of that topic, the tutor lets the learner return to the simulation to continue triaging the victim or to search for another victim (Fig. 16.4) [42].

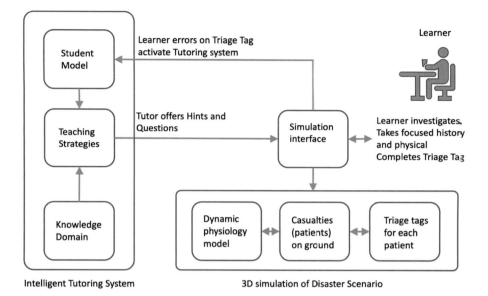

Fig. 16.4 The components of an Intelligent Tutoring System as applied to the V-CAEST program

Question Generation

Question answering is a common form of learner's mental assessment. Understanding assessment depends on understanding the process by which the learner generates the responses to the questions. However, generation of good questions with least amount of ambiguity, is time-consuming and prone to errors. Multiple choice questions (MCQ), in particular, are widely used as learning tools, for evaluating learner knowledge, and to assess efficacy of the instructional activity. Automatic MCQ generation from medical text has been shown to produce questions that are, for the most part, equivalent to traditionally developed items from the perspective of expert medical reviewers [43]. Leo and colleagues [44] present a system for generating case scenario-based questions using knowledge in a medical ontology system, Elsevier Merged Medical Taxonomy (EMMeT). They selected four MCQ question formats that are representative of scenario questions in texts for preparation for medical board examinations. Using these formats as question templates, and EMMeT as a content resource, they generated over three million questions of which a sample was evaluated by experts for appropriateness and difficulty. An important result in this evaluation was that review of generated MCQ questions was far faster than the process of generating each question by a human.

Dynamic Assessment, Feedback, and Guidance

AI has multiple applications within educational assessment, ranging from support of the learning process, to assessing whether learning was achieved [45]. The embedding of data collection within digital education products, paired with computational techniques, makes automated education data analytics feasible and useful. The most common use of analytics is for summative feedback and grading, including AI-based scoring of assignments. While this automation of a manual process is very helpful, an interesting approach is the application of AI-based assessment to support the learning process itself.

AI-based analytics can support dynamic assessment for continuous feedback and guidance for each individual learner. The role of assessment then shifts from one of assigning a final grade to that of being a coach, guiding the learner by supportive and corrective feedback. By shifting the emphasis from summative assessment to coaching for mastery learning, the educational system moves from assessment of learning to assessment for learning [46]. Realistically, this mode of assessment is possible only though the use of big data, that is, data obtained by digital observation of each step of the learner's progress through the instructional material. As described above, in the section on "Computable Representations", this approach requires that the representation of the knowledge to be learnt is in a computable format, to support algorithms that can identify the steps to guide the learner from a current state to the destination of goal state of knowledge.

Very few such AI-based dynamic, personalized assessment systems exist in medical education, except as experimental products. A particularly interesting one, albeit in computer science education, was deployed in a course on computer programming. This massive on-line course, taken by 12,000 students around the world, used an AI feedback system to detect and critique errors in code for individual students [47]. Over 16,000 such critiques were offered and, in 97.9% of the cases, the students agreed with the AI system's assessment. Guidance systems such as this are still in an early development stage, but could be applied in many areas, including medical diagnosis and patient treatment.

Machine Learning and Neural Networks

Machine learning has been applied extensively in using data from learning management systems to make the education delivery process more efficient [48]. For the individual learner, machine learning has the potential to be used to guide optimal learning based on the performance of a cohort of similar learners.

An early study [49] used neural nets to identify information gathering behavior of medical students as they worked through a clinical immunology case. Students with successful solutions demonstrated successful acquisition of the results of relevant diagnostic tests and clinical data. Unsuccessful solutions showed two patterns of performance. One showed extensive searching using a range of tests, demonstrating lack of recognition of relevant data. Another unsuccessful approach showed data collection biased towards solving an unrelated problem, that is, the students had the correct solution but to the wrong problem.

Some examples of the use of big data and analytics are discussed in the section on "Artificial Intelligence Systems and the Education Enterprise".

Affect and Emotion Aware ITS

Emotions are closely related to cognition and are an essential component of learning. Yet, the generation and measurement of emotion is not usually included in the development of technology-rich learning systems [50].

Pekrun [51] postulated a **control-value theory** of achievement emotions. He considered that activity-related emotions such as enjoyment, boredom and frustration, as well as outcome-related emotions such as pride, hopelessness, and danger, related to success or failure, needed to be considered when evaluating education systems. In a systematic meta-analysis of studies on technology-based educational systems, Loderer et al. [52] found that the emotion-level evoked differed across systems, but the relationship between emotions evoked and learning correlated with Pekrun's control-value theory.

Virtual and Augmented Reality

3D graphics and interaction add a dimension of realism that immerses the learner in the learning environment. **Virtual Reality** (VR) moves the 3D experience from the computer or tablet screen into a 3D environment that surrounds the learner. The experience can feel so real that moving through the visual environment, using gestures, while staying physically in one location, can induce motion sickness. **Augmented Reality** (AR) differs from virtual reality in that the real 3D environment remains visible but is overlaid with labels, pointers, or even a semi-transparent 3D virtual environment. Multi-user environments add collaboration capability by bringing others into the environment seen by the user, whether it is in VR, AR, or the computer screen. The use of AI tools and technology can be added to any aspect of 3D interactive simulations, VR or AR. This application of AI is not yet in wide use, so examples of possible new uses are presented.

Interaction within a VR or AR environment, while moving one's head, requires deep understanding of this environment. The incoming camera imagery is transformed into a 3D representation so that the controller in the user's hand (or the representation of the hand itself) recognizes the object's distance and touches it accurately. This capability is present in many 3D games. However, the interaction

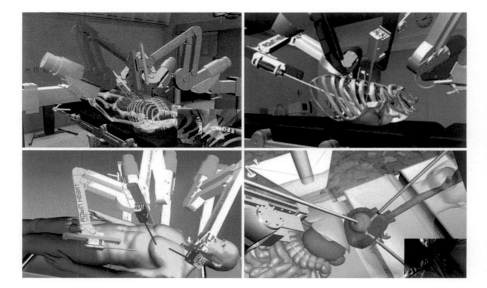

Fig. 16.5 This simulation (Virtual Reality operating room) is used for planning operations using Robin Heart robots (examples are for heart surgery) and for testing robots (in the conceptual phase), and training surgeons. The program was tested for use: (1) on a computer stand; (2) in the Robin Heart Shell 2 robot control console; (3) VR goggles (Oculus). The images are examples of how to visualize simulated operations. The last image outlines the green workspace available for the tool chosen by the surgeon. (Published with permission from [53])

between the hand and the object can be increasingly sophisticated, based on intelligent information about the object and the hand. Sculpting in 3D is an early example of sophisticated interaction between virtual hands and a virtual mass.

Extending this example into surgery, advanced advisory systems can be developed that bring together knowledge about surgical tools and the target tissue. Nawrat [53] demonstrates a prototype VR system for robotic surgery on the heart where the space available for tool movement is visualized relative to the heart and its surrounding anatomy. Aside from the geometric information available in the imagery, intelligence that can be embedded in the advice includes data about typical hand movements, resilience or fragility of the tissue, and common decision and movement errors (Fig. 16.5).

Simulations and Serious Games

Simulations and Serious Games have been shown to increase engagement in the learning process. The use of a Virtual Patient (VP), a simulated patient presented on the computer screen or in VR approximates the real-world experience of patient care, engages the learner, and focuses the learner's attention on the subject being presented [54, 55]. Screen-based virtual patients, with scripted reaction and

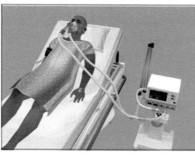

User view –
VR of patient and hospital,
Or screen view of patient in 3D

Dialog –
Speech recognition
Natural Language Processing
Conversational dialog / trialog
Data base of utterances

User actions –
Gestures, controller,
Haptic gloves, mouse

Physiology / Pharmacology mode –
Mathematical or rule-based mode,
with continuous updating based on
user queries

Equipment, fluids, medications –
AI-managed interaction
Inventory/availability

Tracking, Assessment, Feedback –
Usage analytics
Performance assessment
Feedback based on critical actions

Fig. 16.6 The numerous ways in which AI could augment the use of Virtual Patients in medical learning. The figure shows a virtual patient undergoing ventilation. AI could improve the user interface (natural language input, haptic sensation), augment the physiology model, make the simulated equipment and instruments aware of their interaction with the simulated patient, and track all interaction to provide guidance to the user in the learning process

feedback, are in wide use in medical and nursing curricula today (Fig. 16.6). However, the potential for introduction of AI technology is immense.

SimSTAT Anesthesia [56] is an example of a simulation that uses a rule-based AI model of patient physiology, for Maintenance of Certification by the American Society of Anesthesiologists. The simulation is viewed by the learner on a computer screen while the learner plays the role of the anesthesiologist. The learner guides the on-screen anesthesiologist to care for the unconscious patient by clicking on desired interactions, such as the equipment in the room or the icons at the bottom of the screen. Through these interactions, the learner can control the level of sedation, give medications, fluids, and gases, and monitor the patient's physiologic status in dynamic stability. The branching scenario, or story, makes the case appear different from learner to learner, based on their actions, and allows multiple passes through the case to experience the many possible outcomes for the patient. The learner's actions are recorded, and the simulation provides detailed summative feedback at the end of the case. The feedback evaluates whether key clinical actions were taken on time, and whether the ongoing status of the patient was held in a safe zone or allowed to deteriorate too dangerously, even if the patient finally was brought safely through the surgery.

Artificial Intelligence Systems and the Education Enterprise

Learning Analytics

Learning analytics is the measurement, collection, analysis and reporting of data about learners and their contexts, in order to understand and optimize learning. Ellaway et al. [57] point out that if health professional education is to be accountable for how its programs run and are developed, then health professional educators will need to be ready to deal with analytics and 'big data'. Analytic methodologies include descriptive analytics which examines past data to analyze all stages of the student life cycle, and to detect trends; diagnostic analytics, which focuses on the question "why did it happen"; and prescriptive analytics, for recommendations and advice on possible outcomes.[1]

As **Competency-Based Medical Education** (CBME) is introduced in graduate medical education, the volume of assessment data imposes a significant burden on faculty and supervisors. Learning analytics has the potential to process this data and provide insight that will support the assessment process. Chan et al. [58] review learning analytic techniques, with potential application for use by Clinical Competency Committees. In subsequent work, they present design-based research to investigate what issues may arise as faculty consider the use of learning analytics, as well as the importance of user input to the design of 'dashboard' or visualization methods that condense and present this data, when analyzing data on the progress of emergency medicine residents towards completion of Entrustable Professional Activities. Their research identified three sets of issues: challenges in implementation of data collection, such as changing international practices regarding data gathering; challenges in the processing of data, such as data security, analysis, access and governance; and challenges in the presentation of the analytics results, such as efficacy and ethical requirements. They also found that residents and faculty required significantly different visualizations in order to derive utility from the learning analytics 'dashboard' [59]. As design prototypes, these studies utilized a significant amount of manual data processing. However, they show the need for, and provide guidance on future research for more automated, AI approaches to medical education data analytics while retaining the role of the human instructor.

Continuous quality improvement of the medical education system. Boulet and Durning [60] point out that electronic medical records, unique provider identifiers and access to patient records, make it easier to conduct studies that link learning analytics data from medical schools and residency programs to quality of care by individual physicians (assuming appropriate care for the privacy of both patients and the physician). It is possible, therefore, to identify opportunities and flaws in medical education systems. Tsugawa et al. [61] combined graduation data, from medical school records, with clinical performance data from Doximity, the professional network for physicians, to study one possible relationship, in this case, the relationship between country of graduation and practice outcomes. They found that, on their measures of 30-day mortality and re-admission rates, there was no difference between US and foreign graduates, thus allowing them to address concerns that admitting foreign medical graduates to train and practice in the US might worsen US medical care.

Going further, Triola et al. [62] suggest continuous improvement of the educational process itself by linking curriculum and curriculum delivery data to clinical

---

[1] https://www.solaresearch.org/about/what-is-learning-analytics/ (accessed August19, 2022).

outcomes data. This can be very effective in the early clinical years, identifying gaps in the curriculum that result in poor clinical performance and clinical outcome. Once such analysis is incorporated into a continuous quality improvement process, it could become routine for education systems to have intelligently responsive curricula that teach students to be as well-prepared as possible for the real world of medical practice.

As Chan et al. [58] point out, development and application of learning analytics will be complex and expensive. Therefore, it is important that this should have a significant impact on the efficiency of the learning process, the quality of learning achieved, and the safety and quality of patient outcomes.

Ethics and Regulation

AI technology depends on the use of large datasets, statistical techniques, machine learning and deep learning. The neural networks that implement the resulting algorithms can be inherently complex or, even unknowable because of the process of machine learning. The resulting situation is the creation of "black box medicine" [63].

The algorithms underlying black box medicine can improve the process of care, deliver medical recommendations tailored to the individual, and increase hospital efficiency. However, these algorithms are only as good as the data on which they were trained. Much of this data is derived from the electronic health record (EHR) and related databases, data that was often entered with no regard to the potential of introduction of bias. Currently, the care provider uses the EHR as a replacement to capturing the information on paper, without understanding the long-term potential impact on the use of this data [64]. Algorithms generated with data that can reflect existing racial or gender health disparities, if unexamined, can contribute to perpetuating bias and existing inequalities in healthcare. Therefore, education on how to input unbiased data into the EHR is essential.

The above is an example of the need for understanding the ethical implications of AI systems (Chap. 18). Because many of these systems have been designed by non-medical personnel, who may not have deep understanding of the sources that created the data they use, it is essential for physicians and other health professionals to develop an understanding both of medical AI technology and how to create the content that will populate the databases used by this technology. Meanwhile, AI-based devices are being regulated and authorized for use by the United States Food and Drug Administration [65, 66] even while there is considerable variation in the quality of data used by manufacturers to test their AI software. The physicians of the future must have the underlying knowledge of both the power and the limitations of AI, so that they are prepared to deal with the potential need to bypass the recommendations from the AI products they use.

Technology Acceptance and Implementation

Implementation of technology systems, and learner or faculty acceptance of these systems after they are installed for use, have proven to be very difficult. In a review of AI applications in medical education, Chan and Zary [67] analyze the many reasons that make implementation difficult. The major difficulty in implementation was found to be difficulty in assessing effectiveness. Other factors included the difficulty in creating the domain model, the need for content specialists who understood the AI authoring process, the knowledge gap between the physicians and the engineers creating the system, and the difficulty in scaling the system because of the narrow domain of application of each intelligent system. They conclude that, to implement AI in medical education, two challenges need to be overcome—how best to assess the effectiveness of AI in learning and in curriculum design, and how to manage the technical difficulties associated with development of an effective AI system.

The expense of software development is being approached through the open-source movement. The US Army Research Laboratory provides the open-source design framework and authoring system, Generalized Intelligent Framework for Tutoring (GIFT) [68]. Other sources include AutoTutor and AutoTutor Lite (http://ace.autotutor.org/IISAutotutor/index.html). Another expense is the high cost of knowledge content representation, with estimates of 200 or more hours of development for one hour of instruction. Therefore, intelligent tutoring systems are cost-efficient only when deployed over a very large number of learners.

Artificial Intelligence Systems in the Future Workplace

Given that AI-augmented systems will be increasingly available for health care, the education of students, residents and professionals about AI will be essential for acceptance and safe use of these systems. In fact, insufficient knowledge of AI has been found to be key in current resistance to AI acceptance [69], in addition to the system's inability to explain its decisions (see Chap. 8). Aside from lack of understanding of AI methods and explainability, a further barrier to acceptance is the perceived assault on the clinician's professional identity. Education about the optimal use of AI systems, and their role in the support of clinicians, will be an essential step in acceptance and use of AI. Clinicians with an understanding of the foundations and methods of AI will be in a good position to influence the development of the next generation of AI tools, as well as to evaluate these tools and prevent unfounded reliance on exciting but unproven technology [70]. At the same time, the AI systems should be developed with the nature of the user and the workplace environment in mind, as described earlier in this chapter.

Image-based medical disciplines, such as radiology [1], ophthalmology [71–73] and dermatology [74], will be the earliest to experience the use of AI-augmented diagnostic equipment (Chap. 12). In step with this need, an introductory curriculum about AI methods, named AI-RADS, has been piloted for education of radiology residents [32]. A monthly lecture on an AI method was followed by a journal club discussion of an article that required some knowledge of the topic of the lecture. Assessment was conducted using pre-and post-intervention surveys. The residents demonstrated increased confidence in their ability to read AI-related articles in radiology journals, and in their ability to explain key concepts. More such courses and curricula will be needed, across medical disciplines, to familiarize physicians with significant changes expected in the near future.

Some examples of artificial intelligence technologies that the learner can expect to encounter in the clinical workplace include:

- Medical diagnosis, with underlying AI technologies such as pattern detection, knowledge representation, ontologies and reasoning (see Chap. 5); [75]
- Natural language interaction for patient-facing applications based on speech recognition. sentiment understanding, speech synthesis, and chatbots (see Chap. 7); [76]
- Virtual and augmented reality for diagnosis, interventional procedures, and team communication (see Chap. 9);
- Robotic sensing and manipulation, based on object recognition, and path planning and avoidance, for surgery as well as for hospital logistics and materials movement, and
- Predictive analytics for hospital process optimization and for public health, based on large data sets, machine and deep learning, and neural nets (see Chaps. 11, 13, and 15.

Besides learning about AI, these technologies can increase the impact of what physicians learn. Continuing medical education is considered essential for practicing physicians. Their choice of courses usually depends on credentialling requirements or on keeping abreast of the latest medical knowledge in their field. Correction of knowledge or skill deficits is desirable. However, individual practitioners are not always aware of their deficits or may choose to ignore these deficits, to the detriment of their patients. AI methods that are used in ITS are appropriate for evaluating a practitioner's current knowledge and generating a recommended syllabus, both as a remedial course and as a guide toward their new learning goals.

The Road Ahead: Opportunities and Challenges for Intelligent Systems in Training, Learning and Practice

Education today is taking big leaps towards embracing intelligent systems and its applications in the teaching and learning methodologies. As Coiera [77] points out AI-driven tools will define the way medicine will be practiced in twenty-first century. What might the medical practice in the future look like? The hypothetical scenario below, *A typical day in a future physician's life*, says well that intelligent systems will be a critical part of our daily lives in future healthcare. This will require doctors to be knowledgeable about and skillful at using these intelligent systems, creating opportunities for education and training programs for the new age. However, there are also challenges. In the hypothetical future scenario, there is not much room for doctors to use human judgment, when caring for patients. There is a critical need to develop systems and training programs that complement and extend human intellect to foster human-AI collaboration. Future physicians and patients are sometimes challenged to build trust with machines since AI systems are often viewed as competing against human intelligence, as reflected in various Games (*humans vs. machines*).

A Typical Day in a Physician's Practice of the Future

As Dr. X prepares in the morning, her Smart Glass shows her the day's case load. The hospital's Smart Support System (SSS) has reviewed the schedule for the day. It has prepared a simulated Digital Twin of each patient for Dr. X to review before each appointment. The Digital Twin includes an annotated three-dimensional view of anatomy and pathology to the level of detail that Dr. X wishes to explore, including genetic analysis if needed. For those areas where SSS has uncertainty about the data or the inferences, it indicates this with a cloud, and is able to explain its reasoning that leads to its uncertainty. The medical team begins the morning with a huddle to review each Digital Twin and raise issues that SSS can investigate before the actual patient meeting. A nurse queries the ethics of a difficult decision and SSS presents a few prior examples, how they were handled, and the medico-social outcomes of each decision.

Meanwhile, Dr. X notices that one case involves an unusual genetic mutation and she requests SSS to prepare a micro-course for her to study before the appointment. SSS is aware of Dr. X's knowledge status, and uses its ITS to collect the necessary content to fill in the gaps in her knowledge. The micro-course includes subtle problems and choices to assess whether Dr. X has correctly understood the complex new information.

During the course of the day, SSS observes under which situations, Dr. X had to request additional information or get additional consults. It uses this to prepare a refresher summary and course for the close of the day. SSS may also send information back to the medical schools, indicating where there are gaps in the training and education.

In order to foster an AI-human collaborative education program, it is necessary to know the strengths of AI systems, and those of human beings. AI systems' strengths in changing a physician's practice and patient outcomes are already known. So, what are the physicians' strengths? In a 2019 NEJM Catalyst conversation hour, Nirav R. Shah, described the four Cs, which he considered physicians' strengths in dealing with patients: critical thinking, communication, collaboration, and creativity [78]. These four Cs, which are patient-centered, were identied by Shah as the most essential human skills that will need to be augmented in the age of AI. It is necessary to make sure that intelligent systems for training and education are developed with human-centered design strategies in mind to empower us to collaborate in teams, develop understanding, innovate, and solve new problems creatively.

As this chapter highlights, advances in intelligent systems have brought technology-supported education in healthcare to a new era, changing the nature of work towards creating a more efficient, effective, and safe practice environment. By incorporating human intelligence, a machine could serve as an intelligent tutor, tool, and facilitator of clinical decision-making in educational and clinical settings. Using intelligent systems in medical and health education has created new opportunities for designing productive clinical learning activities and developing better technology-enhanced learning applications and environments. The healthcare team is more likely to be multidisciplinary in the future. However, the interdisciplinary nature of AI-based education involving researchers and practitioners from different disciplines raises the unique challenge of building trust. These also include collaborations among computer scientists, engineers, cognitive and social scientists, and health care practitioners. Thus, understanding team-based collaborations will be essential and challenging for developing intelligent collaborative systems for training and education.

Healthcare systems are complex, requiring different ways of implementing ideas and assessing the AI systems as compared to the established approaches [79]. Challenges in a complex environment with uncertainty is seen as embracing the opportunities to adapt, stimulating innovative solutions, and leveraging the sociocultural system to enable ideas to emerge and spread. Training in such an ill-structured environment will be necessary, using instructional materials that do not oversimplify the content or the structure to reflect the reality of complex clinical practice.

Finally, with technological advancements the role of intelligent systems or AI in medical education will increase. Medical schools need to consider curricular reforms, including content related to AI as part of their curriculum and emphasize empathy and integrity. There will be many obstacles in implementing AI in medical education, including insufficient time in curricular hours and difficulties in developing AI applications that are usable, clinically relevant, and safe. At the same time, the potential for a collaborative, even symbiotic, relationship among learner, teacher, education enterprise, and AI system is immense, and points to new, efficient, and enjoyable future learning methods.

Questions for Discussion

- What would Osler say about today's intelligence-based education?
- How can learning with intelligence-based tools augment cognitive limitations of human abilities?
- What user-centered design issues need to be considered before implementing intelligence-based tools for health professionals' education?

- Evaluate the scenario of *a day in a life of a future physician* presented in the chapter. What are some missing aspects of clinical practice?
- Describe some of the challenges and possible solutions of using AI-tools for learning and instruction as we move to the future?
- Design a curriculum for medical education which you believe we will need 10 years in the future.

Further Reading

Patel VL, Yoskowitz NA, Arocha JF, Shortliffe EH. Cognitive and learning sciences in biomedical and health instructional design: a review with lessons for biomedical informatics education. J Biomed Inform. 2009;42(1):176–97.

- This review illustrates how formal methods and theories from cognitive and learning sciences would prove useful in development of assessment criteria and design of instructional tools that match the competencies to be acquired by the trainees. The methodologies and theories discussed are oriented toward understanding and characterizing the cognitive, and to some extent the social impact of technology, on learning and instruction.

Silverman ME, Murray TJ, Bryan CS. The quotable Osler. Philadelphia, PA: American College of Physicians; 2008.

- This book is a collection of quotations compiled from Sir William Osler's various publications by three American editors. The book is divided into themes such as personal qualities, the art and practice of medicine, diagnosis and science and truth. The selected quotes portray Osler as a deeply moral, committed and enthusiastic doctor who believed 'that the practice of medicine is an art, not a trade; a calling, not a business; a calling in which your heart will be exercised equally with your head'.

Rosenberg L. Metaverse 101: defining the key components. n.d. https://venturebeat.com/2022/02/05/metaverse-101-defining-the-key-components/. Accessed August 19, 2022.

- This is short article which puts together some of the useful definitions of concepts related to metaverse. It defines metaverse as a persistent and immersive simulated world (Virtual Reality and Augmented Reality) that is experienced in the first person by large groups of simultaneous users who share a strong sense of mutual presence.

Patel VL, Groen GJ, Norman GR. Reasoning and instruction in medical curricula. Cogn Instr. 1993;10(4):335–78.

- This original research paper examines the knowledge and explanatory processes of students in two medical schools with different modes of instruction. The results presented show the impact of instructional methods on the trainees' organization of knowledge, development of specific reasoning strategies, and generation of coherent explanations for diagnostic hypotheses. The paper presents the importance of process-based assessment of learning and instruction.

Cohen T, Blatter B, Patel VL. Simulating expert clinical comprehension: adapting latent semantic analysis to accurately extract clinical concepts from psychiatric narrative. J Biomed Inform. 2008;41(6):1070–87.

- This manuscript presents cognitively motivated methodology for the simulation of expert ability to organize relevant findings supporting intermediate diagnostic hypotheses, an important psychological construct. Latent Semantic Analysis (LSA) is shown to be a powerful tool for automatic extraction and classification of relevant text segments that is evaluated against expert annotation.

Yu KH, Beam AL, Kohane IS. Artificial intelligence in healthcare. Nat Biomed Eng. 2018;2(10):719–31.

- This review outlines recent breakthroughs in AI technologies and their biomedical applications, identifies the challenges for further progress in medical AI systems, and summarizes the economic, legal and social implications of AI in healthcare.

Dev P, Schleyer T. Digital technology in health sciences education, Chapter 25. In: Shortliffe EH, Cimino J, editors. Biomedical informatics. 5th ed. New York, NY: Springer; 2021.

- This chapter reviews learning theory and digital technology approaches in health sciences education, including classroom technologies, intelligent tutors, simulations, augmented/virtual reality, and collaboration tools.

McGrath JL, Taekman JM, Dev P, Danforth DR, Mohan D, Kman N, Crichlow A Bond WF. Using virtual reality simulation environments to assess competence for emergency medicine learners. Acad Emerg Med. 2018;25(2):186–95. https://doi.org/10.1111/acem.13308. PMID: 28888070.

- This paper examines the current uses of virtual simulation (VS) in training and assessment, including limitations and challenges in implementing VS into medical education curricula. It also provides insights into the needs for determination of areas of focus for VS training and assessment, development and exploration of virtual platforms, automated feedback within such platforms, and evaluation of effectiveness and validity of VS education.

References

1. Yu KH, Beam AL, Kohane IS. Artificial intelligence in healthcare. Nat Biomed Eng. 2018;2(10):719–31.
2. Wartman SA, Combs CD. Medical education must move from the information age to the age of artificial intelligence. Acad Med. 2018;93(8):1107–9. https://doi.org/10.1097/ACM.0000000000002044. PMID: 29095704.
3. Alrassi J, Katsufrakis PJ, Chandran L. Technology can augment, but not replace, critical human skills needed for patient care. Acad Med. 2021;96(1):37–43.

4. Bliss M. William Osler: a life in medicine. New York, NY: Oxford University Press; 1999.
5. Garibaldi B. Residency 2050: what is the future of medical training? In: Perspective. Medscape; 2019. https://www.medscape.com/viewarticle/918613_2.
6. Flexner A. Medical education in the United States and Canada. Washington, DC: Science and Health Publications, Inc.; 1910. Google Scholar.
7. Wartman SA, Combs CD. Medical Education Must Move From the Information Age to the Age of Artificial Intelligence. Acad Med. 2018;93(8):1107–1109. https://doi.org/10.1097/ACM.0000000000002044. PMID: 29095704.
8. Bloom BS, Engelhart MD, Furst EJ, Hill WH, Krathwohl DR. Taxonomy of educational objectives: the classification of educational goals. In: Handbook 1: Cognitive domain. New York, NY: David McKay; 1956.
9. Anderson LW, Krathwohl DR. A taxonomy for learning, teaching, and assessing: a revision of Bloom's taxonomy of educational objectives. New York, NY: Longman; 2001.
10. Krathwohl DR. A revision of bloom's taxonomy: an overview. Theory Pract. 2002;41:212–8.
11. Franklin A, Liu Y, Li Z, Nguyen V, Johnson TR, Robinson D, Okafor N, King B, Patel VL, Zhang J. Opportunistic decision making and complexity in emergency care. J Biomed Inform. 2011;44(3):469–76.
12. Zheng K, Hanauer DA, Weibel N, Agha Z. Computational ethnography: automated and unobtrusive means for collecting data in situ in human–computer interaction evaluation studies. In: Patel VL, Kannampallil TG, Kaufman DR, editors. Cognitive informatics for biomedicine: human computer interaction in healthcare. Cham: Springer International Publishing; 2015. p. 111–40.
13. Churches A. Bloom's digital taxonomy. 2007. http://burtonslifelearning.pbworks.com/w/file/fetch/26327358/BloomDigitalTaxonomy2001.pdf.
14. National Research Council. Advancing scientific research in education. Ottawa, ON: National Research Council; 2005.
15. Patel VL, Groen GJ, Norman GR. Reasoning and instruction in medical curricula. Cogn Instr. 1993;10(4):335–78.
16. Patel VL, Arocha JF, Kaufman DR. Diagnostic reasoning and expertise. Psychol Learn Motiv Adv Res Theory. 1994;31:137–252.
17. Anderson JR, Reder LM, Simon HA. Situated learning and education. Educ Res. 1996;25(4):5–11. https://doi.org/10.3102/0013189x025004005.S2CID54548451. CiteSeerX 10.1.1.556.7550.
18. Sweller J. Cognitive load during problem solving: effects on learning. Cogn Sci. 1988;12:257–85.
19. Sweller J, Chandler P. Evidence for cognitive load theory. Cogn Instr. 1991;8:351–62.
20. Roth WM, Jornet A. Situated cognition. Wiley Interdiscip Rev Cogn Sci. 2013;4(5):463–78.
21. Spiro RJ, Feltovich PJ, Jacobson MJ, Coulson RL. Cognitive flexibility, constructivism and hypertext: random access instruction for advanced knowledge acquisition in ill-structured domains. In: Duffy T, Jonassen D, editors. Constructivism and the technology of instruction. Hillsdale, NJ: Erlbaum; 1992.
22. Anderson JR, Greeno JG, Reder LM, Simon HA. Perspectives on learning, thinking, and activity. Educ Res. 2000;29:11–3.
23. Patel VL, Yoskowitz NA, Arocha JF, Shortliffe EH. (2009). Cognitive and learning sciences in biomedical and health instructional design: a review with lessons for biomedical informatics education. J Biomed Inform. 2009;42(1):176–97. https://doi.org/10.1016/j.jbi.2008.12.002.
24. Patel VL, Kaufman DR, Arocha JF. Steering through the murky waters of a scientific conflict: Situated and symbolic models of clinical cognition. Artif Intell Med. 1995;7:413–38.
25. Greeno JG. A perspective on thinking. Am Psychol. 1989;44:134–41.
26. Rasmussen J, Pejtersen AM, Goodstein LP. Cognitive systems engineering. New York, NY: John Wiley and Sons; 1994.
27. Winograd T, Flores F. Understanding computers and cognition: a new foundation for design. Norwood, NJ: Ablex Publishing Corporation; 1986.
28. Norman DA. Cognition in the head and in the world: an introduction to the special issue on situated action. Cogn Sci. 1993;17:1–6.

29. Patel VL, Kaufman DR. Chapter 4: Cognitive science, and biomedical informatics. In: Shortliffe EH, Cimino JJ, editors. Biomedical informatics. 4th ed. Basel: Springer Nature Switzerland AG; 2021. p. 122–53. https://doi.org/10.1007/978-3-030-58721-5_4.

30. Patel VL, Kaufman DR, Magder SA. The acquisition of medical expertise in complex dynamic environments. In: Ericsson A, editor. The road to excellence: the acquisition of expert performance in the arts and sciences, sports, and games. Mahwah, NJ: Lawrence Erlbaum Associates; 1996. p. 369.

31. Margolis J. Three-year MAP growth at schools using "teach to one": math. 2019. http://margrady.com/wp-content/uploads/2019/02/Three-Year-MAP-Growth-at-TtO-Schools.pdf. Accessed 11 Mar 2021.

32. Lindqwister AL, Hassanpour S, Lewis PJ, Sin JM. AI-RADS: an artificial intelligence curriculum for residents. Acad Radiol. 2020;S1076-6332(20):30556. https://doi.org/10.1016/j.acra.2020.09.017.

33. Kulik JA, Fletcher JD. Effectiveness of intelligent tutoring systems: a meta-analytic review. Rev Educ Res. 2016;86(1):42–78.

34. Fletcher JD, Morrison JE. DARPA digital tutor: assessment data (IDA Document D-4686). Alexandria, VA: Institute for Defense Analyses; 2012.

35. Anderson JR, Corbett AT, Koedinger KR, Pelletier R. Cognitive tutors: lessons learned. J Learn Sci. 1995;4:167–207.

36. Pek P-K, Poh K-L. Making decisions in an intelligent tutoring system. Int J Inf Technol Decis Mak. 2005;4:207–33.

37. Ma W, Adesope OO, Nesbit JC, Liu Q. Intelligent tutoring systems and learning outcomes: a meta-analysis. J Educ Psychol. 2014;106(4):901–18.

38. Nye BD, Graesser AC, Hu X. AutoTutor and family: a review of 17 years of natural language tutoring. Int J Artif Intell Educ. 2014;24:427–69.

39. Graesser AC, Wiemer-Hastings K, Wiemer-Hastings P, Kreuz R, the Tutoring Research Group. Auto tutor: a simulation of a human tutor. J Cogn Syst Res. 1999;1:35–51.

40. Hu X. Virtual civilian aeromedical evacuation sustainment training (V-CAEST). Memphis, TN: University of Memphis; 2015. https://apps.dtic.mil/dtic/tr/fulltext/u2/1002332.pdf. Accessed 11 Mar 2021.

41. Shubeck KT, Craig SD, Hu X. Live-action mass-casualty training and virtual world training: a comparison. Proc Hum Fact Ergonom Soc Ann Meet. 2016;60:2103–017.

42. Lineberry M, Dev P, Lane HC, Talbot TB. Learner-adaptive educational technology for simulation in healthcare: foundations and opportunities. Simul Healthc. 2018;13(3S Suppl 1):S21–7

43. Gierl MJ, Lai H. Evaluating the quality of medical multiple-choice items created with automated processes. Med Educ. 2013;47(7):726–33. https://doi.org/10.1111/medu.12202.

44. Leo J, Kurdi G, Matentzoglu N, et al. Ontology-based generation of medical, multi-term MCQs. Int J Artif Intell Educ. 2019;29:145–88. https://doi.org/10.1007/s40593-018-00172-w.

45. Luan H, Geczy P, Lai H, Gobert J, Yang SJH, Ogata H, Baltes J, Guerra R, Li P, Tsai C-C. Challenges and future directions of big data and artificial intelligence in education. Front Psychol. 2020;11:580820.

46. Lentz A, Siy JO, Carraccio C. AI-assessment: towards assessment as a sociotechnical system for learning. Acad Med. 2021;96:S87–8.

47. Metz C. Can A.I. grade your next test? New York Times. 2021. https://www.nytimes.com/2021/07/20/technology/ai-education-neural-networks.html.

48. Ball R, Duhadway L, Feuz K, Jensen J, Rague B, Weidman D. Applying machine learning to improve curriculum design. In: Proceedings of the 50th ACM Technical Symposium on Computer Science Education; 2019. p. 787–93.

49. Stevens RH, Najafi K. Can artificial neural networks provide an "expert's" view of medical students' performances on computer-based simulations? Proc Annu Symp Comput Appl Med Care. 1992:179–83. https://www.ncbi.nlm.nih.gov/pmc/articles/PMC2248084/pdf/procas-camc00003-0194.pdf. Accessed 16 Jul 2021

50. Graesser AC. Emotions are the experiential glue of learning environments in the 21st century. Learn Instr. 2020;70:101212.

51. Pekrun R. The control-value theory of achievement emotions: assumptions, corollaries, and implications for educational research and practice. Educ Psychol Rev. 2006;18:315–41.
52. Loderer K, Pekrun R, Lester JC. Beyond cold technology: a systematic review and meta-analysis on emotions in technology-based learning environments. Learn Instr. 2020;70:101162.
53. Nawrat Z. MIS AI - artificial intelligence application in minimally invasive surgery. Mini Invas Surg. 2020;4(28). https://doi.org/10.20517/2574-1225.2020.08.
54. Aebersold M. Simulation-based learning: no longer a novelty in undergraduate education. Online J Issues Nurs. 2018;23(2):14.
55. Huang G, Reynolds R, Candler C. Virtual patient simulation at U.S. and Canadian Medical Schools. Acad Med. 2007;82(5):446–51.
56. ASA. Navigate anesthesia emergencies through realistic simulations. Washington, DC: ASA; 2021. https://www.asahq.org/education-and-career/educational-and-cme-offerings/simulation-education/anesthesia-simstat. Accessed 11 Mar 2021.
57. Ellaway RH, Pusic MV, Galbraith RM, Cameron T. Developing the role of big data and analytics in health professional education. Med Teach. 2014;36(3):216–22.
58. Chan T, Sebok-Syer S, Thoma B, Wise A, Sherbino J, Pusic M. Learning analytics in medical education assessment: the past, the present and the future. Acad Emerg Med Educ Train. 2018;2(2):178–87.
59. Thoma B, Bandi V, Carey R, Mondal D, Woods R, Martin L, Chan T. Developing a dashboard to meet Competence Committee needs: a design-based research project. Can Med Educ J. 2020;11(1):e16–34.
60. Boulet JR, Durning SJ. What we measure … and what we should measure in medical education. Med Educ. 2019;53(1):86–94.
61. Tsugawa Y, Jena AB, Orav EJ, Jha AK. Quality of care delivered by general internists in US hospitals who graduated from foreign versus US medical schools: observational study. BMJ. 2017;356:j273. https://doi.org/10.1136/bmj.j273. PMID: 28153977; PMCID: PMC5415101.
62. Triola MM, Hawkins RE, Skochelak SE. The time is now: using graduates' practice data to drive medical education reform. Acad Med. 2018;93(6):826–8. https://doi.org/10.1097/ACM.0000000000002176. PMID: 29443719.
63. Nicholson WN II. Black-box medicine. Harv J Law Technol. 2015;28(2):421–67.
64. Paranjape K, Schinkel M, Nannan Panday R, Car J, Nanayakkara P. Introducing artificial intelligence training in medical education. JMIR Med Educ. 2019;5(2):e16048.
65. Hills B, Nguyen J. FDA'S plan for AI/ML-based software as medical devices: progress and concerns. Morrison Foerster. 2021. https://www.jdsupra.com/legalnews/fda-s-plan-for-ai-ml-based-software-as-1499376/.
66. United States Food and Drug Administration. Artificial intelligence and machine learning in software as a medical device. Silver Spring, MD: FDA; 2021. https://www.fda.gov/medical-devices/software-medical-device-samd/artificial-intelligence-and-machine-learning-software-medical-device.
67. Chan KS, Zary N. Applications and challenges of implementing artificial intelligence in medical education: integrative review. JMIR Med Educ. 2019;5(1):e13930. https://doi.org/10.2196/13930.
68. Sottilare RA, Brawner KW, Goldberg BS, Holden HK. The generalized intelligent framework for tutoring (GIFT). Orlando, FL: U.S. Army Research Laboratory – Human Research & Engineering Directorate (ARL-HRED); 2012. https://scholar.google.com/citations?user=Gs6R8SsAAAAJ&hl=en&oi=sra.
69. Strohm L, Hehakaya C, Ranschaert ER, Boon WPC, Moors EHM. Implementation of artificial intelligence (AI) applications in radiology: hindering and facilitating factors. Eur Radiol. 2020;30(10):5525–32. https://doi.org/10.1007/s00330-020-06946-y. PMID: 32458173; PMCID: PMC7476917.
70. Rubin DL. Artificial intelligence in imaging: the radiologist's role. J Am Coll Radiol. 2019;16(9 Pt B):1309–17. https://doi.org/10.1016/j.jacr.2019.05.036. PMID: 31492409; PMCID: PMC6733578.

71. Du XL, Li WB, Hu BJ. Application of artificial intelligence in ophthalmology. Int J Ophthalmol. 2018;11(9):1555–61.
72. Chartrand G, Cheng PM, Vorontsov E, Drozdzal M, Turcotte S, Pal CJ, Kadoury S, Targ A. Deep learning: a primer for radiologists. Radiographics. 2017;37(7):2113–31. https://doi.org/10.1148/rg.2017170077. PMID: 29131760.
73. EDUCAUSE. Artificial intelligence. In: EDUCAUSE Horizon report: teaching and learning edition; 2021. p. 13–5. https://library.educause.edu/resources/2021/4/2021-educause-horizon-report-teaching-and-learning-edition. Accessed 16 Jul 2021.
74. Esteva A, Kuprel B, Novoa RA, Ko J, Swetter SM, Blau HM, Thrun S. Dermatologist-level classification of skin cancer with deep neural networks. Nature. 2017;542(7639):115–8. https://doi.org/10.1038/nature21056. Erratum in: Nature. 2017;546(7660):686. PMID: 28117445.
75. Rubin DL, Dameron O, Bashir Y, Grossman D, Dev P, Musen MA. Using ontologies linked with geometric models to reason about penetrating injuries. Artif Intell Med. 2006;37(3):167–76. https://doi.org/10.1016/j.artmed.2006.03.006. PMID: 16730959.
76. Reiswich A, Haag M. Evaluation of chatbot prototypes for taking the virtual patient's history. In: Hayn D, et al., editors. dHealth 2019 – from eHealth to dHealth. Amsterdam: IOS Press; 2019. p. 73–80.
77. Coiera E. The fate of medicine in the time of AI. Lancet. 2018;392(10162):2331–32. https://doi.org/10.1016/S0140-6736(18)31925-1. Epub 2018 Oct 11. PMID: 30318263.
78. NEJM. Catalyst group conversation with Nirav H. Shah, MD, MPH on What AI Means for Doctors and Doctoring. 2019. https://catalyst.nejm.org/doi/full/10.1056/CAT.19.0622. Accessed 31 Jan 2022.
79. Kannampallil TG, Schauer GF, Cohen T, Patel VL. Considering complexity in healthcare systems. J Biomed Inform. 2011;44(6):943–7.

Part IV
The Future of AI in Medicine: Prospects and Challenges

Chapter 17
Framework for the Evaluation of Clinical AI Systems

Edward H. Shortliffe, Martìn-Josè Sepùlveda, and Vimla L. Patel

After reading this chapter, you should know the answers to these questions:

- What is a desirable relationship between the evaluation of a system and its design and implementation?
- What is the notion of *iterative design* and how does it influence evaluations developed for laboratory testing and subsequent real-world environments?
- What elements of an AIM system need to be evaluated, and how do the characteristics of the system influence how such evaluations should be undertaken?
- What is *team science* and what is its relevance to the evaluation of AIM systems?
- What special questions arise in the evaluation of commercial systems that are intended for a competitive marketplace?
- What is *usability testing* and how does it influence the design, implementation, and evaluation of AIM systems?
- What are the metrics by which the medical community is likely to assess the success and appeal of a newly developed AIM system?
- What is the role of cognitive informatics, not only in the design of systems but also in their assessment in laboratory and real-world implementations?

E. H. Shortliffe (✉)
Columbia University, New York, NY, USA
e-mail: ted@shortliffe.net

M.-J. Sepùlveda
Florida International University, Miami, FL, USA
e-mail: msepulve@fiu.edu

V. L. Patel
New York Academy of Medicine, New York, NY, USA
e-mail: vpatel@nyam.org

© The Author(s), under exclusive license to Springer Nature Switzerland AG 2022
T. A. Cohen et al. (eds.), *Intelligent Systems in Medicine and Health*, Cognitive Informatics in Biomedicine and Healthcare,
https://doi.org/10.1007/978-3-031-09108-7_17

The Role of Evaluation: Why It Is Important

Observers often note that few areas of endeavor progress more rapidly than bio-medicine and health care—new drugs, new procedures, new fundamental dis-coveries, and new devices, as well as new practices that are introduced in response to enhanced understanding of psychosocial issues that affect human health and disease progression. The medical literature is vast, and it has required a computational approach to citation management and search that was intro-duced much earlier than it was in other areas of science[1]—including in computer science itself.

The biomedical scientific literature, including clinical books and journals, is deeply embedded in the culture of medicine. Clinicians look to journals for evi-dence to support new therapies or approaches, and they learn to respect some jour-nals more than others. The key is peer review and rigorous evaluation before an article, and the underlying study design or research data, are accepted as guidance for a change in how medicine should be practiced. Similarly, relevant regulatory agencies, such as the US Food and Drug Administration (FDA), look to the pub-lished literature and to the underlying data before they approve new medications. They also look to the literature, and research data, when evaluating new medical devices for approval.

But what about software? If new computer programs or systems are developed for use in biomedical or clinical settings, who approves them and how should deci-sions be reached about their validity, quality, and adoption? Chapter 18 discusses some of these regulatory issues in the context of ethics and policy. Currently the FDA is struggling with the development of suitable criteria or guidelines for the approval of AIM systems. In 2021 the FDA published an action plan for "Artificial Intelligence and Machine Learning in Software as a Medical Device",[2] but the over-sight task is complicated by many considerations. How should such programs be evaluated? Should the emphasis be on safety and efficacy (as it is for new pharma-ceuticals), or are there other pertinent considerations? How often should they be re-assessed, given that they evolve and updated versions may be released with some frequency? What are the elements that determine efficacy and software safety? Accurate assessments? Acceptance by clinicians? Changes in practice? Benefits for patients and populations? Cost-effectiveness?

---

[1] MEDLARS (Medical Literature Analysis and Retrieval System) was launched by the U.S. National Library of Medicine in 1964 and was the first large scale, computer based, retrospective search service available to the general public. It expanded to support online search (MEDLINE, for "MEDLARS Online") in 1971 and evolved further to support free literature search (PubMed) for the global community on the Internet in 1997.

[2] Available at https://www.fda.gov/medical-devices/software-medical-device-samd/artificial-intel-ligence-and-machine-learning-software-medical-device. (accessed August 14, 2022)

Regardless of how these regulatory deliberations advance and are resolved (and it is not the purpose of this chapter to guess about what may happen), it is safe to assume that clinicians, as key users of many AIM systems, will again turn to the literature for evidence that will support the adoption of such software tools. Have they been well studied, with resulting peer-reviewed papers published in top journals? Are the results convincing? What would it mean to introduce such tools into a specific clinician's practice environment? Would it be worth it?

Accordingly, this chapter looks at the general issue of how to evaluate AIM systems and other similar software tools intended for use in clinical settings. It is not the goal to tell readers how to design formal studies and to obtain funding to carry them out, or otherwise to provide an evaluation handbook. There are excellent resources available that address such matters [1–3]. Rather the chapter offers a framework for anticipating and addressing the complex mix of issues that arise when designing and undertaking an evaluation plan for a medical software product such as AIM decision support tools. For details, interested readers may want to delve into the subject of **implementation science** [4, 5] as well as Friedman, Wyatt, and Ash's excellent summary of informatics evaluation methods, including formal clinical trials [1], or Herasevich and Pickering's recently revised handbook [3]. There is also a relevant literature that deals with statistical issues in clinical trials [6] and the assessment of cost-effectiveness [7]. Chapter 18 in this volume is focused on ethical issues in the application and evaluation of AI methods and medical applications, and there are many other thoughtful analyses of ethical issues in research, including arguments that ethical considerations should be more explicitly addressed even before research projects are initiated and funded [8].

Framing Questions for Assessing an Evaluation Plan

AIM systems are generally developed in response to some human need. It might therefore be logical to emphasize the system's response to that need in assessing whether it is successful. The AIM literature is accordingly replete with evaluation articles in which the primary focus is the system's performance on the analytic task for which it was designed. Too often other aspects warranting formal evaluation are ignored, even though those issues are typically integral to the overall success and acceptance of the system.

The previous section focused on the "why?" of such evaluations. This section provides a framework for the production of state-of-the-art evaluation data for AIM systems that can both meet performance and outcome goals and, ideally, establish a benchmark against which other similar systems can be evaluated. The framework addresses the needs for formative and normative (naturalistic) data and evidence. The initial formative work occurs in laboratories or controlled collaborative settings. The naturalistic work occurs in the actual intended work setting, where routine usability can be assessed and formal experimental trials can be undertaken. A rigorous implementation and execution of the framework and process could then generate peer-reviewed quality science for top tier clinical, health services, health policy, and informatics journals. The suggested framework outlined in this section guides the discussions in the remainder of this chapter. It generally reflects similar evaluation frameworks that have been published elsewhere [9, 10].

In the early days of AIM research, perhaps most visibly in the medical expert systems community, developers realized that evaluation was not only important for documenting a system's performance but that design and development should start with informal assessments that feed back iteratively into the ongoing evolution of the system [11]. **Iterative design** has accordingly become an accepted approach to system development that allows early tests to influence the subsequent design process, addressing concerns that had been unanticipated but that turn out to be crucial for successful performance, utility, or acceptance. This interplay between design of a system or application and the ongoing assessment of the developing solution is discussed in greater detail in the next section in this chapter ("Design and Iteration").

Here we begin by considering the fundamental questions that guide the process of evaluation for AIM systems (as well as many other health information technology applications) [12]. It is important to start by considering the "what?" as it relates to evaluation—an issue that is entwined with thinking about the nature of the development effort and the ultimate goals. If the focus is on experimenting with a new methodology, then an emphasis on decision making performance is natural—an observation that no doubt accounts for the dominant types of assessments in the literature (accuracy or "correctness" of the results generated by a novel software system). But demonstrating the validity of a system's decisions or advice is often only a small component of a much larger set of questions, especially as the system moves into clinical use or is part of a commercial product that will ultimately be sold to customers. It must be remembered that these systems will need to be incorporated into users' work environments—typically in hospitals, clinics, or office practices.

Many systems ultimately fail to be adopted even though they produce accurate decisions, and the other factors that determine success accordingly need to be part of both the design and the evaluation plan. These evaluation steps must be anticipated at the outset, since they imply design features that may not feasibly be added to a product in the later stages. In AI systems, for example, if explainability and transparency are viewed as necessary components of the ultimate system, it is folly to ignore the issue at the beginning and to assume it will be possible to graft those capabilities onto an otherwise accurate system in the later stages. Features that will ultimately be needed may radically influence the design of the novel methods that are the primary focus. The implication is that the research and development process should begin with a clear sense of what the ultimate system will look like and how it will be used, even though the details will likely evolve as the system itself does. The various evaluation requirements, which typically need to be addressed in a stepwise fashion, will then become clear and can be anticipated throughout. Subsequent sections on "Design and Iteration" and "Naturalistic Studies" address this issue in more detail.

Evaluation plans need to be well matched both to the issue being addressed and to the maturity of the system when it is being studied. Early studies are often informal since they are intended to help to expose unexpected limitations or failures of the developing tool. Later the process becomes more formal, controlled, and labor intensive. As is discussed in the section on "Cognitive Evaluation Methods", the evaluation approach often requires cognitive studies (which can be crucial during the early design process but also are needed to ascertain just how users interact with systems, how they may be confused, and what they feel is helpful or extraneous). Epidemiologists and sociologists may be needed to help to assess the generalizability of the results and the adequacy of the design with regards to potential biases. Statisticians and clinical trial experts are needed when the evaluations become more formal and extensive, typically in the later stages. And economists may need to be involved when cost-effectiveness studies are being designed or carried out. The implication is that, when optimally addressed, the evaluation of AIM systems is a collaborative effort that will benefit from the engagement of people with a variety of types of expertise.

Viewing AIM evaluation as a collaborative effort may sound overwhelming to the single researcher who has more modest goals when building an exploratory system using innovative methods. "Certainly," they might argue, "it is possible for me to demonstrate that my program makes good decisions without bringing in a panoply of evaluation experts!" To some extent this is true, although the design and construction of an exploratory program will benefit from considering the kinds of issues that would need to be incorporated and assessed if the system were to advance to real-world use. It is never too early, for example, to worry about potential biasing in the selection of machine-learning datasets, algorithms, or the need for transparency and interpretability if the use model envisioned would eventually require direct interactions with users.[3]

The majority of published studies of AIM systems have emerged from academic research settings. The culture in academia tends to demand rigorous demonstration of an innovative technology or intervention, often in a series of studies that address more than one dimension of performance. The costs of such studies can vary greatly (with randomized controlled trials typically being the most lengthy, complex, and

---

[3] Recognition of this issue in the medical machine learning community has led to the notion of "silent deployment" of new algorithms after initial training has occurred. Such efforts can help to determine how well any final system might perform in the context of the information ecosystem in which it may eventually be applied (see, for example, recommendations on this subject that have appeared in the clinical literature [13]).

expensive), but AIM investigators and developers have learned to incorporate evaluation plans into their funding proposals so that formal assessments can be rigorously pursued.

Curiously, commercial AIM products too often do not undergo the same kind of formal assessments.[4] As a result, many observers have encouraged companies that are introducing software systems to work formally with collaborating academic units that can undertake unbiased studies and publish the results on behalf of the company. That is the model that dominates in the pharmaceutical industry, where university researchers and clinicians often carry out the evaluation of new drugs and publish the results, perhaps with developers from the company as secondary authors. It would enhance acceptance and validation of commercial software products if they were similarly assessed in an objective manner. Yet there is great variation among companies in how seriously they take such formal assessments, which one can argue are even more important throughout the development cycle of a commercial product than may be the case for a purely academic research project.

Design and Iteration

The design of an AIM system or solution should begin with a clear view of the goals and use models that will drive the development. In large development efforts, even the design phase will ideally involve an integrated multidisciplinary team of researchers, developers, designers, subject matter experts, informaticians, and potential users. Their goal is to collaborate synchronously to develop, validate, and deliver prototypes to field testing. This is the "create" phase of the iterative design and development process (see Fig. 17.1).

Initial field testing is eventually undertaken in controlled real world settings—the "demonstrate" phase in the process (Fig. 17.1). Such studies typically involve small-scale but rapid-cycle implementations and refinement. The focus is on safety, usability, user acceptance, integration with data sources (e.g., EHRs), impact on workflow, and the utility and acceptance of decisions or advice offered by the system.

When the demonstration phase has led to a stable system, it is time to undertake large-scale, real-world, confirmatory experimental studies. Ideally these are randomized controlled trials (RCTs), potentially in community settings (controlled clinical trials, or CCTs), undertaken by independent high quality investigators. The goal is to produce rigorous peer-reviewed publications (the "prove" phase in Fig. 17.1). Even at this late stage there may be lessons learned that feed back to

---

[4] To complicate matters further, there is a need to continue to evaluate both research and commercial systems even after their initial approval and deployment. It is important to verify that their performance remains consistent as knowledge advances or (especially in the case of machine learning applications) as data become available for subpopulations that may have been underrepresented in initial training and evaluation.

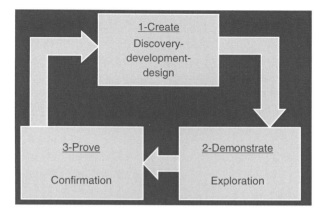

Fig. 17.1 Experiments and studies should be undertaken in a stepwise fashion (see text). Initial activities include the integrated discovery-design-development phase. This leads to the demonstration phase, involving small studies in real-world user environments. Subsequently experimental randomized controlled trials can be undertaken to confirm impacts in routine user environments. However, as technology evolves and real-world experience builds, the cycle typically begins again

stimulate design and development adjustments for the next version of the AIM system or tool.

The individual steps within the three phases depicted in Fig. 17.1 need to be well understood, following the frameworks summarized in the section on "Framing Questions for Assessing an Evaluation Plan" and in other cited articles [9, 10]. In the earliest design stages it is necessary to identify the users who are likely to find value in the system being developed. What are their needs precisely? Will they acknowledge the need for the envisioned system? How varied are the individual users envisioned? Do subgroups have special psychological or acceptance considerations? To answer such questions, it may be necessary to carry out observational studies, fully exploring the need for the envisioned system and potential barriers to its acceptance (see "Cognitive Evaluation Methods"). Formal **focus groups** can also be useful in gaining insights about needs and attitudes of potential users. Workflow considerations are especially important. Valuable systems are often rejected if they are too time consuming or they interrupt processes that are central to the user's responsibilities. It is also useful to define a robust set of user scenarios so that the developing system can adapt to a variety of use cases, thereby enhancing its utility and acceptance.

Such questions imply the early engagement of collaborators who can represent the perspectives and needs of potential users and stakeholders. In this sense the development of AIM systems falls squarely within the notion of **team science**.[5] Although traditional single-investigator driven approaches are ideal for many scientific endeavors, coordinated teams of investigators with diverse skills and

---

[5] See https://www.nationalacademies.org/our-work/the-science-of-team-science. (accessed August 14, 2022)

knowledge are generally required for tackling complex scientific and societal problems such as the development of functional and accepted AIM systems.

For most systems, informal **usability testing** is part of the design and early implementation process, influencing the iterative formative development by providing early reactions that may lead to revised plans for the interface and the way the system offers advice. Over time, however, more formal and rigorous usability testing is required. The test subjects cannot be collaborators and should be drawn from the range of implementation settings in which the developing system is intended to be used. Furthermore, experience has shown that it is folly to attempt to add an interface to a system at the end of the development process since ongoing usability testing often leads to changes in the underlying system, not just to the interface itself.

There is a robust field of usability, **human-computer interaction (HCI)** [14–16] and **human factors engineering (HFE)** [17], combining formal technical computing skills with cognitive science expertise and an ability to anticipate how a given system will be perceived (see "Cognitive Evaluation Methods"). Subfields exist, some of which are derived from a specific application domain. Although general principles of usability apply in health care interface design, optimal systems generally require the engagement of individuals with specialized expertise in working with clinical systems. In addition, such work always requires interactions with real potential users before a system can be judged ready for implementation in the field or, for commercial systems, delivery to the marketplace.

Testing the validity of an AIM system generally requires assessing its decision-making performance. Such work may employ retrospective, cross sectional or prospective methods. Initial testing of the system's capabilities is generally done using retrospective cases due to the speed, lower level of complexity, simplicity from a human subjects' perspective, and modest cost. It is of course also natural that the system should first demonstrate the quality of its advice before it is made available for prospective use with real patients.

Even in these early evaluation stages, study design for assessing the validity of conclusions should optimally provide for blinding of subjects, which eliminates a particularly important source of bias (making judgments about a computer's advice when you know the decision is coming from a computer; see, for example, an early blinded study of therapeutic recommendations carried out by developers of the MYCIN system [18]). As a system matures and is ready for more extensive use in the real world, it also becomes important to assess whether there are differences based on country, region, level of training, and practice setting, generally using a standard set of real world cases. In academic settings where decision-support research has occurred, positive studies of this type have generally been required before a system can be made available for use with real patients prospectively. This type of study is commonly published in the peer-reviewed literature, as previously mentioned. This can help to provide the most rigorous and persuasive evidence of the quality of a system's advice and, in turn, the validity of the methodology that has been developed and implemented. The goal should be publishing results in top scientific or clinical journals.

Cognitive Evaluation Methods

The field of **human computer interaction (HCI)** intersects cognitive-behavioral, computer, and information science. The major focus of HCI is with the evaluation of interactive computer systems for human use with the goal to deploy usable, useful, and safe systems. Theories of cognitive science meaningfully inform and shape design, development, and assessment of health-care information systems by providing insight into principles of system **usability**, as well as the design of a safer workplace. Usability includes five attributes: (1) *learnability*: system should be easy to learn, (2) *efficiency*: a user should be able to attain a high level of productivity, (3) *memorability*: features supported by the system should be easy to remember once learned, (4) *errors*: system should be designed to minimize errors, and (5) *satisfaction*: the user should experience satisfaction.

In the earlier sections of this chapter, we have discussed very broadly a range of approaches that are generally used for evaluating a system's usability. These are classified into field or observational studies, and usability evaluation methods that can be used in both field and laboratory settings. Formal **usability testing** is typically conducted in laboratory settings with user performance evaluated based on pre-selected tasks. Evaluation techniques where actual users are involved in the assessment process are often leveraged in naturalistic field studies.

Verbal **think aloud** methods are often used to capture rich verbal data on the thought processes that underlie human actions [19]. Several studies using verbal think aloud that investigated the nature of reasoning using clinical systems (and EHRs in particular), including the effects of expertise and decision-making, have been conducted by Patel and colleagues [20, 21]. During the think aloud process, the subjects' statements regarding what they are thinking as they are doing their tasks are audio recorded, transcribed, and analyzed using methods of natural language coding.

We have classified cognitive evaluation methods into two categories: analytic evaluation approaches and usability testing. Analytic evaluation studies use experts as participants—usability experts, domain experts, or software designers (see Fig. 17.2). Usability testing includes several approaches to capture data: interviews and focus groups, usability surveys and questionnaires, naturalistic observational approaches, and investigations of clinical workflow. Usability evaluation can be expensive in terms of time and human resources, and automation is a promising way to augment existing approaches. Automated capture of user data and automated analysis of these data can be achieved using modern **computational methods** for

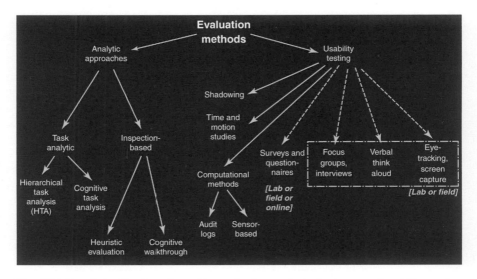

Fig. 17.2 Broad classification of cognitive evaluation methods. In the case of usability testing, some methods are applied in the naturalistic setting (solid lines) whereas others may also be carried out in experimental settings (dashed lines). (Adapted from [22], with permission)

evaluation such as sensor-based technology (e.g., **RFID**) and **audit data logs** (see Fig. 17.2).

When considering HCI, the interplay between technology and clinical cognition is important, as highlighted by an example drawn from a study in which an overdose of potassium chloride was administered through a commercial **computerized provider order-entry (CPOE)** system in an ICU [23]. The authors' analysis of the error included the inspection of system logs, interviews with clinicians, and a cognitive evaluation of the CPOE system involved. In this case, the system provided screen order-entry forms for medications with both intravenous drip (gradual administration) and bolus (rapid administration) orders for a patient – forms that appeared superficially similar. However, they required very different mental calculations to estimate dosage. Through the use of audit data logs, the authors found that the interface did not provide tools to assist the clinicians in their calculation of the proper current dosage. This overdosing case study exemplifies a larger problem: Decision support systems, as intelligent as they may be, too often fail to align with the mental processes underlying clinical decisions.

While there has been a significant recent focus on the usability of decision support systems, one of the less-explored aspects of usability is its impact on clinical workflow [24]. Using a combination of methods, we can categorize the specific aspects of EHR use that potentially deviate from the normal work activities of the clinicians and develop an understanding of how any negative deviations can potentially be mitigated (see Table 17.1). By combining the richness of **ethnographical** methods with the strength of automated computational approaches for collecting data, Zheng and colleagues showed a mismatch between the EHRs designed to support clinicians and those clinicians' actual day-to-day practice [25]. This type of analysis creates opportunities to calibrate the user interface design to align better with clinical workflow and with the clinicians' (users') model when solving medical problems.

The challenges associated with the clinicians' use of EHRs are magnified in a dynamic, information-intensive, and collaborative setting due to the emergent nature of clinical work, characterized by uncertainty of patient conditions, and the frequent interruptions with multitasking in their work environment. As a result, small perturbations through external interventions (such as the introduction of EHRs) can have

Table 17.1 Evaluative data collection approaches and analytic methods to assess clinical workflow in the setting of EHR use

Method	Method rationale	Collected data	Expected outcomes
Clinician Shadowing (Observation)	• To understand ED workflow, roles, EHR use and team interactions in a temporal manner	• Frequency of access of a patient file	• Characterization of ED workflow elements within the context of EHR use, including the general sequence of steps and transition patterns in patient care delivery activities and interaction with EHR
	• To evaluate the degree of coherence or fragmentation of clinicians' activities	• Average time spent per patient file	• Assessment of how the EHR system use changed (positive/ negative) clinicians' information seeking, team interactions, and decision making
	• To identify critical bottle necks in the workflow	• Frequency of additional activities (multitasking) physicians engage in while interacting with EHR	
		• Frequency and average time spent on transitions between clinician activities and EHR use	
Log-file data of EHR use [computational method]	• To assess clinicians' use and interaction with EHR	• Clinicians' interactions with EHR	• Estimation of the time spent viewing and authoring EHR-related clinical documentation
	• To identify rate and time of authoring and viewing EHR clinical documentation	• Rate of viewing and authoring files/notes	• Assessment of patterns of EHR usage in ED by various clinicians
		• Time spent viewing and authoring notes	
		• Frequency of access to new vs. old data	

(continued)

Table 17.1 (continued)

Method	Method rationale	Collected data	Expected outcomes
RFID Sensor-based Location data [computational method]	• To identify instances of team interactions (e.g., team formation and team dissipation) and work activities in the ED throughout stages of implementation	• Frequency and duration of team formations and dissipations (number of contacts)	• Analysis of interactivity patterns among clinicians and among clinicians and patients within the context of EHR implementations
	• To identify drivers of inefficiency in clinicians' workflow processes in the ED	• Time-stamped locations of clinicians at 3–5 second intervals • RFID distance traveled between clinicians' activities	• Change in this pattern over time

significant detrimental effects not only on the timeliness and efficiency of the daily care activities, but also on the occurrence of medical errors and other adverse events. The methods illustrated in Fig. 17.1, for the case of EHR use, generalize for cognitive analytic approaches with other types of technologies, including AIM systems implemented in clinical settings.

Delivery of Decision Support

Given the common emphasis on AIM systems as clinical decision-support tools, it is useful to consider different types of models for offering assessments or advice. Depending on the envisioned use model, the evaluation requirements may be somewhat different.

Medical Device Data-Interpretation

Consider, for example, an area of AIM system development and testing that has been particularly successful in recent years. In this volume, Chap. 12 focuses on systems that use AI methods to interpret medical images (e.g., digital radiology, retinal photographs, and microscopic views of blood smears or pathological sections). Similar methods have been used in interpreting other non-visual signals, such as electrocardiograms (ECGs), electroencephalograms (EEGs), or alternate sources of physiological data. As depicted in Fig. 17.3, these kinds of programs are used to analyze streams of clinical data. Their output is an interpretive report, which is ultimately provided to the clinical team caring for the patient. Typically the clinicians do not interact with the computer themselves; they order a test and wait for the result to be reported to them.

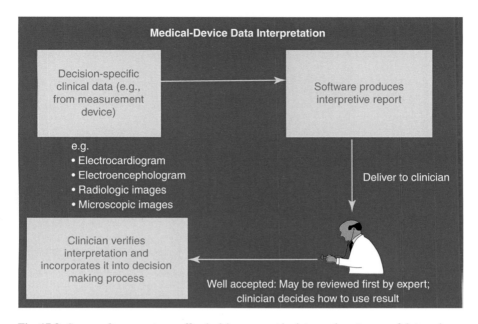

Fig. 17.3 Some software systems offer decision-support by interpreting streams of data and providing written interpretations to the clinical team. Since this workflow corresponds to a familiar process (order a test and get a result that can be verified by examining the data), such applications tend to be well accepted and there are no major usability issues

In such applications, in addition to the interpretive report, there is a depiction of the primary data (the X-ray film itself, a retinal photograph, a 12-lead ECG tracing, etc.) and clinicians (or their expert consultants) have a natural mechanism for assessing whether the report from the computer is persuasive. They can look at the primary data (i.e., look at the film or the ECG tracing) and ask themselves whether the computer's assessment is well aligned with their own sense of what is going on with the patient and the data stream being assessed. In many settings, an expert in the discipline (e.g., a radiologist in the case of chest X-ray interpretation, or a cardiologist for ECG reports) will sign off on the computer's interpretation before the report is provided to the ordering clinical team. In such settings, the use model for the clinicians is not radically different from what they experienced before computer interpretations were introduced. Thus evaluations of usability and acceptance are different—and much more limited—than they need to be when the clinicians are directly using the program themselves.

Event Monitoring and Alerts

A second decision-support model is commonly used in medicine today, especially in settings where EHRs and order-entry systems are in routine use by clinicians. Event monitoring applications, which lead to alerts or warnings, are simple in their

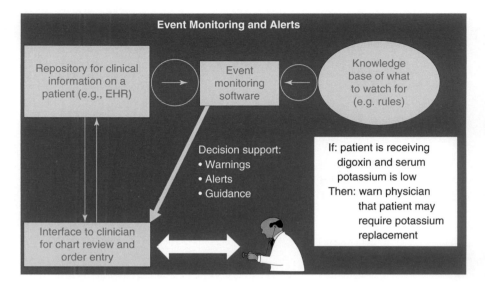

Fig. 17.4 A commonly available decision-support approach is the embedding of logical criteria for generating warnings, alerts, or guidance. These are delivered to clinicians when they are using the EHR to review patient data, to write notes, or to enter orders (e.g., for lab tests, medications, or diagnostic studies). A knowledge base of simple rules is applied prospectively as new data enter a patient's record. When the conditions in a monitoring rule are met (see a simple example for advising potassium replacement in the figure), a warning or alert is generated and delivered to the responsible clinician (generally during a routine interaction with the computer system, although there are methods for delivering urgent warnings by other means such as text messages to the clinician's mobile phone)

logic but can be useful if implemented well (see Fig. 17.4). In these cases, the software system (which typically uses an encoding scheme such as the Arden Syntax[6]—a standard method for representing knowledge in brief rules and inferring decisions) is tightly integrated with the clinician's use of existing software systems. As new information is recorded in the patient's record, monitoring software checks to see if any of the rules' conditions are satisfied. If so, the system responds by generating a suitable alert or warning that is delivered to the responsible clinician. Simple examples include alerting a physician to the implications of a lab result (see the white box example in Fig. 17.4) or warning the physician about an allergy to a newly prescribed medication or a potential interaction between a new drug and other medications that the patient is receiving. When an alert needs to be delivered urgently, the system may not wait until the physician is next using the EHR but may send a warning message to the clinician's mobile phone or to other staff members.

The implementation and evaluation of alerting applications are quite different in their implications than is the case for most advanced, and more complex, AIM

---

[6]The Arden Syntax: https://www.hl7.org/implement/standards/product_brief.cfm?product_id=2. (accessed August 14, 2022)

systems. However, the design and testing of such capabilities clearly involves many of the steps discussed earlier in this chapter: assessing clinical need, determining usability and acceptance of the delivery of such warnings, validating the decision-making content of the rule-set, and considering the value and impact of such warnings when they are delivered.

Direct Consultation with Clinical User

A third model of decision-support delivery was the dominant approach in the early development of AIM systems. Programs such as MYCIN and INTERNIST-1 (see Chap. 2) were conceived as consultation systems, i.e., as programs to which a physician would come for expert consultation. Although developing the knowledge bases and reasoning engines was complex, the use model was very simple: enter into a computer-based (keyboard) interaction with a clinician who would present the case and ask for the program's advice or assessment. In the 1970s, before the introduction of EHRs, personal computers, local area networking, or data standards, there was no other realistic model for developing and testing such decision-support capabilities. Furthermore, graphical interfaces had not been introduced yet, so the interaction was dependent on having users type at a keyboard rather than using pointing devices (e.g., a mouse). This consultation model continued in the AIM development community for several years (see Chap. 2), as depicted in Fig. 17.5.

The consultation model as shown in the figure was ultimately discarded as computational capabilities and human-computer interaction approaches naturally evolved in subsequent decades. Clinicians questioned why they should need to provide data to the computer system when they knew that the answers to most of the questions were available on other computers in the hospital or clinic. They felt that "smart" advisory programs ought to be much more aware of that environment and of the additional data sources on which they could draw. The original consultation model was viewed as being akin to a Greek Oracle approach,[7] which by 1990 was viewed as unrealistic for busy clinicians and had been largely rejected [26]. What replaced it was a growing sense that decision support should be offered as a byproduct of ongoing workflow with other existing computational tools, such as EHRs and order-entry systems, much like the view implemented for event monitoring applications (Fig. 17.4). A cooperative interplay between clinicians and advisory programs that anticipated physicians' needs, and respected their time, became the dominant model (see Fig. 17.6).

Much of the discussion in this chapter has envisioned AIM systems of the type shown in Fig. 17.6. As is shown in the list at the right side of the figure, a number of issues are crucial considerations in the design and implementation of such advisory tools that are intended to function collaboratively and respectfully with clinician

---

[7] https://www.historyanswers.co.uk/ancient/oracle-of-delphi/. (accessed August 14, 2022)

Fig. 17.5 Early AIM systems typically offered consultative advice to clinicians. The interaction required data entry by the clinician, sometimes in direct response to queries from the computer, and culminated in an assessment, diagnosis, or therapeutic recommendation

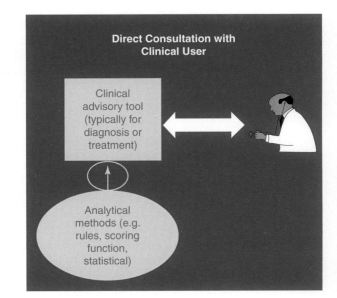

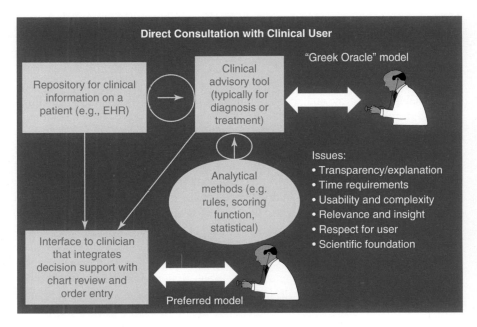

Fig. 17.6 Today the dominant model for AIM systems that interact directly with clinicians is to integrate such guidance with the normal workflow as the physician interacts with EHRs and order-entry systems. Pertinent data to support the advice or guidance can largely be derived from the patient's data available in the EHR or other clinical systems. The "Greek Oracle" model of Fig. 17.5, shown at the upper right of this diagram, has largely been discarded. A number of issues affect the success of applications that follow the current model, as shown in the bulleted list

users. Many of those issues have been mentioned earlier and have been discussed by us in greater detail elsewhere [27].

In summary, the envisioned delivery mechanism for an AIM system's advice or analysis is a crucial element in designing an evaluation plan and testing all pertinent aspects of the program's performance. Although much of this work can initially proceed in controlled test environments, leading to the iterative feedback process described in the section on "Design and Iteration", ultimate rigorous evaluation needs to move to a real-world use environment. As is described in the next section, such work needs to proceed in a step-wise fashion because of the dependencies that exist among the features and characteristics that need to be assessed. This process is outlined in the following section.

Naturalistic Studies

Much of the preceding discussion has focused on the need for iterative evaluation and development in a controlled or laboratory setting. As has been emphasized, the development of use scenarios is part of the early design and implementation work because such efforts can help to predict capabilities that may be crucial to acceptance of a system by intended users. Early informal usability testing can assist this process. Thus there are several development and evaluation steps that must be completed before a system is put into clinical use. These are reflected in the "initial work" portion of the step-wise process outlined in Fig. 17.7.

However, once a system is implemented for routine use in an experimental clinical setting, summary evaluations of its usability and acceptability are needed. Formal usability testing, with real users who are going about their routine duties,

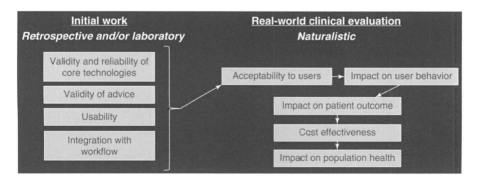

Fig. 17.7 The initial work on an AIM system involves several evaluation steps in a laboratory or controlled setting (see the sections on "Framing Questions for Assessing an Evaluation Plan", "Design and Iteration", and "Cognitive Evaluation Methods"). These include validation of the methodology (decision-making performance) and assessments of usability and impact on workflow. When the system moves into real-world clinical use (i.e., a naturalistic setting), there are a series of step-wise evaluation questions, each of which depends on encouraging results from the previous stage (see text). Among these, the system's impact on patients and their clinical outcome is paramount

is key and often uncovers issues not previously anticipated. Thus usability and workflow assessment is a process that begins in the laboratory environment prior to implementation (through work with collaborating representatives of the intended user community, who can help to anticipate and assess how the system will be used and integrated when moved into routine use). However, such work ultimately needs to be continued, validated, and solidified in real world clinical settings.

Is the System Accepted by Users?

In the naturalistic setting, with introduction of a system for routine use on real patients, the first question that needs to be assessed is whether the intended users will actually accept and utilize the decision support being offered. A negative assessment of this issue clearly requires a return to the development process so that a revised version can be made available and subsequently evaluated to see if the system now is embraced by the users. There is no need to look for beneficial behavioral change on the part of users if they have already ignored or otherwise refused to use the system.

Does the System Have a Positive Impact on User Behavior?

Once a system's acceptability from a usability perspective has been demonstrated in the clinical environment, it becomes necessary to assess how it is actually used by busy clinicians. Do they use it routinely? If not, when do they choose to use it? When it offers advice, are the recommendations accepted and acted upon? When its advice is not followed, what is the explanation offered by the user?

Answering such questions requires formal experimental (including cognitive) work. The results of such studies may be disturbing and may uncover problems that require changes in the system's design or implementation. The goal of such evaluation work is to discover whether physicians or other users actually follow the advice that it offers, or whether they change their approach in some other way.

Such concerns are not hypothetical. Implementers of clinical systems often bemoan the failure of their carefully developed decision-support capabilities to influence the actual decisions of clinicians. For example, consider the alerting systems previously discussed (Fig. 17.4). These systems warn clinicians about potentially significant concerns such as pertinent drug allergies or abnormal lab tests (suggesting that a given treatment should be avoided). Yet studies show that a large percentage of such alerts (well over half in most studies) are ignored by clinicians [28, 29]. Sometimes they ignore the warnings for good reasons, but sometimes they appear to have been simply too busy or too distracted to pay attention. Thus, it cannot be assumed that clinicians will be influenced by a system's advice, even if they regularly use it as part of their routine assessment of a patient. Unless the system is actually affecting user's decisions, there is little point in undertaking studies at the next stage (Fig. 17.7) to determine its impact on patient outcome.

Do Patients Benefit When the System Is Used?

Once formal studies have shown that a system is used and accepted by clinician users, and that user behaviors (decisions) have been influenced positively, it is time to assess whether patients are benefitting from the introduction of the AIM tool into their care environment. A formal randomized control trial (RCT) is the preferred standard for validating new clinical interventions, but the approach was conceived to deal with conventional medical treatments (usually new drugs or devices) and is not easily matched to the evaluation of a decision-support tool. RCTs require careful design, avoidance of bias, and control for potentially confounding variables. They also require approval by human subjects committees (also known as **Institutional Review Boards**, or IRBs), where risk to subjects is considered, along with attention to patient privacy and informed consent. They can be expensive to carry out and, depending on the end points of interest, can take years to complete.

In the area of clinical decision support, remarkably few prospective RCTs of a computer system have been carried out or published. In fact, it is difficult to find any such trials in the literature (there are a handful but they were performed in very limited settings). Even the notion of randomization can be difficult to include in the design of such evaluations. Since the subject of study is as much the clinician as the system itself, it is generally not feasible to design an effective evaluation protocol that randomizes patients being seen by that clinician. Random assignment of clinicians can be attempted (i.e., those who do or do not receive access to the system), but there are substantial opportunities for undesirable crossover effects as physicians using the system may well share their experiences and reactions with other physicians who are not assigned to the study group. As a result, the design of AIM system evaluations may not permit formal RCTs, but great care has to be given to designing protocols that avoid biasing or crossover effects. Even comparing two institutions (one with the system and one without) may not work well since no two organizations are identical and there are many other factors that may prevent them from being comparable (e.g., patient mix, accepted insurance, staffing issues, and the like).

As has been noted, such trials cannot be initiated until prior studies have been done to demonstrate the quality of other aspects of the system's capabilities. This provides reassurance to IRBs that the system is ready for a prospective trial with real patients and helps to assure investigators that a formal trial has a chance of demonstrating a positive impact of the computer program. Results of the prior studies undertaken, as have been previously described in this chapter, will generally be required by IRBs as they seek to address various concerns regarding the decision-support program (Box 17.1).

Box 17.1 Evidence Typically Required Before Human-Subjects Committees (IRBs) Will Approve Trials of AIM Systems on Real Patients

- Evidence of the precision, accuracy and reliability of its key component technologies (e.g., the system's ability to identify and retrieve relevant evidence, its medical logic, and its underlying technical capabilities such as machine learning or natural language processing)
- Evidence that the program gives advice that is similar to or better than the usual standard of care (tests of system *validity* on test cases, where often the standard for comparison is what expert clinicians think about the same cases)
- Evidence that the program is ready to be used in the ongoing care of actual patients in practice settings
- Evidence that the intended users (typically physicians) will find the system helpful, transparent, acceptably usable, and effectively integrated with their workflow and with other systems that they use
- Evidence that, when used, the system in turn positively influences the decisions that users make about a patient

Finally, once such trials are initiated, it should be noted that it may take a long time before sufficient statistical power can be achieved to document differences in end points depending on whether the system was or was not used. And the end points themselves may be highly variable. For example, it may not take long to determine if a patient has recovered from an acute illness when treated in accordance with an AIM system's recommendation, but patient remission or survival when they are being managed with the aid of an AIM tool in oncology, for example, may take much longer to assess.

Is Any Positive Outcome Worth the Associated Expense?

Note that *after* a positive trial, there will typically still be a need for cost-effectiveness analyses to demonstrate that the benefit provided by the system justifies the financial cost associated with its use. Similarly, as competing systems enter the marketplace, comparative-effectiveness studies may also be required to establish whether one provides superior benefit, either overall or in specific settings or circumstances.

Do All Patients Benefit? What Is the Impact on the Population as a Whole?

Policy makers must generally make decisions based on the overall impact of a technology on population health—especially if use of a system or capability is likely to become the standard of care and to be reimbursed by insurance providers. The associated analyses to answer such questions are not typically undertaken by the developers of an AIM system, but they may affect the ability of the population, and the health system as a whole, to benefit from the innovations they have developed. See the discussions of regulation and ethics in Chap. 18 for more details on these issues.

In summary, evaluation experiments and formal studies need to be undertaken in an order that will eliminate confounding variables in a stepwise fashion (Fig. 17.7). The early studies should be undertaken in controlled "laboratory" settings and may be retrospective. Laboratory settings include the iterative design phase as well the demonstration phase of the technology in small studies in real world user environments. After positive results are obtained in the controlled setting, experimental trials can be undertaken to confirm the system's impact in client environments (usability acceptance, impact on behavior, and benefit to patients).

Additional Considerations

The discussion in this chapter has tended to focus on AIM systems designed to provide decision support to health professionals in clinical settings. However, as this book illustrates, there are many other potential use settings and models for AI programs designed to assist in biomedical research and clinical practice. Furthermore, not all users of AIM systems are health professionals. There is also a burgeoning set of research projects and commercial products that are focused more on use by patients and the public. The telehealth phenomenon has provided opportunities to use AI methods to handle the interface with patients, managing the interview and even offering guidance to the clinician at the other end of the link. With various wearable health monitors, there is also a rapidly growing set of opportunities to use AI methods to analyze such data streams and to provide "intelligent" feedback to the individual. In clinical environments, wearable data sources are becoming just another data stream, with opportunities for AI tools to merge information from EHRs with these new data sources in order to provide novel kinds of assessments and advice.

Although these additional opportunities for AIM systems exist, the need for formal evaluation remains. The principles outlined in this chapter can be adapted to address this need, and it is accordingly important for all AIM researchers and developers to carry out well designed evaluations. Anecdotes and impressive demonstrations are not enough. Rigorous assessment and publication will continue to be crucial as the field further matures and seeks to demonstrate its role in the care of individual patients and the overall health of the population.

Questions for Discussion

- What approaches will best guide a system's design and implementation so that the eventual naturalistic requirements for acceptance and impact are considered from the outset?
- How should the individual AIM researcher, or a small group, deal with the *team science* implications that are discussed in this chapter as being pertinent for coordinated design, implementation, evaluation, and feedback?
- After reading the FDA action plan, "Artificial Intelligence and Machine Learning in Software as a Medical Device", referenced in a footnote early in the chapter, how would you characterize the proposal, its utility, and potential barriers to its successful implementation?
- How does a poorly designed EHR implementation contribute to disruptions to clinical workflow? What approaches are most appropriate to study EHR implementation and clinical workflow?
- Why have commercial AIM systems tended to be evaluated less formally and rigorously than systems developed by academic AIM researchers? What are the implications of your observations?
- Consider the three large categories of decision-support systems discussed in the section on "Delivery of Decision Support". The need for explanation capabilities was stressed for the third category (Direct consultation with the clinician user). Would the first two categories benefit from incorporation of explanation capabilities? What are the implications for the underlying analytical methods that would need to be explained?
- Can you develop a summary diagram that would summarize the steps in AIM design, development, testing, introduction, and evaluation that also accounts for the feedback and iterative aspects of the process?

Further Reading

Friedman CP, Wyatt JC, Ash JS. Evaluation methods in biomedical and health informatics. 3rd ed. Cham: Springer; 2022. 557 p.

- This volume has become a standard reference on the broad range of issues that arise when designing and undertaking both formal and informal studies of health information technology applications. The content is broadly applicable to AIM systems evaluation as well.

Herasevich V, Pickering BW. Health information technology evaluation handbook: from meaningful use to meaningful outcomes. 2nd ed. London: Productivity Press, Taylor & Francis; 2021. 200 p.

- A useful and practical guide to the evaluation of clinically oriented technological tools. Using case studies to illustrate key points, the volume covers study structure and design, measurement fundamentals, results analysis, communicating results, guidelines development, and reference standards.

Buchanan BG, Cooper GE, Friedman CP, Gardner R, Haynes RB, Schoolman HM, et al. Evaluation of knowledge-based systems: report of a workshop at the National

Library of Medicine. Bethesda, MD: National Library of Medicine; 1995. p. 35. http://www.shortliffe.net/docs/Evaluation-of-Knowledge-Based-Systems-1995.pdf.

- Although never formally published and for only a few years available online from the NLM as a workshop report, this document is an excellent summary of recurring issues, and resulting approaches, that help to define a framework for the evaluation of AIM systems. As noted (see above URL), a copy has been made available on the Internet for general access.

Clarke K, O'Moore R, Smeets R, Talmon J, Brender J, McNair P, et al. A methodology for evaluation of knowledge-based systems in medicine. Artif Intell Med. 1994;6(2):107–21.

- In this journal paper, which focuses specifically on knowledge-based AIM systems, the authors describe an iterative, four-phased development evaluation cycle framework that covers: (i) early prototype development, (ii) validity of the system, (iii) functionality of the system, and (iv) impact of the system.

Park Y, Jackson GP, Foreman MA, Gruen D, Hu J, Das AK. Evaluating artificial intelligence in medicine: phases of clinical research. JAMIA Open. 2020;3(3): 326–31.

- This paper proposes an interdisciplinary, phased research framework for evaluation of AI implementations in health care. It draws analogies to, and highlights differences from, the clinical trial phases for drugs and medical devices, presenting a study design and methodological guidance for each stage.

Reddy S, Rogers W, Makinen V-P, Coiera E, Brown P, Wenzel M, et al. Evaluation framework to guide implementation of AI systems into healthcare settings. BMJ Health Care Inform. 2021;28(1):e100444.

- This recent paper, like the paper by Park, Jackson, et al., is motivated by the need for a general framework that can guide the evaluation of AIM systems. It provides useful suggestions that complement those offered in the previous paper.

Fox J, Das S. Safe and sound: Artificial Intelligence in hazardous applications. Cambridge, MA: AAAI Press; 2000. 325 p. (American Association for Artificial Intelligence).

- This book describes, from both practical and theoretical perspectives, an AI technology for supporting sound clinical decision making and safe patient management. Fox and Das insist that the same intelligence (artificial and human) must be applied to guaranteeing safety as to assuring acceptable task performance.

Patel VL, Kannampallil T, Kaufman D, editors. Cognitive informatics in health and biomedicine: human computer interaction. London: Springer; 2015.

- This edited book addresses the key gaps in the applicability of theories, models, and evaluation frameworks of HCI and human factors for developing safer system design in biomedical informatics.

Norman DA. Things that make us smart: defending human attributes in the age of the machine. Reading, MA: Addison-Wesley Pub. Co; 1993.

- This book addresses the complex interactions between human thought and the technology it creates, arguing for the development of machines that fit our minds rather than accepting the notion that minds must conform to the machine.

References

1. Friedman CP, Wyatt JC, Ash JS. Evaluation Methods in Biomedical and Health Informatics. 3rd ed. Cham: Springer; 2022. 557 p.
2. Clarke K, O'Moore R, Smeets R, Talmon J, Brender J, McNair P, et al. A methodology for evaluation of knowledge-based systems in medicine. Artif Intell Med. 1994;6(2):107–21.
3. Herasevich V, Pickering BW. Health information technology evaluation handbook: from meaningful use to meaningful outcomes. 2nd ed. London: Productivity Press, Taylor & Francis; 2021. 200 p.
4. Bauer MS, Damschroder L, Hagedorn H, Smith J, Kilbourne AM. An introduction to implementation science for the non-specialist. BMC Psychol. 2015;3(1):32.
5. Eccles MP, Mittman BS. Welcome to Implementation Science. Implement Sci. 2006;1(1):1.
6. Pocock SJ, McMurray JJV, Collier TJ. Making sense of statistics in clinical trial reports: part 1 of a 4-part series on statistics for clinical trials. J Am Coll Cardiol. 2015;66(22):2536–49.
7. Jamison DT, Breman JG, Measham AR, Alleyne G, Claeson M, Evans DB, et al. Chapter 3: Cost-effectiveness analysis. In: Priorities in health. Washington, DC: The International Bank for Reconstruction and Development, The World Bank; 2006. https://www.ncbi.nlm.nih.gov/books/NBK10253/. Accessed 25 Jan 2022.
8. Bernstein MS, Levi M, Magnus D, Rajala BA, Satz D, Waeiss C. Ethics and society review: ethics reflection as a precondition to research funding. Proc Natl Acad Sci. 2021;118(52):e2117261118. https://www.pnas.org/content/118/52/e2117261118. Accessed 25 Jan 2022.
9. Neame MT, Sefton G, Roberts M, Harkness D, Sinha IP, Hawcutt DB. Evaluating health information technologies: a systematic review of framework recommendations. Int J Med Inform. 2020;142:104247.
10. Park Y, Jackson GP, Foreman MA, Gruen D, Hu J, Das AK. Evaluating artificial intelligence in medicine: phases of clinical research. JAMIA Open. 2020;3(3):326–31.
11. Shortliffe T, Davis R. Some considerations for the implementation of knowledge-based expert systems. ACM SIGART Bull. 1975;55:9–12.
12. Buchanan BG, Cooper GE, Friedman CP, Gardner R, Haynes RB, Schoolman HM, et al. Evaluation of knowledge-based systems: report of a workshop at the National Library of Medicine. Bethesda, MD: National Library of Medicine; 1995. p. 35. http://www.shortliffe.net/docs/Evaluation-of-Knowledge-Based-Systems-1995.pdf.
13. Verma AA, Murray J, Greiner R, Cohen JP, Shojania KG, Ghassemi M, et al. Implementing machine learning in medicine. CMAJ. 2021;193(34):E1351–7.
14. Shneiderman B, Plaisant C, Cohen M, Jacobs S, Elmqvist N, Diakopoulos N. Designing the user interface: strategies for effective human-computer interaction. 6th ed. Boston, MA: Pearson; 2016. 616 p.
15. Patel VL, Kannampallil TG, Kaufman DR. Cognitive informatics for biomedicine: human computer interaction in healthcare. 1st ed. Cham: Springer; 2015. 351 p.
16. Shneiderman B. Human-centered AI. New York, NY: Oxford University Press; 2022. 400 p.

17. Lee JD, Wickens CD, Liu Y, Boyle LN. Designing for people: an introduction to human factors engineering. 3rd ed. Charleston, SC: CreateSpace Independent Publishing Platform; 2017. 692 p.
18. Yu VL, Fagan LM, Wraith SM, Clancey WJ, Scott AC, Hannigan J, et al. Antimicrobial selection by a computer. A blinded evaluation by infectious diseases experts. JAMA. 1979;242(12):1279–82.
19. Ericsson KA, Simon HA. Protocol analysis: verbal reports as data. Cambridge, MA: A Bradford Book; 1993. 500 p. Revised Edition.
20. Patel V, Arocha JF, Kaufman D. Diagnostic reasoning and medical expertise. Psychol Learn Motiv Adv Res Theory. 1994;31(C):187–252.
21. Patel VL, Groen GJ. The general and specific nature of medical expertise: a critical look. In: Ericsson KA, Smith J, editors. Toward a general theory of expertise: prospects and limits. New York, NY: Cambridge University Press; 1991. p. 93–125.
22. Patel VL, Kaufman DR, Kannampallil T. Human-computer interaction, usability, and workflow. In: Shortliffe EH, Cimino JJ, editors. Biomedical informatics: computer applications in health care and biomedicine. Cham: Springer International Publishing; 2021. p. 153–75. https://doi.org/10.1007/978-3-030-58721-5_5. Accessed 17 Feb 2022.
23. Horsky J, Kuperman GJ, Patel VL. Comprehensive analysis of a medication dosing error related to CPOE. J Am Med Inform Assoc JAMIA. 2005;12(4):377–82.
24. Carayon P, Karsh B-T, Cartmill R. 2010 Incorporating health information technology into workflow redesign. Digital Healthcare Research. Report No.: AHRQ Publication No. 10-0098-EF. Center for Quality and Productivity Improvement, University of Wisconsin Madison. https://digital.ahrq.gov/sites/default/files/docs/citation/workflowsummaryreport. pdf. Accessed 17 Feb 2022.
25. Zheng K, Hanauer DA, Weibel N, Agha Z. Computational ethnography: automated and unobtrusive means for collecting data in situ for human–computer interaction evaluation studies. In: Patel VL, Kannampallil TG, Kaufman DR, editors. Cognitive informatics for biomedicine: human computer interaction in healthcare. Cham: Springer International Publishing; 2015. p. 111–40. https://doi.org/10.1007/978-3-319-17272-9_6. Accessed 17 Feb 2022. Health Informatics.
26. Miller RA, Masarie FE. The demise of the "Greek Oracle" model for medical diagnostic systems. Methods Inf Med. 1990;29(1):1–2.
27. Shortliffe EH, Sepuveda MJ. Clinical decision support in the era of artificial intelligence. JAMA. 2018;320(21):2199. https://pubmed.ncbi.nlm.nih.gov/30398550/. Accessed 21 Dec 2021.
28. Cho I, Slight SP, Nanji KC, Seger DL, Maniam N, Fiskio JM, et al. The effect of provider characteristics on the responses to medication-related decision support alerts. Int J Med Inform 2015;84(9):630–9.
29. Horsky J, Phansalkar S, Desai A, Bell D, Middleton B. Design of decision support interventions for medication prescribing. Int J Med Inform. 2013;82(6):492–503.

Chapter 18
Ethical and Policy Issues

Diane M. Korngiebel, Anthony Solomonides, and Kenneth W. Goodman

After reading this chapter, you should be able to offer answers to these questions:
- Why is it important to employ an ethics-sensitive approach throughout the development and evaluation of artificial intelligence (AI)?
- What are some of the tangible benefits of incorporating applied ethics when creating AI products and systems?
- Who are stakeholders and why are they important for ethical AI development?
- What are the key components to consider when assessing fairness?
- What are some critical elements of good governance?

Artificial Intelligence (AI) is one of the most exciting technologies to emerge from computer, logic, and cognitive sciences. It has also engendered unprecedented public, professional, and official debate. In its application to health and medicine, it has been paralleled by an extraordinary effort to identify and address complex ethical issues. It has become clear that the success of AI in patient care and research is dependent on the success of this effort to address software quality and standards, governance, explainability and interpretability, transparency and accountability, human control, and bias and fairness. The tools of applied ethics are identified as

D. M. Korngiebel
Department of Biomedical Informatics and Medical Education, University of Washington, Seattle, WA, USA
e-mail: dianemk@uw.edu

A. Solomonides
Research Institute, NorthShore University HealthSystem, Evanston, IL, USA

K. W. Goodman (✉)
Institute for Bioethics and Health Policy, University of Miami, Miami, FL, USA
e-mail: KGoodman@med.miami.edu

© The Author(s), under exclusive license to Springer Nature Switzerland AG 2022
T. A. Cohen et al. (eds.), *Intelligent Systems in Medicine and Health*, Cognitive Informatics in Biomedicine and Healthcare,
https://doi.org/10.1007/978-3-031-09108-7_18

essential if the growing use of AI is to be trusted and trustworthy and therefore to achieve the benefits for which its promoters, developers, and users hope.

This chapter provides an overview of the most important ethical issues that arise when intelligent machines are used in health care; suggests a number of stances and practices to ethically optimize those uses; and addresses some of the leading public policy issues.

Introduction to the Utility of Applied Ethics

Applied ethics is the practical application of critical thinking about values to address and resolve real-world moral issues. For half a century, the tools of applied ethics have helped guide the world's health institutions and practitioners in efforts to address challenges arising in the design and use of new technologies. From organ transplantation and gene therapy to extracorporeal membrane oxygenation and artificial intelligence, the questions about whether, by whom, and under what circumstances a new technology should be used have been guided by applied ethics.

The skills used by scholars to address these issues are akin to those we teach students of medicine and nursing when we introduce the concept of a differential diagnosis. All must answer these questions: What are the facts, what explains them, what more do you want to know, what can be done, what should be done? Ethics is unlike clinical practice, however, because there is no experiment or test that can give the right or best answer. Rather, a suite of analytic skills is required to identify the issue at hand and to derive the most appropriate course of action. In the case of artificial intelligence in health care, a key step—identify the issues—has already been taken. Indeed, in a strikingly short time, the world's scholars have done an extraordinary job of identifying the ethical issues raised by computer algorithms that revise themselves in response to new data and information. In an AI world, we have come swiftly to know that machine learning tools can be biased, make "decisions" that are difficult or impossible to explain, and alter traditional human relationships. We also learned, nearly a half-century ago, that it might be blameworthy *not* to use a tool that can improve health, reduce suffering, or prolong life [1]. The challenge is to identify appropriate uses and users of the tools to achieve the most good without collateral damage, and much of the **bioethics** literature consists of analyses of benefits, risks and harms, and attempts to balance them.

Software Engineering Principles, Standards and Best Practices

We begin with a brief review of the role of sound software engineering practice and describe an ethics approach to the engineering of artifacts, including intangible products such as software. Though AI systems may include substantial hardware components, as in robotics, their most important feature is often the software that encapsulates their "intelligence."

Software Engineering of Dependable Systems

The software development process begins with an assessment of needs, wants, and feasibility of a technical solution, followed by a comprehensive requirements analysis that reflects all stakeholder roles, including inanimate participants, such as the environment, and expected interactions with users, bystanders, and other actors. Agreed requirements and boundaries of the proposed system will lead to design alternatives, depending on the preferred development methodology. For more complex systems, components and their interactions must be determined and prototyped before full-scale translation into code. Good systems development principles encompass built-in protection and security-by-design, consistency of version control, and thorough documentation with traceability of design and development decisions. The design of the "surfaces" of the system—the user interfaces—should be based on sound human-computer interaction principles, with due attention to different users' cognitive styles and to accessibility.

Ethics in Good Engineering Practice

Several branches of applied ethics touch on the software development process just described. The analysts, designers, developers, testers, and deployment and integration engineers are all bound by one or more codes of **professional ethics**, often tied to a professional association or society through which they receive initial and continuing accreditation. **Data ethics**, including principles of privacy (such as a "minimum necessary" precept), confidentiality (e.g., an "only need-to-know" basis for disclosure), and protection ("do no harm"), will also apply throughout. A fair system would also not privilege one group of users over another without good cause, such as a transparently made and disseminated decision to address healthcare inequity or disparities, nor will a fair system restrict users' choices unnecessarily. With an increasing trend in the sharing of code developed in communities of practice, respect for **intellectual property** rights also becomes a focal issue. This extends to acknowledgement of reuse of another group's program code, sharing enhancements as promised under a Creative Commons license, and not importing ideas or artifacts "borrowed" from a previous employer unless they are published openly and can be acknowledged as a source.

Why Context Matters

Knowledge-based and machine learning AI systems are conceived, developed, and deployed to perform useful functions, even when they are created merely as a proof of concept. What makes such a system fit for purpose? By its very nature, AI would not be effective if not trusted, would not be readily trusted if it issues obscure or implausible decisions, or is suspected of built-in undisclosed interests or biases. The human operator of any such AI system therefore plays a crucial role.

Trust and Trustworthiness

It is difficult to earn trust and very easy to lose it. Trust cannot be earned without trustworthiness being established first. Three main areas are crucial for fostering trust in the development of an AI system. First, the importance of stakeholder engagement: stakeholders should be defined broadly to include those who have an impact on the choice and development of the AI tool or system and those who are affected by it, keeping in mind that these two groups may not be discrete [2]. For example, clinicians may assist in AI development and comprise the group using the system [3]. When there are many stakeholders to consider, it may be necessary to prioritize those whose influence should be greatest (e.g., those with much-needed expertise) as well as those likely to be affected the most (e.g., departments expected to implement the AI system, and the different profession-als—physicians, nurses, etc.—in those departments). The perspectives of patients and their advocates must also be considered. For example, if one is designing a mortality prediction AI system, then one should gather insights from family, caregivers, and social workers, as well as from palliative care clinicians and specialists in hospital medicine. Of course, not all stakeholder groups can be consulted, but it is part of a developer's due diligence to identify and engage key stakeholders.

Second, all decisions and their rationales must be documented, beginning with why the development of the AI system is important in the first place. Whether the model is **black box** (e.g., deep learning), **white box** (e.g., a fully curated decision tree), or **gray box** (e.g., a machine learning model with some handcrafted features), everything that can be documented should be documented (see also the section on Transparency and Chap. 8's discussion of explainability). This is vitally important to support and foster accountability, a key priority for AI implementation [4], and one that should be as much of a focus as transparency [5].

Third, the boundaries of the AI system must be carefully considered and the purpose of the AI tool should be made clear. Examples and use cases should be included, with conditions under which the system might be repurposed, and instances where the system should not be repurposed [6]. In documenting these important limitations, examples of uses that are out-of-scope are also of value. This detailed attention will ultimately support liability regulations as they evolve. Although the widespread use of automated intelligence may be on the horizon, AI in health and healthcare delivery is best served by designing AI systems to support human decision-making [7]—at least until better governance mechanisms are in place, informed by a range of complementary studies—including additional research in ethics and implementation.

Explainability and Interpretability

Classical, knowledge-based AI systems are rule-based and deterministic, incorporating lexicons, ontologies and inferences embodying the knowledge of human experts (see Chaps. 4 and 10). In particular, it is possible in such systems to reverse-engineer the trail of inferences to provide an explanation of the machine-generated decision. More recently, **deep learning**-based and connectionist AI systems incorporate or develop knowledge from large volumes of labelled examples, so that rules cannot easily be derived and expressed in simple terms. For such systems, the related concepts of **explainability** and **interpretability** are less direct and are defined differently [8]. Explainability is the ability to provide a reasonably complete logical explanation of the outcomes of an AI system (e.g., a diagnosis or prediction) through an understanding of its decision process [9]. One concern of black box, deep learning models is that complete explainability is only achievable at the most abstract of levels, and requires understanding the principles of deep learning. Interpretability, on the other hand, reflects how intuitive an AI system's outcomes are to its users. One can think of it as simplifying explainability to the point that those with non-technical expertise can follow, or infer, the "why" of an AI model's outcome. Subject to certain caveats, complete explainability—expert understanding—may not be necessary for clinicians to benefit from the appropriate integration of AI into healthcare delivery; however, interpretability is a necessity. If AI developers have documented all the steps in the AI creation process, then a pared-down explanation in language accessible to non-specialists should be achievable. A more detailed description for experts must also be created, drawing on the documentation and audit trail created during the development process.

Efforts to merge or link knowledge-based and machine learning approaches are the focus of ongoing research. Indeed, more research is needed to understand stakeholder needs regarding both explainability and interpretability, but at the minimum (and until we know more) developers should provide documentation both to meet the anticipated needs of experts (e.g., other biomedical AI specialists) and non-specialists, such as clinicians and patients.

Transparency

Transparency should be a key feature throughout the AI creation process, demonstrating that the development team has considered the ethical implications of their product throughout its design [10]. Transparency is closely related to fairness—without transparency during the AI design process, one cannot sufficiently assess fairness [11] and some recommend making information about predictive algorithms fully available [12]. One simple way to support transparency is to document every step, decision, and major action in the development pipeline, starting with the rationale for developing an AI model in the first place. Is the model intended to address a specific need or because it seems like an interesting idea to explore? The purpose for designing a specific AI system should be explicitly stated at the outset, in this conceptualization stage. Defining expected in-scope and out-of-scope uses will help ensure that the development team is mindful of the system's purpose throughout the process.

Early consideration of scope also helps identify stakeholders. For example, if the system is intended to predict mortality, those knowledgeable about the clinical workflow can provide valuable insight [13]; risk managers and compliance officers might help guide appropriate deployment [14]. In particularly sensitive areas such as end-of-life care, the healthcare institution's ethics committee and any patient engagement or stakeholder advisory boards should weigh in on critical decisions [15]. Transparency should be a design feature from the outset [16]. Conducting and documenting stakeholder engagement also demonstrates thoughtful deliberation and commitment to providing appropriate stakeholders with a means to judge the robustness of the development process. Articulating appropriate uses and users of the system could prove critical to AI development and use as a "standard of care" tool; this is especially important as AI system oversight, governance, and liability evolve [17–19].

Furthermore, many AI products today are designed to emulate human interactions (e.g., chatbots, personal assistants—see Chap. 9) or evoke human emotional responses (e.g., robotic animal companions for the elderly) [20]. Human beings are inclined to anthropomorphism, the attribution of human characteristics or behavior to non-humans and objects, to make sense of interactions [21]. There can be benefits from leveraging the propensity of humans to anthropomorphize—doing so can make some interactions, such as basic information gathering or conveyance, easier and more satisfying [22] but there can also be harms, such as misplaced trust [23] and in circumstances in which human users have expectations of reciprocal emotions and those expectations are not met [24, 25].

It should nevertheless always be clear to human users when an interaction is with a non-human entity. Without this clarity, there is a risk that humans will impose human expectations on non-human systems; these include the ability to understand vocal tone or facial expression and to respond with, or actually feel, sympathy or empathy. Imagine a suicide prevention system that a vulnerable individual interacts with as a friend. When the AI friend is not able to understand or engage in empathetic interactions indicative of friendship, the human user might feel further alienated or abandoned, affecting the risk of self-harm. AI tools used to provide companionship for adults with cognitive impairment are exceptionally complicated because affected individuals might not understand or appreciate the concept of AI interactions [26].

The Need for Human Control

Biomedical AI should always be conceptualized as a human-centered tool that prioritizes improved human health [27]. Seeing AI systems as support for human expertise, so-called augmented intelligence, encourages design decisions that emphasize enabling human review of AI-generated recommendations, diagnoses, prognoses, or other actions [28, 29]. Put differently, computers should support humans, not replace them [1]. It is an old lesson.

This insight is captured by the idea of the **human in the loop**, sometimes cast as a counterpoint to unsupervised machine learning and sometimes as a demand for a human expert to be available to review a system's performance and to evaluate the aptness or accuracy of system output, especially about diagnostic recommendations or prognoses.

Moving forward, as regulatory and legal systems struggle to understand and codify liability in decision-making (mediated) by AI tools, it will be increasingly important to document human decision-making in the development and deployment of these tools. In addition, due attention must be paid during AI development to the possibility of automation bias, which is the assumption that a recommendation presented in the presumed context of objective data and analysis must be more correct than human judgment [30–32], and compares with what has been called "the computational fallacy" [33]. Finally, data creation, collection, and curation as well as AI development, deployment, and evaluation do not occur in a value-free vacuum. Biases can enter at any point in the process, which brings us back to the primary recommendation: document all steps, including the rationale for all choices made, during AI system development.

Taking the Long View

Throughout the AI system design process, developers should envision the future effects of their AI tool or product, including the introduction or exacerbation of healthcare disparities [34]. This broad, proactive imagining of future consequences is best completed with the help of diverse stakeholders. It may be easiest to envision immediate or short-term effects (e.g., more accurate prediction of patients at risk of hospital readmission), but medium- and long-term impact must also be considered, especially in the context of indirect influences that a system might have during and after implementation. Such downstream effects might include operational changes, such as reallocation of hospital resources, including personnel reassignments, or the development of specific recommendations for interventions to reduce patient readmission risk. Although these types of concerns may seem to be outside the immediate influence of system developers, that does not give developers license to neglect potential implementation pitfalls. AI tools will never constitute or provide a complete solution to clinical, research, or public health problems or questions. Even the most carefully developed AI tool, accompanied by detailed documentation of the development process (e.g., how and at what points was bias addressed?) [35–37], will be deployed in a value-laden context with its own biases. Responsible developers must consider non-technical challenges, from clinic workflow issues all the way to social consequences and issues of equitable access to, and allocation of, healthcare resources [38, 39]—all of which will affect the use, usefulness, and ethical, social, and legal implications of their AI tools.

Fairness and Sources of Bias

There are several stages in the development of knowledge-based or machine learning systems where human cognitive or other biases may translate into an unfair imbalance or bias in the system's decision-making processes. We consider three phases: the preparatory or problem-formulation phase in which prior knowledge or data are selected; the development phase, in which technical and other choices are made by human designers; and deployment, wherein human cognitive biases might reinforce biased decision-making. To be sure, bias might also be introduced when system output is interpreted by users.

Fairness, Bias, Equality, Equity

Fairness is often discussed in terms of *distributive justice*: if there is a good to be shared or divided up between individuals—or between nations, communities, or corporations—what would be a fair, i.e., a just way of sharing or making that division? In other words, how is it possible to ensure that the distribution is *equitable, impartial, free of favoritism, unbiased, nondiscriminatory,* or *even handed*? However, some of these terms conflate the notion of equality with equity. "Fair shares" does not mean equal shares if there is a notion of *deserving*—e.g., a greater share to go to those who have done more work, made a greater contribution, or made a larger sacrifice. Similarly, shares may not be equal if there is a notion of *equity,* e.g., when we are dealing with social, common, or moral goods, such as health, access to clean air, affordable, healthful food, living-wage employment, education and childcare, and the list goes on—where there is a presumption that everyone has the right to be served equitably. Equity may reflect level of need as much as fundamental rights: a person with a chronic condition will need more health care; an individual with learning difficulties may need educational support.

In an AI context, concern for fairness has focused mainly on **machine learning** (ML; see Chap. 6), where the ML system is "trained" or conditioned to differentiate among inputs. Such systems may either classify them by some degree of similarity without external intervention ("unsupervised learning") or accept or reject instances once it has encountered a significant number of correctly labelled instances presented to it as its initial training ("supervised learning"). It is well known that the "training set," i.e., the data used to condition the ML system, may include biased conjunctions that may end up being interpreted as inferences. For example, if a certain category of patients has shorter stays in hospital (perhaps because economic circumstances lead them to avoid lengthy stays), the ML system may draw the unwarranted conclusion that patients in that category *do not need* a longer stay in hospital. As a result they may be discharged prematurely.

As in this example, the potential implicit *un*fairness lies in what some patients do or do not receive compared to others in a *systematic* way, meaning that patients who fall into certain categories are apparently treated differently, as if their category determined the treatment they would receive. This may or may not be justified, and thus be explainable, depending on context. If it is not, then it may represent a form of harm to one group or the other, or, conversely, privilege one group above the other. In this way, healthcare disparities persist and exacerbate health disparities.

Data Sets

Many forms of AI use reference data sets of various kinds (see Chap. 3). Many AI systems have relied on formalizing and incorporating human knowledge, beginning with a process of knowledge elicitation that employs a variety of methods to absorb knowledge and experience into distinctions, assertions, and inferences. Certain kinds of operational knowledge, such as of the issues that arise frequently at a helpdesk or in making a clinical diagnosis, could be collected into an expert system (see Chap. 4). Cases represented in data sets that are amenable to classification along certain quantifiable dimensions and could be organized according to a notion of distance. In an experimental breast-cancer screening project, it was suggested that on encountering a worrisome mammogram, a radiologist might ask the system to find the "nearest ten cases" to the one under review. This followed from the notion that the subsequent histories of those ten might give an accurate prognosis as well as possible directions for treatment [40]. Indeed, larger data sets were used to drive diagnostic expert systems and prognostic scoring systems, some of which were highly accurate.

Machine learning relies on very large volumes of data, so large that—in the language of the field—the signal can overwhelm the noise and emerge loud and clear. Given the pivotal role of data in ML systems, human biases have been encoded via unrepresentative data sets, flawed assessments, or even non-catastrophic misdiagnoses, and these data are then used to train an algorithm, that algorithm is liable to exhibit the same biases. Bias detection and mitigation are areas of continuing research, with a number of prominent methods under consideration. Among these, methods that challenge the neutrality of the data—so-called adversarial methods [41]—show promise.

In assessing the utility of data in training an **artificial neural network**, it is useful to think of it not as a monolith (or even as a "data lake") but to consider the broad structure of raw data, computed data, stored data, and a range of data *about* the data. These are often called "metadata" but these types of data can in fact be differentiated into categories that represent different kinds of information: where, when, and how the data were sourced, how were they structured, and how credible are they? We represent this information using a concept termed the **data manifold** (Fig. 18.1).

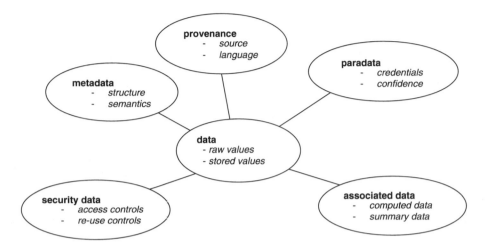

Fig. 18.1 The data manifold. Data are characterized not only by their values, but also by what is loosely termed their "metadata", which can be analyzed into metadata proper, provenance data, paradata (e.g., concerning the credibility of the data), security data, various computed summaries, and so on. (Reprinted by permission from Solomonides, A. Chapter 14—Research Data Governance, Roles, and Infrastructure. In R Richesson and J Andrews (eds). Clinical Research Informatics. Springer Nature. 2019 [42])

Among the issues to be considered is whether the data were fairly and transparently sourced, with due respect for the rights, privacy, and **security** of the data subjects. Data collected surreptitiously or by a process lacking transparency, may be flawed with no opportunity to be checked and verified or corrected in its flow from source to use, e.g., in the creation of an AI system.

Algorithmic Design

Can good design of machine-learning algorithms mitigate some of these dataset problems? The design of complex artefacts presents problems beyond the challenge of devising the isolated component parts and their interconnections, difficult though these may be. A system with hard-to-predict mutual influences and unanticipated firing patterns among its subunits will almost certainly spring surprises, and the more abstract the function of a system is, the more difficult it will be to envision, predict, and control all these interactions. Subject to sound software engineering practice, algorithmic design involves human choices, including how much adaptive capacity any suggested solution should allow. Scientists and technologists are not immune to the countless biases that have been chronicled—preferences, hopes, predilections [43]. ML systems are most effective when they have parametric leeway to adapt and improve their performance, but, as some disastrous examples have shown, this also provides space to become toxic, as proved to be the case with Microsoft's Tay chatbot. Designed to learn language from interaction with other users on Twitter, Tay was overwhelmed by extremist language and within hours began to make misogynistic, anti-Semitic, and other offensive comments. It was withdrawn for a post-mortem just 16 hours after launch [44].

In terms of fairness, there is an additional complexity: sometimes a factor that may lead to biased results (e.g., race) may also be associated with a characteristic that has a real differential impact on certain outcomes. An example in the COVID-19 pandemic concerns level of vitamin D, which appears to confer some protection from COVID-19, and where vitamin D absorption may be lower in African Americans, an effect also confounded by environmental and socioeconomic factors, such as the opportunity to be exposed to the sun [45, 46].

Implementation and Algorithmovigilance

Allowing that an AI system may have been designed in good faith and developed by a team of well-intentioned experts, it is still possible that their product will exhibit biases when implemented. Drugs are developed under stricter conditions than software, yet are sometimes found to be harmful after release to the market; so it may be with software. The idea behind **algorithmovigilance** [47] is similar to that of post-market "pharmacovigilance," the philosophy and the practice of monitoring and notifying any "adverse events" when a drug is adopted: this does not necessarily avoid all harm, but it serves to limit such harm and leads to a reassessment of the safety of a drug. A similar approach to clinical decision support (CDS) systems (see Chap. 10) post-implementation has been cogently advocated to ensure that any clinical harm is limited to as few cases as possible [48], but recognition of a moral harm—such as race-based discrimination—that a biased system may be causing may be harder to uncover.

Organizational and Economic Dimensions

There is no AI ethics without ethics [49]. An organization whose business model is unethical, whether explicitly or implicitly, cannot introduce ethical AI into its operations simply by checking off a list of putative criteria. Moreover, even a moral organization may find itself having to function in an ecosystem of similar, and potentially less moral, entities whose aggregate behavior patterns could shape everyone's conduct. Both intra- and inter-organizational complexity shape the forces that lead to development, adoption, and scaling of technological solutions; the more abstract the technology, the more complexity obscures the conditions of decision-making. In a similar vein Olivia Gambelin [50] discusses the paradoxical

D. M. Korngiebel et al.

position of the AI ethicist in any competitive organization and concludes that, of all virtues, *bravery* is the determining characteristic of the effective AI ethicist. High profile dismissals of AI ethicists from companies such as Google have underscored her argument. They suggest that a conflict between morals and business models creates a greater threat to ethics than to the business. The greatest risk to an AI ethicist in an organization is isolation: the more recognition of the need for an ethical voice and the more integrated that voice is, the more effective the program is likely to be.

Recommendations for Identifying Bias

Bias may be subtle or blatant but deniable. Subtle forms of bias may occur when proxy variables are used for others that are harder to assess. A case in point is that of the health services firm Optum's algorithm to predict future medical need. The proxy for health status is past expenditure on medical care. African Americans spend less for reasons of access and cost, but the algorithm downgrades their medical needs in consequence. Oddly, this also provides an example of a blatant but deniable bias. When this bias was disclosed [39], the firm defended its position by claiming that researchers had misconstrued the purpose of the algorithm and that numerous other factors were taken into consideration to adjust for any misalignment. The lesson would appear to be that bias can be identified through meticulous scholarship and yet remain through a sheer denial that it exists.

In social studies of science and technology, a distinction is drawn between what may be termed "use/abuse" and "immanent values" theories. Are technologies value free, or at least value neutral, such that what goes wrong with them is due to abuse—as opposed to "appropriate" use? Or are the values that informed the very conception so embedded in the technology and its artefacts that neither can be separated from those values, and they are mutually constitutive? In 2015, the Future of Life Institute organized an open letter on *Research Priorities for Robust and Beneficial Artificial Intelligence* with signatories including prominent critics, such as the physicist Stephen Hawking and entrepreneur Elon Musk, but also a stellar array of AI scientists. The potential for AI systems to improve healthcare and further our scientific knowledge in medicine seems undeniable. The underlying science is being developed concurrently in academic labs, in university spinoffs, and—preeminently—in major "big tech" divisions and subsidiaries. It may be more fruitful to address the question *how should AI research be done?* than to anticipate every possible wrong turn.

Insurance companies are developing AI applications to nudge or support patients towards healthier lifestyles. Yet from their poor reputation, if not poor record, for denials, these companies have an obvious conflict of interest. Perhaps a similar technology in the hands of an advocacy organization would help patients overcome their difficulties with insurance benefits. From a researcher's point of view, the question might be more *Are these the right contexts and organizations to work with to develop this cool AI system, or should I be looking elsewhere?* But there are cases where an AI application's development should be reconsidered. Facial recognition software that seeks to identify sexual orientation is an example. It may be an interesting project to a researcher, and the research might even receive IRB approval and be published in a peer-reviewed journal [51], but that does not stop human rights organizations from protesting the project and its "findings." [52] In this example, if a broad range of stakeholders had been involved from the start, including representation from those most likely to be affected by the AI work, the research team might have made a different choice of focus for their facial recognition project. This of course poses the challenging question whether there are certain kinds of empirical inquiry that are inherently out of bounds.

Governance and Oversight

"**Governance**," the term, is best seen as an overarching approach to ensuring that standards are met, values are adhered to, and accountability maintained. Though governance might be by governments, the law alone is sometimes inadequate to ensure best practice, especially in some professions. Nurses and physicians, for instance, though licensed to practice by governments, are most closely overseen by peers, their adherence to standards, and a certification by professional organizations. There is now broad agreement that computer systems (including both those that use AI software and those that do not) and the organizations that use them should be subject to some form of governance. This is a basic requirement to ensure patient and public safety and that systems are appropriately used by appropriate users. A system of governance or oversight must first be clear about exactly what is being governed and to what end. It is for this reason that the identification of ethical issues is so important. We have in this chapter so far identified the following foci of oversight:

- Software quality and standards
- Explainability and interpretability
- Transparency and accountability
- Human control
- Bias and fairness

The value of this list is that it is uncontroversial; there is no good reason to oppose the inclusion of any item, although controversy might arise regarding the kind or scope of governance for each item.

The development of, and adherence to, standards are ethical issues [15]. In a better world, we might be able to assume that all professionals would govern themselves by planning and documenting carefully, evaluating continuously, and always ensuring computer systems are used for legitimate purposes by appropriately trained people. Governance mechanisms and key actors are seen in Box 18.1, where the items in the left column will have arrows pointing to one or more entities on the right:

Box 18.1 Governance Mechanisms and Actors. The Mechanisms in the Left Column Will Map to Various Actors in the Column on the Right

Law (statutes and case law)	Administrators
Governments (FDA, EMA, Health Canada, etc.)	Clinical practices
Institutions (leadership, ethics committees, etc.)	Clinicians
Professional organizations	System developers
Corporations and trade groups	Software
Patient organizations	Corporations
Health NGOs (WHO, UNESCO, etc.)	Institutions (hospitals, systems, etc.)

Some entities will need to exercise self-government. Every "arrow" will engender debate, which is necessary to reach agreed-upon standards. If, for instance, each entity on the left prioritizes or weighs values differently, the result will be a hash of potentially contradictory rules and guidance. It seems therefore to be a very positive development that the "foci of oversight" itemized here represent a distillation of what seems to be broad agreement of that which should be governed. This is apparent in the burgeoning literature on AI governance [53, 54].

Though it is in some circles fashionable to denigrate the role and responsibility of government in ensuring public safety, such a libertarian fetish is inapt and fatuous in the context of computational healthcare. For example, the uncontroversial right of patients to easily view their health records online required, in the United States, a federal mandate to eliminate "information blocking" [55]. Most hospitals would not do this, clinicians were reluctant, and some EHR system vendors had to scramble to comply. The free market saw no traction, no advantage, in ensuring this right. This is not to say that governmental regulation is the only or best solution—rather, it is to argue that an overarching policy framework should be able to make use of all the tools available.

Even when software is regarded as a medical device [56, 57], it is likely to be impossible for a government or legal system to regulate it to be, say, free of error. For this reason, there should be a renewed effort to explore the utility of recommendations emerging in the 1990s to shape the role of the U.S. Food and Drug Administration and otherwise to regulate clinical systems [58, 59]. An especially interesting idea called for local oversight of clinical software by autonomous oversight committees akin to Institutional Review Boards. Various forms of certification (the idea of medical software certification also dates to the 1990s [60, 61]) provide another potentially useful tool: governments and other entities can certify systems as adhering to certain quality standards, as the U.S. Office of the National Coordinator for Health Information Technology does for EHRs.

AI governance is as urgent as it is difficult. It ranges from the granularity of lines of code to a system's success in a global health emergency. What is needed is the recognition that new technology always raises ethical, legal, and social issues, and that they are best addressed, in the first instance, by the tools of applied ethics, and, in the second, by the engines of fair and just civil society.

AI at Large

We conclude our assessment of the ethical and policy issues surrounding AI with a brief review of some broader social and professional implications, not least the rare if not unprecedented public attention devoted to this evolving technology.

AI, Humanity, and Society

The very idea of "artificial intelligence" has intrigued and provoked concern from its very inception. John McCarthy invented the term in the 1950s because the subject of Automata Studies, on which he was co-editing a special collection, failed to attract any visionary contributions on the potential of computational problem solving. Nearly two decades later, in a debate at the Royal Institution in London, he and two British colleagues faced off with Sir James Lighthill, one of the fiercest scientific critics of the project. Introducing the subject of the debate, "The General Purpose Robot is a Mirage," the chair commented, "Tonight we are going to enter a world where some of the oldest visions that have stirred man's imagination blend into the latest achievements of his time" [62]. Sir James had recently submitted a report to the UK Science Research Council in which he discouraged any further investment in AI, arguing that what had already been successful was better described as "automation"—an engineering discipline—while the wilder shores of general purpose AI was a distracting mirage. McCarthy acknowledged that the project had proved much more difficult than he had anticipated, but remained optimistic. In the popular imagination, and in its reception in the lay press, it would appear that the question is settled: in 1997 IBM Deep Blue defeated the reigning world champion at chess and in 2011, IBM Watson defeated the all-time best Jeopardy! player at that game: what more could there be to say? The philosopher John Searle, deeply critical of claims for AI, wrote in *The Wall Street Journal*, "Watson Doesn't Know It Won on 'Jeopardy!'. IBM invented an ingenious program—not a computer that can think." On the other hand, Garry Kasparov, the defeated chess grandmaster, produced a thoughtful reflection on the nature of intelligence in his book, *Deep Thinking* [63]. In 2015, literary agent John Brockman posed the question, "What to Think

About Machines that Think?" [64] to which more than 180 prominent thinkers were invited to contribute short-essay answers. In 2019, returning to the topic, Brockman edited 25 more positions on the question [65]. Evidently, in popular science, as in popular culture, there is much to be said on this subject.

AI and the Healthcare Professions

STAT, an online publication on health care and biomedicine, published a collection of articles on AI from late 2019 to early 2021 under the title "Promise and Peril: How artificial intelligence is transforming health care." Publications in nearly every discipline, from radiology to primary practice to ophthalmology, have had special issues on AI and its anticipated impact on the specialty. Concerns focus on what AI might entail in terms of work patterns, relationships with patients, burden and burn-out—issues that have figured large since the advent of electronic health records and, even more so, clinical decision support, but so far only minimally associated with AI. Questions of professional liability and legal implications have led law firms to offer advice blogs [66, 67], adopting a cautious stance and emphasizing the need for physicians to remain in ultimate control of decision-making. Policy insti-tutes have also weighed in on this issue [68, 69], recognizing that the time is fast approaching, if it is not already here, for definitive legislation, if not regulation, of AI in medicine and healthcare. Among learned publications, attention should be drawn to reviews by a team that has for some time focused on this issue and on AI explainability in healthcare [18, 70, 71]. The cautionary tone of this work may be a useful counterpoint to the persistent optimism of the field [72–74].

Questions for Discussion

- When considering which stakeholders to consult as an AI system is developed, one cannot possibly consult everyone who might be involved or who might be affected. What criteria might and should AI system developers use to prioritize whom to consult? When stakeholder feedback is received, it might be in conflict with recommendations from other stakeholders, or even with the approaches of the development team. When these situations occur, how might dissonant feed-back be resolved?
- Machine Learning-based AI (ML/AI) has the potential to introduce bias at three stages: through training data that incorporate bias, in the development phase where the developers' preconceptions and preferences may bias the product, and in deployment, where human cognitive biases may be reinforced by flawed decisions by the AI system. Consider three common cognitive biases: anchoring (focusing on a single trait or variable at the expense of all others), availability heuristic (focusing on recent or familiar observations), and confir-mation bias (preferring advice or solutions that confirm a preconceived idea). How may each of these figure in the introduction of bias in the three stages of ML/AI?

- Future electronic health records will include point-of-care, AI-based decision-support tools for diagnosis and prognose\is. Should all clinicians have access to such tools? Should education be required before such use? Should computergen-erated advice be reviewed by others before it is acted upon?
- Who ought to be responsible for oversight and governance of clinical health AI development and use? Imagine and describe an institutional policy to guide – and enforce? – such governance.

Further Reading

Miller RA, Schaffner KF, Meisel A. Ethical and legal issues related to the use of computer programs in clinical medicine. Ann Intern Med. 1985;102(4):529–36.

- This article is a landmark in efforts to identify and analyze ethical issues in health information technology. It emphasizes the issues of appropriate use, confidenti-ality, and validation, among others

Mitchell M, Wu S, Zaldivar A, Barnes P, Vasserman L, Hutchinson B, Spitzer E, Raji ID, Gebru T. Model cards for model reporting. In: Proceedings of the Conference on Fairness, Accountability, and Transparency, Atlanta, GA, USA; 2019.

- This work provides a handy tool to help support documentation to accompany model development, thus fostering key goals of transparency and explainability.

Nielsen A. Practical fairness: achieving fair and secure data models. Sebastopol, CA: O'Reilly Media, Inc; 2020.

- Nielsen takes a practical view of fairness, organizing her categories under three questions borrowed from Shoshana Zuboff [75]: Who gets what? (Rules of allo-cation); How do we decide who gets what? (Rules of decision); and Who decides who decides? (Rules of political authority). The focus is on the practical, built on a comprehensive analysis of the problem of fairness in Machine Learning

Obermeyer Z, Powers B, Vogeli C, Mullainathan S. Dissecting racial bias in an algorithm used to manage the health of populations. Science. 2019;366(6464): 447–53.

- This is a watershed study on how misinformed data labeling meant to improve access to care for those patients who need it most did the exact opposite, instead further exacerbating healthcare disparities among already underserved African-American patients

Vayena E, Blasimme A, Cohen IG. Machine learning in medicine: addressing ethi-cal challenges. PLoS Med. 2018;15(11):e1002689. https://doi.org/10.1371/journal. pmed.1002689.

- This report identifies and organizes main ethical and regulatory "concerns," and makes clear that successfully addressing them is necessary for machine learning in healthcare

World Health Organization. Ethics and governance of artificial intelligence for health. Geneva: WHO; 2021. https://www.who.int/publications/i/item/9789240029200.

- A guidance document drafted by an international group of scholars and government representatives. It includes a number of consensus principles and recommendations to "ensure the governance of artificial intelligence for health maximizes the promise of the technology ..."

Zuboff S. Big other: surveillance capitalism and the prospects of an information civilization. J Inf Technol. 2015;30(1):75–89.

- At the dawn of the modern information age there was an optimism and a promise in the air that we would soon achieve "Athens without slaves." The extent to which this vision has fallen short is documented in Zuboff's careful economic analysis of the "information surplus." This provides a sobering contrast to the evergreen optimism of the AI community

References

1. Miller RA, Schaffner KF, Meisel A. Ethical and legal issues related to the use of computer programs in clinical medicine. Ann Intern Med. 1985;102(4):529–36.
2. Arnold MH. Teasing out artificial intelligence in medicine: an ethical critique of artificial intelligence and machine learning in medicine. J Bioeth Inq. 2021;18(1):121–39.
3. Asan O, Bayrak AE, Choudhury A. Artificial intelligence and human trust in healthcare: focus on clinicians. J Med Internet Res. 2020;22(6):e15154.
4. Murphy K, Di Ruggiero E, Upshur R, Willison DJ, Malhotra N, Cai JC, et al. Artificial intelligence for good health: a scoping review of the ethics literature. BMC Med Ethics. 2021;22(1):14.
5. Shah H. Algorithmic accountability. Phi Trans Ser A Math Phys Eng Sci. 2018;376(2128):20170362.
6. Weber C. Engineering bias in AI. IEEE Pulse. 2019;10(1):15–7.
7. Matheny ME, Whicher D, Thadaney IS. Artificial intelligence in health care: a report from the National Academy of Medicine. JAMA. 2020;323(6):509–10.
8. Markus AF, Kors JA, Rijnbeek PR. The role of explainability in creating trustworthy artificial intelligence for health care: a comprehensive survey of the terminology, design choices, and evaluation strategies. J Biomed Inform. 2021;113:103655.
9. Amann J, Blasimme A, Vayena E, Frey D, Madai VI. Explainability for artificial intelligence in healthcare: a multidisciplinary perspective. BMC Med Inform Decis Mak. 2020;20(1):310.
10. Wiens J, Saria S, Sendak M, Ghassemi M, Liu VX, Doshi-Velez F, et al. Do no harm: a roadmap for responsible machine learning for health care. Nat Med. 2019;25(9):1337–40.
11. Vayena E, Blasimme A, Cohen IG. Machine learning in medicine: addressing ethical challenges. PLoS Med. 2018;15(11):e1002689.
12. Van Calster B, Wynants L, Timmerman D, Steyerberg EW, Collins GS. Predictive analytics in health care: how can we know it works? J Am Med Inform Assoc. 2019;26(12):1651–4.
13. Coiera E. The last mile: where artificial intelligence meets reality. J Med Internet Res. 2019;21(11):e16323.
14. Alami H, Lehoux P, Denis JL, Motulsky A, Petitgand C, Savoldelli M, et al. Organizational readiness for artificial intelligence in health care: insights for decision-making and practice. J Health Organ Manag. 2020; https://doi.org/10.1108/JHOM-03-2020-0074.

15. Goodman KW. Ethics, medicine, and information technology: intelligent machines and the transformation of health care. Cambridge: Cambridge University Press; 2016.
16. Felzmann H, Fosch-Villaronga E, Lutz C, Tamò-Larrieux A. Towards transparency by design for artificial intelligence. Sci Eng Ethics. 2020;26(6):3333–61.
17. Sullivan HR, Schweikart SJ. Are current tort liability doctrines adequate for addressing injury caused by AI? AMA J Ethics. 2019;21(2):E160–6.
18. Price WN II, Gerke S, Cohen IG. Potential liability for physicians using artificial intelligence. JAMA. 2019;322(18):1765–6.
19. Price WN II, Gerke S, Cohen IG. How much can potential jurors tell us about liability for medical artificial intelligence? J Nucl Med. 2021;62(1):15–6.
20. Broadbent E. Interactions with robots: the truths we reveal about ourselves. Annu Rev Psychol. 2017;68:627–52.
21. Epley N, Waytz A, Akalis S, Cacioppo JT. When we need a human: motivational determinants of anthropomorphism. Soc Cogn. 2008;26(2):143–55.
22. Waytz A, Morewedge CK, Epley N, Monteleone G, Gao JH, Cacioppo JT. Making sense by making sentient: effectance motivation increases anthropomorphism. J Pers Soc Psychol. 2010;99(3):410–35.
23. Weizenbaum J. ELIZA—a computer program for the study of natural language communication between man and machine. Commun ACM. 1966;9(1):36–45.
24. Salles A, Evers K, Farisco M. Anthropomorphism in AI. AJOB Neurosci. 2020;11(2):88–95.
25. Fiske A, Henningsen P, Buyx A. Your robot therapist will see you now: ethical implications of embodied artificial intelligence in psychiatry, psychology, and psychotherapy. J Med Internet Res. 2019;21(5):e13216.
26. Wangmo T, Lipps M, Kressig RW, Ienca M. Ethical concerns with the use of intelligent assistive technology: findings from a qualitative study with professional stakeholders. BMC Med Ethics. 2019;20(1):98.
27. Jotterand F, Bosco C. Keeping the "human in the loop" in the age of artificial intelligence: accompanying commentary for "correcting the brain?" by Rainey and Erden. Sci Eng Ethics. 2020;26(5):2455–60.
28. Topol EJ. High-performance medicine: the convergence of human and artificial intelligence. Nat Med. 2019;25(1):44–56.
29. Rajkomar A, Dean J, Kohane I. Machine learning in medicine. NEJM. 2019;380(14):1347–58.
30. Goddard K, Roudsari A, Wyatt JC. Automation bias - a hidden issue for clinical decision support system use. Stud Health Technol Inform. 2011;164:17–22.
31. Anderson M, Anderson SL. How should AI be developed, validated, and implemented in patient care? AMA J Ethics. 2019;21(2):E125–30.
32. Sujan M, Furniss D, Grundy K, Grundy H, Nelson D, Elliott M, et al. Human factors challenges for the safe use of artificial intelligence in patient care. BMJ Health Care. Inform. 2019;26(1):e100081.
33. Kwinter S. The computational fallacy. Thresholds. 2003;26:90–2.
34. Rajkomar A, Hardt M, Howell MD, Corrado G, Chin MH. Ensuring fairness in machine learning to advance health equity. Ann Intern Med. 2018;169(12):866–72.
35. Mitchell C, Ploem C. Legal challenges for the implementation of advanced clinical digital decision support systems in Europe. J Clin Transl Res. 2018;3(Suppl 3):424–30.
36. Liu X, Cruz Rivera S, Moher D, Calvert MJ, Denniston AK. Reporting guidelines for clinical trial reports for interventions involving artificial intelligence: the CONSORT-AI extension. Nat Med. 2020;26(9):1364–74.
37. Sendak MP, Gao M, Brajer N, Balu S. Presenting machine learning model information to clinical end users with model facts labels. NPJ Digit Med. 2020;3:41.
38. Pham Q, Gamble A, Hearn J, Cafazzo JA. The need for ethnoracial equity in artificial intelligence for diabetes management: review and recommendations. J Med Internet Res. 2021;23(2):e22320.
39. Obermeyer Z, Powers B, Vogeli C, Mullainathan S. Dissecting racial bias in an algorithm used to manage the health of populations. Science. 2019;366(6464):447–53.

40. Warren R, Solomonides AE, del Frate C, Warsi I, Ding J, Odeh M, et al. MammoGrid--a prototype distributed mammographic database for Europe. Clin Radiol. 2007;62(11):1044–51.
41. Beutel A, Chen J, Zhao Z, Chi EH. Data decisions and theoretical implications when adversarially learning fair representations. arXiv. 2017:170700075.
42. Solomonides A. Research data governance, roles, and infrastructure: methods and applications. In: Richesson RL, Andrews JE, editors. Clinical research informatics. Cham: Springer; 2019. p. 291–310.
43. Pohl R. Cognitive illusions: intriguing phenomena in thinking, judgment and memory. New York, NY: Routledge; 2016.
44. Leetaru K. How Twitter corrupted Microsoft's Tay: a crash course in the dangers of AI in the real world. 2016. https://www.forbes.com/sites/kalevleetaru/2016/03/24/how-twitter-corrupted-microsofts-tay-a-crash-course-in-the-dangers-of-ai-in-the-real-world/#5553441c26d2.
45. Meltzer DO, Best TJ, Zhang H, Vokes T, Arora V, Solway J. Association of vitamin D status and other clinical characteristics with COVID-19 test results. JAMA Netw Open. 2020;3(9):e2019722.
46. Meltzer DO, Best TJ, Zhang H, Vokes T, Arora VM, Solway J. Association of vitamin D levels, race/ethnicity, and clinical characteristics with COVID-19 test results. JAMA Netw Open. 2021;4(3):e214117.
47. Embi PJ. Algorithmovigilance-advancing methods to analyze and monitor artificial intelligence-driven health care for effectiveness and equity. JAMA Netw Open. 2021;4(4):e214622.
48. Petersen C, Smith J, Freimuth RR, Goodman KW, Jackson GP, Kannry J, et al. Recommendations for the safe, effective use of adaptive CDS in the US healthcare system: an AMIA position paper. J Am Med Inform Assoc. 2021;28(4):677–84.
49. Lauer D. You cannot have AI ethics without ethics. AI Ethics. 2021;1(1):21–5.
50. Gambelin O. Brave: what it means to be an AI Ethicist. AI Ethics. 2021;1(1):87–91.
51. Wang Y, Kosinski M. Deep neural networks are more accurate than humans at detecting sexual orientation from facial images. J Pers Soc Psychol. 2018;114(2):246–57.
52. Murphy H. Why Stanford researchers tried to create a 'Gaydar' machine. 2017. https://www.nytimes.com/2017/10/09/science/stanford-sexual-orientation-study.html.
53. Cath C. Governing artificial intelligence: ethical, legal and technical opportunities and challenges. Phi Trans Ser A Math Phys Eng Sci. 2018;376(2133):20180080.
54. Macrae C. Governing the safety of artificial intelligence in healthcare. BMJ Qual Saf. 2019;28(6):495–8.
55. Everson J, Patel V, Adler-Milstein J. Information blocking remains prevalent at the start of 21st Century Cures Act: results from a survey of health information exchange organizations. J Am Med Inform Assoc. 2021;28(4):727–32.
56. Pelayo S, Bras Da Costa S, Leroy N, Loiseau S, Beuscart-Zephir MC. Software as a medical device: regulatory critical issues. Stud Health Technol Inform. 2013;183:337–42.
57. Gordon WJ, Stern AD. Challenges and opportunities in software-driven medical devices. Nat Biomed Eng. 2019;3(7):493–7.
58. Miller RA, Gardner RM. Summary recommendations for responsible monitoring and regulation of clinical software systems. American Medical Informatics Association, The Computer-based Patient Record Institute, The Medical Library Association, The Association of Academic Health Science Libraries, The American Health Information Management Association, and The American Nurses Association. Ann Intern Med. 1997;127(9):842–5.
59. Miller RA, Gardner RM. Recommendations for responsible monitoring and regulation of clinical software systems. American Medical Informatics Association, Computer-based Patient Record Institute, Medical Library Association, Association of Academic Health Science Libraries, American Health Information Management Association, American Nurses Association. J Am Med Inform Assoc. 1997;4(6):442–57.
60. Denvir T. An overview of software assessment. Comput Methods Prog Biomed. 1994;44(1):55–60.
61. Forsström J. Why certification of medical software would be useful? Int J Med Inform. 1997;47(3):143–51.

62. BBC. TV Lighthill Controversy Debate at the Royal Institution. 1973. http://www.aiai.ed.ac. uk/events/lighthill1973/.
63. Kasparov GK, Greengard M. Deep thinking: where machine intelligence ends and human creativity begins. New York, NY: Perseus Books; 2017.
64. Brockman J. What to think about machines that think: today's leading thinkers on the. New York, NY: HarperCollins; 2015.
65. Brockman J. Possible minds: twenty-five ways of looking at AI. New York, NY: Penguin Random House; 2019.
66. Crowell & Moring. Shifting liability: AI in medical devices. Crowell & Moring. 2020. https:// www.crowell.com/NewsEvents/AlertsNewsletters/all/Shifting-Liability-AI-in-Medical-Devices.
67. Sankey P. AI medical diagnosis and liability when something goes wrong. Enable Law. 2021. https://www.enablelaw.com/news/expert-opinion/ai-medical-diagnosis-and-liability-when-something-goes-wrong/.
68. Ordish J. Legal liability for machine learning in healthcare. Cambridge: PHG Foundation; 2021. https://www.phgfoundation.org/briefing/legal-liability-machine-learning-in-healthcare.
69. Maliha G, Parikh R. Artificial intelligence and medical liability: system reforms. Philadelphia, PA: Leonard Davis Institute of Health Economics; 2019. https://ldi.upenn.edu/our-work/research-updates/artificial-intelligence-and-medical-liability-system-reforms/.
70. Babic B, Gerke S, Evgeniou T, Cohen IG. Beware explanations from AI in health care. Science (New York, NY). 2021;373(6552):284–6.
71. Maliha G, Gerke S, Cohen IG, Parikh RB. Artificial intelligence and liability in medicine: balancing safety and innovation. Milbank Q. 2021; https://doi.org/10.1111/1468-0009.12504.
72. Topol EJ. Deep medicine: how artificial intelligence can make healthcare human again. New York, NY: Basic Books; 2019.
73. Topol EJ. The patient will see you now: the future of medicine is in your hands. New York, NY: Basic Books; 2015.
74. Topol EJ. The creative destruction of medicine. New York, NY: Basic Books; 2012.
75. Zuboff S. The age of surveillance capitalism: the fight for a human future at the new frontier of power. New York, NY: Public Affairs; 2019.

Chapter 19
Anticipating the Future of Artificial Intelligence in Medicine and Health Care: A Clinical Data Science Perspective

Anthony C. Chang

After reading this chapter, you should know the answers to these questions:

- How will a future of "intelligence-based medicine" be different than the current evidence-based medicine in terms of clinical practice and patient outcome?
- What are several promising artificial intelligence tools that are being explored for future application in clinical medicine and health care?
- How might artificial intelligence tools be deployed in ways that are analogous to the human central and peripheral nervous systems?
- What is the current relationship between artificial intelligence technology and health care stakeholders, and how might this relationship need to change in the future?

If we do it right, we might be able to evolve a form of work that taps into our uniquely human capabilities and restores our humanity. The ultimate paradox is that this technology may become a powerful catalyst that we need to reclaim our humanity.
    —John Hagel, author and consultant in Silicon Valley

A. C. Chang (✉)
Medical Intelligence and Innovation Institute (MI3), Children's Health of Orange County, Orange, CA, USA

© The Author(s), under exclusive license to Springer Nature Switzerland AG 2022
T. A. Cohen et al. (eds.), *Intelligent Systems in Medicine and Health*, Cognitive Informatics in Biomedicine and Healthcare,
https://doi.org/10.1007/978-3-031-09108-7_19

Introduction

Artificial intelligence and its panoply of technological tools have had an impact in medicine and healthcare in several domains, especially in medical imaging [1] and decision support [2]. As the COVID-19 pandemic demonstrated, however, there is much more work that needs to be done in deploying artificial intelligence in health care. To be fair, this observation is probably more true in the domains of healthcare data, databases, and information technology infrastructure than it is for AI itself. Despite this observation, the future of AI in clinical medicine and health care is promising and expectations remain high that it and its technological tools will deliver in the long term [3]. As we head toward a future of "intelligence-based" rather than evidence-based medicine, the gap between the latter and an AI-centric future form of medicine is increasingly large (see Fig. 19.1).

The future of AIM and health care can be strategically deconstructed first into *two main categories* of technology (and its exponential rise) and stakeholders (and their gap to technology) that are further separated into *three states* in order to understand the present and forecast the future: current state, near future state (this coming decade), and future state (beyond this decade). The second category, stakeholders, delineates the special human-machine synergy in the form of three separate dyads that are essential for AI to be promulgated into the future era of precision medicine and population health.

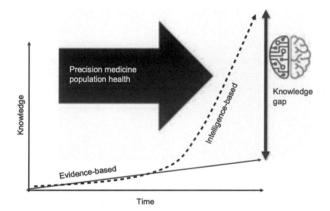

Time

Fig. 19.1 Intelligence-Based Medicine. The graph shows knowledge on the vertical axis plotted over time. While evidence-based medicine has increased medical knowledge in past decades, this alone does not meet the need for an increase in knowledge necessary for both precision medicine and population health. This knowledge gap requires a paradigm shift with a much steeper trajectory using both data and artificial intelligence. (From Chang AC. *Intelligence-Based Medicine*. Elsevier, 2020)

AI in Medicine Technology: An Exponential Rise

Current State

There is an impressive portfolio of technological tools that are available or soon to be so in the domain of artificial intelligence in medicine. The most advanced appears to be deep learning in the form of convolutional neural networks (CNN) in medical imaging (see Chap. 12). Deep learning applied to fundus photographs from ophthalmological examinations have now been shown to be screening tools for not only diabetes but also other conditions. The Cambrian explosion of CNN tools have made progress in static imaging but are now starting to make inroads into moving images such as ultrasound studies, endoscopic imaging, and even echocardiograms. Machine and even deep learning has made progress in electronic medical records in projects on readmission prediction or decision support (see Chaps. 10 and 11), but these have not been nearly as productive as CNN and medical imaging due to the records being fragmented in location and complex in nature. There is some promising work in the area of drug design [4] or repurposing in treatment for cancer patients and even for COVID-19 patients during the pandemic as a result of machine and deep learning, especially with protein structure determination based on genomic sequencing. More recently, natural language processing (NLP) capabilities with transformer architectures such as Generative Pre-trained Transformer 3 (GPT-3) and Bidirectional Encoder Representations from Transformers (BERT) have started to be considered for their deployment in healthcare (see Chap. 7), especially with their relative ease of use and expansive libraries. NLP continues to advance at an exponential pace, with a recent architectural development being the Google Brain's Switch Transformer language model named after yet another Sesame Street character, MoE (Mixture of Experts). The future prediction models will incorporate both structured data (vital signs, laboratory values, etc) and proportionally more unstructured data (clinician notes, radiology reports, etc.) so the model will have the best of both of these data and information worlds. **Unsupervised learning** also holds great promise for discovery of new phenotypic expressions of disease subtypes and treatment responses [5] (see Chap. 14). Lastly, healthcare is starting to embrace an older AI technology of **robotic process automation (RPA)** for administrative tasks that can be automated by algorithms rather than completed by humans.

Near Future State

There are other AI technologies that will be very useful for clinical medicine in the near future.

There is exciting work on pushing AI "peripherally" to devices even at the microprocessor level. This **artificial intelligence of things**, or AIoT, provides a portfolio of "intelligent" devices for the future of chronic disease management as well as population health strategies. The internet of things becoming **internet of everything** (IoE) with edge AI will be invaluable for chronic disease management and population health in the future. There is already discussion about how neural nets can be located on a microprocessor (termed **"tinyAI"** by MIT researchers). The future development of AI in healthcare will be in two directions: Towards a centralized cloud for analytics and concomitantly towards a peripheral network with AI embedded in many devices and sensors. This will be the AI equivalent of a brain and peripheral nervous system. In addition, the limitations and nuances of existing electronic medical records in current state demands a disruptive technology in the future. One such promising technology is **graph databases** coupled with **knowledge graphs** to create a paradigm shift in how electronic medical records are structured and curated. Both IoE and graph databases will be particularly useful when **federated learning** becomes more common as a methodology to collect and share data. Federated learning consists of edge devices with local data that can train their own copy of the model from a central server, and only the parameters/weights from these models (but not the data) are sent to the global model. **Multimodal AI**, such as combining perception and linguistic capabilities of machines, can increase the potential for AI to deal with the complexities of healthcare (see Fig. 19.2). The advent of GPT-3 will be an asset to a more sophisticated AI to better understand and adapt to the world. In the area of medical education and clinical training, not only AI in and of itself but also in combination with extended reality can be extraordinarily effective in educating and training clinicians; adding an AI dimension to extended reality can be termed **intelligent reality**. Along with this virtualization of clinical medicine and healthcare can be AI imbued in the **digital twin** concept for both the patient as well as the health system (see Fig. 19.3) [6]. All of this demand for artificial intelligence will warrant the availability of **quantum computing**.

Future State

There will be significant needs and advances for AI in medicine in the coming decades. First, means of decreasing the human burden of labeling in supervised learning in the form of **few shot learning** or **generative adversarial networks** can enable more automated interpretation in the future. In addition, there need to be AI systems that can perform real-time AI. For this to occur, AI architectures will need to be even more robust and will need to include **anytime algorithms** as well as incorporate the nuances of **complexity** and **chaos theory** as biomedical phenomena often have complex rather than complicated elements. Furthermore, **deep reinforcement learning** may have succeeded at the game Go but will be less spectacular in clinical medicine as the nuances and complexities as well as the fuzziness of

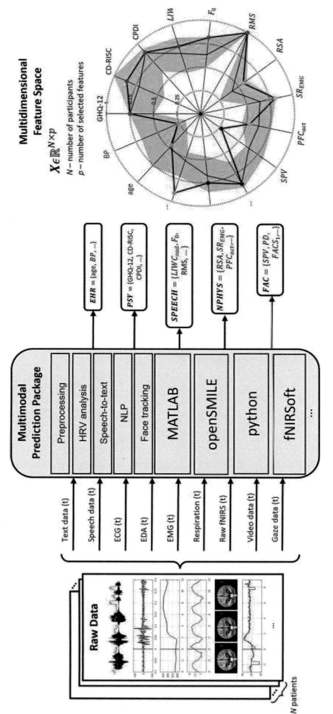

Fig. 19.2 Multimodal Artificial Intelligence. Multimodal data acquisition in real-time is the input with feature computation after collection of data from several different sources in patients with COVID-19. General Health Questionnaire (GHQ-12), Connor-Davidson Resilience Scale (CD-RISC), COVID-19 Peritraumatic Distress Index (CPDI); NLP feature LIWC "sad," voice fundamental frequency (F0), voice root mean square (RMS); respiratory sinus arrhythmia (RSA), EMG-based startle reactivity (SREMG), prefrontal cortex activity (PFCact); saccadic peak velocity (SPV); pupil dilation (PD), a feature related to facial action coding system (FACS). (From Cosic K et al. AI-Based Prediction and Prevention of Psychological and Behavioral Changes in Ex COVID-19 Patients. Front Psychol 2121; 12:782866)

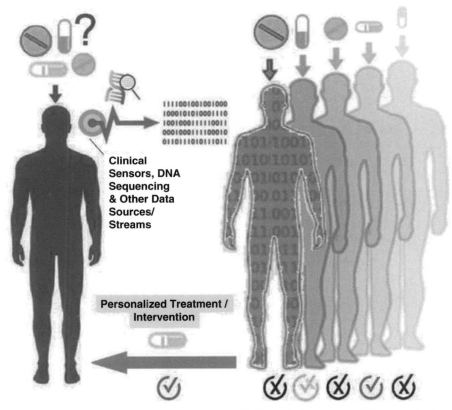

Fig. 19.3 Digital Twins and Artificial Intelligence. Digital twin copies or instances of the index patient is shown with data streaming in from clinical sensors, DNA sequencing, and other data sources and streams. All of these data create an index patient for *in silico* testing to determine which therapy is best for the medical condition. (From Boulos MNK et al. Digital Twins: From Personalized Medicine to Precision Public Health. *J Pers Med* 2021; 11 (8): 745–756)

biomedicine will be daunting challenges for its execution [7]. The entire learning portfolio will need to be explored and orchestrated for biomedical work: **transfer learning**, unsupervised and **self-supervised learning**, **predictive learning**, **apprenticeship learning** and other types of learning to come in the future. Lastly, cognitive elements of artificial intelligence such as (1) **cognitive architecture** (declarative and procedure learning and memory, perception, action selection, etc.), (2) Geoff Hinton's "**capsule networks**" [8], or (3) Jeff Hawkins' "**reference frames**" described in his book *A Thousand Brains: A New Theory of Intelligence* [9], will need to be increasingly a motif in artificial intelligence in medicine and healthcare that will incorporate cognitive elements such as the insights, intuition, and intelligence of our clinicians (see Fig. 19.4).

Fig. 19.4 Cognitive Artificial Intelligence Era. The third wave of AI with more cognitive elements will enable artificial general intelligence (AGI) which will be more human-like with intuition and common sense (see Chap. 5). (From Chang AC. *Intelligence-Based Medicine*. Elsevier, 2020)

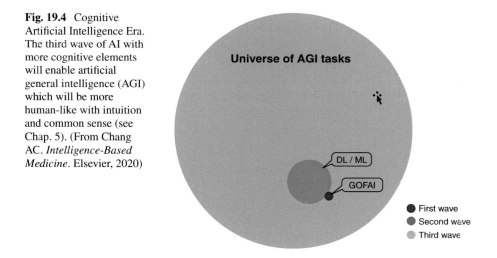

The AI in Medicine Stakeholders: Increasing Gap to Technology

Current State

For many data scientists, this past decade has been an interesting journey into healthcare with mixed dividends. While the aspiration to help improve patients' lives and/or create a viable business venture was a driving force for artificial intelligence experts, the nuances of access to healthcare data and inadequacies of databases was a deterrent for some. The future gain for AI in healthcare is not only in helping clinicians make better and faster decisions in urgent, complex situations but also in ensuring clinicians not make simple, avoidable mistakes. In short, AI can raise practitioner's decision quality, accuracy, and velocity.

For clinicians at all levels of education and training, there is an escalating need to learn about the basics of AI as it is becoming more evident that those clinicians who understand AI will have a growing advantage over those who do not. In addition, clinicians are still grappling with explainability and interpretability of AI, especially more sophisticated AI methodologies like deep learning. While clinicians need to be more accepting of not being enlightened about every technical detail of AI, these caretakers do need to be able to assure themselves the accuracy and functionality of the technology by serial testing and continual learning. AI in healthcare and its myriad of forms changes the dynamics of the traditional paternalistic clinician-patient dyad to a much more complex clinician-AI-patient triad. This dramatically alters the trust and accountability aspects with ethical, legal, and financial implications.

The myriad of issues and challenges in ethical, legal, regulatory, and financial domains focused on AI technology usually have a linear trajectory whereas emerging and disruptive AI technologies have mostly an exponential trajectory. The mismatch of these two curves creates both challenges and opportunities. In addition, for all those involved in AI in medicine, everyone will need to hold each other accountable in the validity and the accuracy of AI algorithms and models [10]. The best AI in medicine and healthcare projects have a special synergy between data scientists and clinicians in order to couple good data science with high clinical relevance for overall impact on health outcome. Without the necessary clinical relevance, a model or a project can be just good data science in healthcare.

Near Future State

For AI experts, there is a dire need for more talent especially at the PhD level to work in healthcare. There is a concomitant requirement for these AI experts to gain expertise in healthcare data and databases and therefore stretching their domain beyond machine and deep learning. In addition, AI alone in medicine is not going to make impact long term unless it is applied "intelligently" with human clinician insight and intuition to render it truly meaningful. If not, we have essentially an AI in medicine type III error (providing the right answer to the wrong problem).

For the clinicians, adoption will need to be accelerated to accommodate the technology that is available. A small cohort of clinicians will need to be champions of AI by learning a minimal amount of knowledge to be able to be conversant with a data scientist. An even smaller number of clinicians may decide to get formal education about data science and AI to gain a special insight having dual education; this insight can be geometric, not merely additive. For the rest of the clinicians, the advent of **automated machine learning** (autoML) can facilitate the use of machine and deep learning for clinical projects. In addition, creative uses of AI in the future can include embedding knowledge into the EHR while gaining continuing medical education (CME) credits.

Future State

The stakeholders of AI in medicine in the future will have a much closer interactional relationship that is continual and collaborative. In the healthcare systems, there will be a growing number of chief intelligence officers who are stewards of both clinical and administrative projects using AI tools. Some of these officers will be clinicians with an AI background, while others will be AI-focused experts who are interested in working in healthcare. Professional schools in nursing, pharmacy, dental, and medical domains will routinely include AI in the curriculum, with a few school having dual degree programs that include both a doctorate in the profession and a masters or doctorate degree in data science and AI. The overall focus of AI in medicine will be on the patients' outcomes and well-being. Ethics of AI in medicine will reach a new height of discussion and interest as increasing number of cases become controversial and demand expertise in all three areas to converge for discussions. Other issues such as regulation, legal, and entrepreneurship in AI will be regularly discussed and have national and international committees and working groups actively collaborate on policies for guidance and consistency. The gap between these domains and the exponential rise of AI technology will start to narrow after much work and focus from passionate advocates, as well as opponents, of AI.

The AI in Medicine Dyads: Synergy and Beyond

The Human-Human Dyad

While the present and near future states of AI in medicine will evolve from symbiosis to synergy, the future state will be an artificial intelligence-clinical medicine and healthcare **convolution**: a distinctly different third function as a direct result of convergence of two functions. Clinicians, most with education and training in data science and AI, will work closely with data scientists on a daily basis on hospital rounds and clinical settings and provide clinical insights and intuition. Clinicians will be fully indoctrinated in AI in healthcare, which will be less about learning to code, but much more about understanding the principles of AI tools, the designing of AI solutions to clinical problems, and acquiring knowledge about data and databases, biostatistics, information technology infrastructure, and digital health. Data scientists will reciprocate by pointing out possible biases and heuristics of the decision-making process while expounding on data science tenets. The AI domain experts will also learn to accommodate the complexities, chaos and fuzzy nature of biomedicine. The deep mutual respect and close real-time synergy between Formula One racers and their engineering teams is good to appreciate and perhaps emulate. If clinicians and data scientists can foster such an ideal relationship, the patients will all win as a result of these special dyads. This collaboration will evolve into cultural transformation as the philosophy fosters **swarm intelligence** across many healthcare organizations.

The Machine-Machine Dyad

In this era, the regulatory process is greatly facilitated by algorithms that focus on various aspects of the machine and deep learning workflow, as part of the algorithm bundle that overlooks data integrity and the machine and deep learning procedural integrity. Of course, this preliminary screening process will always need human oversight. In addition, machines will become more sophisticated with hybrids such as **graph neural networks** and **transformers** becoming part of other AI tools. Finally, the internet of everything will be in full deployment, with over a trillion intelligent devices with neural networks connected as a huge network and feeding information (without the data) into the cloud resembling an AI nervous system. This AI health hub overlooks the health of entire populations of residents from birth onward with focus on social determinants of health. These approaches are consistent with Alan Turing's prescient philosophy of "machine, not human, to deal with machine".

The Human-Machine Dyad

The experiences with algorithms in deploying vaccinations around the world during the COVID-19 pandemic show very clearly that human insight and common sense are very much needed, especially to monitor equity of vaccine distribution. In addition, health systems will develop this human-machine synergy in the form of an AI center of excellence that incorporates both clinical and AI expertise. With data and information more accessible and organized in health systems, endeavors such as quality improvement, peer review, clinical research, and business intelligence can potentially all be supported by a single "intelligence" resource for special multi-dimensional insights. Again, human-machine synergy is preferred over either humans or machines alone.

Conclusion: Convolution to Consilience

In several decades, there is no longer labeling any process in clinical medicine and healthcare as "artificial intelligence" as AI becomes embedded into a myriad of processes and devices. Intelligence-based medicine permanently becomes standard of care and practice for the previously impossible goals of precision medicine and population health. Medical intelligence is widely practiced as a convolution of clinical medicine and artificial intelligence, and medicine and healthcare gradually evolves into Edward Wilson's paradigm of *consilience*: the convergence of natural and social sciences along with other sciences into a unity of knowledge [11].

Leonardo da Vinci wrote "Knowing is not enough; we must apply. Being willing is not enough; we must do." With the pandemic raging on and the virus undergoing mutations with worrisome frequency, we need to be resilient and retaliate with not only with our collective human intellect but also any good artificial intelligence tool we can summon. This will give us the hope we all need. Finally, perhaps the most valuable dividend for AI in clinical medicine and healthcare is that during the future decades long process of working with patient data as well as machines and algorithms, we have the opportunity to learn more about not only ourselves but also our biases so we can decrease healthcare inequities and finally bring social justice to all. The best dividend in the future of artificial intelligence in medicine, therefore, is a reclaiming of humanity in medicine.

Questions for Discussion

- Consider some technological advances expected to improve the outcomes of patients with the advances in AI in the biomedical domain. What challenges do you perceive to achieving these improvements?

- What are potential obstacles for artificial intelligence to reach the paradigm of precision medicine and population health?
- What are means through which new medical knowledge will be discovered in patients with diseases, and how will this help to improve patient outcome?
- What is in store for the future practicing clinicians and their interface with AI in clinical medicine and healthcare?
- How will the upcoming generations of clinicians be educated and trained in AI in clinical medicine and healthcare?
- Consider the following dyads: (1) human to human, (2) human to machine, and (3) machine to machine. What are some issues with each dyad as it relates to the future of AIM? Think beyond those that are discussed in the chapter as well.

Further Reading

Chang AC. Section IV: The future of artificial intelligence and application in medicine. In: Intelligence-based medicine: artificial intelligence and human cognition in clinical medicine and healthcare. London: Elsevier; 2020.

- The section of the book is devoted to future technologies and issues of artificial intelligence in clinical medicine and health care and is relevant for both the clinician as well as the artificial intelligence expert.

Russell S, Norvig P. Artificial intelligence: a modern approach. 4th ed. New York: Pearson Education; 2021.

- The "bible" of artificial intelligence that is now updated relatively soon after the last edition given how fast this field has evolved in just the past few years.

Stanford University Human-Centered Artificial Intelligence (HAI). Artificial Intelligence Index Report 2021. https://aiindex.stanford.edu/wp-content/uploads/2021/11/2021-AI-Index-Report_Master.pdf.

- This is an excellent report of the state of the art of artificial intelligence with projections into the future decades with all the nuances to be expected.

References

1. Esteva A, Chou K, Yeung S, et al. Deep learning enabled medical computer vision. NPJ Digit Med. 2021;4(1):5.
2. Loeb GE. A new approach to medical diagnostic decision support. J Biomed Inform. 2021;9:103723.
3. Stanford University Human-Centered Artificial Intelligence (HAI). Artificial Intelligence Index Report 2021.
4. Xiong J, Xiong Z, Chen K, et al. Graph neural networks for automated de novo drug design. Drug Discov Today. 2021;21:S1359–6446.
5. Sweatt AJ, Hedlin HK, Balasubramanian V, et al. Discovery of distinct immune phenotypes using machine learning in pulmonary arterial hypertension. Circ Res. 2019;124(6):904–19.
6. Peirlinck M, Costabal FS, Yao J, et al. Precision Medicine in human heart modeling. In: Biomechanics and modeling in mechanobiology. 2021; online ahead of print.

7. Komorowski M, Celi LA, Badawi O, et al. The artificial intelligence clinician learns optimal treatment strategies for sepsis in intensive care. Nat Med. 2018;24:1716–20.
8. Sabour S, Frosst N, Hinton GE. Dynamic routing between capsules. In: Advances in neural information processing systems (NIPS); 2017. p. 30.
9. Hawkins J. A thousand brains: a new theory of intelligence. New York: Basic Books; 2021.
10. Norgeot B, Quer G, Beaulieu-Jones BK, et al. Minimum information about clinical artificial intelligence modeling: the MI-CLAIM checklist. Nat Med. 2020;26(9):1320–4.
11. Wilson EO. Consilience: the Unity of knowledge. New York: First Vintage Books; 1998.

Chapter 20
Reflections and Projections

Trevor A. Cohen, Vimla L. Patel, and Edward H. Shortliffe

After reading this chapter, you should know the answers to these questions:
- How might explainable models influence human/AI team performance?
- What are some potential advantages of integrating formal knowledge with deep learning?
- What clinical applications of AIM technologies—other than predictive models of diagnoses or outcomes—show potential as growth areas in the near future?
- How might one obtain additional training in, and exposure to, AIM?

Introduction

At the conclusion of the volume, we would like to reconsider some key themes that feature prominently in the development of AIM, including some that were introduced in Chap. 1. While most of these themes are not new to the field, it is informative to revisit them in the light of recent developments (including a few that were reported in the literature only recently, after discussions provided in the earlier chapters were completed). These developments include both the current

T. A. Cohen (✉)
University of Washington, Seattle, WA, USA
e-mail: cohenta@uw.edu

V. L. Patel
The New York Academy of Medicine, New York, NY, USA

E. H. Shortliffe
Columbia University, New York, NY, USA

© The Author(s), under exclusive license to Springer Nature
Switzerland AG 2022
T. A. Cohen et al. (eds.), *Intelligent Systems in Medicine and Health*, Cognitive
Informatics in Biomedicine and Healthcare,
https://doi.org/10.1007/978-3-031-09108-7_20

predominance of models that prioritize accuracy over interpretability, and the related tendency to prioritize accuracy over other factors—including human factors—when evaluating AIM systems (see Chap. 17). As readers will have surmised from earlier discussions in this volume, we are concerned by some of these recent developments and propose some revisions in emphasis, suggesting the corresponding research that is required.

Explainability and Complementarity

One recurring theme concerns the desire for explainable models (see Chap. 8). In a 1981 study, physicians rated the capacity for explanation in decision support systems as the single most important design feature for future automated advisory tools [1], even more important than the accuracy of the advice. Yet the general trend in recent AIM work has involved sacrificing or downplaying interpretability in exchange for the accuracy that comes with heavily parameterized data-driven models such as deep neural networks. Some recent work has bucked this trend. For example, the Prescience system provides a visual summary explaining its predictions of the onset of hypoxemia (low blood oxygen levels) to guide anesthetists during surgery by listing interpretable features (such as reduced tidal volume) that drive its predictions [2]. The underlying model used in this work, **Shapley Additive Explanations (SHAP)**, is based on cooperative game theory [3], extending ideas developed by a Nobel prize winning economist, Lloyd Stowell Shapley, to quantify the relative contributions of members of a coalition [4]. The open source SHAP library provides approaches to establishing the importance of features across a range of machine learning models, including deep learning models such as pre-trained transformers for text categorization (Fig. 20.1). This can offer intuitive explanations of the importance of individual features for specific predictions made by complex models [5].

However, while the contributions of individual features do provide a form of interpretability, this is far removed from the structured reasoning provided by

base value		f(x)
-9.682003 -6.730298 -3.778594 -0.826890 2.124815 **4.397537**.519		

))))))))))))))))) (

mhm well she ' s spilling the water from from it ' s it ' s running over rather in the the youngsters are are getting the jam and in the meantime he ' s tilting his stool hm he is he ' s he ' s trying to get the cake down and then and the mother is the water is and his stool is slipping out from

Fig. 20.1 SHAP visualization for a decision from a deep learning model trained to detect transcripts of participants with Alzheimer's disease dementia responding to a picture description task, using data from the Alzheimer's Dementia Recognition through Spontaneous Speech (ADReSS) challenge [6]. The visualization suggests (shaded emphasis reflecting chunks of text with a positive influence on the prediction) that the model is predicting this transcript came from a participant with dementia in part because of the frequent repetition ("it's it's", "he's he's") that is known to occur in this condition

physicians to explain their diagnostic decision making in cognitive studies [7]. It is also very different from the virtuosic explanations, weaving together observable signs and symptoms with detailed accounts of the pathophysiology underlying a suspected disease process, that those with clinical training may remember receiving from experienced diagnosticians on teaching rounds. A justification for a diagnostic decision that points out *which* signs and symptoms were considered, without explaining *why* they lead to the identified diagnosis, suggests a superficial understanding of the problem. Cognitive studies of diagnostic reasoning also show that there are conditions under which explanations are needed during a problem solving process [8].

Furthermore, recent evidence suggests that providing explanations at the level of feature importance may increase the likelihood that *both accurate and inaccurate model predictions* are accepted [9]. These authors also note a number of prior studies—including the hypoxemia prediction work previously mentioned—in which the improvements in team performance demonstrated with explanations could be further enhanced by eliminating the human in the loop entirely. There are counterexamples in which human/AI teams are truly complementary, such as those discussed in Chap. 5 [10, 11]. However, this is not always the case (at least not for classification accuracy). Note, however, that providing explanations may have other potential benefits, such as enhancing the speed of human decision making [9] and drawing attention to salient patient data. One way to encourage such complementarity involves deliberately optimizing machine learning models to maximize human/AI team performance, explicitly modeling the ability of a human decision maker to accept or override a prediction on the basis of model confidence (e.g. the probability assigned to a particular category, such as "COVID-19 +ve"). Such approaches can balance the amount of human effort required against overall system accuracy [12]. Intriguingly, models trained in this fashion may exhibit changes in behavior that include trading the accuracy of low-confidence predictions (predictions that are more likely to be overridden), for greater accuracy in high-confidence predictions. While such results have emerged from experiments conducted in simulation, they are reminiscent of the observation that the accuracy of a radiological deep learning system to diagnose pneumonia was improved by human evaluation of low-confidence predictions [11]. A system focused on optimizing the accuracy of its high-confidence predictions would likely further improve human/AI team accuracy in this context. In effect, the system would incorporate a model of human behavior in response to the confidence of its predictions.

A complementary approach to having AI systems model human behavior involves equipping flesh-and-blood team members with useful mental models of their digital collaborators. In order to understand the role of such mental models, Bansal and colleagues have investigated the role of the complexity of the **error boundary**, which demarcates the inputs for which an AI model is likely to fail, in human/AI team performance [13]. In this work, participants were crowdsourced users of a platform for AI-supported decision making, and were tasked with deciding whether to take an automated recommendation for particular problems. Accurate decisions were rewarded monetarily, irrespective of whether or not the automated recommendations were followed, and the task was constructed such that its success was contingent upon learning the error boundary of the model correctly. The authors conclude that error boundaries that are parsimonious (achieved by constraining the number of features visible to users) and predictable (achieved by pushing models toward deterministic decisions and ensuring that they remain consistent in their decisions on previously-encountered examples as they learn) are easier for users to model mentally, and consequently lead to better human/AI team decisions. In short, the human component of the team needs to know *when to trust* the AI component, and when to second-guess it (see Chap. 18).

Taken together, this work suggests that team performance improves when AI and human team members are aware of one another's strengths and weaknesses—just as is the case with teams of human beings [14]. This requires more than an explanatory mechanism, and is not an inevitable consequence of model transparency. Rather, the respective capabilities and vulnerabilities of AI and human team members must be learned from their observed behavior. As we have argued previously [15], methods of cognitive informatics are ideally suited to the task of identifying human vulnerabilities to medical error, and there is a long track record of the application of such methods to characterize mental models in medicine [16, 17]. We anticipate that the characterization of both human and machine error boundaries will be a fruitful area of investigation and system design to be addressed by cognitive informatics researchers in the future, as will the development of methods of explanation that make such error boundaries apparent.

Restoring Knowledge to AIM

Another recurring theme throughout this volume concerns the relative neglect of knowledge-based methods in recent AIM work. While it is understandable that deep learning methods would attract attention because of their recent successes, the aphorism "knowledge is power"—as applied to AI by Feigenbaum—has been an axiom of AIM since the inception of the field (see Chap. 2). Bengio, LeCun and Hinton, joint recipients of the prestigious Turing Award in 2018 for their work on deep learning, acknowledge that the successes of deep learning have largely involved perceptual tasks (such as radiologic image analysis in the case of medicine, as is discussed in Chap. 12) [18]. Drawing on Kahneman's influential dual systems theory [19], they note that these successes involve so-called "**System 1**" tasks—tasks that we accomplish without conscious effort. In contrast "**System 2**" tasks, such as formal reasoning, require deliberate conscious effort to execute a sequence of steps. The "System 2" symbolic systems that were developed at the inception of AIM were well positioned to explain their diagnostic decisions to human interrogators because these decisions were produced through a deliberate series of steps traversing atomic units of interpretable knowledge (see also Chap. 5). However, neither the acquisition of formal knowledge, nor automated reasoning of this sort, have been the main focus of deep learning research to date. Bengio, LeCun and Hinton conclude by expressing their collective desire to develop neural network models that retain their desirable learning and generalization capabilities while also supporting the "System 2" tasks, such as reasoning through recombination of knowledge components, that were the focus of the symbolic AI research initiative.

The idea of integrating symbolic and distributed representations (such as neural network weights) is not new. Integrative approaches, such as Harnad's three-level representational system and Gärdenfors' Conceptual Spaces framework [20, 21], propose unified models with the capacity for both perception and reasoning. Functional implementations of neuro-symbolic reasoning, such as Smolensky's tensor product binding [22] and a set of related approaches collectively known as Vector Symbolic Architectures [23–27], use deliberate transformations of the high-dimensional vector representations that underlie neural network models to encode the nature of the relationships among entities, permitting approximate inference. Of late, there has been a resurgence of interest in the development of integrated models, as illustrated by the identification of Neuro-Symbolic AI as a focus area for the 2021 Association for the Advancement of Artificial Intelligence (AAAI) Conference on Artificial Intelligence.[1] Such models have already been applied to represent and draw inference from tens of millions of assertions extracted from the biomedical literature using natural language processing [28–30], and to represent general knowledge expressed in the form of a graph (see Chap. 4) [31]. Recent work has also provided methods that can augment the representations learned by neural networks with information from formal knowledge structures such as taxonomies [32–34] (see also the concluding section of Chap. 4), and has shown how formal logical operators used in quantum physics can apply to neural-network-derived vector representations [35, 36]. We anticipate that methods to augment deep neural network models with formal knowledge and explicit reasoning capabilities will be an important focus of research in the immediate future, with the potential to support the ability of AIM models to learn how to draw accurate conclusions from relatively small amounts of data, to advance approaches to interpretability beyond an exclusive focus on feature weights, and to compensate for biases inherent in data used for training.

Forward-Thinking Clinical Applications

Diagnostic and therapeutic decision support has been the primary focus of AIM system development since the field's inception, with imaging implications being particularly prominent at present because of their alignment with technological

---

[1] https://aaai.org/Conferences/AAAI-21/aaai21focusareacalls/. (accessed August 17, 2022).

developments in image processing. Other applications that have attracted attention include the prediction of future patient states (such as sepsis [37]). However, there are many other aspects of medical practice that could benefit from the application of AIM methods, and we anticipate that the scope of applications will broaden as healthcare professionals become better acquainted with them.

Recent innovative applications of AIM methods include using sensors to permit physical environments to respond to the presence of human agents [38]. Examples of work in this area include automated measurement of hand-hygiene dispenser use, with the goal of reducing hospital-acquired infections [39], and measurement of patient mobilization in the intensive care unit, which can reduce related complications and improve long-term functional outcomes [40]. Another promising direction concerns using AIM to anticipate medical error. In recent work by King et al., machine learning models trained on a large dataset of physician orders with relevant contextual information were able to predict voided medication orders—orders in which clinicians correct or reconsider a previous prescribing decision [41]. While further improvements in accuracy would be a prerequisite for deployment of such a system to mitigate errors, interpretation of the factors associated with prediction—such as student-entered orders and lack of predefined dosage options—reveal opportunities for system-level changes to enhance patient safety.

Another area that is attracting considerable interest concerns the use of AIM methods to reduce the documentation burden of physicians, which constrains the time available for doctor-patient interaction and has been associated with increased risk of physician burnout [42]. That AIM can be applied to recover time from clerical documentation, allowing more focus on human interaction in medicine, is one of the central arguments in Topol's recent book, *Deep Medicine: How Artificial Intelligence Can Make Healthcare Human Again* [43]. One pragmatic approach to reducing this burden concerns using contextual information to enhance the utility of autocomplete suggestions [44]. Another proposal concerns the development of "digital scribes", ambient agents that can pre-populate a clinical note with information detected while continuously monitoring discussion and movement during a clinical encounter [45]. Realizing this ambitious goal will require both negotiation of technological challenges, such as speaker identification and compensation for ambient noise, and addressing privacy concerns, particularly if speech recognition is to leverage deep learning models that are hosted on commercial servers. However, the potential of an application of this sort to restore physicians' attention to patient care has already attracted considerable commercial investment, both from large technology companies such as Google and Microsoft, and from speech recognition solution developers such as Nuance Communications (and their recent acquisition, Seattle-based startup Saykara[2]) [46].

Others have called for a shift in emphasis from *decision* support to *cognitive* support [47–49]. That is, rather than predicting diagnostic labels or suggesting therapies, AIM methods could mediate the aggregation and organization of clinical

---

[2] https://medcitynews.com/2021/02/nuance-buys-healthcare-voice-assistant-startup-saykara/. (accessed August 17, 2022).

information to support clinical decision making. Investigators have explored the use of both machine learning and encoded expert knowledge as a means to support the management and navigation of information that is pertinent to specific decision-making processes [47, 48]. Along similar lines, Adler-Milstein and colleagues have developed an analogy between clinical diagnosis and navigation ("wayfinding"), and argue that AIM methods should learn from physician information-seeking behavior to aggregate information in support of cognitive tasks and provide cues along the path to a diagnostic conclusion [49]. These proposals suggest fruitful and largely unexplored areas of application of AIM methods to support clinical care by synthesizing information to support decisions. Systems of this sort would supple-ment existing decisions and workflows, rather than attempting to redefine them by offering automated recommendations.

Workflow, and the Workforce

Designing technology to fit the current workflow requires a thorough understand-ing of the practice environment. Li and his colleagues propose a "delivery science" of AIM to ensure (a) that the development of algorithmic approaches is rooted in stakeholder-identified priority problems, and (b) that these stakeholders and their existing workflows inform the design, rollout and evaluation of the resulting inter-ventions [50]. Such stakeholder engagement is also integral to the design and evaluation framework offered in Chap. 17. It follows that those wishing to imple-ment successful AIM solutions at the point of care may be best positioned to do so from within the institution in which these solutions will be deployed. To this end, Cosgriff et al. argue the need for dedicated departments of clinical AI, to drive the development and implementation of AI models with demonstrated healthcare ben-efits, and to train future leaders in the field [51]. New York's Icahn School of Medicine at Mount Sinai has already taken this initiative, with their establishment of a Department of Artificial Intelligence and Human Health.[3] Of course, many such AIM solutions for pressing clinical problems have emerged over the years from departments of biomedical informatics. These departments, particularly when supporting healthcare operations, already fulfill some of the proposed func-tions of a medical AI department, including the development of models that apply to patient care using real-time data, and the facilitation of interoperability of institutional data. However, Cosgriff et al. argue for a scaling up of such efforts in order to expedite the development and deployment of predictive models that sup-port clinical care, with problem formulation, model development, local optimiza-tion, workflow integration and continuous evaluation as core departmental functions.

---

[3] https://icahn.mssm.edu/about/departments/ai-human-health. (accessed August 17, 2022).

Intertwined with the need for principled integration of AI models into care is the need to educate practitioners with the broad knowledge base required to do this effectively. In addition to specialists in AIM who will require advanced and focused graduate-level training, there are already avenues through which practicing physicians can advance their knowledge in the field. As Langlotz (a radiologist and AIM researcher) puts it, "AI won't replace radiologists, but radiologists who use AI will replace radiologists who don't" [52]. The same could be said of other subdisciplines. Avenues available to medical practitioners interested in learning more about AIM include clinical informatics fellowship programs,[4] the clinical informatics subspecialty board certification [53], the American Board of Artificial Intelligence in Medicine (ABAIM)'s certification program,[5] and a range of educational activities supported by the AIMed organization.[6] All these efforts were created for those with clinical training who wish to expand their knowledge of AIM and related informatics topics. Thus, we envision a narrowing of the knowledge gap between specialists in AIM and specialists in medicine, establishing the common core of shared understanding required to support effective teamwork [14].

Evaluation

Another recurring theme involves the evaluation of AIM systems. Assertions of superhuman AIM performance and the predictions of physician displacement that accompany them[7] have predictably attracted a degree of backlash [54], with a recent review of 81 such "AI vs. clinicians" evaluations in medical imaging drawing attention to the sparse representation of randomized clinical trials among them [55]. This reflects a cultural difference in the estimation of the utility of different forms of evidence. As is discussed in Chap. 17, while assessment of the accuracy of performance of a predictive model using a reference set is clearly important, it is just one component of a series of evaluations required to assess system usability, performance in practice, healthcare benefits, and return on investment. Without this more extensive view of evaluation, AIM systems will not meet the standards of scrutiny applied to other medical interventions and are likely to be greeted with skepticism by clinicians accustomed to basing their practice on evidence from meta-reviews of clinical

---

[4] https://amia.org/careers-certifications/informatics-academic-programs. (accessed August 17, 2022).

[5] https://abaim.org/certification. (accessed August 17, 2022).

[6] Available from: https://ai-med.io/. (accessed August 17, 2022).

[7] This was perhaps most controversially claimed by neural network pioneer Geoffrey Hinton, who compared radiologists to a cartoon character (Wile E. Coyote) 'treading air' after stepping off a cliff before the inevitable drop. It was recounted in an interview with Siddhartha Mukherjee for an article for the New Yorker (https://www.newyorker.com/magazine/2017/04/03/ai-versus-md). (accessed August 17, 2022). Hinton subsequently reframed the likely impact on radiologists as shifting their work from purely perceptual to more cognitively demanding tasks.

trials. Furthermore—and as noted by the FDA[8]—evaluation should not terminate at the point of deployment. Continued assessment of real-world performance of AIM models is required to understand how well they perform locally, as well as with particular subpopulations to offset the potential for AIM to exacerbate healthcare disparities by performing better in some populations than others [56]. Also, knowledge and conventions evolve over time, requiring ongoing assessment and updating of AIM functionality. We view addressing these gaps in typical approaches to evaluation of AIM systems as crucial to realizing their potential to improve healthcare effectiveness and quality and, accordingly, to being accepted.

Concluding Remarks

This concluding chapter has highlighted themes that are of particular importance for the further development of the field. It is undoubtedly an exciting time to be working in the area of AIM, and our book is intended to provide readers not only with a sense of well-justified enthusiasm for the proximal future of the field, but also with a grounding in the as-yet-unresolved issues that may threaten the realization of AIM's potential to improve health care and biomedical research. Over a decade ago, a panel of AIM experts discussed the opportunities that AI in medicine had afforded and outlined challenges for the future [57]. Now we have new and different opportunities for AIM, bringing with them unique challenges that we need to address. The concluding sentence to Alan Turing's seminal paper, *Computing Machinery and Intelligence*, reads: "We can only see a short distance ahead, but we can see plenty there that needs to be done." [58] Accordingly, this volume has sought to provide readers with a suitable vantage point from which to consider how best to engage with ongoing efforts to advance these remarkable technologies and, in turn, their potential to improve health care and biomedicine.

Questions for Discussion

- How might one investigate the role of explainability in human/AI teams operating in clinical environments? Is it possible to provide cognitively satisfying explanations of conclusions that are drawn using machine learning methods?
- Which emerging application areas for AIM have the greatest near-term potential to improve the quality and safety of health care?
- What are some currently available resources for computable knowledge, and how might the knowledge they contain inform the development of deep learning models?

---

[8] https://www.fda.gov/medical-devices/software-medical-device-samd/artificial-intelligence-and-machine-learning-software-medical-device. (accessed August 17, 2022).

- Given what you have learned about AI systems in health care, what do you see as some of the biggest challenges in real-world applications and in education for the future?

Further Reading

Bansal G, Wu T, Zhou J, Fok R, Nushi B, Kamar E, Ribeiro MT, Weld D. Does the whole exceed its parts? The effect of AI explanations on complementary team performance. In: Proceedings of the 2021 CHI Conference on Human Factors in Computing Systems 2021 May 6. pp. 1–16.

- This is a thought-provoking paper that describes an empirical investigation into the effects of explanations in human/AI team performance. It doesn't concern medical AI applications, but raises a number of important issues that are relevant to AIM applications, and provides a template for their empirical investigation.

Cosgriff CV, Stone DJ, Weissman G, Pirracchio R, Celi LA. The clinical artificial intelligence department: a prerequisite for success. BMJ Health Care Inform. 2020;27(1).

- This paper presents an argument for dedicated medical AI departments that are tightly integrated with institutional infrastructure to support the integration and evaluation of AIM models for deployment, as well as to serve as entities that lead AIM research.

Li RC, Asch SM, Shah NH. Developing a delivery science for artificial intelligence in healthcare. NPJ Digital Med. 2020;3(1):1–3.

- This paper outlines a multidisciplinary process for integration of AIM applications into clinical care. It includes consideration of stakeholder perspectives, local information infrastructure and engagement of institutional leadership.

References

1. Teach RL, Shortliffe EH. An analysis of physician attitudes regarding computer-based clinical consultation systems. Comput Biomed Res. 1981;14(6):542–58. PMID: 7035062.
2. Lundberg SM, Nair B, Vavilala MS, Horibe M, Eisses MJ, Adams T, Liston DE, Low DK-W, Newman S-F, Kim J, Lee S-I. Explainable machine-learning predictions for the prevention of hypoxaemia during surgery. Nat Biomed Eng. 2018;2(10):749–60.
3. Lundberg SM, Lee S-I. A unified approach to interpreting model predictions. In: Proceedings of the 31st International conference on neural information processing systems; 2017. p. 4768–77.
4. Roth AE. The Shapley value: essays in honor of Lloyd S. Shapley. Cambridge: Cambridge University Press; 1988. http://public.ebookcentral.proquest.com/choice/publicfullrecord.aspx?p=1578960.
5. Chen H, Lundberg S, Lee S-I. Explaining models by propagating Shapley values of local components. In: Shaban-Nejad A, Michalowski M, Buckeridge DL, editors. Explainable AI in healthcare and medicine: building a culture of transparency and accountability [internet]. Cham: Springer International; 2021. p. 261–70. https://doi.org/10.1007/978-3-030-53352-6_24.

6. Luz S, Haider F, de la Fuente S, Fromm D, MacWhinney B. Alzheimer's Dementia recognition through spontaneous speech: the ADReSS challenge. In: Proceedings of Interspeech; 2020. p. 2172–6. 10.21437/Interspeech.2020-2571.

7. Arocha JF, Patel VL, Patel YC. Hypothesis generation and the coordination of theory and evidence in medical diagnostic reasoning. Med Decis Making. 1993;13:198–211.

8. Patel VL, Arocha JF, Groen GJ. Medical expertise as a function of task difficulty. Mem Cognit. 1990;18:394–406.

9. Bansal G, Wu T, Zhou J, Fok R, Nushi B, Kamar E, Ribeiro MT, Weld D. Does the whole exceed its parts? The effect of AI explanations on complementary team performance. In: Proceedings of the 2021 CHI conference on human factors in computing systems. New York: Association for Computing Machinery; 2021. p. 1–16. https://doi.org/10.1145/3411764.3445717.

10. Lakhani P, Sundaram B. Deep learning at chest radiography: automated classification of pulmonary tuberculosis by using convolutional neural networks. Radiology. 2017;284(2):574–82.

11. Patel BN, Rosenberg L, Willcox G, Baltaxe D, Lyons M, Irvin J, Rajpurkar P, Amrhein T, Gupta R, Halabi S, Langlotz C, Lo E, Mammarappallil J, Mariano AJ, Riley G, Seekins J, Shen L, Zucker E, Lungren MP. Human–machine partnership with artificial intelligence for chest radiograph diagnosis. NPJ Digit Med. 2019;2(1):1–10.

12. Bansal G, Nushi B, Kamar E, Horvitz E, Weld DS. Is the most accurate AI the best teammate? Optimizing AI for teamwork. In: Proceedings of the AAAI Conference on Artificial Intelligence, vol. 35(13); 2021. p. 11405–14.

13. Bansal G, Nushi B, Kamar E, Lasecki WS, Weld DS, Horvitz E. Beyond accuracy: the role of mental models in human-AI team performance. In: Proceedings of the AAAI Conference on human computation and crowdsourcing, vol. 7; 2019. p. 2–11.

14. Mathieu JE, Heffner TS, Goodwin GF, Salas E, Cannon-Bowers JA. The influence of shared mental models on team process and performance. J Appl Psychol. 2000;85(2):273–83.

15. Patel VL, Kaufman DR, Cohen T, editors. Cognitive informatics in health and biomedicine: case studies on critical care, complexity and errors. London: Springer; 2014. https://www.springer.com/gp/book/9781447154891.

16. Kaufman DR, Patel VL. Progressions of mental models in understanding circulation physiology. In: Singh I, Parasaruman R, editors. Human cognition: a multidisciplinary perspective. London: SAGE; 1999. p. 300–46.

17. Morgan GM, Fischhoff B, Bostrom A, Atman CJ. A mental models approach to HIV/AIDS. In: Risk communication: a mental models approach. Cambridge: Cambridge University Press; 2002. p. 160–78.

18. Bengio Y, Lecun Y, Hinton G. Deep learning for AI. Communications of the ACM. ACM New York; 2021;64(7):58–65.

19. Kahneman D. Thinking, fast and slow. London: Macmillan; 2011.

20. Harnad S. Category induction and representation. Cambridge: Cambridge University Press; 1987.

21. Gärdenfors P. Conceptual spaces: the geometry of thought. Cambridge, MA: MIT Press; 2000.

22. Smolensky P. Tensor product variable binding and the representation of symbolic structures in connectionist systems. Artif Intell. 1990;46(1–2):159–216.

23. Gayler RW. Vector Symbolic Architectures answer Jackendoff's challenges for cognitive neuroscience. In: Slezak P, editor. ICCS/ASCS International Conference on Cognitive Science. Sydney: University of New South Wales; 2004. p. 133–8.

24. Plate TA. Holographic reduced representation: distributed representation for cognitive structures. Stanford, CA: CSLI; 2003.

25. Kanerva P. Hyperdimensional computing: an introduction to computing in distributed representation with high-dimensional random vectors. Cogn Comput. 2009;1(2):139–59.

26. Rachkovskij DA, Kussul EM. Binding and normalization of binary sparse distributed representations by context-dependent thinning. Neural Comput. 2001;13(2):411–52.

27. Kleyko D, Rachkovskij DA, Osipov E, Rahimi A. A survey on hyperdimensional computing aka vector symbolic architectures, Part I: Models and data transformations. arXiv:211106077; http://arxiv.org/abs/2111.06077.

28. Widdows D, Cohen T. Reasoning with vectors: a continuous model for fast robust inference. Logic J IGPL. 2015;23(2):141–73.
29. Cohen T, Widdows D. Embedding of semantic predications. J Biomed Inform. 2017;68:150–66. PMID: 28284761.
30. Kilicoglu H, Shin D, Fiszman M, Rosemblat G, Rindflesch TC. SemMedDB: a PubMed-scale repository of biomedical semantic predications. Bioinformatics. 2012;28(23):3158–60.
31. Nickel M, Rosasco L, Poggio T. Holographic embeddings of knowledge graphs. In: Proceedings of the AAAI Conference on artificial intelligence, vol. 30; 2016. https://ojs.aaai. org/index.php/AAAI/article/view/10314.
32. Faruqui M, Dodge J, Jauhar SK, Dyer C, Hovy E, Smith NA. Retrofitting word vectors to semantic lexicons. In: Proceedings of the 2015 Conference of the North American Chapter of the Association for Computational Linguistics: human language technologies. Denver, CO: Association for Computational Linguistics; 2015. p. 1606–15. https://aclanthology.org/ N15-1184.
33. Peters ME, Neumann M, Logan R, Schwartz R, Joshi V, Singh S, Smith NA. Knowledge enhanced contextual word representations. In: Proceedings of the 2019 Conference on Empirical Methods in Natural Language Processing and the 9th International Joint Conference on Natural Language Processing (EMNLP-IJCNLP). Hong Kong, China: Association for Computational Linguistics; 2019. p. 43–54. https://aclanthology.org/D19-1005.
34. Colon-Hernandez P, Havasi C, Alonso J, Huggins M, Breazeal C. Combining pre-trained language models and structured knowledge. arXiv:210112294. 2021. http://arxiv.org/ abs/2101.12294.
35. Birkhoff G, Von Neumann J. The logic of quantum mechanics. Ann Math. 1936;37(4):823–43.
36. Widdows D, Kitto K, Cohen T. Quantum mathematics in artificial intelligence. J Artif Intell Res. 2021;72:1307.
37. Fleuren LM, Klausch TLT, Zwager CL, Schoonmade LJ, Guo T, Roggeveen LF, Swart EL, Girbes ARJ, Thoral P, Ercole A, Hoogendoorn M, Elbers PWG. Machine learning for the prediction of sepsis: a systematic review and meta-analysis of diagnostic test accuracy. Intensive Care Med. 2020;46(3):383–400.
38. Haque A, Milstein A, Fei-Fei L. Illuminating the dark spaces of healthcare with ambient intelligence. Nature. 2020;585(7824):193–202. PMID: 32908264.
39. Singh A, Haque A, Alahi A, Yeung S, Guo M, Glassman JR, Beninati W, Platchek T, Fei-Fei L, Milstein A. Automatic detection of hand hygiene using computer vision technology. J Am Med Inform Assoc. 2020;27(8):1316–20. PMCID: PMC7481030.
40. Yeung S, Rinaldo F, Jopling J, Liu B, Mehra R, Downing NL, Guo M, Bianconi GM, Alahi A, Lee J, Campbell B, Deru K, Beninati W, Fei-Fei L, Milstein A. A computer vision system for deep learning-based detection of patient mobilization activities in the ICU. NPJ Digit Med. 2019;2(1):1–5.
41. King CR, Abraham J, Fritz BA, Cui Z, Galanter W, Chen Y, Kannampallil T. Predicting self-intercepted medication ordering errors using machine learning. PLoS One. 2021;16(7):e0254358.
42. Shanafelt TD, Dyrbye LN, Sinsky C, Hasan O, Satele D, Sloan J, West CP. Relationship between clerical burden and characteristics of the electronic environment with physician burnout and professional satisfaction. Mayo Clin Proc. 2016;91(7):836–48.
43. Topol E. Deep medicine. How artificial intelligence can make healthcare human again. New York: Basic Books; 2019.
44. Greenbaum NR, Jernite Y, Halpern Y, Calder S, Nathanson LA, Sontag DA, Horng S. Improving documentation of presenting problems in the emergency department using a domain-specific ontology and machine learning-driven user interfaces. Int J Med Inform. 2019;132:103981.
45. Coiera E, Kocaballi B, Halamka J, Laranjo L. The digital scribe. NPJ Digit Med. 2018;1(1):1–5.
46. Lin SY, Mahoney MR, Sinsky CA. Ten ways artificial intelligence will transform primary care. J Gen Intern Med. 2019;34(8):1626–30. PMCID: PMC6667610.

47. Dalai VV, Khalid S, Gottipati D, Kannampallil T, John V, Blatter B, Patel VL, Cohen T. Evaluating the effects of cognitive support on psychiatric clinical comprehension. Artif Intell Med. 2014;62(2):91–104. PMID: 25179216.
48. Cohen T, Kannampallil TG, Patel VL. Cognitive support for clinical comprehension. In: Zhang J, Walji M, editors. Better EHR: usability, workflow and cognitive support in electronic health records. New York: National Center for Cognitive Informatics and Decision Making in Healthcare; 2014. p. 319–42. https://sbmi.uth.edu/nccd/better-ehr/.
49. Adler-Milstein J, Chen JH, Dhaliwal G. Next-generation artificial intelligence for diagnosis: from predicting diagnostic labels to "Wayfinding". JAMA. 2021;326(24):2467–8. https://doi.org/10.1001/jama.2021.22396.
50. Li RC, Asch SM, Shah NH. Developing a delivery science for artificial intelligence in healthcare. NPJ Digit Med. 2020;3(1):1–3.
51. Cosgriff CV, Stone DJ, Weissman G, Pirracchio R, Celi LA. The clinical artificial intelligence department: a prerequisite for success. BMJ Health Care Inform. 2020;27(1):e100133. PMCID: PMC7368506.
52. Reardon S. Rise of robot radiologists. Nature. 2019;576(7787):S54–8.
53. Detmer D, Munger B, Lehmann C. Clinical informatics board certification: history, current status, and predicted impact on the clinical informatics workforce. Appl Clin Inform. 2010;01(1):11–8.
54. Thamba A, Gunderman RB. For Watson, solving cancer wasn't so elementary: prospects for artificial intelligence in radiology. Acad Radiol. 2021;29(2):312–4. PMID: 34933804.
55. Nagendran M, Chen Y, Lovejoy CA, Gordon AC, Komorowski M, Harvey H, Topol EJ, Ioannidis JPA, Collins GS, Maruthappu M. Artificial intelligence versus clinicians: systematic review of design, reporting standards, and claims of deep learning studies. BMJ. 2020;368:m689. PMCID: PMC7190037.
56. Goyal M, Knackstedt T, Yan S, Hassanpour S. Artificial intelligence-based image classification methods for diagnosis of skin cancer: challenges and opportunities. Comput Biol Med. 2020;127:104065.
57. Patel VL, Shortliffe EH, Stefanelli M, Szolovits P, Berthold MR, Bellazzi R, Abu-Hanna A. The coming of age of artificial intelligence in medicine. Artif Intell Med. 2009;46(1):5–17. PMCID: PMC2752210.
58. Turing AM. Computing machinery and intelligence. Mind. 1950;LIX:433.

Terms and Definitions

10× genomics (10×) 10× genomics is a popular technique to perform single-cell RNA sequencing. The technique is named after 10× Genomics Inc, the company who developed and owned the technique intellectual property (Chap. 14).

Abductive reasoning A cyclical process of generating possible explanations or a set of hypotheses that are able to account for the available data and then each of these hypotheses is evaluated on the basis of its potential consequences. In this regard, abductive reasoning is a data-driven process that relies heavily on the domain expertise of the person (Chaps. 3 and 5).

Accessibility The characteristic of data that allows research teams to pool data and conduct analyses so that they can have greater confidence in the results (e.g., greater statistical power because the size of the dataset is larger) (Chap. 3).

Acoustic coupler An interface device for coupling electrical signals by acoustical means—usually into and out of a telephone. Such devices were frequently used to connect computer terminals with computers at a distance, often through terminal interface processors (TIPs) (Chap. 2).

Activation function In a neural network, an activation function (such as the sigmoid function) determines the output of a node, given the weighted sum of inputs to the node (Chaps. 1, 6 and 12).

Active learning A human-in-the-loop form of machine learning (ML) where the ML model is re-trained after batches of human annotation and then used to select the next set of data for the human to annotate, often drastically reducing the amount of human annotation needed (Chap. 7).

ACT-R A cognitive architecture offering a theory for simulating and understanding human cognition. Researchers working on ACT-R strive to understand how people organize knowledge and produce intelligent behavior (Chap. 16).

Adaptive artificial intelligence-based clinical decision support An artificial intelligence-based clinical decision support system in which the knowledge base or model is dynamic and is updated with new data and new methods for learning from data (Chap. 10).

Adjacency matrix A square matrix that describes a graph's connectivity where each element (i, j) in the matrix is a 1 if an edge exists between node i and node j and 0 otherwise (Chap. 4).

Advanced Research Projects Agency (ARPA) U.S. Department of Defense Advanced Research Projects Agency (also known as DARPA) (Chap. 2).

Affordances Attributes of objects that enable individuals to know how to use them (e.g., a door handle affords turning or pushing downward to open a door). Well-designed technologies (Chap. 16).

AI winter A period of reduced funding and interest in artificial intelligence research (Chap. 2).

AI-CDS See artificial intelligence-based clinical decision support (Chap. 10).

AI-CDS system See: artificial intelligence-based clinical decision support system (Chap. 10).

AlexNet The name of a convolutional neural network (CNN) architecture, designed by Alex Krizhevsky in collaboration with Ilya Sutskever and Geoffrey Hinton. AlexNet competed in the ImageNet Large Scale Visual Recognition Challenge, achieving a top-5 error of 15.3%, more than 10.8 percentage points lower than that of the runner up (Chap. 12).

Algorithmovigilance A term (coined by Peter Embi) to describe systems or processes for scrutinizing AI algorithms. It is analogous to post-market "pharmacovigilance," the philosophy and practice of monitoring pharmaceutical products to identify adverse events or other harms after they are approved and in use (Chap. 18).

Annotation The process of labeling or classifying an image using text, annotation tools, or both, to describe its type, subject matter, and other attributes (Chap. 12).

Anonymization The process by which data is irreversibly altered in such a way that a data subject can no longer be identified directly or indirectly, either by the data controller alone or in collaboration with any other party (Chaps. 2 and 3).

Anti-factor Xa (anti-Xa) A laboratory test of blood that measures the inhibition of factor Xa activity, is part of the clotting process (Chap. 15).

Anytime algorithm A class of algorithms that continuously searches for a better and better answer to a problem (so that you can query the algorithm for the best solution at "anytime") rather than the typical algorithm that produces a final answer (Chap. 19).

Applied ethics The practical application of critical thinking about values to address and resolve real-world moral issues (Chap. 18).

Apprenticeship learning In this type of learning, a human expert defines a goal by demonstrating how to attain this goal so that the artificial intelligence system can mimic this behavior of reaching this goal (Chap. 19).

Approximation error In machine learning, this is an error caused by limits on the amount of data available for training. For example, few examples of a category of interest may be available, making it difficult for the model to make accurate predictions for it (Chap. 6).

ARPA See Advanced Research Projects Agency

ARPAnet A large wide-area network (also known as the ARPA Network) created in the 1960s by the U.S. Department of Defense Advanced Research Projects Agency (DARPA) for the free exchange of information among universities and research organizations; the precursor to today's Internet (Chap. 2).

Artificial intelligence (AI) The field of study concerned with endowing computers with the ability to produce behavior and outcomes that are considered to require intelligence when produced by humans (Chaps. 3 and 10).

Artificial intelligence of things (AIoT) Two complementary technologies of artificial intelligence and internet of things (IoT) to enable rapid decisions with analytics from massive volumes of data derived from IoT- (Chap. 19).

Artificial intelligence-based clinical decision support (AI-CDS) A computer-based system that uses artificial intelligence to render clinical decision support (Chap. 10).

Artificial neural network A computer program that performs classification by taking as input a set of findings that describe a given situation, propagating calculated weights through a network of several layers of interconnected nodes, and generating as output a set of numbers, where each output corresponds to the likelihood of a particular classification that could explain the findings (Chaps. 1, 2, 11, and 15).

ASCVD Atherosclerotic cardiovascular disease, defined as acute coronary syndrome, history of myocardial infarction, stable or unstable angina, coronary or other arterial revascularization, stroke, transient ischemic attack, or peripheral arterial disease presumed to be of atherosclerotic origin (Chap. 8).

Attention A mechanism used in neural networks to focus on ("attend to") specific aspects of a complex input (Chap. 4).

Audit data logs A detailed record of every action or activity taken related to data or reports. While paper audit trails were originally kept manually, now digital records can be tracked automatically via audit trail if you have the right software platform capable of data auditing (Chap. 17).

Augmented intelligence A design pattern for a human-centered partnership model of people and AI working together to enhance cognitive performance, including learning, decision making, and new experiences (Chap. 5).

Augmented reality An interactive experience of a real-world environment where the objects that reside in the real world are enhanced by computer-generated perceptual information, which may include visual, auditory, haptic, somatosensory and olfactory modalities (Chap. 16).

Autoencoder A type of artificial neural network that has an hourglass-shaped architecture. The input and output layers have the same number of nodes as the number of dimensions in the data. One layer has the smallest number of nodes, which is called the 'encode' layer. The size of the middle layer decreases from the input to the encode layer and increases from the encode layer to the output layer. The data in the output layer, which is a type of synthetic data, is very similar to the data in the input layer. This means that another classification model could not accurately differentiate the data between the input and the output layer.

If so, the encode layer represents the original data so well that it can create a very similar synthetic dataset (Chaps. 4 and 14).

Automated ML (AutoML) Automating the modeling process that facilitates processes such as data preprocessing, features engineering, model selection, and meta-learning for hyperparameters optimization (Chap. 19).

AutoTutor An intelligent tutoring system that simulates the discourse patterns of human tutors, based on analysis of human-to-human tutoring sessions, and theoretically-grounded tutoring strategies based on cognitive learning principles (Chap. 16).

Backward chaining The computational process of seeking to determine the truth of a goal statement by tracing out potential paths of inference using logical rules that can assert that statement as fact (Chaps. 3 and 4).

Backward reasoning The process of reasoning in the opposite fashion to forward reasoning, where the purpose is to determine the initial facts and information with the help of the given conclusions. It is often referred to as bottom-up reasoning (Chap. 5).

Basis function expansion A technique through which a feature vector for machine learning is expanded into a longer vector containing individual component combinations, using mathematical transformations (Chap. 6).

Bayes' Theorem An algebraic expression often used in clinical diagnosis for calculating posttest probability of a condition (a disease, for example) if the pretest probability (prevalence) of the condition, as well as the sensitivity and specificity of the test, are known (also called Bayes' rule). Bayes' theorem also has broad applicability in other areas of biomedical informatics where probabilistic inference is pertinent, including the interpretation of data in bioinformatics (Chap. 4).

Bayesian belief network A probabilistic model based on known or computed conditional independence of variables, based on Bayes' theorem (Chap. 15).

Bayesian probability theory An approach to probabilistic reasoning that applies an algebraic expression, often used in clinical diagnosis, for calculating posttest probability of a condition (a disease, for example) if the pretest probability (prevalence) of the condition, as well as the sensitivity and specificity of the test, are known (also called Bayes' theorem or Bayes' rule) (Chap. 2).

Bidirectional Encoder Representations from Transformers (BERT) A methodology that applies the bidirectional training of a transformer, which is an attention model, to language modeling with a deeper sense of language context and fluidity (Chap. 19).

Big data A field that treats ways to analyze, systematically extract information from, or otherwise deal with data sets that are too large or complex to be dealt with by traditional data-processing application software (Chaps. 10 and 12).

Binary classification A special case of classification involving only two classes (Chap. 6).

Binding affinity Binding affinity measures the strength of interaction between a protein and another protein or chemical (Chap. 14).

Bioethics A branch of applied ethics addressing healthcare and its professions, as well as issues arising in human and animal research, clinical care, and public health (Chap. 18).

Bioinformatics A subfield of biomedical informatics that involves the study of how information is represented and transmitted in biological systems, starting at the molecular level (Chap. 2).

Biomedical informatics The interdisciplinary field that studies and pursues the effective uses of biomedical data, information, and knowledge for scientific inquiry, problem solving, and decision making, driven by efforts to improve human health (Chap. 2).

Black box A computer or computer system in which the processes that generate output are opaque or inscrutable (Chap. 18).

Bootstrapping A resampling method that mimics the sampling process by using random sampling with replacement. Bootstrapping estimates the properties of an estimator (such as its variance) by measuring those properties when sampling from an approximating distribution. Given a dataset with N samples, bootstrapping repeatedly creates datasets of size N (known as *bootstrap samples*) by resampling with replacement N instances of the original dataset. Each bootstrap sample can include repeated instances of the original dataset. The bootstrap sample is used to train the desired model. The samples that are not selected for the bootstrap sample are used as a test set. The described procedure is repeated B times, and the final performance of the model is computed as an average over the B samples (Chap. 11).

Canonical correlation analysis A way of inferring information from cross-covariance matrices. If we have two vectors X and Y of random variables, which do not need to have the same dimension, and there exist correlations among the variables (for example, in brain cancer, the patients' survival time and the patients' time for a recurrent tumor to occur), then canonical-correlation analysis will find linear transformation of X (denote: X_t) and Y (denote: Y_t) such that X_t and Y_t have maximum correlation with each other (Chap. 14).

Capsular network A relatively new deep learning concept promulgated by Geoff Hinton that is based on human brain modules called "capsules" that are good for routing visual images to the appropriate capsule for improved hierarchical relationships (Chap. 19).

Carotid arterial intimal-medial thickness (CIMT) A widely used and validated imaging technique whereby the thickness of the inner two layers of the carotid artery—the intima and media—are measured, typically by ultrasound or MRI, to detect subclinical vascular disease (Chap. 12).

Causal reasoning The process of identifying causality. i.e., the relationship between a cause and its effect (Chaps. 2 and 3).

Certainty factor An early method of assigning likelihoods to facts and conclusions of rules, and then subsequently accumulating evidence, introduced in the MYCIN system and subsequently adopted in many other systems, including neural networks (Chap. 4).

Chaos theory The study of nonlinear dynamics in mathematics in which seemingly random events are predictable from simple deterministic equations in complex systems, such as weather, migratory patterns of birds, and pandemics (see also Butterfly Effect) (Chap. 19).

Chatbot A computer system that supports a synchronous mode of text-based communication (Chaps. 2 and 9).

Chemical structure The three-dimensional arrangement of atoms in a chemical (Chap. 14).

Chromatin immunoprecipitation (ChIP) Chromatin immunoprecipitation is a technique to investigate the interaction between proteins and DNA in the cell. It aims to determine whether specific proteins are associated with specific genomic regions, such as transcription factors on promoters or other DNA binding sites (Chap. 14).

Chunking A process by which individual pieces of information are grouped together in a meaningful whole, to improve short-term retention of the material, thus bypassing the limited capacity of working memory and allowing the working memory to be more efficient (Chap. 5).

Citizen data scientist A person who works in fields other than those supporting data science (e.g., statistics and analytics) yet creates models using artificial intelligence. The benefit of a citizen data scientist is in adding to the workforce performing analysis, as well as applying knowledge from the other fields to the analysis process (Chap. 15).

Classification As an example: does this patient belong in (i.e., is classifiable into) the group of patients with Type 2 diabetes? (Chaps. 3 and 6).

Clinical decision support Any process that provides healthcare workers and patients with situation-specific knowledge that can inform their decisions regarding health and health care (Chap. 10).

Clinical decision support system (CDSS) A computer-based system that assists physicians in making decisions about patient care (Chap. 10).

Clinomic The study of clinotype. It is also used as an adjective to refer to clinotype (Chap. 14).

Clinotype Refers to the measures and characteristics of the living subject, which are useful for medical research and interventions (Chap. 14).

Cloud computing An approach to computing that uses computing resources, such as processors, data, or files, that are located in a remote location ("in the cloud") (Chap. 2).

Cognitive architecture Sometimes used to describe the third and upcoming wave of AI (the first being programming and the second being current deep learning) with attention to more inter-object relationships such as attention and memory as well as reasoning and other capabilities that are akin to how humans think (Chap. 19).

Cognitive informatics The interdisciplinary domain, comprising the cognitive and information sciences, that focuses on human information processing, mechanisms and processes within the context of computing and computer applications (Chaps. 5 and 8).

Cognitive load theory Cognitive load refers to the used amount of working memory resources. The fundamental tenet of cognitive load theory is that the quality of instructional design will be higher if greater consideration is given to the role and limitations of working memory (Chap. 16).

Cognitive task analysis The analysis of both the information-processing demands of a task and the kinds of domain-specific knowledge required performing it, used to study human performance (Chap. 5).

Competency-based education An approach that allows trainees to distinguish between the skills and knowledge that they already have and those for which they need more education and training. This is contrasted to time-based educational methods (Chap. 16).

Complexity Used to describe a situation that cannot easily be deconstructed meaningfully into separate component parts as each part is interdependent with the other parts (therefore "holistic" with dynamic relationships) and the process is therefore nonlinear and the outcome is highly unpredictable or stochastic (Chap. 19).

Comprehension An understanding and interpretation of what is read, heard, and seen (Chap. 5).

Computable representation A method for storing knowledge in a computer so that it can be manipulated computationally, e.g., to draw inferences (Chap. 16).

Computational linguistics The subfield of linguistics focused on the modeling of language using computational methods, often used as a synonymous term of NLP (Chap. 7).

Computational methods In evaluation work, use of computational tools for capturing and analyzing qualitative data in attempts to find solutions for real-life problems (Chap. 17).

Computerized provider order-entry (CPOE) The process of providers (e.g., physicians) entering and sending treatment instructions—including medication, laboratory, and radiology orders—via a computer application rather than paper, fax, or telephone (Chap. 17).

Concatenation-based integration A method that involves combining data sets from different data types at the raw or processed data level before modelling and analysis (Chap. 3).

Concept normalization (CN) NLP task involving the mapping of a concept in text to a standardized form in a lexicon, terminology, or ontology (a concept-level equivalent of word sense disambiguation) (Chap. 7).

Concept recognition NLP task involving the identification of phrases in text that describe an abstract concept from a particular semantic category (e.g., name of a disease or anatomical region) (Chap. 7).

Conditional independence Formally, two manifestations of a disease, A and B, are conditionally independent when $P(A,B|D)=P(A|D)P(B|D)$, i.e., when their joint probability is simply the product of their individual probabilities given disease D (Chap. 4).

Connectionism A movement in cognitive science that works to explain intellectual abilities using artificial neural networks (Chap. 2).

Consilience A unified theory of knowledge espoused by biologist Edward O. Wilson that involves many disciplines from biology to physics as well as social sciences and the humanities to create a domain where sciences and the arts meet (Chap. 19).

Context mechanism MYCIN's mechanism to allow rules to mention various entities such as cultures and organisms without needing to relate them explicitly (Chap. 4).

Continual learning A concept to learn a model for a large number of tasks sequentially without forgetting knowledge obtained from the preceding tasks, where the data in the old tasks are not available anymore during the training of new ones (Chap. 12).

Control value theory The theory implies that trainees and instructors' achievement emotions can be influenced by changing subjective control and values relating to achievement activities and their outcomes (Chap. 16).

Conversational agent An intelligent agent that converses with humans via a dialog system interface (Chap. 9).

Conversational assistant A conversational agent that uses speech input and output to perform a wide range of tasks, as exemplified by the now ubiquitous Siri, Amazon Alexa, and Google Home products (Chap. 9).

Convex function A real-valued function in which the y value for points on the line segment between two x values always falls beneath the y values of the function at these points. The quadratic $y=x^2$ is a classic example of a convex function (Chap. 6).

Convex hull The convex hull of a set of datapoints is the smallest polygon that both encloses all of them, and does not bend inward upon itself (Chap. 6).

Convolution A mathematical function derived from two given functions by integration to derive a third function, or an integral that blends one function with another function (or simply as an integral of the convolution) (Chap. 19).

Convolution (in image analysis) A linear operation of a filter or kernel to local neighborhoods of points in an input. Since a feature may occur anywhere in the image, the filter weights are shared across all the image positions. Thus, image features can be extracted with fewer parameters, increasing model efficiency (Chap. 12).

Convolutional neural network (CNN) A form of deep neural network used in image processing, which learns translation invariant features across an image. It does so by applying the same set of parameters (called a filter) in different positions within an image, providing the capability to recognize informative features irrespective of their location. The filters slide along input features to summarize sections of the image. They are typically used in multiple layers to abstract features of the entire image (Chaps. 4 and 6).

Copy-number variation (CNV) A phenomenon in which sections of the genome are repeated and the number of repeats in the genome varies among individuals (Chap. 14).

Co-reference resolution NLP task involving the identification of co-referring textual elements—each element often being referred to a "mention" in a "chain" of elements—such that all mentions refer to the same real-world object, such as identifying which named entity a pronoun refers to (Chap. 7).

Cross sectional imaging A discipline of radiology that encompasses the use of a number of advanced imaging techniques (typically CT, MRI, and ultrasound, and occasionally some nuclear medicine techniques) that view the body in cross-section (i.e., as axial) slices (Chap. 12).

Cross-modal application An application that involves information obtained from more than one modality (e.g. image and text data or EHR and genomic data) (Chap. 4).

Cybernetics The science of communications and automatic control systems in both machines and living things (Chap. 2).

DARPA See Advanced Research Projects Agency (D refers to Defense)

Data augmentation The process of augmenting the training dataset with transformations of the input data with the goal of inducing the model to be invariant to the transformation (Chap. 4).

Data ethics A branch of applied ethics that examines issues associated with data collection, storage, and sharing; privacy and confidentiality; appropriate use; etc. (Chap. 18).

Data manifold The different kinds of information attached to data in addition to what is generally termed "metadata": where, when, and how the data was sourced, how was it structured, and how credible is it. (Chap. 18).

Data programming The programmatic creation of training datasets via noisy labelling functions (Chap. 4).

Data-derived artificial intelligence-based clinical decision support An artificial intelligence-based clinical decision support system in which a key component is a model that is typically derived from data (Chap. 10).

Decision tree A diagrammatic representation of the outcomes associated with chance events and voluntary actions. Also a supervised learning method that predicts the value of a target variable by learning simple decision rules inferred from the data features (Chaps. 4 and 11).

Decision tree classifier A flowchart-like structure in which each internal node represents a "test" on an attribute (e.g. whether the value of that attribute is below a certain threshold), each branch represents the outcome of the test, and each leaf node represents a class label. The tree is built in an iterative way, by selecting at each step the best feature to split the data. Having found the best split, data are partitioned into the two resulting regions, and the splitting process is repeated on each of the two regions. Then, this process is repeated on all the resulting regions. For classification trees, splitting is determined on the basis of the "impurity" of the considered node, which can be quantified using different criteria, such as misclassification error, Information Gain, Gain Ratio, and Gini Index. The paths from root to leaf represent classification rules. Similarly, in regression trees, given the continuous nature of the outcome, "impurity" is computed as the Sum of Squared Errors at the node (Chap. 11).

Deductive reasoning An hypothesis-based logical reasoning process that deduces conclusions from test results. It moves from the general rule to the specific application (Chap. 5).

Deep feedforward neural networks Neural networks with an input layer, multiple hidden layers and an output layer that are fully connected to one another, in the sense that every node in one layer connects to every node in the subsequent layer (Chap. 6).

Deep learning A class of machine learning algorithms that uses multiple layers in an artificial neural network to extract higher-level features progressively from raw input. Deep learning can be used both for classification and regression, using architectures that include convolutional and recurrent neural networks as well as deep reinforcement learning. In image interpretation, the approach progressively learns a composition of features to reflect a hierarchy of structures in the data. An end-to-end approach, it learns simple features (such as signal intensity, edges, and textures) as components of more complex features such as shapes, lesions, or organs, thereby leveraging the compositional nature of images (Chaps. 1, 2, 10, 11, 12, 18, and 19).

Deep reinforcement learning A combination of traditional reinforcement learning and an artificial neural network to enable software agents to maximize the reward from various states and actions in the environment. The AlphaGo model from DeepMind is an example of this AI tool (Chap. 19).

De-identification The process by which data are altered to reduce the likelihood that a data subject's identity can be revealed (Chap. 3).

Department of Defense (DOD) In the USA, the largest government agency. It provides military forces and capabilities needed to deter war and ensure the nation's security, including by supporting research. The DOD has been a major source of support for the development of AI methods and applications through its Advanced Research Projects Agency (Chap. 2).

Dependency parsing A syntactic NLP task involving the identification of syntactic structures as represented by word-word relations (instead of embedded phrases as in treebank) (Chap. 7).

Dialog A conversational exchange between two or more entities (Chap. 9).

Dialog system A computational artifact designed to engage humans in dialog (Chap. 9).

Digital taxonomy A structure guiding how to organize and classify digital content. For example, Bloom's Digital Taxonomy helps one to navigate through the myriad digital tools and to make choices based on the kinds of learning experiences in which students should be engaged (Chap. 16).

Digital transformation An approach that draws upon user-centered design to re-imagine how essential functions can be improved by exploiting AI methods and other digital technologies (Chap. 13).

Digital twin The virtual model of a physical system for learning from real world processes and experiences to achieve a closed-loop of the virtual and real world physical systems in order to improve efficiency and to increase innovation (Chap. 19).

Discourse segments The components of a discourse, comprising one or more utterances (Chap. 9).

Discriminative model in machine learning, a model that learns the conditional distribution of the labels given observed features. That is, it assigns the probability of a label based on the observed features of a data point, without considering how these features are distributed in other examples (Chap. 6).

Distributed cognition A process in which cognitive resources are shared socially to extend individual cognitive resources or to accomplish something that an individual agent could not achieve alone. It emphasizes the ways that cognition is off-loaded into the environment through social and technological means. It is a framework for studying cognition rather than a type of cognition (Chap. 5).

Division of Research Resources (DRR) Prior to 1990, DRR was a Division at the National Institutes of Health (NIH) that funded shared research facilities, among other activities. In 1990 it merged with the Division of Research Services to form that National Center for Research Resources (NCRR). It was abolished in 2011 when NIH was reorganized to create a new National Center for Advancing Translational Sciences (NCATS) (Chap. 2).

Domain model A domain model is a conceptual model of a domain that incorporates both behavior and data. It may partially represent the entire domain. It may also contain a formal, computable representation of the knowledge, skills and strategies (Chap. 16).

Doublet In single-cell RNA sequencing, a 'drop', which is identified by a barcode, or a datapoint, is expected to contain the genome from only one cell. A doublet occurs when a drop contains the genome of more than one cell (Chap. 14).

Dynamic Bayesian network A probabilistic causal network that relates variables to each other over adjacent time steps. At any point in time T, the value of a variable can be calculated from the internal regressors and the immediate prior value at T-1 (Chap. 11).

Dynamic differential equations A class of algorithms that represent a continuous process by one or more differential equations. There must be at least one equation that has a derivative with respect to time (Chap. 14).

Dynamic imaging An amalgam of digital imaging, image editing, and workflow automation. It is used to automate the creation of images by zooming, panning, colorizing, and performing other image processing and color management operations on a copy of a digital master. In radiology, dynamic imaging refers to sequential imaging of a volume of tissue over time, which often implies scanning the same area during the passage of intravenous contrast over time (Chap. 12).

ECG (electrocardiogram) A standardized tracing of the heart's electrical activity—voltage/time as recorded from multiple electrodes (Chap. 8).

Electronic health record (EHR) A repository of electronically maintained information about an individual's lifetime health status and health care, stored so that it can serve the multiple legitimate users of the record. Also sometimes termed electronic medical record (EMR) and, historically, computer-based patient record (CPR) (Chaps. 1, 7, and 10).

Embedding A low-dimensional representation of a word, object, or concept that encodes certain topological, algebraic, or other properties (Chap. 4).

Embodied conversational agent An agent that includes the ability to use human-like conversational nonverbal behavior in a dialog, such as a hand gesture and facial display (Chap. 9).

Emergent properties Properties a collection of systems or members have which individuals within those systems or members lack (Chap. 8).

Entropy A measure of the uncertainty represented by a probability distribution. A distribution in which one possibility is certain and others have been ruled out has zero entropy, and one in which all possibilities are equally likely has maximal entropy (Chap. 4).

Epistemology The investigation of what distinguishes justified belief or knowledge from opinion (Chap. 3).

Equity Allocation of resources and opportunities in a manner that achieves an equal outcome (Chap. 13).

Error boundary In work on human/AI teams, used to describe human team members' knowledge of the limits of AI performance, manifesting as their ability to identify examples in which the model is likely to be wrong (Chap. 20).

Ethnographical Relating to ethnography, which is a qualitative research approach used to study people and cultures. It can provide an in-depth understanding of the socio-technological realities surrounding everyday software development practice (Chap. 17).

Expectation-maximization (EM) In statistics and machine learning, a class of algorithms to infer the data distribution and to train the machine learning model. The algorithm is initiated by a set of default distributions (or models) parameters and the default likelihood assignment of datapoints to each distribution (or model). Then, the expectation step (E step) recomputes the distributions (or models) parameters such that they are the best fit according to the datapoints likelihood assignment. After the E step, the maximization step (M step) recomputes the datapoints' likelihood assignment according to the new distributions (or models) parameters. These two steps are repeatedly executed, one after the other, until all distributions (or models) and datapoints' likelihood assignment do not significantly change (Chap. 14).

Expert system Software that uses AI methods to combine data and expert knowledge to offer advice or make decisions in an area of human activity (Chaps. 1 and 2).

Explainability The ability to provide a reasonably complete explanation of an AI system's output (e.g., a diagnosis or prediction) based on an understanding of its decision process (Chaps. 8 and 18).

Explanation A summary of the basis for a statement that is purported to be true. In decision support, the line of reasoning, pertinent data, and accepted factual knowledge that together justify an interpretation or recommendation (Chap. 3).

Extended reality (XR) The immersive technologies of virtual reality (simulated digital environment with full immersion), augmented reality (virtual objects and/or information are overlaid on real world objects and places), and mixed (or hybrid) reality (real-world and digital objects co-exist) (Chap. 19).

External representation A representation of information on a physical medium (Chap. 5).

Fairness Related to "justice," the concept that goods/benefits and burdens/harms are or should be equitably shared by individuals and groups (Chap. 18).

FDA See Food and Drug Administration.

Feature engineering A process of using domain knowledge to extract features from raw data that can better represent the underlying problem to the predictive models, resulting in improved model accuracy on unseen data (Chap. 12).

Federated learning A decentralized form of machine learning in which the model is centralized while the data are not, thereby assuring that the privacy and security concerns of the data are no longer an issue since the data are kept and secured locally (Chaps. 7 and 19).

Federated query model A way to send a query statement to an external database and get the result back as a temporary table (Chap. 3).

Few shot learning An innovative machine learning method that can make predictions based on a small number of labeled samples for training so that the machines can learn rare cases. Variations of few shot learning include one-shot and zero-shot learning (Chap. 19).

Findability The ease with which information contained in a location or set of locations can be found, both from outside those sites (using search engines and the like) and by users already on the site (Chap. 3).

Focus group A form of group interview that capitalizes on communication among research participants in order to generate data and insights. The idea behind the focus group method is that group processes can help people to explore and clarify their views in ways that would be less easily accessible in a one-on-one interview (Chap. 17).

Food and Drug Administration (FDA) A US federal agency tasked with monitoring various foods, biopharmaceuticals, medical devices, cosmetics and veterinary products (Chap. 8).

Forward chaining The computational process of inferring new facts from what is previously known, using inference rules that state an implication from known facts to new facts (Chap. 4).

Forward reasoning The process of reasoning with initial data towards the goal, which is usually uncertain. It is often referred to as top down reasoning (Chap. 5).

Fourier transform A mathematical transform that decomposes functions depending on space or time into functions depending on spatial or temporal frequency, such as the expression of a musical chord in terms of the volumes and frequencies of its constituent notes (Chap. 12).

Frame An abstract representation of a concept or entity that consists of a set of attributes, called slots, each of which can have one or more values to represent knowledge about the entity or concept (Chap. 4).

Fuzzy logic A logic in which a proposition is not necessarily true or false but can be (believed to be) true to some degree. Its semantics differs from probabilistic methods because fuzzy values are subjective and independence is typically not assumed (Chap. 4).

Gabor filter A linear filter used for image texture analysis, which essentially means that it analyzes whether there is any specific image frequency content in specific directions in a localized region around the point or region of analysis (Chap. 12).

Gaussian discriminant analysis A supervised machine learning algorithm that attempts to fit a Gaussian distribution to each data category (Chap. 6).

GDPR (general data protection regulation) A European Union (EU) law designed to set guidelines for information privacy, applicable to EU member countries and the European Economic Area (Chap. 8).

Generative adversarial network (GAN) A class of machine learning frameworks designed by Ian Goodfellow and colleagues. It involves having two neural networks (called the generator and the discriminator) compete with one another in a game (in the form of a zero-sum game, where one agent's gain is the other agent's loss) in order recursively to create and improve new content (Chaps. 12 and 19).

Generative model In machine learning, a model that learns the joint distribution over observed features and labels for the training set. That is, it considers the observed features for a particular data point in relation to their underlying distribution across the entire training set (Chap. 6).

Generative pre-trained transformer (GPT-3) An unsupervised learner and language prediction model created by OpenAI with 175 billion parameters. It deploys deep learning to perform natural language processing tasks (Chap. 19).

Genome All genetic information of an organism (Chap. 14).

Genomics A branch of molecular biology concerned with the structure, function, evolution, and mapping of an organism's genetic material (Chap. 2).

Governance The processes to ensure the appropriate use of resources (e.g., information technology) in order to ensure standards are met, values adhered to, and accountability ensured. Governance might or might not entail regulation by governments (Chaps. 15 and 18).

Gradient boosting A supervised method for classification and regression built from an ensemble of weak classifiers (typically, decision trees), which are combined into a single strong learner in an iterative fashion (Chap. 11).

Gradient boosted decision tree A gradient boosting algorithm which produces a sequential ensemble (or committee) of decision trees. Each tree is associated with a voting weight, and the final decision of the ensemble is a weighted majority vote of its members. Each decision tree in the sequence is optimized to correct errors made by the previously added members of the ensemble (Chap. 6).

Gradient descent A widely-used optimization algorithm that makes multiple small corrections to model parameters in accordance with their influence on the error of a model, bringing it closer to an optimization objective (Chap. 6).

Graph database A (NoSQL) type of database that uses graph structures for semantic queries with nodes and edges to represent and store data. The nodes are the entities in the graph and the relationships provide connections between two node entities (Chap. 19).

Graph neural networks A class of neural network models that learn representations of graph structure and work on optimizing transformation on all the attributes of the graph including nodes and edges. These networks accept a graph as input and transform these embeddings while maintaining the input graph connectivity (Chaps. 4 and 19).

Graphical processing unit (GPU) A specialized electronic circuit designed to manipulate and alter digital memory rapidly to accelerate the creation of images for internal storage and delivery on a display device (Chap. 2).

Gray box Machine learning model with some hand-crafted features or, generally, some (but incomplete) knowledge of system processes (Chap. 18).

Gray-level co-occurrence matrices (GLCM) A matrix that is defined over an image to be the distribution of co-occurring pixel values (grayscale values, or colors) at a given offset. It is used as an approach to texture analysis with various applications, especially in medical image analysis (Chap. 12).

HbA1c Hemoglobin A1c, a measure of average blood sugar over the past 3 months (Chap. 3).

Health Evaluation and Logical Processing [HELP] One of the first electronic health record systems, developed at LDS Hospital in Salt Lake City, Utah. Still in use today, it was innovative for its introduction of automated alerts (Chap. 10).

Health Insurance Portability and Accountability Act (HIPAA) A privacy rule established by the US Congress in 1996, that established national standards to protect individuals' medical records and other personal health information. It applies to health plans, health care clearinghouses, and those health care providers that conduct certain health care transactions electronically (Chaps. 2 and 7).

Heuristic A strategy derived from previous experiences with a similar problem, often described as a "rule of thumb". In computer science, a technique for solving a problem more quickly when classic methods are too slow or cumbersome (Chap. 2).

Heuristic classification Any technique or approach to classification problem solving that employs a practical method that is not guaranteed to be optimal, perfect, or rational, but is nevertheless sufficient for reaching an immediate, short-term goal or approximation (Chap. 5).

Hidden Markov Model (HMM) A statistical Markov model in which the system being modeled is assumed to be a Markov process with unobservable ("*hidden*") states X. An HMM assumes that there is another process Y whose behavior "depends" on X. By observing Y, the goal of an HMM is to learn about X (Chap. 11).

Hierarchical clustering Hierarchical clustering is a method of cluster analysis which seeks to build a hierarchy of clusters. For example, a dataset could be first clustered into two clusters, C1 and C2. Then, we can further cluster the data into C11, C12, C13, C21, and C22. Here, C11, C12, and C13 are children clusters from C1; meanwhile, C21 and C22 are children clusters from C2 (Chap. 14).

HIPAA See Health Insurance Portability and Accountability Act.

HITECH Health Information Technology for Economics and Clinical Health Act, enacted as part of the American Recovery and Reinvestment Act of 2009. It was designed to promote the adoption and meaningful use of health information technology, with an emphasis on electronic health records (Chap. 2).

Hold-out A validation strategy for machine learning models that consists of randomly splitting a dataset into training and test set. Usually, 2/3 of the data are used for training and 1/3 for test, but other proportions can be used depending on the size of the available dataset. The model is then trained on the training set and its performance is measured on the test set. The procedure can be repeated several times (repeated hold-out) (Chap. 11).

Human computer interaction (HCI) A multidisciplinary field of study focusing on the design of computer technology and, in particular, the interaction between human beings (the users) and computers (Chaps. 10 and 17).

Human factors engineering (HFE) The field dealing with the integration of human factors requirements into design. The objective is to provide systems that reduce the potential for human error, increase system availability, lower lifecycle costs, improve safety, and enhance overall system performance (Chap. 17).

Human-in-the loop The idea or requirement that human experts should (be available to) review and/or assess system performance and output. Human beings may be involved in a live and virtuous cycle where they train, tune, and test a particular algorithm (Chaps. 12 and 18).

Hyperparameters In machine learning and AI, a hyperparameter is a parameter whose value must be preset before executing the algorithm to train the learning model. In statistics, a hyperparameter is a parameter of a prior distribution (Chaps. 6 and 14).

Hyperplane A subspace with dimensionality one less than the space that encloses it. For example, in a three-dimensional space, a hyperplane would be a two-dimensional plane (Chap. 6).

Hypothesis-driven reasoning In medical reasoning, a pattern of reasoning in which information is reviewed in an attempt to reconcile it with a pre-existing hypothesis that may be generated under uncertainty without being fully grounded in observed signs or symptoms (Chap. 5).

Hypothetico-deductive approach In medical reasoning, a method of inquiry that proceeds by formulating a hypothesis (such as a diagnostic explanation for a patient's symptoms) in a form that can be falsifiable (e.g., through a test outcome that runs contrary to predictions expected if the hypothesis were true). Results that are consistent with the hypothesis can corroborate the theory. Thus repeated questions or tests can guide the reasoner to accept the hypothesis or to pursue competing explanations for the results (Chaps. 2 and 5).

ICell8 A well-known technique to perform single-cell RNA sequencing. The technique was developed and owned by Takara Bio Inc (https://www.takarabio.com/products/automation-systems/icell8-system-and-software) (Chap. 14).

ImageNet A large visual database designed for use in visual object recognition software research. More than 14 million images have been hand-annotated by the project to indicate what objects are pictured, and in at least one million of the images, bounding boxes are also provided. ImageNet contains more than 20,000 categories with a typical category, such as "balloon" or "strawberry," consisting of several hundred images (Chap. 12).

IMDRF (International Medical Device Regulators Forum) A group of world-wide regulators tasked with reconciling regulatory requirements for medical devices (Chap. 8).

Implementation science The scientific study of methods to promote the systematic uptake of research findings and other evidence-based practices into routine practice, and, hence, to improve the quality and effectiveness of health services (Chap. 17).

Inductive bias Any design decision that provides a basis for choosing one generalization over another (Chap. 4).

Inductive reasoning A method for drawing conclusions by making inferences from the specific to the general (in contrast with deductive reasoning) (Chaps. 3 and 5).

Inference A conclusion reached on the basis of evidence and reasoning (Chap. 3).

Influence diagram A graphical representation that combines chance, choice, and outcome nodes in a probabilistic framework (Chap. 4).

Infobutton A context-specific link from healthcare application to some information resource that anticipates users' needs and provides targeted information (Chap. 10).

Information extraction (IE) An application of NLP focusing on the extraction of specific structured information from free text (Chap. 7).

Information retrieval (IR) An application of NLP focusing on the identification of information (usually in the form of a natural language document) relevant to a particular query (e.g., set keywords or a natural language question), generally in the context of a significant amount of potential information (the "corpus"). The preeminent IR use case is a search engine such as Google or PubMed (Chap. 7).

Information theory The scientific study of the quantification, storage, and communication of digital information (Chap. 2).

Institutional Review Board (IRB) A committee within a university or other organization receiving federal funds to conduct research that reviews research proposals involving human subjects. The IRB reviews the proposals before a project is submitted to a funding agency to determine if the research project follows the ethical principles and federal regulations for the protection of human subjects. The committee has the authority to approve, disapprove or require modifications of these projects or proposals (Chap. 17).

Intelligence-based medicine Another term for artificial intelligence in medicine, it tends to be used to focus on clinical medicine practiced using data with machine learning, and especially deep learning, for improving diagnosis and therapy rather than solely relying on the conventional evidence-based medicine (Chap. 19).

Intelligent agent An autonomous, goal-directed computational artifact (Chap. 9).

Intelligent reality The integration of machine learning algorithms with smart interactive devices (including sensors and wearable devices) and immersive technologies to enable the user to have real-time decision support (Chap. 19).

Intelligent tutor A computational system that incrementally presents content relevant to a learning goal using different teaching strategies for different types of content and student ability. It also intervenes when the student requests help or makes serious mistakes.

Interface model A combination of a system's multimedia presentation and a user's input interface. In the case of teaching and learning content, systems, such models may range from simple screen display and mouse input to virtual reality (VR), haptics, and affect detection.

Internal representation A representation of information in the human mind (Chap. 5).

Internet of everything (IoE) The intelligent connection (embedded AI) of people, process, data, and things to make networked connections from the internet of things (IoT) to render the devices more relevant and valuable (Chap. 19).

INTERNIST-1 An early computer-based diagnostic program trained on clinical pathological conference cases, able to diagnose cases with multiple disorders (Chaps. 2 and 4).

Interoperability The ability of computer systems or software to exchange and make use of information (Chap. 3 and 13).

Interpretability A measure of how intuitive an AI system's outcomes are to its users. One can think of it as simplifying explainability to the point that those with non-technical expertise can follow, or infer, the "why" of an AI system's output (Chap. 18).

Intravenous unfractionated heparin (IV-UFH) A medication administered through a vein that affects blot clot formation (Chap. 15).

Intron Any nucleotide sequence within a gene (also called an intragenic region) that is removed by RNA splicing. An intron does not encode to the final mature RNA; therefore, an intron does not encode protein (Chap. 14).

Iterative design An approach that designers, developers, educators, and others use to continually improve a design or product. People create a prototype and test it, then tweak and test the revised prototype, and repeat this cycle until they reach a solution that appears to be optimal (Chap. 17).

KDD See knowledge discovery in databases.

Kernel methods Methods through which data points are represented in terms of their similarity to other data points in a set (Chap. 6).

Kernel regression/kernelized logistic regression The application of a linear or logistic regression model to features that have been transformed using kernel methods (Chap. 6).

k-fold cross validation A strategy for machine learning models. To perform cross-validation, the dataset is randomly split into k subsets (folds). Iteratively, the model is built on k-1 folds and performance are tested on the remaining fold. The procedure is repeated k times and the average performance is computed. The average error on the k test folds approximates the true error on independent data of the model that is built on all the k folds (Chap. 11).

k-nearest neighbor algorithm A machine learning algorithm that assigns labels to unseen examples by generalizing from the labels of the most similar examples in a training set (Chap. 6).

Klein's data-frame theory A theory on how people start with an initial idea that informs what kinds of data they seek through an iterative process to modify their initial 'frame' (Chap. 8).

Knowledge base A collection of stored facts, heuristics, and models that can be used for problem solving (Chaps. 4 and 10).

Knowledge discovery in databases (KDD) The process of finding knowledge in data, emphasizing the application of particular data mining methods from the general field of machine learning (Chap. 2).

Knowledge distillation The process of transferring knowledge from a larger model to a smaller model (Chap. 4).

Knowledge engineering The term for all the technical, scientific, and social aspects involved in building, maintaining, and using knowledge-based systems (Chap. 2).

Knowledge graph Also known as a semantic network, represents a network of real-world entities—i.e. objects, events, situations, or concepts—and illustrates the relationship between them. This information is usually stored in a graph database and visualized as a graph structure, prompting the term knowledge "graph" (Chaps. 3 and 19).

Knowledge representation The field of AI that is dedicated to representing information about the world in a form that a computer system can use to solve complex tasks such as diagnosing a medical condition or having a dialog in natural language (Chap. 3).

Knowledge-based artificial intelligence-based clinical decision support An artificial intelligence-based clinical decision support system in which a key component is a knowledge base that is typically manually constructed (Chap. 10).

Knowledge-based system A program that symbolically encodes, in a knowledge base, facts, heuristics, and models derived from experts in a field and uses that knowledge to provide problem analysis or advice that the expert might have provided if asked the same question (Chap. 4).

Laplace smoothing A regularization process performed on probability estimates in which counts start at one (or some other small constant), so that no conditional probability is ever estimated at zero (Chap. 6).

Lasso regression A form of regularized linear regression that tends to drive the coefficients of redundant features toward zero (Chap. 6).

Latent semantic analysis A mathematical method for computer modeling and simulation of the meaning of words and passages by analysis of representative corpora of natural text. It closely approximates many aspects of human language, learning and understanding (Chap. 16).

Learner model A model that represents the learner's current state in the domain space, and is updated in real-time as the learner progresses through the learning exercises. It is a structured representation of a learner's knowledge, misconceptions, and difficulties (Chap. 16).

Left-ventricular assist device (LVAD) A battery-operated mechanical pump that is surgically implanted to help the heart's left ventricle pump blood to the rest of the body (Chap. 15).

LISP A family of programming languages, originally specified in 1958 (and thus second only to Fortran among old computer languages still in use), that uses a distinctive, fully parenthesized prefix notation. The name LISP derives from "LISt Processor", reflecting LISP's use of linked lists as a major data structure. It has been used extensively in the AI community (Chap. 2).

Literature-based discovery (LBD) An application of NLP focusing on hypothesis generation by discovering links between previously un-connected biomedical concepts, the canonical example being Swanson's discovery of the link between Raynaud's disease and fish oil via intermediate terms (Chap. 7).

Local area networking (LAN) A computer network that comprises a collection of devices connected together in one physical location, such as a building, office, or home (Chap. 2).

Local data store Keeping information on a disk, tape drive, or similar technology that is directly attached to the computer or device (as opposed to being elsewhere on a network or in the cloud) (Chap. 3).

Logic Programming A programming paradigm, also called rule-based programming, which is largely based on formal logic. Any program written in a logic programming language is a set of sentences in logical form: IF (AND, OR), THEN (Chap. 14).

Logistic regression A supervised machine learning algorithm that transforms the output of a linear regression model into a value between 0 and 1 that can be interpreted as a class probability (Chap. 6).

Loss function A function that measures how far a machine learning model is from achieving a desired optimization objective. Typically, the loss function estimates how far a prediction is from the true label of a data point, or a set of data points (Chap. 6).

Machine intelligence An early synonym for artificial intelligence, favored especially in the United Kingdom (Chap. 2).

Machine learning (ML) A branch of AI and computer science that focuses on the use of data and algorithms to imitate the way the human beings learn, gradually improving its accuracy at classification or prediction (Chaps. 2, 3, 6, and 10).

Machine translation NLP task involving the automatic translation from one natural language to another (e.g., from French to English) (Chap. 7).

Markov model A mathematical model of a set of strings in which the probability of a given symbol occurring depends on the identity of the immediately preceding symbol or the two immediately preceding symbols. Processes modeled in this way are often called Markov processes (Chap. 11).

Mass spectroscopy An analytical technique that is used to measure the mass-to-charge ratio of ions. The results are typically presented as a mass spectrum, a plot of intensity as a function of the mass-to-charge ratio. The technique is used in a variety of fields and may be applied to pure samples of complex mixtures (Chap. 2).

Matrix factorization An approach for generating embeddings by decomposing a matrix into the product of two lower dimensionality rectangular matrices (Chap. 4).

MEDLINE Online implementation of MEDLARS, accessible by public via the Internet. The currently dominant version of MEDLINE is known as PubMed.

MEDLARS (Medical Literature Analysis and Retrieval System) The National Library of Medicine's electronic catalog of the biomedical literature, which includes information abstracted from journal articles, including author names, article title, journal source, publication date, abstract, and medical subject headings (Chap. 7).

Mental representations Also known as *cognitive representations*, the mental imagery of things that are not currently seen or sensed by the sense organs. It is a hypothetical internal cognitive symbol that represents external reality (Chap. 5).

Metaverse A persistent and immersive simulated world in which users can interact with a computer-generated environment and with other users (Chap. 16).

Microarray See gene expression microarray.

MINIMAR standards A set of standards put forth to ensure that the interpretability of a model is helpful for end users, in an attempt to mitigate inherent biases (Chap. 8).

miRNA Abbreviation for microRNA, refers to a small single-stranded non-coding RNA molecule (containing about 22 nucleotides) found in plants, animals and some viruses, that functions in RNA silencing and post-transcriptional regulation of gene expression (Chap. 14).

Model-based integration A process for performing analysis on each data type independently, followed by integration of the resultant models to generate knowledge about the trait of interest (Chap. 3).

Modeling The act or realization of making a model (Chap. 3).

Modus ponens The logic rule that allows deriving the conclusion of an implication when seeing its premises (Chap. 4).

Modus tollens The logic rule that allows deriving the negation of the premise of an implication if its conclusion is known to be false (Chap. 4).

Monte Carlo simulations Computational algorithms that rely on repeated random sampling to obtain numerical results. Monte Carlo simulation uses randomness to solve problems that might be deterministic in principle. Monte Carlo methods are mainly used for optimization, numerical integration and to generate draws from a probability distribution (Chap. 11).

Multimodal artificial intelligence An AI paradigm in which a myriad of data types (such as EHR data, image data, and wearable device data) are gathered and analyzed via algorithms for higher performance in predictions (Chap. 19).

MYCIN An early expert system that used rules to encode knowledge of infectious disease diagnosis and therapy selection. The program served as a consultant to offer advice to clinicians caring for patients with serious bacterial or fungal infections (Chaps. 2–4).

Naive Bayes model/classifier A machine learning classifier using Bayes Theorem in a way that assumes conditional independence of variables that may in fact be linked statistically (Chaps. 4 and 15).

Naive Bayes A method that uses Bayes Theorem while making the simplifying assumption that variables are conditionally independent of one another. Also used in supervised machine learning making the same independence assumption regarding features in the input vector, given the class (Chap. 6).

Named entity recognition (NER) NLP task involving the identification of phrases in text that describe a specific object from a particular semantic category (e.g., name of a specific person or location) (Chap. 7).

National Institutes of Health (NIH) The national medical research agency for the USA, located in Bethesda, MD, supporting scientific studies that seek to turn discovery into improved health (Chap. 2).

Natural history The typical progression of a disease process in an individual over time, in the absence of treatment (Chap. 3).

Natural language generation (NLG) The subfield of NLP that deals with generating coherent language as an output by translating a semantic representation (e.g., a data structure) into natural language text (Chaps. 7 and 9).

Natural language processing (NLP) The branch of computer science—and more specifically, the branch of artificial intelligence or AI—concerned with giving computers the ability to understand text and spoken words in much the same way human beings can (Chap. 1).

Natural language understanding (NLU) The subfield of NLP that deals with understanding the meaning of language as it is input to a system (Chaps. 7 and 9).

Nearest neighbor search A form of proximity search to find a number of data points in a given set that are closest to a new point of interest (Chap. 12).

Nested k-fold cross validation Strategy for hyperparameter selection and model evaluation, in which two loops of cross validation are performed. The outer loop is used to select the best performing model and it consists of a k-fold cross validation procedure. However, for each iteration of the outer loop, an inner loop of cross validation is performed by randomly splitting the training folds into L folds and by performing an L-fold cross validation. The inner loop is usually exploited to evaluate different combinations of hyperparameters (Chaps. 6 and 11).

Neural architecture search (NAS) A technique for automating the design of artificial neural networks (Chap. 12).

NLP See natural language processing.

Noisy-or assumption In Bayes networks, where a node may have multiple parents, a simplifying assumption that the presence of each parent contributes independently to the likelihood of the node (Chap. 4).

Non-coding RNA (ncRNA) An RNA molecule that is not translated into a protein (Chap. 14).

Non-negative matrix factorization A group of algorithms in multivariate analysis and linear algebra where a matrix V is factorized into two (and more) matrices W and H ($V \gg W \times H$), with the property that all three matrices have no negative elements (Chap. 14).

Non-parametric model In machine learning, a model making minimal assumptions about the structure of the underlying data, rather than defining a function a priori (such as a linear function). A classic example is the k-nearest neighbor algorithm, where new data are compared to examples in the training set directly at the point of prediction (Chap. 6).

Norman's Theory of Action A seven stage model of human action designed to explain the thought process of a person performing a task, as put forward by Norman (Chap. 8).

Observational Medical Outcomes Partnership (OMOP) A large collaborative consortium formed to facilitate and inform studies using large, often multi-institutional, observational health care data sets. OMOP efforts continue under the auspices of the Observational Health Data Sciences and Informatics (OHDSI) consortium (Chap. 6).

One single centralized datastore A database that is located, stored, and maintained in a single location (Chap. 3).

One-shot learning Instead of hundreds or thousands of annotated data elements, one-shot learning acquires information about object categories from one, or only a few, training examples (Chap. 12).

Ontology A description (like a formal specification of a program) of the concepts and relationships that can exist for an agent or a community of agents. In biomedicine, such ontologies typically specify the meanings and hierarchical relationships among terms and concepts in a domain. Note that philosophers use "ontology" as the study of what exists, which is a broader concept than what computer science has adopted (Chaps. 2–4).

Open domain question answering A natural language processing task in which a model is asked to produce an answer to a question without being provided the document containing the answer (Chap. 4).

Optical character recognition (OCR) A computer vision/NLP task of converting an image containing text to its string representation (e.g., generating a Word file from a photograph of a text document) (Chap. 7).

Optimization problem Involves finding the values of a parameter for a given function (called the optimization objective) at which the function achieves a maximum or a minimum value (Chap. 6).

Overfitting In machine learning, occurs when a model conforms too closely to its training data, reducing its ability to generalize to unseen examples (Chap. 6).

Packet switching A method for transmitting a data stream across digital networks by breaking it down into small segments or packets for more efficient transfer. Adjacent packets may be sent over different routes to assure efficiency and then reassembled when they reach their destination (Chap. 2).

Parametric model In machine learning, a model with a fixed number of parameters that are updated during training to improve the accuracy of model predictions. The choice of model (e.g. linear vs. non-linear) is based on assumptions about the structure of the function to be learned (Chap. 6).

Parenchyma In reference to normal lung, parenchyma denotes a gas-exchanging part of the lung, consisting of the alveoli and their capillaries. Some definitions may also include the connective tissue framework supporting gas exchanging tissue. The term may also be applied to other organs beside the lung (Chap. 12).

Partial thromboplastin time (PTT) A laboratory test of blood that measures the time it takes for a blood clot to form. Common therapeutic range is 60–100 s for clotting (Chap. 15).

Part-of-speech The syntactic (or grammatical) category of a word (e.g., noun, verb, adjective), often one of the first tasks performed in a pipeline of NLP models (Chap. 7).

Pathophysiological explanations Those that draw on knowledge of disease processes and their impact on human physiology (Chap. 5).

Patient-derived xenograft (PDX) Patient derived xenografts are models of cancer where the tissue or cells from a patient's tumor are implanted into an immunodeficient or humanized mouse (Chap. 14).

Pedagogical Model Represents what effective teachers do to engage students at each step of a teaching and learning session. It includes changes in teaching strategy if the student makes errors or is unable to progress adequately.

Personalized machine learning A machine learning approach where the model is tailored to the characteristics of the current person and is optimized to perform especially well for that person. See also population machine learning (Chap. 10).

Polygenic risk scoring A polygenic score (PGS), also called a polygenic risk score (PRS), genetic risk score, or genome-wide score, is a number that summarizes the estimated effect of many genetic variants on an individual's phenotype (Chap. 14).

Pooled cohort equations Clinical decision support tool requiring multiple inputs including age, gender, race, patient history elements, certain lab and vital sign values designed to estimate 10 year absolute rate of ASCVD events (Chap. 8).

Pooling An operation that groups feature map activations into a lower resolution feature map to enlarge the receptive field of deep neural networks and to reduce the model's sensitivity to small shifts of the objects (Chap. 12).

Population health monitoring An approach that systematically collects data on health status, usually to inform longer-term planning and evaluation of programs (Chap. 13).

Population machine learning A machine learning approach where the model is optimized to perform well on the average of all future individuals. See also personalized machine learning (Chap. 10).

Prediction A statement about what will happen or might happen in the future (Chap. 3).

Predictive learning The ability of a machine to model the environment, to predict the possible futures, and to understand how the world works by observing it and acting in it—in short, a predictive model of the world (Chap. 19).

Premature closure A type of cognitive error in the reasoning process in which a physician prematurely stops considering other alternative diagnostic possibilities once an initial tentative diagnosis is made (Chap. 3).

Present Illness Program (PIP) An early computer-based diagnostic program that incorporated insights from the study of human clinical reasoning (Chap. 4).

Principal component analysis (PCA) A technique for reducing the dimensionality of large datasets by transforming a large set of variables into a smaller one while still containing most of the information in the larger set (Chap. 12).

Principle of rationality A principle typically adopted in economics that decision makers choose actions that maximize their expected utility (Chap. 4).

Privacy A concept that applies to people, rather than documents, in which there is a presumed right to protect that individual from unauthorized divulging of personal data of any kind (Chap. 3).

Professional ethics Standards or rules for correct behavior by members of a (generally) learned profession, and often tied to a professional association or society through codes, oaths, guidelines, etc. (Chap. 18).

Propositions An expression, generally in language or other symbolic form, that can be believed, doubted, or denied or is either true or false (Chap. 5).

Protein physical structure (protein structure) The three-dimensional arrangement of atoms and amino-acids in a protein (Chap. 14).

Protocol analysis Method in which transcripts of think-aloud sessions, which generate think-aloud protocols are analyzed to investigate the cognitive processes underlying performance of the task. Also called verbal protocol analysis (Chap. 5).

Provenance The place where something originally came from or began, or a record tracing the history of certain elements or items that helps to confirm their authenticity and validity (Chap. 3).

Pseudogenes Nonfunctional segments of DNA that resemble functional genes. They cannot encode functional protein (Chap. 14).

Public health informatics A sub-discipline of biomedical informatics, this is the systematic application of information and computer science and technology to public health practice, research, and learning (Chap. 13).

Public health surveillance The systematic, ongoing collection and analysis of data to detect and guide actions to control hazards such as infectious disease outbreaks. It includes indicator-based surveillance (IBS) and event-based surveillance (EBS) (Chap. 13).

Public health The science and the art of preventing disease, prolonging life, and promoting health through organized community efforts (Chap. 13).

Quantum computing Use of quantum mechanics to calculate outputs by harnessing the power of atoms and molecules to perform memory and processing tasks with qubits (basic unit of information in quantum computing that can hold a superposition of possible states) (Chap. 19).

Question answering (QA) An application of NLP focusing on automatically providing the user with an answer to a natural language question, with answers typically coming from either a large corpus (possibly also involving an information retrieval step) or a large ontology/database (requiring the question be converted to a structured query via an NLP task known as semantic parsing) (Chap. 7).

Radial basis function (RBF) A function widely-used in kernel methods to measure the similarity between data points (Chap. 6).

Radio frequency identification (RFID) A technology that uses radio waves passively to identify a tagged object. An RFID tag stores information that can be read wirelessly by an RFID reader (Chap. 17).

Radiology report A document that describes radiologist's highest level of synthesis and insight into a patient's condition. It is the most important product that radiologists generate to help direct patient care (Chap. 12).

Radiomics features A method that extracts a large number of features from radiographic images. These features have the potential to uncover disease characteristics that fail to be appreciated by the naked eye (Chap. 12).

Random forest An ensemble of decision trees. Bagging is applied to train each tree learner, by randomly selecting with replacement a subset of the training set, and by training a single tree on this selected subset. The final prediction for a classification problem is the class predicted by the majority of trees. For a regression problem the final prediction is the average prediction (Chap. 11).

Random walk A process consisting of a sequence of steps taken in a randomized fashion (Chap. 4).

Rasmussen's decision ladder A tool put forth by Rasmussen that aids in visualizing the multiple steps required for decision making, often involving multiple chains and pathways (Chap. 8).

Recurrent neural network An ANN architecture often used to summarize sequential data such as time series or natural language text (Chap. 4).

Reference frame Grids of a number of dimensions that keep the brain organized in terms of knowledge in the context of a learning model (Chap. 19).

Reflective thinking Thinking that encompasses a set of abilities that people use to examine their own thoughts processes and those of others analytically, thereby allowing themselves to question and challenge their own thoughts and those of others (Chap. 16).

Regularization In machine learning, imposing a penalty to prevent a model from fitting too tightly to its training data (see overfitting), in order to improve its ability to generalize to unseen examples (Chap. 6).

Reinforcement learning A method of determining the optimal policy for what actions to take under different circumstances, learnable from past experience (Chap. 4).

Relation extraction (RE) NLP task involving the recognition of a semantic relationship between two or more phrases in text (e.g., in a *part-whole* relation, one phrase is identified as the *part* while the other phrase is the *whole*) (Chap. 7).

Repeated hold-out Validation strategy for machine learning techniques that consists of repeating hold-out validation N times. Therefore, the prediction error will be estimated as the average error on the N test sets (Chap. 11).

Representation learning The process of learning an informative representation of data to make it easier to extract useful information for a downstream task, often applied to machine learning models (Chaps. 1 and 4).

Retrospective think-aloud A think-aloud session about an event after the event has occurred to discuss and reflect what happened during the event (Chap. 5).

Reusability In computer science and software engineering, the use of existing assets in some form within the software product development process (Chap. 3).

RFID See radio frequency identification (Chap. 17).

Ridge regression A form of regularized linear regression that uses the L2 norm of the parameter vector as a penalty term, to constrain the growth of coefficients for each feature (Chap. 6).

RNA sequencing (RNA-seq) See next generation sequencing methods.

Robotic process automation (RPA) A portfolio of software tools that builds and manages software robots that will mimic and automate what humans do with digital systems so that workflows can be streamlined as part of a digital transformation (Chap. 19).

Rule-based system A system that applied human-made rules to store, sort, and manipulate knowledge. A classic example is a domain-specific expert system such as MYCIN that uses rules to simulate expert decision making (Chap. 3).

SaMD (software as a medical device) Software intended to be used for one or more medical purposes that performs these purposes without being implemented as part of a hardware medical device" (Chap. 8).

Scale-invariant feature transform (SIFT) A feature detection algorithm in computer vision to detect and describe local features in images (Chap. 12).

Schema In a database-management system, a machine-readable definition of the contents and organization of a database (Chap. 5).

Security The process of protecting information from destruction, unauthorized access, or misuse, including both physical and computer-based mechanisms (Chap. 3).

Cover and differentiate A set of candidate explanations for the events or states that need to be explained (or covered), combined with differentiating among the candidates to pick those that best explain the specified events or states (Chap. 5).

SEIPS model A model of work system and patient safety that provides a framework for understanding the structures, processes, and outcomes in health care and their interrelationships (Chap. 8).

Self supervised learning A method of machine learning that can be regarded as an intermediate form of supervised and unsupervised learning. It is a type of autonomous learning that does not necessarily require annotated data. The approach predicts an unobserved part of the input from observed parts of the input and has had a profound impact on natural language processing and computer vision by obviating the need for data labeling (Chaps. 12 and 19).

Semantic interoperability The ability of computer systems to exchange data with unambiguous, shared meaning. It is a requirement to enable machine computable logic, inferencing, knowledge discovery, and data federation among information systems (Chap. 3).

Semantic network A graph structure in which, typically, nodes correspond to concepts and links to relationships between concepts (Chap. 4).

Semi-supervised learning A machine learning algorithm that is a hybrid of supervised and unsupervised learning that utilizes a small amount of labeled data and then a relatively large amount of unlabeled data so that the latter can become labeled (Chaps. 10 and 19).

Shapley additive explanations (SHAP) A method to explain the influence of features on individual predictions made by machine learning models, based on ideas from game theory (Chap. 20).

Situated learning A theory that defines learning that takes place in the same context in which it is applied. For example, the workplace is considered as a community of practice, where workers acquire and assimilate norms, behavior, values, relationships, and beliefs of that community (Chap. 16).

Situational awareness theory The perception of elements of the environment within a volume of time and space, including the comprehension of their meaning and the projection of their status in the near future (Chap. 8).

Situational model A mental representation built to capture the underlying situation described in the text. It integrates textual information with relevant aspects of the comprehender's knowledge (Chap. 5).

Social determinants of health (SDH or SDOH) The non-medical factors that influence health outcomes (Chap. 13).

Sociotechnical systems Work systems that involve a complex set of interactions among humans, technologies, and the work environment (Chap. 8).

Speech synthesis See text-to-speech.

Static artificial intelligence-based clinical decision support An artificial intelligence-based clinical decision support system in which the knowledge base or model is static and does not evolve over time (Chap. 10).

Stemming The process of removing inflectional forms of a word to its base (stem) form (Chap. 7).

Structural error In machine learning, error caused by limits on the classes of model available to conform to a training set. For example, a linear model lacks the expressiveness to model a non-linear function accurately (Chap. 6).

Supervised machine learning An ML approach in which an algorithm uses a set of inputs and corresponding outputs to try to learn a model that will enable the prediction of an output when faced with a previously unseen input (Chaps. 1, 3, 6, and 10).

Support vector machines A supervised machine learning approach that maps data points into a geometric space while attempting to maximize the distance between the data points from each class that are most similar to those from another class. These marginal data points are then used as a basis for classification (Chap. 6).

Swarm intelligence An artificial intelligence strategy designed to solve complex problems with the internet of things that is inspired by decentralized systems with no centralized leader but with individuals that interact with one another locally (such as flocks of birds or schools of fish) (Chap. 19).

Symbolic representations The process of mentally representing objects and experiences through the use of symbols (including linguistic symbols) (Chap. 5).

Syntactic interoperability The ability of two systems to communicate with one another. See also semantic interoperability (Chap. 3).

System 1/System 2 These terms distinguish between rapid, intuitive thought processes (system 1—e.g. making a spot diagnosis from a radiological image) and a more deliberate, laborious analytical process (System 2—e.g. deriving the chain of physiological causal relationships that led to the lesion observed) (Chap. 20).

t-distributed stochastic neighbor embedding (tSNE, or t-SNE) A statistical method for visualizing high-dimensional data by giving each data element a location in a two or three-dimensional map (Chap. 14).

Team science A collaborative effort to address a scientific challenge that leverages the strengths and expertise of professionals, typically trained in different fields (Chap. 17).

Test set In machine learning, this refers to data that were not used during model development or training, but are held out from these processes in order to evaluate the model's ability to generalize to unseen examples (Chap. 6).

Text-based model A mental representation that contains textual information built in the process of text comprehension (Chap. 5).

Text classification (TC) Application of NLP focusing on classifying whether a specific span of text (e.g., document or sentence) contains information relevant to the target need (Chap. 7).

Text comprehension Process of developing a mental representation of text during reading; the ability to process text, understand its *meaning*, and to integrate with what the reader already knows (Chap. 5).

Text mining The subfield of data mining that is concerned with textual data, often used as a synonymous term for NLP (Chap. 7).

Text summarization NLP task involving automatically generating short, coherent summaries of one (or many) long text documents (Chap. 7).

Text-to-speech (TTS) The conversion of utterance text into an acoustic signal that people would recognize as human speech (Chap. 9).

Think aloud A method used to gather data in usability testing for product design and development, in psychology, and in a range of social sciences (e.g., reading, writing, translation research, decision making, and process tracing). Research protocols involve participants thinking aloud as they are performing a set of specified tasks. Participants are asked to say whatever comes into their mind as they complete the task, which is usually recorded and transcribed for analysis (Chaps. 1, 5, and 17).

Time-series machine learning methods An AI approach that involves developing models from data to describe a sequence of observations occurring at regular time intervals (Chap. 15).

Tiny AI The new technology of specialized AI chips that has more computational power in smaller physical spaces combined with new algorithms that miniaturize existing deep learning models without loss of capability so that AI can become distributed and localized (Chap. 19).

Topological data analysis (TDA) An approach to the analysis of datasets using techniques from topology. TDA provides a general framework to analyze high-dimensional, incomplete, and noisy data and provides dimensionality reduction and robustness to noise (Chap. 11).

Training set In supervised machine learning, the data represented as features, with labels for each data point. This set is used to train the model to make predictions (Chap. 6).

Transcript count The total number of RNA transcripts for a given gene, either inside a cell or inside a tissue, after performing next generation sequencing (NGS) (Chap. 14).

Transcriptome The set of all RNA transcripts, including coding and non-coding, in an individual or a population of cells (Chap. 14).

Transcriptomics The study of RNA transcript (Chap. 14).

Transfer learning Machine learning approach that focuses on storing knowledge gained from solving one problem (a pre-trained model) and then applying this knowledge to solve another problem so that relatively few data are needed to train neural networks (Chaps. 1, 7, and 19).

Transformation-based integration A method that involves performing mapping or data transformation of the underlying data sets before analysis. The modelling approach is applied at the level of transformed matrices (Chap. 3).

Transformer A deep learning architecture popularized with NLP models that is capable of maintaining an attention mechanism while processing sequences in parallel so that sequences do not have to be processed sequentially (as in recurrent neural networks) (Chap. 19).

Translational invariance In image processing, a model with translational invariance responds in the same way to an informative feature (such as a lung abscess) irrespective of where it occurs in an image (Chap. 6).

Transparency The value or virtue that openness is superior or preferable to secrecy or opacity. A transparent device, program, or system is one whose structure and workings are available for or accessible to review or scrutiny (Chap. 18).

Treebank parsing A syntactic NLP task involving the identification of the tree-based grammatical structure of a sentence, such as noun phrases, verb phrases, preposition phrases, and the phrases that may be recursively embedded within these (Chap. 7).

Underfitted model In machine learning, a model that fits poorly to its training data, often on account of strong assumptions (e.g. linear relationships). This will result in poor performance on both training and test sets (Chap. 6).

Unified medical language system (UMLS) A terminology system, developed under the direction of the National Library of Medicine, to produce a common structure that ties together the various diverse vocabularies that have been created for biomedical domains (Chaps. 4 and 7).

Uniform manifold approximation and projection (UMAP) A nonlinear dimensionality reduction technique. After performing UMAP, the low-dimensional datapoint Euclidean distance reflects the high-dimensional datapoint similarity (Chap. 14).

Unsupervised machine learning A machine learning approach that learns patterns from the data without labeled training sets (Chaps. 3, 6, and 10).

Usability A quality attribute that assesses how easy user interfaces are to use. The word also refers to methods for improving ease-of-use during the design process (Chaps. 1 and 17).

Usability testing Evaluating a product or service by testing it with representative users. Typically participants will try to complete tasks while observers watch, listen and take notes. The goal is to identify any usability problems, to collect qualitative and quantitative data, and to determine the participant's satisfaction with the product (Chap. 17).

Utterance An isolated message from one entity within a dialog (Chap. 9).

Validation set In machine learning, a held-out subset of the training data that is often used to identify optimal hyperparameters, such as the number of neighbors to consider in a k-nearest neighbor algorithm, or the regularization parameter in a regression model (Chap. 6).

Vanishing gradient problem In deep neural networks, this problem arises because of chains of multiplication of fractional numbers during backpropagation, resulting in a cumulative gradient that is too small to permit further learning (Chap. 6).

Virtual reality A collection of interface methods that simulate reality more closely than does the standard display monitor, generally with a response to user maneuvers that heighten the sense of being connected to the simulation (Chap. 16).

Volumetric stack A series of individual two-dimensional images from a cross sectional imaging study, "stacked" together to form a volume, typically oriented in a cephalo-caudad ("head-to-toe") orientation, and displayed sequentially to provide a three-dimensional depiction of anatomy (Chap. 12).

Western blotting (Western blot) Western blotting is a technique in molecular biology and immunogenetics to detect specific proteins in a tissue sample (Chap. 14).

White box A transparent system, e.g., one based on a fully curated decision tree, useful for testing or validation (Chap. 18).

Word error rate (WER) An evaluation metric for speech recognition systems (Chap. 9).

Word sense disambiguation (WSD) NLP task involving the identification of a specific meaning of a word based on its context, particularly for polysemous words with multiple potential meanings (Chap. 7).

Index